Nutrition for the
Food Service Professional

Nutrition for the
Food Service Professional

Third Edition

Karen Eich Drummond

MS, RD, FADA, FMP, AHCFA

VAN NOSTRAND REINHOLD

I⊤P® A Division of International Thomson Publishing Inc.

New York • Albany • Bonn • Boston • Detroit • London • Madrid • Melbourne
Mexico City • Paris • San Francisco • Singapore • Tokyo • Toronto

For more information, contact:

Van Nostrand Reinhold
115 Fifth Avenue
New York, NY 10003

Chapman & Hall GmbH
Pappelallee 3
69469 Weinheim
Germany

Chapman & Hall
2-6 Boundary Row
London SE1 8HN
United Kingdom

International Thomson Publishing Asia
221 Henderson Road #05-10
Henderson Building
Singapore 0315

Thomas Nelson Australia
102 Dodds Street
South Melbourne, 3205
Victoria, Australia

International Thomson Publishing Japan
Hirakawacho Kyowa Building, 3F
2-2-1 Hirakawacho
Chiyoda-ku, 102 Tokyo
Japan

Nelson Canada
1120 Birchmount Road
Scarborough, Ontario
Canada M1K 5G4

International Thomson Editores
Seneca 53
Col. Polanco
11560 Mexico D.F. Mexico

4 5 6 7 8 9 10   RRD-HB   01 00 99 98

Library of Congress Cataloging-in-Publication Data

Drummond, Karen Eich.
    Nutrition for the food service professional / Karen Eich Drummond—3rd ed.
        p.   cm.
    Includes bibliographical references and index.
    ISBN 0-442-02114-3
    1. Nutrition. 2. Food service.   I. Title
    TX353.D78   1996   96-16756
    613.2—dc20   CIP

http://www.vnr.com
product discounts • free email newsletters
software demos • online resources

email: info@vnr.com

A service of I(T)P®

In memory of my father,
Frank J. Eich

Contents

Preface

This book is written primarily for students in foodservice management, hospitality management, and culinary programs. Practicing foodservice professionals may find it useful as well. Its content focuses on personal nutrition, selected nutrition topics such as vegetarian eating, and nutrition in restaurants and foodservices.

This third edition of *Nutrition for the Foodservice Professional* includes 15 chapters covering the fundamentals of personal nutrition (Chapters 1–7), selected nutrition topics (Chapters 8–11), and nutrition in restaurants and foodservices (Chapters 12–15).

The latest nutrition information has been used to update and revise each chapter, including:

1. the fourth edition of the *Dietary Guidelines for Americans* (1995)
2. the United States Department of Agriculture's *Food Guide Pyramid*
3. the new food and nutrition labels

The latest nutrition research on many other topics is also included.

This third edition uses many of the features from the prior edition as well as new features.

1. Each chapter now begins with an **Outline** to help students get the big picture first.
2. The outline is followed by a list of **Key Questions** and a **Quiz** to stimulate interest and help students assess what they already know about the topic.
3. **Food Facts** and **Hot Topics** continue to appear in each chapter. Food Facts discusses relevant food-related topics, such as fat substitutes and the 5-a-Day program to increase fruit and vegetable consumption. Hot Topics discuss controversial topics in nutrition, such as biotechnology and trans fatty acids. Many of the Food Facts and Hot Topics have been changed to address more pertinent food and nutrition issues.

4. A new boxed feature, **Label Reading Questions and Answers**, appears in the first six chapters. Each feature uses a question-and-answer format to show how to read the new food labels with regard to the nutrient(s) discussed in that chapter.

5. **Sidebars** appears in all chapters to highlight important points, give definitions, and add interesting tidbits of information.

6. Instead of a summary at the end of each chapter, a **Mini-Summary** is given after each chapter heading. This is intended to help students see what is important in each section.

7. At the end of each chapter, **Key Terms** are listed, each of which can be found in the Glossary at the back of the book.

8. Two types of exercises are now given at the end of each chapter: **Review Questions** and **Activities and Applications**. Review Questions are just that—questions that help students review the chapter material. They also ask students to use information-processing skills such as comparing and classifying. Activities and Applications encourage students to analyze, evaluate, create, problem-solve, and apply chapter concepts. They encompass activities that might normally go into a separate workbook, but are put here for ease of use.

9. **References** are listed in the text, when appropriate, and at the end of each chapter.

I hope that both old and new features will make *Nutrition for the Foodservice Professional* easier to use and more fun as well.

Part I, The Fundamentals of Personal Nutrition, uses the same format as previously, with an introductory chapter followed by chapters on specific nutrients: carbohydrates, lipids, proteins, vitamins, and water and minerals. The final chapter in Part I, "Putting It All Together," discusses the new **Dietary Guidelines** and the **Food Guide Pyramid**. Part II contains four chapters on additional nutrition topics: nutrition over the life cycle, weight management and exercise, vegetarian menu-planning, and nutrition and disease. With four chapters, Part III discusses nutrition and menu planning, developing healthy recipes, marketing healthy menu options, and light beverages and foods for the beverage operation. These chapters have been extensively revised to help readers develop as well as market healthy menus and recipes.

As with the second edition, the third edition is meant to be a practical, how-to book tailored to the needs of current and future foodservice, hospitality, and culinary professional. It is written for those who need to use nutritional principles to evaluate and modify menus and recipes, as well as to respond knowledgeably to customers' questions and needs. Please direct any comments and suggestions to me at Van Nostrand Reinhold.

Karen Drummond, MS, RD, FADA, FMP, AHCFA

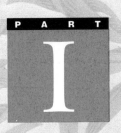

PART

I

The

Fundamentals

of

Personal Nutrition

CHAPTER

1

Introduction to Nutrition

KEY QUESTIONS

1. How do you define *nutrition* and *nutrient*? What are the six groups of nutrients?
2. What are your daily calorie needs based on?
3. What are the characteristics of a nutritious diet?
4. How do you decide which foods to eat?
5. How do taste and smell affect eating?
6. Once you have eaten, how is the food digested in the digestive tract and then absorbed and metabolized in the body?
7. What does RDA mean, and what is the purpose of RDAs?

QUIZ

Directions: Circle *True* if you agree with the statement and *False* if you disagree.

1. Fat is a nutrient.	*True*	*False*
2. Calories measure energy in a food.	*True*	*False*
3. Women have higher basal metabolic needs than men.	*True*	*False*
4. The larger the body, the more energy expended in physical activity.	*True*	*False*
5. Cost and convenience are factors affecting food selection.	*True*	*False*
6. Most of what we call taste is really smell.	*True*	*False*
7. Food empties from the stomach into the large intestine.	*True*	*False*
8. Enzymes help break down food into smaller units.	*True*	*False*
9. Metabolism refers to the building up and breaking down of substances in the body.	*True*	*False*
10. RDA means "Recommended Daily Allowance."	*True*	*False*

NUTRITION AND NUTRIENTS

Nutrients nourish the body.

To begin this first chapter, let's explore what nutrition is. **Nutrition** is a science, which means that it is a branch of knowledge dealing with a body of facts. Compared to other scientific fields such as chemistry, nutrition is a young science. Many nutritional facts revolve around nutrients, such as sugar. **Nutrients** are the nourishing substances in food, providing energy and promoting the growth and maintenance of your body. In addition, nutrients regulate the many body processes, such as heart rate and digestion, and support the body's optimum health and growth.

Nutrition also encompasses how nutrients relate to health and disease. Almost daily we are bombarded with news reports that something in the food we eat, such as fat, is not good for us—that it may indeed cause or complicate diseases such as heart disease or cancer. Nutrition, also, looks closely at the relationships between nutrients and disease. Last, nutrition examines the processes by which you choose different kinds and amounts of foods and the balance of foods and nutrients in your diet.

In summation, nutrition is a science that studies nutrients in foods and in the body and how these nutrients relate to health and disease. Nutrition also deals with food selection, and the type of diet you eat. Because it has so many meanings, let us take a look at the word *diet*. Anyone who has tried to lose weight has no doubt been on a diet. In this sense, *diet* means weight-reducing diet. But a more general definition of *diet* is: the foods and beverages you normally eat and drink. At times, you may change what you normally eat in order, for example, to lose weight.

Nutrition is a science that studies nutrients in foods and in the body and how these nutrients are related to health and disease. Nutrition also looks at how you select foods and the type of diet you eat.

There are about 50 nutrients that can be arranged into six groups as follows.

1. Carbohydrates
2. Lipids (include fats and oils)
3. Proteins
4. Vitamins
5. Minerals
6. Water

The first three nutrients, called **energy-yielding nutrients**, can be burned as fuel to provide energy for the body. Vitamins, minerals, and water cannot be used to provide energy.

Most, but not all, nutrients are considered **essential nutrients**. Essential nutrients either cannot be made in the body or cannot be made in the quantities needed by the body; therefore, we must obtain them through food. Carbohydrates, vitamins, minerals, water, and some parts of lipids and proteins are considered essential.

You have to take in essential nutrients by eating.

It's been said many times, "You are what you eat." This is certainly true; the nutrients you eat can be found in your body. Water is the most plentiful nutrient in the body, accounting for about 60 percent of your weight. Protein accounts for about 15 percent of your weight, whereas fat accounts for 20 to 25 percent, and carbohydrates only 0.5 percent. The remainder of your weight includes minerals, such as calcium in bones, and traces of vitamins.

MINI-SUMMARY Nutrition is the science that studies nutrients in foods and in the body and how these nutrients relate to health and disease. Nutrition also looks at how you select foods and the type of diet you eat.

The six groups of nutrients are carbohydrates, lipids, proteins, vitamins, minerals, and water, of which the first three are energy-yielding nutrients. Lipids contain the most calories per gram—9 calories per gram compared to 4 calories per gram for carbohydrates and proteins. Carbohydrates, vitamins, minerals, water, and some parts of lipids and proteins are considered essential nutrients.

CALORIES

Calories measure energy.

Food energy and the energy needs of the body are measured in units called **calories**. The number of calories in a particular food can be determined by burning a weighed portion of the food and measuring the amount of heat (or calories) it produces. Although we use the term *calorie* in our speech, and will use it in this book, the correct term is *kilocalorie*, a unit of 1000 calories. Of the nutrients, only carbohydrates, lipids, and proteins provide calories as follows.

Per gram, fat contains the most calories.

Carbohydrates: 4 calories per gram
Lipids: 9 calories per gram
Proteins: 4 calories per gram

A **gram** is a unit of weight; there are 28 grams in 1 ounce. Alcohol, although not a nutrient because it does not promote the growth and maintenance of the body, provides 7 calories per gram.

The number of calories you need each day is based on your basal metabolic needs, level of physical activity, and thermic effect of food.

The number of calories you need is based on three factors: your energy needs when your body is at rest and awake (referred to as **basal metabolism**), your level of physical activity, and the energy you need to digest and absorb food (referred to as the **thermic effect of food**). Basal metabolic needs include energy needed for vital bodily functions when the body is at rest but awake. For example, your heart is pumping blood to all parts of your body, your cells are making proteins, and so on. Your basal metabolic rate (BMR) depends on the following factors.

1. Gender.   Men have a higher BMR than women because men have a higher proportion of muscle tissue (muscle requires more energy for metabolism than fat). The BMR for women is about 10 percent lower than for men.
2. Age.   As people age, they generally gain fat tissue and lose muscle tissue, so BMR declines about 2 to 3 percent per decade after age 30.
3. Growth.   Children, pregnant women, and lactating women have higher BMRs.
4. Height.   Tall, thin people have more body surface and lose body heat quicker. Their BMR is therefore higher.

TABLE 1-1 **Calories spent per hour in physical activity.**

Activity	Calories Burned*
Bicycling, 6 mph	240 calories
Bicycling, 12 mph	410 calories
Cross-country skiing	700 calories
Jogging, 5-1/2 mph	740 calories
Jogging, 7 mph	920 calories
Jumping rope	750 calories
Running in place	650 calories
Running, 10 mph	1280 calories
Swimming, 25 yards/minute	275 calories
Swimming, 50 yards/minute	500 calories
Tennis, singles	400 calories
Walking, 2 mph	240 calories
Walking, 3 mph	320 calories
Walking, 4-1/2 mph	440 calories

* The calories burned in a particular activity vary in proportion to one's body weight. For example, a 100-pound person burns 1/3 fewer calories, so you would multiply the number of calories by 0.7. For a 200-pound person, multiply by 1.3.

Source: National Heart, Lung, and Blood Institute and the American Heart Association. 1993. Exercise and your heart: A guide to physical activity.

5. Temperature. BMR increases in both hot and cold environments in order to keep the temperature inside the body constant. The BMR increases about 7 percent for each increase of 1 degree Fahrenheit.
6. Fever and stress. Both these circumstances increase BMR.

Basal metabolic rate also decreases when you diet or eat fewer calories than normal. Basal metabolic rate accounts for the largest percentage of energy expended—about two-thirds for individuals who are not very active.

Your level of physical activity strongly influences how many calories you need. Table 1-1 shows the calories burned per hour for a variety of activities. The number of calories burned depends on the type of activity, how long and how hard it is performed, and an individual's size. The larger your body, the more energy you use in physical activity. Aerobic activities such as walking, jogging, cycling, and swimming are excellent ways to burn calories if they are brisk enough to raise heart and breathing rates. Physical activity accounts for 25 to 40 percent of total energy needs.

The thermic effect of food is the smallest contributor to your energy needs: from 5 to 10 percent of the total. In other words, for every 100

Two keys to losing weight are to excercise regularly and eat a low-fat diet.

calories you eat, about 5 to 10 are used for digestion, absorption, and metabolism of nutrients, a topic we explore shortly.

MINI-SUMMARY   Food energy and the body's energy needs are measured in units called **calories**. You burn calories to maintain your basal metabolic rate (about 65 percent), for physical activity (about 25 to 40 percent), and to digest, absorb, and metabolize food (about 5 to 10 percent). Your basal metabolic rate depends on your gender, age, growth, height, outside temperature, and fever or stress.

CHARACTERISTICS OF A NUTRITIOUS DIET

A nutritious diet has the following four characteristics. It is
1. adequate
2. balanced
3. moderate
4. varied

A nutritious diet is adequate, balanced, moderate, and varied.

As we discuss each of these characteristics, think about your own diet.

Your diet must provide enough nutrients, but not too many. This is where adequate and moderate diets fit in. An **adequate diet** provides enough of the essential nutrients and calories, whereas a **moderate diet** avoids excessive amounts of calories and any particular food or nutrient. In the case of calories, for example, consuming too many leads to obesity. The concept of moderation allows you to occasionally indulge in foods that some consider harmful, such as french fries, premium ice cream, or chocolate.

Other examples of nutrient-dense foods are sweet potatoes, oranges, milk, brown rice, red beans, and flounder.

Although it may sound simple to eat enough, but not too much, of the necessary nutrients, surveys show that most adult Americans find this hard to do (Murphy, Rose, Hudes, and Viteri, 1992). This national study showed that only 2 percent of participants ate a nutritionally adequate and calorically moderate diet. One of the best ways to overcome this problem is to select nutrient-dense foods. **Nutrient-dense foods** contain many nutrients for the calories they provide. As Figure 1-1 shows, broccoli offers many nutrients for its few calories. In comparison, the cupcake contains many more calories and few nutrients.

Next, you need a **balanced diet**. A balanced diet does not overemphasize certain foods at the expense of others. For example, if you drink a lot of soft drinks, you may not be drinking much milk, a rich source of the mineral calcium.

Last, you need a **varied diet**—in other words, one that includes many

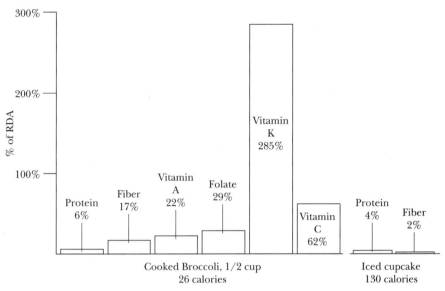

FIGURE 1-1
Nutrient Density
Comparison*

*The nutrients examined were protein, fiber, and vitamins that contributed at least 10% of the RDA.

different foods. If you imagine everything you eat for one week piled in a grocery cart, how much variety is in your cart from week to week? Do you buy (or have someone buy for you) the same bread, the same cereal, the same fresh fruit, and so on, every week? Do you constantly eat favorite foods? Do you try new foods? A varied diet is important because it is more likely to ensure that you get the essential nutrients in the right amounts.

MINI-SUMMARY A nutritious diet is adequate, balanced, moderate, and varied.

FACTORS INFLUENCING FOOD SELECTION[1]

To say that many factors influence food choices is an understatement. In fact, researchers have conservatively enumerated sixteen general categories related to stable food preferences: food characteristics, age, family relations, television, culture, self-concept, socioeconomic status, sex, peer pressure, body weight, race, food familiarity, nutritional knowledge, parental attitudes, food associations, and geography. You could also add religious beliefs, which often restrict certain foods. These factors interact with one another to produce, over space and time, the

[1]Adapted from HEALTHFUL QUANTITY BAKING, Maureen Egan and Susan Davis Allen. Copyright ©1992 by John Wiley & Sons, Inc. Reprinted with permission.

Food Facts: Food Basics

When you go to the supermarket, you find all types of foods: whole foods, fresh foods, organic foods, processed foods, enriched foods, food products, and so on. So many terms can cause much confusion, so let's take a close look at each one. As we examine the terms, think about whether you consume many or few foods from each category.

Whole foods are foods as we get them from nature. Examples include milk, eggs, meats, poultry, fish, fruits, vegetables, dried beans and peas, and grains.

Fresh foods are raw foods that have not been frozen, processed (canned or frozen), or heated. Fresh foods also cannot contain any preservatives. Examples of fresh foods include fresh fruits and vegetables, fresh meats, poultry, and fish.

Organic foods are generally foods that have been grown without synthetic pesticides or fertilizers. Organic farmers use, for example, animal and plant manures to increase soil fertility and crop rotation to decrease pest problems. The goal of organic farming is to preserve the natural fertility and productivity of the land. The exact meaning of the term *organic* varies from one part of the United States to another. By 1997, the United States hopes to implement national standards for organic foods and agriculture as required by the Organic Foods Production Act. These standards prohibit certain materials, such as mostly synthetic fertilizers, and mandate certain practices, such as those that make the soil richer. In addition to fruits and vegetables, other organic foods include meat, dairy products, and processed foods.

Processed foods have been prepared using a certain procedure: cooking (frozen pancakes), freezing (frozen dinners), canning (canned vegetables), dehydrating (dried fruits), milling (white flour), culturing with bacteria (yogurt), or adding vitamins and minerals (enriched foods). In some cases, processing removes and/or adds nutrients.

When processing adds nutrients, the resulting food is either an **enriched** or a **fortified food**. For example, when whole wheat is milled to produce white flour, nutrients are lost. As a result, white flour must be enriched by law with three vitamins and iron to make up for some of these lost nutrients. Milk is often fortified with vitamin D because there are few good food sources of this vitamin. A food is considered enriched when nutrients are added to replace the same nutrients lost in processing. A food is considered fortified when one or more nutrients are added that never were in the food. For example, orange juice does not contain calcium, so when calcium is added, the product is called calcium-fortified orange juice. Probably the most notable fortified food is iodized salt, introduced in 1924 to combat iodine deficiencies.

Whereas the food supply once contained mostly whole, farm-grown foods, today's supermarket shelves are stocked primarily with **food products**. Food products contain parts of whole foods and often have added ingredients such as sugars, sugar or fat substitutes, and nutrients. For instance, cookies are made with white flour from grains and eggs. Then sugar, shortening, and nutrients are added. The supermarket shelves are jammed with food products such as breakfast cereals, cookies, crackers, sauces, soups, baking mixes, frozen entrees, pasta, snack foods, and condiments.

As you can probably guess, your best bet nutritionally is to consume more whole foods and fewer food products.

world of human food choices. Consequently, making food choices implies more than simply eating whatever "tastes good." Yet many people, including those who make the food, never consider this aspect of their daily lives. It is important to understand that this process does exist and to explore what it means.

Let's now look at food availability, palatability, cost, and convenience, as well as the social, psychological, and nutritional factors leading to food choices.

Availability

Food availability plays a fundamental role in determining our food choices because we can eat only the food at hand. For example, people who recall the food rationing and "victory gardens" in the United States during World Wars I and II realize how diets and recipes are altered by availability. On the other hand, no culture eats every edible food available to it. For example, insects might be considered a delicacy by an Indonesian but not by an American.

Until 500 years ago, most humans grew, gathered, hunted, or traded their foods principally within a geographically defined area. Today, the United States enjoys a tremendous variety of foods from around the country and the world. With so many foods available, other factors must explain why we choose one food over another.

Palatability

How well food is accepted depends on its taste, texture, smell, and temperature. Each person has a somewhat different sense of taste. A food that one person finds too salty may seem just right to someone else. The texture of a food also determines whether we find it acceptable. We expect mashed potatoes to be smooth, an apple to be crunchy, and meat to be tender. Fat in foods has an appealing texture and feels good in the mouth. The smell and temperature of food also influence how well the food will be accepted. Adults tend to like their hot foods hot and their cold foods cold.

Although many Americans seem to want reduced-fat foods, if these foods don't taste good, chances are they will not be picked up at the supermarket again.

Cost and Convenience

Cost and convenience also influence food choices. At one time or another, many people find themselves facing tight budgets. During such times, people tend to purchase bargain foods or foods that give the best perceived value. For example, we might spend more than our budget allows for a special-occasion meal, such as a birthday meal. On the other hand, we often purchase items because of their lower price, regardless of any other factor.

Today, as more people work outside the home, less time is available for other activities, including food preparation. Convenience, therefore, becomes yet another factor in food selection, especially when income is high and time for food preparation is low. Individuals or families in these situations typically purchase convenience foods with their additional income, as shown in recent decades by the growth of fast-food chains and the decline of food preparation in the home.

Social Factors

One of the strongest social connections to food exists because people have historically shared food, thereby creating a common bond by the food they have eaten together. This social norm has continued through the ages, and whether formal or informal, eating always has a measure of ritual. This fulfills a social need, one we would hate to stop. Thus we are prone to eat the same kinds of food our friends and neighbors eat. Even today, when it seems we have lost our sense of community, we still tend to share similar dietary habits because food choices are firmly rooted in our culture and typically change slowly.

Another social influence is socioeconomic status. Food can be somewhat of a status symbol, as evidenced by the wide array of foods for banquets, parties, and other social gatherings found at various socioeconomic levels throughout society.

Psychological Factors

Another factor affecting food choice is our psychological perception of different foods. Two important aspects of this factor are familiarity and food associations. We tend to eat foods similar to those we ate as children simply because they are familiar. This is not to say that we can't enjoy new foods, but rather that some learning and sense of adventure are required to do so.

We also associate different foods with different sensations and experiences. We avoid foods associated with unpleasant experiences, whereas the opposite is true for foods associated with pleasant experiences. Moreover, all foods have characteristic flavors, textures, and most important, odors that we associate with and expect. Peanut butter cookies, for example, smell and taste like peanut butter and have a firm, crunchy texture. Any substitute that does not have these characteristics would be rejected as inauthentic.

Food is such a common aspect of our lives that we use it to reward ourselves and others. An extra-rich dessert is appropriate to reward an accomplishment. And, of course, eating foods we find comforting can help relieve tension and calm us.

Nutritional Factors

The nutritional link between food and health is nothing new. For example, in medieval times, certain plants were used to restore health or avoid illness. In recent years, however, this knowledge has become especially focused in the hearts and minds of Americans because of the number of diet-related diseases, such as heart attacks, and various types of cancer. There are also concerns about the potential danger of chemical or "unnatural" food additives.

For health reasons, more and more consumers are basing their food choices not only on the factors mentioned here, but also on nutritional value.

MINI-SUMMARY Factors such as availability, palatability, cost, and convenience, as well as social, psychological, and nutritional considerations affect our food choices.

TASTE AND SMELL

From birth, we have the ability to smell and taste. Most of what we call taste is really smell, a fact we realize when a cold hits our nasal passages. Even though the taste buds are working fine, the smell cells are not, and this dulls much of food's flavor.

Most of what we call taste is really smell. If you don't believe this, try eating with your fingers holding your nose closed! You'll see it's true.

First, let's look at taste. Taste comes from 10,000 **taste buds**—clusters of cells resembling the sections of an orange. Taste buds, found on the tongue, cheeks, throat, and the roof of the mouth, house 60 to 100 receptor cells each. The body regenerates taste buds about every three days. They are most numerous in children under six, which may explain why youngsters are such picky eaters. These cells bind food molecules dissolved in saliva, and alert the brain to interpret them.

Although the tongue is often depicted as having regions that specialize in particular taste sensations—the tip detects sweetness, the front saltiness, the sides sour, and the back bitter—researchers find that taste buds for each sensation are actually scattered everywhere. In fact, a single taste bud can have receptors for all four types of taste.

If you could taste only four things (sweet, salt, sour, and bitter), how could you taste the flavor of cinnamon or chicken or any other food? This is where smell comes in. Your ability to identify the flavors of specific foods requires smell.

The ability to detect the strong scent of a fish market, the antiseptic odor of a hospital, the aroma of a ripe melon—and thousands of other smells—is possible thanks to a yellowish patch of tissue the size of a quarter high up in your nose. This patch is actually a layer of 12 million specialized cells, each sporting ten to twenty hairlike growths called cilia that bind with the smell and send a message to the brain. Our sense of smell may not be as refined as that of dogs, who have billions of olfactory cells, but we can distinguish among about 10,000 scents.

You can smell foods in two different ways. If you smell coffee brewing while you are getting dressed, you smell it directly through the nose. But if you are drinking coffee, the smell of the coffee goes to the back of your mouth and then up into your nose.

The fact that former President George Bush does not like broccoli may be due to his genes.

The senses of smell and taste begin with detection by receptors in the nose and tongue. Nerve impulses generated by the taste buds and olfactory receptors travel to the taste and smell areas of the brain that interpret the messages as smell and taste. To some extent, what you smell or taste is genetically determined.

MINI-SUMMARY Thanks to taste buds and specialized nose cells, we can taste and smell food. You can taste sweet, salt, sour, and bitter, but you need smell in order to taste food's varied flavors.

WHAT HAPPENS WHEN YOU EAT

Once we have smelled and tasted our food, our meal goes on a journey through the **gastrointestinal tract** (also called the digestive tract) a hollow tube running down the middle of the body (Figure 1-2). The top of the tube is your mouth, which connects in turn to your esophagus, stomach, small intestine, large intestine, rectum, and anus, where solid wastes leave the body.

Think of the digestive tract as a hollow tube through which food travels. Whichever food components do not pass through the walls of the digestive tract to be used by the body are excreted in the feces.

The digestive system starts with the mouth, also called the **oral cavity**. Your tongue and teeth help with chewing. The tongue, which extends across the floor of the mouth, moves food around the mouth during chewing. Your 32 permanent teeth grind and break down food. Chewing is important because it breaks up the food into smaller pieces so it can be swallowed. **Saliva**, a fluid secreted into the mouth from the salivary glands, contains important digestive enzymes and lubricates the food so that it may readily pass down the esophagus. **Enzymes** are substances that speed up chemical reactions. Digestive enzymes help break down food into forms of nutrients that can be used by the body. The tongue rolls the

Mouth:	Tastes food.
	Chews food.
	Makes saliva.
Esophagus:	Passes food to stomach.
Stomach:	Makes enzyme that breaks down protein.
	Makes hydrochloric acid.
	Churns and mixes food.
	Acts like holding tank.
Small intestine:	Makes enzymes.
	Digests most of food.
	Absorbs nutrients across villi into blood and lymph.
Large intestine:	Passes waste to be excreted.
	Reabsorbs water and minerals.
Rectum:	Stores feces.

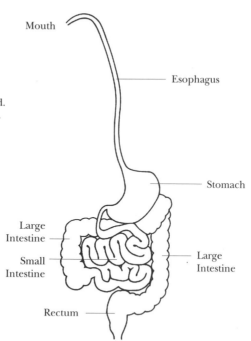

FIGURE 1-2.
Human digestive tract.

chewed food into a **bolus** (or ball) to be swallowed.

When swallowing occurs, a flap of tissue, the **epiglottis**, covers the trachea, or windpipe, so that food does not get into the lungs. Food now enters the **esophagus**, a muscular tube that leads to the stomach. Food is propelled down the esophagus by **peristalsis**, rhythmic muscle contractions in the wall of the esophagus. You might think of this involuntary contraction that forces food through the entire digestive system as squeezing a marble (the bolus) through a rubber tube. Peristalsis also helps break up food into smaller and smaller particles.

Food passes from the esophagus through the **cardiac sphincter**, a muscle that relaxes and contracts (in other words, opens and closes) to move food from the esophagus into the stomach. The **stomach**, a muscular sac that holds about 4 cups or 1 liter of food, is lined with a mucous membrane. Within the folds of the mucous membrane are digestive glands that make **hydrochloric acid** and an enzyme to break down proteins. Hydrochloric acid aids in protein digestion, destroys harmful bacteria, and increases calcium and iron absorption. Because hydrochloric acid can damage the stomach, the stomach protects itself with a thick mucous lining. Also, acid is produced only when we are eating or thinking about eating.

From beginning to end, this is the order in which food travels: mouth, esophagus, stomach, small intestine, large intestine, rectum, and anus.

From the top part of the stomach, food is slowly moved to the lower part, where the stomach churns it with the hydrochloric acid and digestive enzymes. The food is ready to move on when it reaches a liquid consistency known as **chyme**. Food is then passed into the first part of the small intestine in small amounts (the small intestine can't process too much food at one time). Liquids leave the stomach faster than solids, and carbohydrate or protein foods leave faster than fatty foods. The stomach absorbs few nutrients, but it does absorb alcohol. It takes about three hours for the stomach to empty.

The **small intestine**, about 20 feet long, has three parts: the **duodenum**, the **jejunum**, and the **ileum**. The small intestine was so named because its diameter is smaller than the large intestine, not because it is shorter. Actually, the small intestine is longer.

The duodenum, about 1 foot long, receives the digested food from the stomach as well as enzymes from other organs such as the liver and pancreas. The liver provides **bile**, a substance that helps in fat digestion, and the pancreas provides bicarbonate, a substance that neutralizes stomach acid. The small intestine itself produces digestive enzymes.

In the duodenal wall (and throughout the entire small intestine) are tiny, fingerlike projections called **villi**. The muscular walls mix the chyme with the digestive juices and bring the nutrients into contact with the villi. Most nutrients pass through the villi of the duodenum and jejunum into either the blood or lymph vessels where they are transported to the liver and to body cells. The duodenum connects with the second section, the jejunum, which connects to the ileum. Most digestion is completed in the first half of the small intestine; whatever is left goes into the large intestine after about 3 to 10 hours.

The **large intestine** (also called the **colon**) is 4 to 5 feet long and extends from the end of the ileum to a cavity called the rectum. One function of the large intestine is to receive and store the waste products of digestion; in other words, the material that was not absorbed into the body. The large intestine stores this material in the **rectum** until it is released as solid feces through the **anus**, which opens to allow elimination. The large intestine also absorbs water and some minerals.

MINI-SUMMARY The gastrointestinal tract is like a hollow tube running through your body. The top of the tube is your mouth, which connects in turn to your esophagus, stomach, small intestine, large intestine, rectum, and anus. In the mouth, food is ground by the teeth, chewed, and mixed with saliva to make it easier to pass through the esophagus. Peristalsis propels the food down the esophagus into the stomach and through the rest of the digestive tract. The stomach, a muscular sack, holds about 1 liter of food. Within the folds of the stomach's mucous lining are digestive glands that make hydrochloric acid and an enzyme to break down proteins. Hydrochloric acid aids in protein digestion. The stomach churns the food to the liquid consistency of chyme. The duodenum of the small intestine receives the digested food from the stomach as well as enzymes from other organs such as the liver and pancreas. Most nutrients pass through the villi of the duodenum and jejunum into either the blood or lymph vessels. The large intestine stores the waste products of digestion and absorbs water and some minerals.

DIGESTION, ABSORPTION, AND METABOLISM

To become part of the body, food must first be digested and absorbed. **Digestion** is the process by which food is broken down into its components in the mouth, stomach, and small intestine with the help of digestive enzymes. Complex proteins are digested, or broken down, into their building blocks, called amino acids; complicated sugars are reduced to simple sugars such as glucose; and fat molecules are broken down into fatty acids.

Before the body can use any nutrients present in food, they must pass through the walls of the stomach or intestines into the body's tissues, a process called **absorption**. Nutrients are absorbed into either the blood or the lymph, two fluids that circulate throughout the body delivering needed products to the cells and picking up wastes. Blood is composed mostly of water, red blood cells (which carry and deliver oxygen to the cells), white blood cells (which are important in resistance to disease, called immunity), nutrients, and other components. Lymph is similar to blood but has no red blood cells. It travels to areas where there are no blood vessels to feed the cells.

Within each cell, **metabolism** takes place. Metabolism refers to all the chemical processes by which nutrients are used to support life. Metabolism has two functions: the building up of substances (called **anabolism**), and the breaking down of substances (called **catabolism**). Within each cell, nutrients such as glucose are split into smaller units in a catabolic reaction that releases energy. The energy is either converted to heat to maintain body temperature or used to perform work within the cell. During anabolism, substances such as proteins are built from their amino-acid building blocks.

MINI-SUMMARY Before the body can use food nutrients, they must be digested and absorbed through the small intestine (across the villi) into

Food is first digested, then nutrients are absorbed from the digestive tract. Nutrients are transported around the body in the blood or lymph so the body's cells can metabolize them.

either the blood or lymph system. Within each cell, metabolism takes place. Metabolism refers to all the chemical processes by which nutrients are used to support life. Metabolism has two parts: the building up of substances such as protein (anabolism), and the breaking down of substances such as fat (catabolism).

RECOMMENDED DIETARY ALLOWANCES (RDAs)

Since 1941, the **Recommended Dietary Allowances** (Appendix B) have been prepared by the Food and Nutrition Board of the National Academy of Sciences/National Research Council in Washington, D.C. The RDAs include recommendations on nutrient intakes for Americans (Canada has its own recommendations) and are revised about every five years to keep them up to date. The RDAs are defined as

> the levels of intake of essential nutrients that, on the basis of scientific knowledge, are judged by the Food and Nutrition Board to be adequate to meet the known nutrient needs of practically all healthy persons in the United States. (*Recommended Dietary Allowances*, 10th edition, National Research Council, 1989).

RDAs are safe and adequate levels with ample margins of safety (about 30 to 50 percent) designed to meet the needs of practically all of the healthy population.

Individuals with special nutritional needs and/or medical problems are not covered by the RDAs.

RDAs are set for protein, 11 vitamins, and seven minerals (Table 1-2). No RDA is set for either carbohydrate or fat because individuals who are meeting both the calorie and protein RDAs and eating a variety of foods are assumed to be meeting these needs. The RDAs are neither minimal requirements (except for sodium, potassium, and chloride), average requirements, nor optimal requirements; they are adequate levels with ample margins of safety (about 30 to 50 percent) designed to meet the needs of practically all of the healthy population as well as make up for the poor absorption of certain nutrients.

Various RDAs have been set for different groups of people: infants, children, men, women, pregnant women, and lactating women. Most groups (infants, children, men, and women) are further divided by age. In this manner, you can look up your own RDAs by sex and age group. You will notice that a height and weight is given for each category. This is the height and weight of the Reference Individual on which the RDAs are based. For example, the Reference Woman for females (ages 25–50 years) is 5 feet 4 inches, weighs 138 pounds, and is normally active. The heights and weights used are not ideal figures but are the actual medians (midpoints) of Americans within the given age bracket.

TABLE 1-2. The Recommended Dietary Allowances (RDAs).		
RDAs Are Set for	*Estimated Safe and Adequate Daily Dietary Intakes Are Given for*	*Estimated Minimum Requirements Are Given for*
Energy	Vitamins:	Minerals:
Protein	Biotin and pantothenic acid	Sodium, chloride, and potassium
Vitamins:	Minerals:	
A, D, E, K, C,	Chromium, molybdenum,	
thiamin, riboflavin,	copper, manganese, and fluoride	
niacin, B_6, folate, and B_{12}		
Minerals:		
Calcium, phosphorus,		
magnesium, iron, zinc,		
iodine, and selenium		

Although designed primarily for planning and evaluating diets and menus for groups of people (such as children eating school lunches), individuals can use RDAs to examine their own diets. This is possible only if intake is averaged over a long enough period of time. Keep in mind that the "D" in RDA means "dietary," not "daily," and "R" means "recommended," not "required." RDAs are also used to evaluate the quality of the national food supply, provide a standard that can be used on food labels (see chapter 7), and develop guidelines for good eating.

RDAs for Energy

The RDAs for energy were set differently from those for nutrients. If the energy RDAs had an ample safety margin, this could lead to obesity over time. Therefore the energy RDAs are not padded; they represent the average needs of individuals. For each age level, it is estimated that an individual's needs will be met by a range of 20 percent plus or minus the average energy allowance given. Individuals needing more calories are those who, for instance, have a larger body size or are more active. Individuals needing fewer calories are those who are smaller in size, older, or less active.

Estimated Safe and Adequate Daily Dietary Intakes

When there is insufficient scientific evidence to develop an RDA, the Food and Nutrition Board will establish a table of Estimated Safe and Adequate Daily Dietary Intake. This table includes two vitamins and five trace elements or minerals and intake ranges that will meet nutritional needs and avert toxic doses (Table 1-2). Upper levels in the safe and adequate range for trace elements should not be regularly exceeded, because the toxic level may be only several times the usual intake.

Estimated Minimum Requirements

Needs for sodium, chloride, and potassium are found in a separate table that estimates minimum requirements. The minimum requirement is based on what is needed for growth and for replacement of normal daily losses (through sweating, urine, and so forth). Dietary deficiency of these three minerals in healthy individuals is unlikely. In the case of sodium and chloride, there is no evidence that higher intakes are beneficial. In fact, for some individuals, a high sodium intake aggravates problems with high blood pressure. On the other hand, desirable intakes of potassium may significantly exceed the minimum requirement, as higher levels may help individuals suffering from hypertension.

The Next Revision of the RDAs

The next revision of the RDAs will address levels of intake that cause deficiency, average requirements, and maximum safe levels for nutrients that seem to prevent disease.

Since 1993, the Food and Nutrition Board has solicited papers, testimony, opinions, and money to reevaluate the concept of what the RDAs are based on. Up to this point, the RDAs have focused on nutrients necessary to prevent deficiency diseases. The next revision will probably also look at nutrients important for disease prevention. For example, vitamin E may protect against heart disease when taken in amounts far exceeding the RDAs. The Food and Nutrition Board may specify maximum safe levels for these nutrients.

The next revision will probably also set two levels of intake *below* the RDA (Food and Nutrition Board, 1994). Let's compare the RDA with these two new levels.

1. Deficient level of intake: Healthy individuals will, over time, show deficiency symptoms.
2. Average-requirement level of intake: Sufficient to maintain the desired physical functions in a population.
3. RDA intake level: This intake level, which is adequate to meet the known nutritional needs of almost all healthy persons, will remain the same.

The Food and Nutrition Board hopes that the next version of the RDAs will be more flexible and will be used in more situations.

MINI-SUMMARY RDAs are set for protein, 11 vitamins, and 7 minerals and include ample safety margins. The RDAs for energy do not include a safety margin. Estimated safe and adequate daily dietary intakes are given for two vitamins and five minerals, and estimated minimum requirements are given for sodium, chloride, and potassium. Revised RDAs are due soon and will probably include levels at which deficiencies will occur, average requirements, and upper limits for nutrients that may prevent disease.

INTRODUCTION TO READING NUTRITION LABELING

Under the Nutrition Labeling and Education Act of 1990 and regulations from the Food and Drug Administration and the U.S. Department of Agriculture, virtually all food labels must now give information about a food's nutritional content. This wasn't always the case. Until 1994, nutrition information was voluntary; manufacturers had to provide it only when a food contained added nutrients or when nutrition claims appeared on the label. Nearly 40 percent of products didn't carry nutrition information.

FIGURE 1-3
Nutrition Label

Nutrition Facts
Serving Size 1 cup (228g)
Servings Per Container 2

Amount Per Serving
Calories 250 Calories from Fat 110

	% Daily Value*
Total Fat 12g	**18%**
Saturated Fat 3g	**15%**
Cholesterol 30mg	**10%**
Sodium 470mg	**20%**
Total Carbohydrate 31g	**10%**
Dietary Fiber 0g	**0%**
Sugars 5g	
Protein 5g	

Vitamin A 4%	•	Vitamin C 2%	
Calcium 20%	•	Iron 4%	

* Percent Daily Values are based on a 2,000 calorie diet.

Figure 1-3 is a sample nutrition label. Serving size is the first stop when you read the Nutrition Facts, because calorie and nutrient content is given per serving. Just how big is a serving? On the new label, serving sizes are real-life, given in amounts close to what most people really eat. Of course, if you eat more or less than the serving size, you will need to calculate the increase or decrease in calories and nutrients.

If you check serving sizes on similar foods, you'll see that they are similar. That means you don't need to be a math whiz to compare two foods. It's easy to see the calorie and nutrient differences between similar servings of canned fruit packed in syrup versus natural juices. The same is true for two brands of packaged macaroni and cheese.

Look for servings in two measurements—common household and metric measures. A serving of applesauce would read 1/2 cup (114 g).

The household measure is easier to understand, but the metric measure gives a more precise idea of the amount. For example, 114 g means 114 grams, a measure of weight. There are 28 grams in 1 ounce. The label helps you get familiar with metrics, too.

The next stop on the Nutrition Facts panel is the Calories per Serving category, which lists the total calories in one serving, as well as the calories from fat.

Nutrients are listed next. Information about some nutrients is required. These nutrients are total fat, saturated fat, cholesterol, sodium, total carbohydrate, dietary fiber, sugars, protein, vitamin A, vitamin C, calcium, and iron. Others are listed voluntarily. If foods contain insignificant amounts of a required nutrient, they might be omitted from the label.

Information about other nutrients is required if a claim is made about the nutrients on the label or if the nutrients are added to the food. For example, fortified breakfast cereals must give Nutrition Facts for any added vitamins and minerals.

Nutrient amounts actually are listed in two ways—in metric amounts (in grams) or as a percentage of the **Daily Value**. Daily Values are a guide to the total nutrient amount you need for a day based on a 2000-calorie diet. Therefore, the Daily Value may be a little high, a little low, or right on target for you. Percent Daily Values show you how much of the Daily Value is in one serving. For example, in Figure 1-3 the Percent Daily Value for total fat is 18% and for dietary fiber is 10%. The Daily Value for fat (and also carbohydrate and protein) is based on a 2000-calorie-per-day diet. The Daily Value for dietary fiber is 25 grams. Table 1-3 lists the Daily Values for the required nutrients and dietary components.

Reading labels will be discussed further in each of the succeeding chapters in Part 1. Just look for the boxed feature titled "Label-Reading Questions and Answers."

TABLE 1-3. Daily Values.	
Fat	65 grams
Saturated fat	20 grams
Cholesterol	300 milligrams
Total carbohydrates	300 grams
Fiber	25 grams
Sodium	2400 milligrams
Protein	50 grams
Vitamin A	5000 International units
Vitamin C	60 milligrams
Calcium	1000 milligrams
Iron	18 milligrams

REVIEW QUESTIONS

1. Define *nutrition* and *nutrient.*
2. What are the six categories of nutrients?
3. Define essential nutrients and list which are essential.
4. What is meant by calories?
5. Describe the three factors that influence how many calories you need each day.
6. Describe briefly the four characteristics of a nutritious diet.
7. Give two examples of foods that are nutrient dense and two that are not.
8. Give an example of how each of the following factors influence what you eat: food availability, palatability, cost, and convenience, as well as the social, psychological, and nutritional factors.
9. Describe how the senses of taste and smell work.
10. You have just had a fast-food lunch. Describe what happens as these foods go through your gastrointestinal tract from start to finish.
11. Distinguish among digestion, absorption, and metabolism.
12. What is the primary purpose of the RDAs?
13. How is the RDA for energy different from the RDA for protein?

14. When there was not enough scientific evidence to develop an RDA, what did the Food and Nutrition Board do?
15. Why are no RDAs set for sodium, chloride, and potassium?

ACTIVITIES AND APPLICATIONS

1. Quiz

Here are the answers to the quiz at the beginning of the chapter. How did you do?

1. True	6. True
2. True	7. False
3. False	8. True
4. True	9. True
5. True	10. False

2. How Many Calories Do I Need Each Day?

Use the following two steps to calculate the number of calories you need.

a. To determine your basal metabolic needs, multiply your weight in pounds by 10.9 if you are male, 9.8 if you are female. (These numbers are based on a BMR factor of 1.0 calorie per kilogram of body weight per hour for men and 0.9 calorie for women.)

EXAMPLE 150 pound woman x 9.8 = 1470 calories

b. To determine how many calories you use each day for physical activity, first determine your level of activity:

Very light: You spend most of your time seated or standing.

Light activity: You spend part of your day up and about, such as in teaching or cleaning house.

Moderate activity: You engage in an exercise activity for an hour or so at least every other day, or your job requires some physical work.

Heavy activity: You engage in manual labor, such as roofing.

Once you have picked your activity level, multiply your answer in (a) by one of the following numbers.

Very light (men and women): Multiply by 1.3
Light (men): Multiply by 1.6
Light (women): Multiply by 1.5
Moderate (men): Multiply by 1.7
Moderate (women): Multiply by 1.6

Heavy (men): Multiply by 2.1
Heavy women): Multiply by 1.9
(Source: Food & Nutrition Board, 1989)

EXAMPLE A women with light activity.
  1470 calories x 1.5 = 2205 calories needed daily

3. Factors That Influence What Foods You Eat

Determine which of the following factors influence what you eat and why or why not: food taste, your age, your family, television, your culture or ethnic background, your self-concept, your socioeconomic status, your sex, peer pressure, your body weight, your nutritional knowledge, parental food habits and attitudes, food associations, your religion, nutrition and health concerns, food availability, cost, convenience, and familiarity with the food.

4. Taste and Smell

Pick one of your favorite foods, eat it normally, and then take a bite of it while holding your nose closed. How does it taste when you can't smell very well? What influence does smell have on taste?

5. Nutrient-Dense Foods

Pick one food that you ate yesterday that could be considered nutrient dense. Also pick one food that would *not* be considered nutrient dense. Use Appendix A or another resource to look at the nutritional profiles of these foods. Explain why one food is nutrient dense and the other is not.

Hot Topic: Biotechnology

Biotechnology is the use of genetic engineering to change the genetic material of a living cell so it makes new substances or performs new functions. Biotechnology is being used to create an abundant supply of better-tasting and more nutritious foods. To get a better idea of what biotechnology is all about, let's take a peek into the supermarket of the near future. At first glance, products won't seem much different from those you are used to. Cucumbers, peppers, and corn will still be there. But amid all the produce and other kitchen staples, you are apt to find new versions of familiar foods— ones that are custom built to improve quality or remove unwanted traits. Insect-resistant apples, long-lasting raspberries, and potatoes that absorb less fat when fried are among the more than 50 plant products currently under study that are likely to reside on grocers' shelves in the future.

These commodities will arrive courtesy of **genetic engineering**, a process that allows plant breeders to modify the genetic makeup of a plant species precisely and predictably, creating improved varieties faster and easier than can be done using more traditional plant-breeding techniques. New methods allow scientists to identify a gene that produces a particular trait and transfer a copy of it to another plant used for human food or animal feed. Although the notion of tinkering with a plant's traits is thought of as radically new by some people, scientists have been doing it for many years in cruder, less predictable ways. Even in ancient times, farmers practiced a less-refined and more time-consuming version of genetic manipulation by saving seeds from crops that proved the hardiest and most disease resistant. Genetic engineering, though, can do much more than farmers could. Farmers could only incorporate the genes found in closely related plants or animals that interbreed. Genetic engineering can make use of any genes, regardless of their origin. Thus, a useful gene from an animal could be inserted into a plant.

For the last 10 years, genetic engineering has inhabited agricultural research laboratories and is now making its initial appearance in food stores. In 1994, the first genetically engineered whole product went on the market when the Food and Drug Administration (FDA) approved the Flavr Savr tomato, which can be shipped vine-ripened without rotting rapidly. If picked when ripe, tomatoes rot quickly. The Flavr Savr was the first genetically engineered, ready-to-eat food available to the public. The rotting problem was solved by inserting a reversed copy—an "antisense" gene—of the DNA molecules that prompt tomato spoilage. This suppresses the enzyme that results in rotting, allowing the tomato to stay ripe up to 10 days—plenty of time for shipping and sale.

Although genetic engineering promises tastier, more nutritious, more resistant, and less perishable foods, genetically engineered foods have encountered a few obstacles to widespread public acceptance. Some consumers, along with a few advocacy groups, have voiced concern about the safety and environmental impact of these new food products. Some urge an outright ban on any genetically engineered foods. Others support mandatory labeling that discloses the use of genetic engineering. Still others advocate more stringent testing of these products before marketing. The FDA presently suggests a series of safety tests and requires sponsors of genetically engineered products to consult them about any relevant safety questions before marketing new products. Sponsors must also seek permits to grow their plants in controlled areas, such as greenhouses. After proving that the plant will not adversely affect the environment, a permit will be issued by the U.S. Department of Agriculture to grow the plant in open test fields.

Another concern is how far genetic engineering will go. It's one thing to give consumers a tomato that stays ripe longer, but it's quite another to give them a tomato that has higher levels of vitamins that may help reduce the risk of diseases such as heart disease and cancer. Foods such as bread and salt were originally enriched and fortified to prevent nutritional-deficiency diseases. Now we are talking about a new category of foods, called **functional foods**, or **designer foods**, supplemented with ingredients thought to help prevent disease or improve health. In some cases, they are developed through biotechnology. Some of the health-promoting ingredients being touted are a variety of vitamins and **phytochemicals**, substances found in fruits and vegetables that seem to be helpful in preventing cancer. An important question to consider at this point is whether you want to meet your nutrient needs through a healthful diet composed mostly of whole foods (see Food Facts) or by choosing designer foods.

Every day, researchers are testing genetically engineered foods in the hopes of getting them onto supermarket shelves. Ultimately, the choice of selecting or rejecting these foods rests in consumers' hands.

REFERENCES   American Dietetic Association. 1995. Position of The American Dietetic Association: Biotechnology and the future of food. *Journal of The American Dietetic Association* 95(12): 1429–1432.

Chabner, Davi-Ellen. 1991. The *Language of Medicine.* Philadelphia: W. B. Saunders.

Egan, Maureen, and Susan Davis Allen. 1992. *Healthful Quantity Baking.* New York: John Wiley & Sons.

Food and Nutrition Board. 1994. How should the Recommended Dietary Allowances be revised?: A concept paper from the Food and Nutrition Board. *Nutrition Reviews* 52(6): 216–219.

Food and Nutrition Board, National Academy of Sciences/National Research Council. 1989. *Recommended Dietary Allowances.* Washington, DC: National Academy Press.

Monsen, Elaine R. 1989. The 10th edition of the Recommended Dietary Allowances: What's new in the 1989 RDAs? *Journal of the American Dietetic Association* 89(12): 1748–1752.

Murphy, S. P., D. Rose, M. Hudes, & F. Viteri. 1992. Demographic and economic factors associated with dietary quality for adults in the 1987–88 Nationwide Food Consumption Survey. *Journal of The American Dietetic Association* 92(11): 1252–1257.

Signed, certified & organic. 1992. *Nutrition Action Healthletter* 19(9):8–9.

Simko, Margaret D., and Lydia Jarosz. 1990. Organic foods: Are they better? *Journal of The American Dietetic Association* 90(3): 367, 370.

U.S. Department of Health and Human Services, Public Health Service. 1988. *The Surgeon General's Report on Nutrition and Health: Summary and Recommendations.* Washington, DC: U.S. Government Printing Office.

Label Reading Questions and Answers: Calories

What is the Daily Value for calories on the food label?

The Daily Value for calories is 2000 calories. The Percent Daily Values are therefore based on 2000 calories.

Does a "calorie-free" food really have no calories?

"Calorie-free" claims are allowed if the food contains less than 5 calories per serving. These foods may also be labeled "no calories" or "without calories."

What does it really mean if a label says the food is "low-calorie" or "reduced or fewer calories"?

Low-calorie means the food has 40 or fewer calories per serving. *Reduced* or *fewer calories* means the food has at least 25 percent fewer calories per serving than the reference food. For example, diet cola can be labeled "reduced calorie" because it has at least 25 percent fewer calories than regular colas.

If a food label says a food is "light," does that mean it has fewer calories?

If a food is labeled "light," it must contain one-third fewer calories or half the fat of the reference food. For example, a popular brand of light cream cheese states "50% Less Fat and 30% Fewer Calories than Cream Cheese." The word "light" can also be used to refer to other food characteristics, such as light in color or texture.

Carbohydrates

KEY QUESTIONS

1. What are the various types of carbohydrates, and in which foods are they found?
2. What are the health effects of carbohydrates?
3. How are carbohydrates digested, absorbed, and metabolized?
4. What are the functions of carbohydrates in the body?
5. How can you eat less refined sugar and more complex carbohydrates?

QUIZ

Directions: Circle *True* if you agree with the statement and *False* if you disagree.

1. Honey is better for you than sugar.	*True*	*False*
2. Refined sugar is the only carbohydrate that promotes tooth decay.	*True*	*False*
3. High-fructose corn syrup contains sugar.	*True*	*False*
4. Eating too much sugar causes diabetes.	*True*	*False*
5. Eating too much sugar causes hyperactivity in children.	*True*	*False*
6. Fiber is not found in meat or dairy products.	*True*	*False*
7. Beans are an excellent source of fiber.	*True*	*False*
8. Water-soluble fiber lowers blood cholesterol levels.	*True*	*False*
9. If there is not enough carbohydrate for energy, the body burns fat.	*True*	*False*
10. One form of sugar, glucose, is a very important fuel in the body.	*True*	*False*

Directions: Check which foods are significant sources of fiber.

11. Apples	19. Apple juice
12. Milk	20. Peas
13. Corn	21. Brown rice
14. Eggs	22. Baked beans
15. Oranges	23. Hamburger
16. Fish	24. Soft drinks
17. Bran flakes	25. Fried chicken
18. Cheddar cheese	

INTRODUCTION

Carbohydrate literally means hydrate (water) of carbon, a name derived from the investigations of early chemists who found that heating sugars for a long period of time in an open test tube produced droplets of water on the sides of the tube and a black substance, carbon. Later chemical analysis of sugars and other carbohydrates indicated that they all contain at least carbon, hydrogen, and oxygen.

Carbohydrates are the major components of most plants, making up from 60 to 90 percent of their dry weight. In contrast, animals and humans contain a comparatively small amount of carbohydrates. Plants are able to make their own carbohydrates from the carbon dioxide in air and in water taken from the soil in a process known as **photosynthesis**. Photosynthesis converts energy from sunlight into energy stored in carbohydrates. Animals are incapable of photosynthesis and, therefore, depend on plants as a source of carbohydrates. Besides being a food source, carbohydrates are used in clothing (cotton, linen, rayon), shelter, fuel, and paper (wood).

Carbohydrates are separated into two categories: simple and complex. **Simple carbohydrates**, also called **sugars**, include both natural and refined sugars. Carbohydrates are much more than just sugars, though, and includes the **complex carbohydrates** starch and fiber. Another name for complex carbohydrate is **polysaccharide** (*poly* means many), a good name for starch and fiber because both are long chains of many sugars.

Simple carbohydrates include sugars, and complex carbohydrates include starch and fiber.

SUGARS

Simple carbohydrates include **monosaccharides**, or single sugars, and **disaccharides**, or double sugars (*mono* means one and *di* means two). The term *sugar* refers to both monosaccharides and disaccharides collectively. In most cases, sugars taste sweet.

Monosaccharides include the simple sugars glucose, fructose, and galactose, which are the building blocks of other carbohydrates such as disaccharides and starch.

In photosynthesis, plants make glucose, which provides energy for growth and other plant activities. **Glucose**, also called dextrose, is the most significant monosaccharide because, as in plants, it is the human body's number one source of energy. Most of the carbohydrates you eat are converted to glucose in the body. The concentration of glucose in the blood, referred to as the *blood sugar level*, is vital to the proper functioning of the human body. At least 50 to 100 grams of carbohydrates must be

Our bodies must have a certain amount of glucose in the blood at all times in order to function properly.

eaten daily to maintain adequate blood glucose levels. Glucose is found in fruits such as grapes, in honey, and, in trace amounts, in most plant foods.

Fructose, the sweetest natural sugar, is also found in honey as well as in many fruits. Fructose is about 1.5 times as sweet as sucrose. Fructose and glucose are the most common monosaccharides in nature.

The last single sugar, **galactose**, does not occur alone in nature but is linked to glucose to make milk sugar, also called lactose, a disaccharide.

Most naturally occurring carbohydrates contain two or more monosaccharide units linked together. Disaccharides, the double sugars, include sucrose, maltose, and lactose. **Sucrose** is the chemical name for what is commonly called cane sugar, table sugar, granulated sugar, or simply, sugar. It is extracted from sugarcane or sugar beets and used mainly to sweeten foods. As Figure 2-1 indicates, sucrose is simply two common single sugars—glucose and fructose—linked together. Although the primary source of sucrose in the American diet is refined sugar, sucrose does occur naturally in small amounts in many fruits and vegetables. Table sugar is more than 99 percent pure sugar and provides virtually no nutrients for its 16 calories per teaspoon.

Maltose, which consists of two bonded glucose units, does not occur in nature to any appreciable extent. It is fairly abundant in germinating (sprouting) grain and is produced in the manufacture of beer when dried

The chemical name for table sugar is sucrose.

FIGURE 2-1.
Monosaccharides and disaccharides

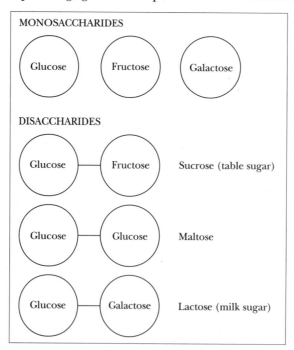

barley soaked in water germinates.

The last disaccharide, **lactose**, is commonly called milk sugar. It is found naturally only in milk, where it occurs to the extent of about 5 percent, and in certain other dairy products. Unlike most carbohydrates, which are in plant products, lactose is one of the few carbohydrates associated exclusively with animal products. Milk is not thought of as sweet because lactose is one of the lowest-ranking sugars in terms of sweetness (Table 2-1). Lactose is removed in the manufacture of some cheeses and added to several nondairy products.

Lactose is the sugar found in milk. It is not very sweet.

TABLE 2-1. Relative sweetness of sugars and alternative sweeteners.	
Name	Sweetness Compared to Sucrose
Sugars	
Fructose	1.5
Sucrose	1.0
Glucose	0.7
Lactose	0.2
Alternative Sweeteners	
Saccharin (Sweet N'Low)	300
Aspartame (Nutrasweet, Equal)	200
Acesulfame–K (Sunette)	200

Sugars in Food

Sugar occurs naturally in some foods, such as fruits and milk. Fruits are an excellent source of natural sugar, but be aware that some canned fruits contain much added sugar. Canned fruits are packed in one of three styles: in fruit juice, light syrup, or heavy syrup. Both light syrup and heavy syrup have added sugar. Heavy syrup contains the most added sugar (about 4 teaspoons of sugar to ½ cup of fruit). Dried fruits, such as raisins, are more concentrated sources of natural sugar than fresh fruits because dried fruits contain much less water.

Although a natural sugar, honey (made by bees) is primarily fructose and glucose, the same two components of table sugar. Therefore, by the time they are absorbed, honey and table sugar are the same thing. Although they are different in flavor and texture, the body can't tell the difference between natural and refined sugars. They both contribute only energy and no other nutrients in significant amounts. Because honey is more concentrated, it has twice as many calories as the same amount of sugar.

Lactose, or milk sugar, is present in large amounts in milk, ice cream,

TABLE 2-2 Common forms of refined sugars.

Form of Sugar	Description
Granulated sugar (sucrose)	Most important and most used sugar product on the market. Made from beet sugar or cane sugar, which are identical in chemical composition.
Powdered or confectioners' sugar	Granulated sugar that has been pulverized. Available in several degrees of fineness, designated by the number of X's following the name. 6X is the standard confectioners' sugar and is used in icing and toppings.
Brown sugar	Sugar crystals contained in a molasses syrup with natural flavor and color—91 to 96 percent sucrose. Sold in 4 grades—the higher the grade, the darker the brown sugar, the more flavor.
Turbinado sugar	Sometimes viewed incorrectly as raw sugar. Produced by separating raw sugar crystals and washing them with steam to remove impurities.
Syrups	
Corn syrup	Made from cornstarch. Mostly glucose. Only 75 percent as sweet as sucrose. Less expensive than sucrose. Used extensively in baked goods. Also used in canned goods.
High-fructose corn syrup	Corn syrup treated with an enzyme that converts glucose to fructose, which results in a sweeter product. Used in soft drinks, baked goods, jelly, syrups, fruits, and desserts.
Maple syrup	Made with mature sugar maple tree sap that flows in the spring. Mostly replaced by pancake syrup—a mixture of sucrose and artificial flavorings.
Molasses	Thick syrup left over after making sugar from sugarcane. Brown in color with a high sugar concentration.

ice milk, sherbet, cottage cheese, cheese spreads and other soft cheeses, eggnog, and cream. Hard cheeses contain only traces of lactose.

Refined sugars, such as table sugar or corn syrup, are added to foods as sweeteners (Table 2-2). Besides sweetening, they prevent spoilage in jams and jellies and perform several functions in baking such as browning the crust and retaining moisture in baked goods so they stay fresh. Sugar also acts as a food for yeast in breads and other baked goods that use yeast for leavening.

High-fructose corn syrup is corn syrup that has been treated with an enzyme that converts part of the glucose it contains to fructose. The reason for changing the glucose to fructose lies in the fact that fructose is twice as sweet as glucose. High-fructose corn syrup is therefore sweeter, ounce for ounce, than corn syrup, so smaller amounts can be used (making it cheaper). It is used to sweeten almost all nondiet soft drinks and is frequently used in canned juices, fruit drinks, sweetened teas, cookies, jams and jellies, syrups, and sweet pickles. Although table sugar consumption has dropped over the past 15 years, consumption of high-fructose corn syrup has increased almost 250 percent, according to figures from the U.S. Department of Agriculture.

Table sugar consumption has dropped, whereas high-fructose corn syrup consumption has increased.

If you chew sugarless gums, you may know that they often contain sorbitol or mannitol for sweetness. These substances are called sugar alcohols. **Sorbitol** is 60 percent as sweet as sucrose with about the same number of calories per gram (that is, 4 calories). Sorbitol is used in such products as sugarless hard and soft candies, chewing gums, jams, and jellies. **Xylitol**, another sugar alcohol, has limited FDA approval for special dietary uses. Xylitol is about as sweet as table sugar and is absorbed very slowly. A third sugar alcohol, **mannitol**, is poorly digested so it does not contribute a full 4 calories per gram. It occurs naturally in pineapple, olives, sweet potatoes, and carrots, and is added to sugarless gums. Both mannitol and sorbitol, when taken in large amounts, can cause diarrhea. Products whose reasonably foreseeable consumption may result in a daily ingestion of 50 grams of sorbitol or 20 grams of mannitol must bear the labeling statement "Excess consumption may have a laxative effect."

The sugar alcohols are mostly found in the dietetic section of the supermarket in sugarless gums and hard candies.

The sugar content of various foods is listed in Table 2-3.

Sugars and Health

The media has connected sugar to any number of different health problems. Fears that sweeteners cause many health problems, such as obesity or diabetes, are unfounded. All in all, sugar likely contributes to only one problem: tooth decay.

OBESITY. Sugar has been said to cause obesity, an idea that probably derives from the fact that high-sugar foods, which are often teamed up with fat (as in many cakes and cookies), are usually high in calories. They are also, by the way, typically low in nutrients and are therefore referred to as **empty calories**. For example, the cupcake pictured in Figure 2-2 supplies 170 calories with virtually no nutrients. Important nutrients can be crowded out of the diet by empty-calorie foods. Excess calories from too many empty calories—or any other food, for that matter—results in extra pounds. Therefore, sugar or any other dietary carbohydrate has no particular role in the cause of obesity. Calorie balance and obesity are covered in Chapter 9.

TABLE 2-3. Sugar content of foods.	
Food/Portion	*Teaspoons of Sugar*
Dairy	
Skim milk, 1 cup	3
Swiss cheese, 1 ounce	Less than 1
Vanilla ice cream, ½ cup	4
Meat, Poultry, and Fish	
Meat, poultry, or fish, 3 ounces	0
Eggs	
Egg, 1	0
Grains	
White bread, 1 slice	Less than 1
English muffin, 1	Less than 1
White rice, cooked, ½ cup	Less than 1
Cheerios cereal, 1 cup	Less than 1
Honey Nut Cheerios, 1 cup	3
Quaker Oatmeal Squares, 1 cup	2
Fruits	
Apple, 1 medium	4.5
Banana, 1 medium	7
Orange, 1 medium	3
Raisins, 14 grams	2.5
Vegetables	
Broccoli, ½ cup raw chopped	Less than 1 gram
Mixed vegetables, ⅛ cup	Less than 1 gram
Beverages	
Cola soft drink, 12 fluid ounces	10
Cakes, Cookies, Candies, and Pudding	
Brownie, 1 average	6
Chocolate graham crackers, 8	2
Chocolate chip cookies, 3	3
Lemon drops, 4 pieces	2.5
M & M candies, 70 pieces	7
Vanilla pudding, ½ cup	6
Sweeteners	
White sugar, 1 tablespoon	3
Honey, 1 tablespoon	4
High-fructose corn syrup, 1 tablespoon	4

Homemade Cupcake with Icing

FIGURE 2-2.
Example of
empty calories.

Information per serving:

Serving Size = 1 Cupcake
Calories   170
Protein   2 grams
Carbohydrates   30 grams
Fat   5 grams
Sodium   110 milligrams

Percentage of U.S. Recommended Daily Allowances

Protein   2
Niacin   *
Thiamin   *
Vitamin A   *
Vitamin C   *
Riboflavin 2
Calcium   *
Iron*

*Less than 2% of USRDA

DIABETES. Researchers do not know why **diabetes** occurs, but they know that sugars do not cause it. Diabetes is a disorder in the way the body handles sugars. People with diabetes do not make enough insulin, or they cannot use the insulin their bodies do make. Insulin gets sugar from the bloodstream into the body's cells, where sugar is used to produce energy. Therefore, untreated diabetics have high blood sugar levels. Treatment for diabetics includes a balanced diet, regular exercise, and medication when prescribed. The diabetic diet is discussed in more detail in Chapter 14.

Diabetes is characterized by high blood sugar levels, hypoglycemia by low blood sugar levels.

HYPOGLYCEMIA. Whereas diabetes is characterized by high blood sugar levels, hypoglycemia is characterized by low blood sugar levels. **Hypoglycemia** refers both to low blood sugar and to diseases that cause low blood sugar. Some health professionals feel that hypoglycemia has been overdiagnosed in the American public. There are, basically, two types of hypoglycemia: postprandial hypoglycemia and fasting hypoglycemia. The most common variety is **postprandial hypoglycemia**, which occurs generally 1 to 4 hours after meals and has symptoms such as quickened heartbeat, shakiness, weakness, anxiety, sweating, and dizziness, mimicking anxiety or stress symptoms. It may be caused when a rapid rise in blood glucose after a meal causes a temporary overproduction of insulin, which pulls too much sugar out of the bloodstream.

A second type of hypoglycemia, **fasting hypoglycemia**, is rare. It has numerous causes, such as drugs, and can be serious. Its symptoms occur after not eating for eight or more hours, so it usually occurs during the night or before breakfast.

Hypoglycemia may be due to cancer, pancreatic diseases, removal of part of the stomach, or other reasons. Hypoglycemia is also seen in people with diabetes as a common side effect of their insulin therapy. A diet for people with hypoglycemia includes regular, well-balanced meals with moderate amounts of refined sugars and sweets.

HYPERACTIVITY IN CHILDREN. During the 1980s two reports came out linking sugar intake with hyperactivity in children. Unfortunately, the study methods were unclear as to whether sugar caused the hyperactivity or the hyperactivity caused the children to eat sugar. Recently, researchers analyzed 23 studies on sugar and behavior involving more than 500 children. Their analysis shows that sugar, in general, does not affect children's behavior or cognitive performance (Wolraich, Wilson, and White, 1995).

Most people with lactose intolerance can drink some milk as long as it is part of a meal.

LACTOSE INTOLERANCE. Lactose (milk sugar) is a problem for certain people who lack, or more commonly, don't have enough of the enzyme **lactase**. Lactase is needed to split lactose into its components in the small intestine. If lactose is not split, it travels to the colon where bacteria ferment it and produce short-chain fatty acids and gas. These by-products do not normally cause any problems or discomfort in small amounts. However, if a lot of lactose travels to the colon, symptoms such as rectal gas, abdominal distention, and diarrhea often occur within about 30 minutes to 2 hours after ingesting milk products. The symptoms are normally cleared up within two to five hours. This problem, called **lactose intolerance**, seems to be an inherited problem especially prevalent among Africans, Greeks, and Asians, as well as other population groups (Saavedra and Perman, 1989).

Treatment for lactose intolerance requires a diet that is limited in lactose, which is present in large amounts in milk, ice cream, ice milk, sherbet, cottage cheese, eggnog, and cream. Most individuals can drink small amounts of milk without any symptoms, especially if eaten with food. Chocolate milk and whole milk are sometimes better tolerated than skim or 2 percent milk due to variations in fat content and the presence of other sugars which may delay emptying of the stomach (Dehkordi, Rao, Warren, and Chawan, 1995). Sweet acidophilus milk (milk containing the bacteria *Lactobacillus acidophilus*) may also help to alleviate lactose intolerance. Lactose-reduced milk and some other lactose-reduced dairy products are available in supermarkets, as is the enzyme lactase (which is also sold in pharmacies). Lactase can be added to milk to reduce the lactose content. Eight fluid ounces of lactose-reduced milk contains only 3 grams of lactose, compared with 12 grams in regular milk. Reducing the lactose content of milk by 50 percent is often adequate to prevent symptoms of lactose intolerance (Brand and Holt, 1991). Although lactose-reduced milk and other lactose-digestive aids are available, they may not be necessary when lactose intake is limited to one cup of milk (or equivalent) or less a day (Suarez, Savaiano, and Levitt, 1995).

Yogurt is usually well tolerated because it is cultured with live bacteria that digest lactose. This is not always the case with frozen yogurt, because most brands do not contain nearly the number of bacteria found in fresh yogurt (there are no federal standards for frozen yogurt at this time). Also, some yogurts have milk solids added to them that can cause problems. Many hard cheeses contain very little lactose and usually do not cause symptoms because most of the lactose is removed during processing or digested by the bacteria used in making cheese.

People who have difficulty digesting lactose report tremendous variation in which lactose-containing foods they can eat and even the time of day they can eat them. For example, one individual may not tolerate milk at all, whereas another can tolerate milk as part of a big meal. The ability to tolerate lactose is not an all-or-nothing phenomenon. As people with lactase deficiency usually decrease their intake of dairy products and thus their calcium intake, they should try different dairy products to see what they can tolerate.

DENTAL CARIES. The only negative health effect of sugar that most health experts agree on is that sugar (and starches too) do contribute to the development of **dental caries**, or cavities. The more often sugars and starches—even small amounts—are eaten and the longer they are in the mouth before teeth are brushed, the greater the risk for tooth decay. Dental caries are a major cause of tooth loss. This is so because every time you eat something sweet, the bacteria living on your teeth ferment the carbohydrate to form acids on the surfaces of the teeth. This acid eats away at the teeth, and cavities eventually develop. The fermentation may continue for hours. The deposit of bacteria, protein, and polysaccharides that forms on the teeth in the absence of toothbrushing during a period of 12 to 24 hours is called **plaque**. Without good tooth brushing habits, plaque may cover all surfaces of the teeth.

Other factors influence how much impact foods will have on the development of dental caries. The sequence of eating foods in a meal, food form (liquid, solid and sticky), and combinations of foods also influence

Certain foods, such as apples and cheese, are helpful in terms of preventing tooth decay.

dental caries. At meals, if unsweetened foods, such as aged cheeses are eaten after a sugared food, the plaque will be less acidic so less acid eats away at the teeth. Cheese also stimulates more saliva to be produced, which helps to wash away acids. This is why eating sugary or starchy foods as frequent between-meal snacks is more harmful to teeth than having them at meals. Sticky carbohydrate foods, such as raisins, cause more problems than liquid carbohydrate foods because they stick to the teeth and provide a constant source of fermentable carbohydrates for the bacteria until washed away. Liquids containing sugars have been considered less harmful to teeth than solid sweets because they clear the mouth quickly.

Food such as dried fruits, breads, cereals, cookies, crackers, and potato chips increase chances of dental caries when eaten frequently. Foods that do not seem to cause cavities include some vegetables, meats, fish, aged cheeses, and nuts. To prevent dental caries, brush your teeth often, floss your teeth once a day, try to limit sweets to mealtime, and see your dentist regularly.

MINI-SUMMARY Carbohydrates are separated into two categories: simple and complex. Simple carbohydrates are sugars and include both natural and refined sugars. Complex carbohydrates are long chains of many sugars. Monosaccharides are the building blocks of other carbohydrates and include glucose (the main source of the body's energy), fructose (found in fruits), and galactose (found in milk sugar). Disaccharides include sucrose (table sugar), maltose, and lactose (milk sugar). Refined sugars, such as high-fructose corn syrup, are used to sweeten soft drinks, break-

FIGURE 2-3.
The structures
of starch and
glycogen.

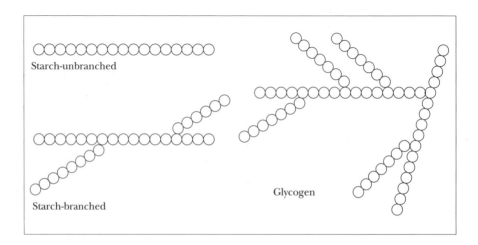

Starch-unbranched

Starch-branched

Glycogen

fast cereals, candy, baked goods such as cakes and pies, syrups, and jams and jellies. The only negative health effect of sugar that most health experts agree on is that sugar and starches contribute to the development of dental caries, or cavities. Lactose (milk sugar) is a problem for people with lactose intolerance. They experience abdominal cramps, bloating, and diarrhea about 30 minutes to 2 hours after ingesting milk products. Lactose-reduced milk, yogurt, and hard cheeses are usually well tolerated.

STARCH

Plants, such as peas, store glucose in the form of **starch**. Starch is made of many chains of hundreds to thousands of linked glucoses. The chains may be straight or may have tree-like branches (Figure 2-3). When you eat starchy foods, digestive enzymes break apart the glucose molecules.

Just as plants store glucose in the form of starch, your body stores glucose in a form called **glycogen**. Like starch, glycogen is a polysaccharide. It is a chain of glucose units, but the chains are longer and have more branches than starch (Figure 2-3). Glycogen is stored in two places in the body: the liver and the muscles. An active 150-pound man has about 350 calories stored in his liver glycogen and about 1400 calories stored in his muscle glycogen. When the blood sugar level starts to dip and more energy is needed, the liver converts glycogen into glucose, which is then delivered by the bloodstream. Muscle glycogen does not supply glucose to the bloodstream but is used strictly to supply energy for exercise.

Read the Food Facts on page 63 for more information on grains.

Starch in Food

Starch is only found in plant foods. Cereal grains, the fruits or seeds of cultivated grasses, are rich sources of starch and include wheat, corn, rice, rye, barley, and oats. Cereal grains are used to make breads, baked goods, breakfast cereals, and pastas. Starches are also found in root vegetables such as potatoes, and dried beans and peas such as navy beans.

Starchy foods in general are not flavorful if eaten raw, so most are cooked to make them taste better and be more digestible. Starch, such as cornstarch, is used extensively as a thickener in cooking, because starch undergoes a process called **gelatinization** when heated in liquid. When starches gelatinize, granules absorb water and swell making the liquid thicken. When this occurs, the liquid becomes thicker because there is less water. Gelatinization is a process unique to starches, so you find them frequently used as thickeners in soups, sauces, gravies, puddings, and other foods. Other thickeners include white flour and arrowroot.

Starch and Health

Starch creates the same problem as sugar in the mouth and therefore contributes to tooth decay and dental caries.

MINI-SUMMARY   Starch is a storage form of glucose in plants. The body stores glucose as glycogen in the liver and muscles. Glycogen is important to maintain normal blood sugar levels. Starches are found in cereal grains, breads, baked goods, cereals, pastas, root vegetables, and dried beans and peas. They are commonly used as thickeners. Like sugar, starch contributes to dental caries.

FIBER

Dietary fiber is mostly material from plant cell walls that resists digestion by our digestive enzymes. Like starch, most fibers are chains of bonded glucose units, but what's different is that the units are linked with a chemical bond our digestive enzymes can't break down. In other words, most fiber passes through the stomach and intestines unchanged and is excreted in the feces. Fiber was called *roughage* a few generations ago.

Fiber is found only in plant foods; it does not appear in animal foods. There are two major types of fiber—water-soluble and water-insoluble. **Water-soluble fiber** swells in water, like a sponge, into a gel-like substance. **Water-insoluble fiber** also swells in water, but not nearly to the extent as soluble fiber.

The water-soluble fibers include gums, mucilages, pectin, and some hemicelluloses. They are generally found around and inside plant cells. The water-insoluble fibers include cellulose, lignin, and the remaining hemicelluloses. They generally form the structural parts of plants. The amount of fiber in a plant varies among plants and may vary within a species or variety depending on growing conditions and the plant's maturity at harvest.

Fiber in Food

Fiber is abundant in plants, so legumes (dried beans, peas, and lentils), fruits, vegetables, whole grains and grain products, nuts, and seeds provide fiber. The values reported in Table 2-4 reflect the dietary fiber, not crude fiber, found in these foods. An older and not very accurate method of determining a food's fiber content measured the crude fiber. Current methods, although still not perfect, measure the dietary fiber, a much more accurate figure. Appendix C contains more extensive information on the fiber content of foods. Fiber is not found in meat,

TABLE 2-4. **Fiber content of selected foods.**

Food/Portion	Grams Fiber	Food/Portion	Grams Fiber
Dairy Group		*Vegetables*	
Milk, 1 cup	0	Broccoli spears, 1/2 cup	2.4
Plain yogurt, 1 cup	0	Carrots, 1/2 cup	2.0
Cheddar cheese, 1 once	0	Green beans, canned, 1/2	2.0
Ice cream, soft serve, 1 cone	0	Lettuce, iceberg, 1 cup	0.5
Meat, Poultry, Fish		Potato, 1/2 cup	1.5
Meat, poultry, and fish	0	*Legumes*	
Eggs		Chick peas, 1/2 cup	4.3
Eggs	0	Kidney beans, 1/2 cup	6.9
Grains		Lentils, 1/2 cup	5.2
White bread, 1 slice	0.6	Split peas, 1/2 cup	3.1
Whole-wheat bread, 1 slice	1.5	*Nuts and seeds*	
Hamburger bun, ½	0.7	Almonds, 6 whole	0.6
Saltine crackers, 6	0.5	Peanuts, 10 large	0.6
Fruits		Peanut butter, smooth,	
Apple, red, 1 small	2.8	1 tablespoon	1.0
Applesauce, ½ cup	2.0		
Banana ½ small	1.1		
Orange, 1 small	2.9		
Orange juice, 1/2 cup	0.1		
Raisins, 2 tablespoons	0.4		

Source: Anderson, James W. 1990. *Plant Fiber in Foods.* Lexington: HCF Nutrition Research Foundation, Inc. Reprinted with permission.

poultry, fish, dairy products, and eggs. Foods containing water-soluble fibers are as follows.

Beans and peas, such as kidney beans, pinto beans, chickpeas, split peas, and lentils

Some cereal grains, such as oats and barley

Some fruits and vegetables, such as apples, grapes, citrus fruits, carrots

Water-insoluble fiber includes the structural parts of plants such as skins and the outer layer of the wheat kernel. You have seen insoluble fiber in the skin of whole-kernel corn and in celery strings. It is found in:

Wheat bran

Whole grains such as whole wheat and brown rice, and products made with whole grains such as whole-wheat or rye bread

Many vegetables, such as potatoes, green beans, and cabbage

Beans and peas are among the highest food sources of dietary fiber.

Most foods contain both water-insoluble and water-soluble fibers.

Whenever the fiber-rich bran and the vitamin-rich germ are left on the endosperm of a grain, the grain is called *whole grain* (see Figure 2-4 in Food Facts). Examples of whole grains include whole wheat, whole rye, bulgur (whole-wheat grains that have been steamed and dried), oatmeal, whole cornmeal, whole hulled barley, popcorn, and brown rice.

The milling of whole wheat in the United States to produce white flour (also called wheat flour) removes the bran and germ and leaves behind mostly starch. By law, white flour must be enriched, meaning that the following four nutrients must be returned to the flour: thiamin, riboflavin, niacin, and iron. Unfortunately, enrichment does not replace the fiber, and it replaces only 4 nutrients out of the 20 removed. Whole-wheat flour (particularly stone-ground) retains most of the original nutrients and has more fiber, vitamin B_6, folacin, magnesium, and zinc than enriched white flour.

Enriched wheat flour still has fewer nutrients than whole-wheat flour.

As a rule, unrefined foods contain more fiber than refined foods because fiber is usually removed in processing. For example, raw apples contain much fiber in the skin, but the skin is removed to make applesauce or canned sliced apples.

Although purified fibers (such as wheat or oat bran) and fiber supplements (some in pill form) are available, they are not generally recommended. Whole foods contain a greater variety of fibers as well as many other nutrients. Purified fibers in large amounts can be harmful, and certain purified fibers may not have the same effect in the body as the actual food fiber.

Fiber and Health

Fiber has many benefits to the body (American Dietetic Association, 1993).

- Water-soluble fibers decrease blood cholesterol levels in most cases (Glore, Van Treeck, Knehans, and Guild, 1994). Studies of people eating oats, oat bran, and beans show that these foods seem to help lower blood cholesterol levels. At the same time, these people were usually consuming a diet with less fat, so this certainly influenced the outcome as well. Eating more soluble fiber may help lower blood cholesterol when part of an overall health plan that includes eating less fat, less cholesterol, and exercising.
- Water-soluble fibers delay emptying of the stomach so that you feel full longer. This can help individuals lose weight or keep weight off. Also, higher-fiber diets contain fewer calories, which can also help these individuals.

- Since water-insoluble fiber speeds the movement of wastes through the intestines, increases fecal bulk, and absorbs some water in the intestinal tract, stool is softer and easier to eliminate. A diet high in insoluble fiber is used in prevention and treatment of hemorrhoids and diverticulosis (Klurfeld, 1987). **Hemorrhoids** are enlarged veins in the lower rectum. **Diverticulosis** is a disease of the large intestine in which the intestinal walls become weakened, bulge out into pockets, and at times become inflamed.

- The water-insoluble fibers may be responsible for reducing the risk of colon cancer, the second most common and most deadly cancer, possibly by decreasing the amount of time the cancer-causing agents remain in the intestines.

- Fiber seems to help diabetics maintain more normal blood sugar levels. Because water-soluble fibers delay emptying of the stomach, glucose from food is absorbed more slowly from the intestinal tract.

Finally, fiber-rich foods usually require more time to chew and provide an increased sense of fullness, or satiety, so they are excellent choices for weight loss or maintaining a healthy weight.

MINI-SUMMARY Dietary fiber is mostly material from plant cell walls that resists digestion. Fiber is found only in plant foods. Water-soluble fibers include gums, mucilages, pectin, and some hemicelluloses. They are found in beans and peas, some cereal grains such as oats, and some fruits and vegetables. Water-soluble fibers tend to decrease blood cholesterol levels and delay stomach emptying. Water-insoluble fibers include cellulose, lignin, and the remaining hemicelluloses. They are found in wheat bran, whole grains, and many vegetables. Water-insoluble fiber makes stool easier to eliminate and may reduce the risk of colon cancer. Fiber-rich foods also help diabetics maintain normal blood sugar levels.

DIGESTION, ABSORPTION, AND METABOLISM

Before carbohydrates can be absorbed through the villi of the small intestine, they must be broken down into monosaccharides, or one-sugar units. Starch digestion begins in the mouth, where enzymes start to break down starch into polysaccharides and **oligosaccharides** (a chain of 4 to 10 glucose units). Then the intestine completes the breakdown of starch into maltose, which is split by an enzyme into 2 glucose units. Glucose is then absorbed.

Through the work of various enzymes, all sugars are broken down into the single sugars: glucose, fructose, and galactose. They are then

TABLE 2-5. Carbohydrate digestion.

Site	Name of Enzyme	Carbohydrate Acted Upon	Products Formed
Mouth	Salivary amylase	Starch	Polysaccharides, Oligosaccharides
Small intestine	Pancreatic amylase Sucrase	Starch Sucrose	Maltose Glucose, fructose
	Lactase	Lactose	Glucose, Galactose
	Maltase	Maltose	Glucose

The most important function of carbohydrates is to provide fuel for your body.

absorbed and enter the bloodstream, which carries them to the tissues and the liver. In the liver, fructose and galactose are converted to glucose or further metabolized. The hormone insulin makes it possible for glucose to enter body cells, where it is used for energy or stored as glycogen.

Table 2-5 summarizes how the various forms of carbohydrates are digested. Don't forget that fiber cannot be digested, or broken down into its components, so it continues down to the large intestine to be excreted.

MINI-SUMMARY During digestion, various enzymes break down starch and sugars into monosaccharides, which are then absorbed. In the liver, fructose and galactose are converted into glucose or further metabolized.

FUNCTIONS OF CARBOHYDRATES

Carbohydrates are the primary source of the body's energy. Protein and fat can be burned for energy by other cells, but the body uses carbohydrates first, in part because it is the most efficient energy source. In fact, the central nervous system, including the brain and nerve cells, relies almost exclusively on glucose for energy.

If there are not enough carbohydrates for energy, the body can burn either fat or protein, but this is not desirable. When fat is burned for energy without any carbohydrates present, the process is incomplete and results in the production of **ketone bodies**, which start to accumulate in the blood. An excessive level of ketone bodies can cause the blood to become too acidic (called **ketosis**), which then interferes with the transport of oxygen in the blood. Ketosis can cause dehydration and may even lead to a fatal coma. Carbohydrates are important to help the body use fat efficiently.

Carbohydrates also spare protein from being burned for energy so protein can be better used to build and repair the body. About 100 grams of carbohydrates are needed daily to spare protein from being burned for fuel, to prevent ketosis, and to provide glucose to the central nervous system. This amount represents what you minimally need, not what is desirable (about two to three times more).

Carbohydrates are part of various materials found in the body such as connective tissues, some hormones and enzymes, and genetic material.

As already discussed, fiber promotes the normal functioning of the intestinal tract.

MINI-SUMMARY Carbohydrates are the primary source of the body's energy. The central nervous system relies almost exclusively on glucose and other simple carbohydrates for energy. Carbohydrates are also important to help the body use fat efficiently. When fat is burned for energy without any carbohydrates present, the process is incomplete and could result in ketosis. Carbohydrates are part of various materials found in the body.

RECOMMENDATIONS AND TIPS FOR NUTRITIOUS FOOD SELECTION

Refined Sugars

The **Dietary Guidelines for Americans** recommends using sugars only in moderation. The World Health Organization suggests a maximum of 10 percent of total calories from refined sugars. According to a report from the RDA Sugars Task Force, the average daily intake of added sugars was 53 grams daily, or about 11 percent of calorie intake (Glinsmann, Irausquin, and Park, 1986). To keep your consumption of refined sugar within the recommendations, try the following.

GENERAL RECOMMENDATIONS

1. Instead of regular soft drinks or powdered drink mixes, choose diet soft drinks, 100 percent pure fruit juices, bottled waters such as seltzer, or iced tea made without added sugar or with artificial sweeteners.
2. Use less refined sugar in coffee, tea, cereals, and so forth, or use sugar substitutes.

MEALTIME

3. Choose 100 percent pure fruit juices, which do not contain added sugars. Products labeled "fruit drinks," "fruit beverages," or "flavored

TABLE 2-6.	Where are the added sugars?		
Food Groups	*Added Sugars (teaspoons)*	*Food Groups*	*Added Sugars (teaspoons)*
Bread, Cereal, Rice, and Pasta		*Milk, Yogurt, and Cheese*	
Bread, 1 slice	0	Milk, plain, 1 cup	0
Muffin, 1 medium	★1	Chocolate milk, 2 percent, 1 cup	★★★3
Cookies, 2 medium	★1	Lowfat yogurt, plain, 8 oz.	0
Danish pastry, 1 medium	★1	Lowfat yogurt, flavored, 8 oz.	★★★★★5
Doughnut, 1 medium	★★2	Lowfat yogurt, fruit, 8 oz.	★★★★★★★7
Ready-to-eat cereal, sweetened, 1 oz.	*	Ice cream, ice milk, or	
Pound cake, no-fat, 1 oz.	★★2	frozen yogurt, 1/2 cup	★★★3
Angelfood cake, 1/12 tube cake	★★★★★5	Chocolate shake, 10 fl. oz.	★★★★★★★★★9
Cake, frosted, 1/16 average	★★★★★★6		
Pie, fruit, 2 crust, 1/6 8" pie	★★★★★★6	*Other*	
		Sugar, jam, or jelly, 1 tsp.	0
Fruit		Syrup or honey, 1 tbsp.	★★★3
Fruit, canned in juice, 1/2 cup	0	Chocolate bar, 1 oz.	★★★3
Fruit, canned in light syrup, 1/2 cup	★★2	Fruit sorbet, 1/2 cup	★★★3
Fruit, canned in heavy syrup, 1/2 cup	★★★★4	Gelatin dessert, 1/2 cup	★★★★4
		Sherbert, 1/2 cup	★★★★★5
		Cola, 12 fl. oz.	★★★★★★★★★9
		Fruit drink, ade, 12 fl. oz.	★★★★★★★★★★★★12

* Check product label.   ★ = 1 teaspoon sugar.   Note: 4 grams of sugar = 1 teaspoon

drinks" usually contain only small amounts of fruit juice and much refined sugar.

4. Choose unsweetened breakfast cereals. For less sugar, choose cereals with less than 4 grams (1 teaspoon) of sugar per serving, unless the sugar comes from a dried fruit such as raisins. Top cereals with fresh fruit.

5. Jams, jellies, and pancake syrup contain much refined sugar. For less refined sugar and calories, select jams, jellies, and fruit spreads made without (or with less) sugar, and pancake syrup labeled "reduced-calorie." Other toppings for toast or pancakes are chopped fresh fruit, applesauce, or part-skim ricotta cheese and fruit.

6. Many fruited yogurts contain much sugar. For less sugar, mix fresh fruit or canned fruit (packed in its own juice) into plain yogurt.

SNACKS

7. Enjoy a fresh apple or banana instead of a candy bar if you want something sweet.
8. Buy cookies that contain less refined sugar, such as graham crackers, vanilla wafers, gingersnaps, and fig bars.
9. Substitute bagels, English muffins, rolls, or fruited muffins for sweetened breakfast pastries such as Danish.

DESSERTS AND BAKING

10. Instead of sweet desserts such as cake, emphasize fruits in desserts. Fresh fruit can be baked (as in baked apples), poached (as in poached pears), broiled, or made into compote. Try baked pears or baked apples with a sprinkle of cinnamon, or a broiled peach or grapefruit half with a sprinkle of nutmeg.
11. Select unsweetened frozen fruits or canned fruits packed in juice, rather than those packed in light or heavy syrup. One-half cup of fruit canned in heavy syrup contains approximately 4 teaspoons of sugar.
12. Select gelatin and pudding mixes without sugar.
13. Make desserts at home so you can better control the amount of sugar you use. When baking from scratch, you can decrease the sugar in many of your recipes by about one-fourth to one-third of the original amount without any significant difference in quality.
14. Add a small amount of vanilla, cinnamon, or nutmeg to sweet baked products to enhance flavor when you reduce sugars.
15. Select baking recipes that use fruit as a sweetener.
16. Use a fruit sauce or a sprinkling of powdered sugar in place of frosting on cake.

Complex Carbohydrates: Starch and Fiber

The *Dietary Guidelines for Americans* recommends that adults eat at least three servings of vegetables and two servings of fruits daily, and at least six servings of grain products (up to eleven), such as breads, cereals, pasta, and rice, with an emphasis on whole grains (U.S. Department of Agriculture, 1995). The World Health Organization (WHO) recommends at least 50 percent (and not more than 75 percent) of total calories from complex carbohydrates.

In a study of 4000 households, the average number of times grain products were eaten was three per day over a two-week period (Albertson and Tobelmann, 1995). Because serving sizes were not recorded, you cannot directly compare this number to the recommendations. With respect to whole-grain consumption, most study participants failed to consume even one whole-grain food each day, and about 20 percent of participants did not eat *any* whole-grain food products.

To eat more starchy foods, eat breads, rolls, and bagels; breakfast cereals (cooked and ready-to-eat); pastas (fresh and dried); whole grains (such as barley and brown rice); dried beans, peas, and lentils (use in soups, casseroles, and as side dishes); and starchy vegetables (such as peas and corn).

With respect to fiber, current research indicates that daily consumption of 20 to 35 grams of dietary fiber from a variety of foods may be helpful in promoting health and managing certain diseases (American Dietetic Association, 1993; Pilch, 1987; U.S. Department of Health and Human Services, 1991). Americans are currently consuming, on average, fewer than 20 grams daily, with perhaps half consuming fewer than 10 grams daily (American Dietetic Association, 1988). Here are some tips to increase your fiber consumption.

GENERAL RECOMMENDATIONS
1. The majority of available breads and baked goods are made with white flour, a poor source of fiber. For more fiber, choose whole-grain breads and baked goods, such as whole-wheat and rye bread, and items made with bran, such as bran muffins. The term "wheat bread" on a food label does not mean whole wheat, and color is not a good indication because colorings are sometimes added to make a product look more like whole wheat. Look for whole-wheat bread (made with 100 percent whole-wheat flour) or another whole grain listed first on the ingredient label. Other whole-grain ingredients include cracked wheat, oatmeal, whole cornmeal, and whole rye.
2. Eat fruits, preferably in their whole form, at any meal or for snacks, at least twice daily.

BREAKFAST
3. Choose whole-grain and bran cereals (good fiber sources), and make sure the cereal contains at least 4 grams of dietary fiber per serving.
4. Whole fruits have more fiber than fruit juice so include whole fruits with your breakfast.
5. Bran muffins are a tasty, high-fiber breakfast food.

LUNCH AND DINNER
6. For fiber, select soups rich in split peas, beans, lentils, and vegetables. Use barley to thicken vegetable soups.
7. Use whole-wheat or other whole-grain pasta instead of refined pasta

products. For example, make macaroni salad with whole-wheat macaroni for added fiber and flavor, or serve whole-wheat spaghetti with homemade tomato sauce with vegetables.

8 Top casseroles with wheat germ.

9. Try recipes using grains (see Food Facts).

10. Use cooked or canned dry beans and peas in main dishes, side dishes, and salads. For example, combine black beans and rice with chili powder or other peppery seasoning for a Caribbean-style dish. Try a mixture of any of these with a vinegar and oil dressing for a three- or four-bean salad: green beans, wax beans, kidney beans, lima beans, great northern beans, or chickpeas. Add kidney beans or chickpeas to a lettuce or spinach salad.

11. Use brown rice instead of white rice.

12. Leave the skin on potatoes.

13. Have a bean salad or mixed green salad with plenty of vegetables such as carrots, broccoli, and cauliflower. Include kidney or garbanzo beans as well.

SNACKS

14. Most commercial cookies contain little fiber, unless made with whole grains, such as oats, or dried fruits, such as raisins, dates, and figs.

15. For fiber in crackers, choose whole-grain crackers, such as whole-wheat crackers, or crackers made with bran.

16. Fresh fruits and popcorn are two high-fiber snacks.

DESSERTS AND BAKING

17. Bake or broil fruits for dessert.

18. Use fresh, frozen, canned, or dried fruits when baking muffins, pancakes, quick breads, or other baked products. Dried apricots, raisins, bananas, blueberries, or apples add extra fiber and variety in flavor.

19. White flour and baking mixes made from white flour contain little fiber. For more fiber, choose whole-grain flours, such as whole wheat, and mixes using whole-grain flour.

20. When baking, use plenty of fresh, frozen, canned, and dried fruits to increase fiber.

21. For puddings, try rice (use brown rice), tapioca, and bread (use whole-wheat bread).

MINI-SUMMARY It is recommended that you get at least 50 percent of your calories in the form of carbohydrates with no more than 10 percent of total calories coming from refined sugars. Daily consumption of 20 to 35 grams of dietary fiber from a variety of foods may be helpful in promoting health and managing certain diseases.

KEY TERMS

Carbohydrates
Complex
  carbohydrates
Dental caries
Diabetes
Dietary fiber
Dietary Guidelines
  for Americans
Disaccharides
Diverticulosis
Fasting
  hypoglycemia
Fructose
Galactose
Gelatinization
Glucose
Glycogen

Hemorrhoids
High-fructose
  corn syrup
Hypoglycemia
Ketone bodies
Ketosis
Lactase
Lactose
Lactose
  intolerance
Maltose
Mannitol
Monosaccharides
Nonnutritive
  sweeteners
Oligosaccharides
Photosynthesis

Plaque
Polysaccharide
Postprandial
  hypoglycemia
Simple
  carbohydrates
Sorbitol
Starch
Sucrose
Sugar
Sugar alcohols
Water-insoluble
  fiber
Water-soluble fiber
Xylitol

REVIEW QUESTIONS

1. What is the difference between simple carbohydrates and complex carbohydrates?
2. Which is the most significant monosaccharide and why is it so important? Which monosaccharide is found in honey and many fruits? Which monosaccharide is found only in milk sugar?
3. Which monosaccharides make up sucrose, maltose, and lactose?
4. Which sugar is being used more to sweeten soft drinks and other sweet foods?
5. Describe the three sugar alcohols, including the foods they are found in.
6. Briefly describe the relationship between sugar and obesity, diabetes, hypoglycemia, hyperactivity in children, and dental caries.
7. Which dairy products can lactose-intolerant people choose to eat?
8. How does sugar and starch contribute to dental caries?
9. Explain the purpose of glycogen and where it is stored.

10. Which foods are starchy?
11. Why are water-soluble fibers so named?
12. Name the water-soluble and the water-insoluble fibers.
13. Which foods contain significant amounts of water-soluble fiber? What are the health effects of water-soluble fiber?
14. Which foods contain significant amounts of water-insoluble fiber? What are the health effects of water-insoluble fiber?
15. Why does whole-wheat flour contain more nutrients than white flour?
16. Describe briefly how carbohydrates are digested, absorbed, and metabolized.
17. List five functions of carbohydrates.
18. What percent of calories should come from carbohydrates? From refined sugars?
19. How much fiber should you eat daily?
20. Do Americans eat recommended amounts of fiber?

**ACTIVITIES
AND
APPLICATIONS**

1. Quiz

Use the following to check your answers on the quiz at the beginning of the chapter.

1.	*False*	6.	*True*
2.	*False*	7.	*True*
3.	*True*	8.	*True*
4.	*False*	9.	*True*
5.	*False*	10.	*True*

These foods are significant sources of fiber: apple, corn, orange, bran flakes, peas, brown rice, and baked beans.

2. Self-Assessment

List how many servings of the following foods you normally eat daily.

Refined Sugars	*Number of Servings*
Sugar in coffee or tea	_____
Sweetened beverages	_____
Sweetened breakfast cereals	_____
Candy	_____
Commercially made baked goods, including cakes, pies, cookies, and doughnuts	_____
Jam, jelly, pancake syrup	_____

Complex Carbohydrates	*Number of Servings*
Breads and rolls	_____
Ready-to-eat and cooked cereals	_____
Pasta, rice, and other grains	_____
Dried beans and peas	_____
Potatoes	_____
Fruits	_____
Vegetables	_____

How do you rate? Do you get at least six servings per day of breads, rolls, cereals, pasta, rice, and other grains? Do you get a daily serving of dried beans and peas? Do you get at least five servings per day of fruits and vegetables combined? If not, you should not be choosing foods from the refined sugar column of the chart until your more important nutritional needs are met. Compare how many servings you have daily of foods high in refined sugars and complex carbohydrates. The idea is to push complex carbohydrate intake and minimize refined sugars.

3. Carbohydrate Basics

Check off under the appropriate column(s) if the food contains significant amounts of sugar, starch, and/or fiber.

Food	*Sugar*	*Starch*	*Fiber*
1. Hamburger	_____	_____	_____
2. Chicken wing	_____	_____	_____
3. Flounder	_____	_____	_____
4. Boiled egg	_____	_____	_____
5. American cheese	_____	_____	_____
6. Sour cream	_____	_____	_____
7. White bread	_____	_____	_____
8. Whole-wheat bread	_____	_____	_____
9. Chocolate cake	_____	_____	_____
10. Macaroni	_____	_____	_____
11. Brown rice	_____	_____	_____
12. Split peas	_____	_____	_____
13. Peanuts	_____	_____	_____
14. Fresh orange	_____	_____	_____
15. Broccoli	_____	_____	_____

4. Whole Grain or Refined Grain?

Read the following bread labels and decide which one is white bread and which one is whole grain bread.

#1 MADE FROM: Unbromated unbleached enriched wheat flour, corn syrup, partially hydrogenated soybean oil, molasses, salt, yeast, raisin juice concentrate, potato flour, wheat gluten, honey, vinegar, mono- and diglycerides, cultured corn syrup, unbleached wheat flour, xanthan gum, and soy lecithin.

#2 MADE FROM: Stoneground 100% whole wheat flour, water, high-fructose corn syrup, wheat gluten, yeast, honey, salt, molasses, partially hydrogenated soybean oil, raisin syrup, soy lecithin, mono- and diglycerides.

5. *How Many Teaspoons of Sugar?*

One teaspoon of sugar weighs 4 grams. Determine how many teaspoons of sugar are in each of the following foods, as described on their nutrition labels. Which food contains more sugar? Which food contains more fiber?

Nutrition Facts	*Nutrition Facts*
Amount per serving	Amount per serving
Calories 230	Calories 140
Calories from fat 140	Calories from fat 20
Total fat 16 g	Total fat 2.5 g
Saturated 6 g	Saturated 0.5 g
Polyunsaturated 1 g	Polyunsaturated 1 g
Monounsaturated 7 g	Monounsaturated 0.5 g
Cholesterol 74 g	Cholesterol 0 g
Sodium 180 mg	Sodium 180 mg
Total carbohydrate 28 g	Total carbohydrate 21 g
Dietary fiber 0 g	Dietary fiber 5 g
Sugar 24 g	Sugar 4 g
Protein 21 g	Protein 8 g

6. *Ranking of Foods by Fiber Content*

Using Appendix C, Fiber Content of Food, look up the dietary fiber content of two foods you like to eat in each category given. The first category is cereals, followed by grains, breads and crackers, fruits and juices, vegetables, legumes, nuts and seeds, and miscellaneous foods. Rank the foods in order of fiber content. Start with the food with the most fiber. Which food categories tend to have the most fiber?

7. *Nonnutritive Sweetener Sleuth*
Check out your refrigerator and cupboards to see what kinds of foods, and how many, contain nonnutritive sweeteners. Look for the words Equal, aspartame, saccharin, acesulfame potassium, Sunette, or Sweet One.

REFERENCES

Albertson, Ann M., and Rosemary C. Tobelmann. 1995. Consumption of grain and whole-grain foods by an American population during the years 1990 to 1992. *Journal of The American Dietetic Association* 95(6): 703–704.

American Dietetic Association. 1993. Position of the American Dietetic Association: Health implications of dietary fiber. *Journal of The American Dietetic Association* 93(12): 1446–1447.

American Dietetic Association. 1996. Position of the American Dietetic Association: Oral health and nutrition. *Journal of The American Dietetic Association* 96(2): 184–189.

American Dietetic Association. 1987. Position of the American Dietetic Association: Appropriate use of nutritive and non-nutritive sweeteners. *Journal of The American Dietetic Association* 87(12): 1689–1694.

American Medical Association. 1985. Aspartame, review of safety issues. *Journal of The American Medical Association* 254(3): 400–402.

American Medical Association. 1985. Saccharin, review of safety issues. *Journal of The American Medical Association* 254(18): 2622–2624.

Anderson, James W. 1985. Health implications of wheat fiber. *American Journal of Clinical Nutrition* 41(5): 1103–1112.

Anderson, James W., and Carol A. Bryant. 1986. Dietary fiber: Diabetes and obesity. *American Journal of Gastroenterology* 81(10): 898–906.

Anderson, James W., Nancy J. Gustafson, Carol A. Bryant and Janet Tietyen-Clark. 1987. Dietary fiber and diabetes: A comprehensive review and practical application. *Journal of The American Dietetic Association* 87(9): 1189–1197.

Anderson, James W., Belinda M. Smith, and Nancy J. Gustafson. 1994. Health benefits and practical aspects of high-fiber diets. *American Journal of Clinical Nutrition* 59(Suppl.): 1242S–1247S.

Asp, Nils-Georg. 1986. Dietary fibre—definition, chemistry and analytical determination. *Molecular Aspects of Medicine* 9: 17–27.

Blundell, J. E., and V. J. Burley. 1987. Satiation, satiety and the action of fibre on food intake. *International Journal of Obesity* 11(Suppl. 1): 9–25.

Brand, Janette C., and Suzanne Holt. 1991. Relative effectiveness of milk with reduced amounts of lactose in alleviating milk intolerance. *American Journal of Clinical Nutrition* 54: 148–151.

Brody, Jane. 1985. *Jane Brody's Good Food Book.* New York: W. W. Norton and Company.

Brown, W. Virgil, and W. Karmally. 1985. Coronary heart disease and the consumption of diets high in wheat and other grains. *American Journal of Clinical Nutrition* 41(5): 1163–1171.

Burley, V. J., A. R. Leeds, and J. E. Blundell. 1987. The effect of high- and low-fibre breakfasts on hunger, satiety, and food intake in a subsequent meal. *International Journal of Obesity* 11(Suppl. 1): 87–93.

Butcho, H. H., and F. N. Kotsonis. 1989. Aspartame: A review of recent research. *Comments Toxicology* 3: 253–78.

Cohen, Samuel M. 1986. Saccharin: Past, present, and future. *Journal of The American Dietetic Association* 86(7): 929–931.

Dehkordi, N., D. R. Rao, A. P. Warren, and C. B Chawan. 1995. Lactose malabsorption as influenced by chocolate milk, skim milk, sucrose, whole milk, and lactic cultures. *Journal of The American Dietetic Association* 95(4): 484–486.

Demark-Wahnefried, Wendy, Jean Bowering, and Paul S. Cohen. 1990. Reduced serum cholesterol with dietary change using fat-modified and oat bran supplemental diets. *Journal of The American Dietetic Association* 90(2): 223–229.

DePaola, D. P., M. P. Faine, and R. I. Vogel. 1994. Nutrition in relation to dental medicine. In: Shils, E. M., J. A. Olson, and M. Shike (eds.) *Modern Nutrition in Health and Disease* (8th ed.) Philadelphia, PA: Lea and Febiger.

Eastwood, Martin. 1987. Dietary fiber and the risk of cancer. *Nutrition Reviews* 45(7): 193–198.

Eastwood, Martin A. 1992. The physiological effect of dietary fiber: An update. *Annual Review of Nutrition* 12: 19–35.

Glinsmann, W. H., H. Irausquin, and Y. K. Park. 1986. Evaluation of health aspects of sugars contained in carbohydrate sweeteners. *Journal of Nutrition* 116(11S): S5–S216.

Glore, Stephen R., Dianne Van Treeck, Allen W. Knehans, and Marinell Guild. 1994. Soluble fiber and serum lipids: A literature review. *Journal of The American Dietetic Association* 94(4): 425–436.

Heaton, K. W. 1987. Cholesterol-rich gallstones. *Molecular Aspects of Medicine* 9: 89–94.

Jenkins, David J. A., Thomas Wolever, Alexandra Jenkins, and Rodney H. Taylor. 1987. Dietary fibre, carbohydrate metabolism and diabetes. *Molecular Aspects of Medicine* 9: 97–109.

Jenkins, David J. A., Alexandra Jenkins, A. V. Rao, and Lillian U. Thompson. 1986. Cancer risk: Possible protective role of high-carbohydrate, high-fiber diets. *American Journal of Gastroenterology* 81(10): 931–935.

Klurfeld, David M. 1987. The role of dietary fiber in gastrointestinal disease. *Journal of The American Dietetic Association* 87(9): 1172–1177.

Kolars, Joseph C., Michael D. Levitt, Mostafa Aouji, and Dennis A. Savaiano. 1984. Yogurt—an autodigesting source of lactose. *New England Journal of Medicine* 310(1): 1–3.

Kritchevsky, D. 1987. Dietary fibre and lipid metabolism. *International Journal of Obesity* 11(Suppl. 1): 33–43.

Lecos, Chris W. 1985. Sweetness Minus Calories = Controversy. *FDA Consumer* 19(1): 18–23.

Leon, A. S., D. B. Hunninghake, C. Bell, D. K. Rassin, and T. R. Tephly. 1989. Safety of long-term large doses of aspartame. *Archives of Internal Medicine* 149: 2318–2324.

Levine, Rachmiel. 1986. Monosaccharides in health and disease. *Annual Review of Nutrition* 6: 211–24.

Macdonald, Ian. 1987. Metabolic requirements for dietary carbohydrate. *American Journal of Clinical Nutrition* 45(5): 1193–1196.

Macdonald, Ian. 1987. Simple and complex carbohydrates. *American Journal of Clinical Nutrition* 45(5): 1039–1040.

Mann, Jim. 1987. Complex carbohydrates: Replacement energy for fat or useful in their own right? *American Journal of Clinical Nutrition* 45(5): 1202–1206.

Martini, Margaret C., Denise Kukielka, and Dennis A. Savaiano. 1991. Lactose digestion from yogurt: Influence of a meal and additional lactose.

American Journal of Clinical Nutrition 53: 1253–1258.

Mesquita, Maria, Miguel Seabra and Manuel J. Halpern. 1987. Simple carbohydrates in the diet. *American Journal of Clinical Nutrition* 45(5): 1197–1201.

Miller, Roger W. 1986. Empty calories: Putting on pounds with poor nutrition. *FDA Consumer* 20(9): 20–23.

Morgan, R. W., and O. Wong. 1985. A review of epidemiological studies on artificial sweeteners and bladder cancer. *Food Chemistry and Toxicology* 23: 529–533.

Morrison, A. S., and J. E. Buring. 1980. Artificial sweeteners and cancer of the lower urinary tract. *New England Journal of Medicine* 302(10): 537–541.

Newberne, Paul M., and Michael W. Conner. 1986. Food additives and contaminants, An update. *Cancer* 58(8): 1851–1862.

Ornstein, M. H., and I. McLean Baird. 1987. Dietary fibre and the colon. *Molecular Aspects of Medicine* 9: 41–56.

Pilch, S. 1987. Physiological effects and health consequences of dietary fiber. Bethesda, MD: Life Sciences Research Office, Federation of American Societies for Experimental Biology.

Powers, Margaret A. 1994. Sweetener blending: How sweet it is! *Journal of The American Dietetic Association* 94(5): 498–499.

Ripsin, C. M., J. M. Keenan, D. R. Jacobs, P. J. Elmer, R. R. Welch, L. Van Horn, K. Liu, W. H. Turnbull, F. W. Thye, M. Kestin, M. Hegstead, D. M. Davidson, M. H. Davidson, L. D. Dugan, W. Demark-Wahnefried, and S. Beling. 1992. Oat products and lipid lowering: A meta-analysis. *Journal of The American Medical Association* 267(24): 3317–3325.

Saavedra, J. M., and J. A. Perman. 1989. Current concepts in lactose malabsorption and intolerance. *Annual Review of Nutrition* 9: 475–502.

Saudek, C. D. 1990. Recurrent hypoglycemia. *Journal of The American Medical Association* 264: 2791–2794.

Shutler, Susan M., Ann F. Walker, and A. Graham Low. 1987. The cholesterol-lowering effects of legumes. I: Effects of the major nutrients. *Human Nutrition: Food Sciences and Nutrition* 41F: 71–86.

Shutler, Susan M., Ann F. Walker, and A. Graham Low. 1987. The cholesterol-lowering effects of legumes. II: Effects of fibre, sterols, saponins and isolavones. *Human Nutrition: Food Sciences and Nutrition* 41F: 87–102.

Slavin, Joanne L. 1987. Dietary fiber: Classification, chemical analyses, and food sources. *Journal of The American Dietetic Association* 87(9): 1164–1171.

Smith, U. 1987. Dietary fibre, diabetes, and obesity. *International Journal of Obesity* 11(Suppl. 1): 27–31.

Suarez, Fabrizis L., Dennis A. Savaiano, and Michael D. Levitt. 1995. A comparison of symptoms after the consumption of milk or lactose-hydrolyzed milk by people with self-reported severe lactose intolerance. *The New England Journal of Medicine* 333(1): 1–4.

Toma, R. B., and D. J. Curtis. 1986. Dietary fiber: Effect on mineral bioavailability. *Food Technology* 40(2): 111–116.

U.S. Department of Agriculture and U.S. Department of Health and Human Services. 1990. Nutrition and Your Health: Dietary Guidelines for Americans. *Home and Garden Bulletin* No. 232.

U.S. Department of Health and Human Services, Public Health Service. 1991. Healthy People 2000: National Health Promotion and Disease Prevention Objectives. Washington, DC: U.S. Government Printing Office.

Walker, A. R. P. 1987. Dietary fibre and mineral metabolism. *Molecular Aspects of Medicine* 9: 69–74.

Wolraich, Mark L., David B. Wilson, and J. Wade White. 1995. The effect of sugar on behavior or cognition in children. *Journal of The American Medical Association* 274(20): 1617–1621.

Yokogoshi, Hidehiko, Carolyn H. Roberts, Benjamin Caballero, and Richard J. Wurtman. 1984. Effects of aspartame and glucose administration on brain and plasma levels of large neutral amino acids and brain 5-hydroxyindoles. *American Journal of Clinical Nutrition* 40(1): 1–7.

Grains, properly called cereal grains, are the seed kernels of cultivated grasses. Examples are wheat, corn, rice, rye, barley, and oats. All cereal grains have a large, high-starch center area known as the *endosperm* (see Figure 2-4). At one end of the endosperm is the germ, the area of the kernel that sprouts into a new plant when allowed to germinate. The bran covers both the endosperm and the germ. The seed contains everything needed to reproduce the plant: the germ is the embryo, the endosperm contains the nutrients for growth, and the bran protects the entire seed.

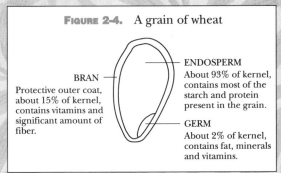

FIGURE 2-4. A grain of wheat

ENDOSPERM
About 93% of kernel, contains most of the starch and protein present in the grain.

BRAN
Protective outer coat, about 15% of kernel, contains vitamins and significant amount of fiber.

GERM
About 2% of kernel, contains fat, minerals and vitamins.

Most grains undergo some type of processing or milling after harvesting to aid cooking, make them less chewy, and lengthen their shelf life. Many grains, such as oats and rice, have a tough, inedible outer husk, or hull, that must be removed. Other processing steps might include polishing the grain to remove the bran and germ (as in white flour), cracking the grain (as in cracked wheat), or steaming the grain (as in bulgur) to shorten the cooking time. The processes of rolling or grinding a grain, such as oatmeal, also shorten the cooking time.

Whole grains are always a more nutritious choice and are good sources of fiber, complex carbohydrates, B vitamins, and minerals. Whole grains are also a good protein choice. And you get all this good nutrition with a minimum of calories and fat. To summarize their nutritional profile, grains are:

Low or moderate in calories
High in complex carbohydrates
High in fiber (if whole grain)
Low in fat
Moderate in protein
Full of vitamins and minerals

Most grains are cooked by stirring into a boiling liquid (water or broth), then reducing the heat to a simmer, covering, and cooking until the liquid is absorbed.

Start putting more grains on your table by serving them as breakfast cereals and side dishes, such as pilaf, and incorporating them into soups, stews, casseroles, stir-fry, breads, and salads. It should be easy, since grains are inexpensive, easy to store, and can be used in countless tasty recipes. Many cook quickly as well: bulgur cooks in under 20 minutes, buckwheat kasha and quinoa in only 15 minutes.

Barley

When the term *barley* is used in a recipe, it usually refers to pearl barley, a white variety that has had the inedible husks or hulls, germ, and bran removed. Pearl barley can be boiled and used in soups, casseroles, stews, stuffings, cooked cereals, as a side dish, or as pilaf. Its taste is mild and nutty, and its texture is chewy.

Buckwheat

Although buckwheat has many grain-like characteristics, it is from an entirely different family and is actually a fruit. Two forms of buckwheat are available for purchase: whole white buckwheat and roasted buckwheat, also called kasha. Kasha can be purchased whole or ground. Roasting gives the buckwheat kernels a distinct, nutty flavor. You will probably have to acquire a taste for roasted buckwheat. Kasha can be used in soups, stuffings, side dishes, and salads. Whole white buckwheat has a mild flavor and can be used to replace rice or pasta.

Millet

Millet, a golden grain, is grown and used in the Far East and China. Although the millet raised in the United States is mostly used to feed animals and birds, millet has been eaten by people in other parts of the world since Old Testament times. Millet is an important dietary component for many Africans, Indians, and Chinese. No wonder, it contains a high-quality protein. It can be purchased in natural food stores as a whole grain. Cooking millet has had the inedible hull (that the birds just love!) removed as well as an outer bran layer that is also inedible. It can be boiled and used in soups, casseroles, meat loaves, porridge, croquettes, pilaf, salads, stuffings, or as a side dish.

Oats

Oats are a unique grain: When they are milled, only the inedible hull is removed and the bran and germ are left with the kernel. Whichever form of oats you buy, you are getting whole-grain nutrition. Rolled oats, or "old-fashioned oats," are made by cutting up raw oats into a product that is then steamed, shaped into flakes, and dried. Rolled oats require only 5 minutes cooking time.

Quick oats start out as rolled oats but are sliced finer and slightly precooked so they cook quicker—in about 1 minute. Instant oats are cut even smaller and result in a product that needs only to be mixed with boiling water.

Rice

Rice, perhaps the first grain ever cultivated by man, is a semiaquatic member of the grass family. Its edible seed is the staple grain for over half the world's population.

Rice is classified by its shape: short-grain, medium-grain, or long-grain. Long-grain rice is four to five times as long as it is wide. Its cooked grains are separate and fluffy, and are used for side dishes, entrees, salads, pilaf, and so on. Medium-grain rice is a little shorter and plumper than long-grain rice. After cooking, the rice is more moist, tender, and has a greater tendency to cling together than long-grains. Both medium-grain and short-grain rice are good choices for making creamy dishes, such as rice pudding, risotto, molds, or croquettes.

Short-grain rice is a little shorter than medium-grain rice. The shorter the grain, the more tender and clinging as it cooks. The boiled rice used in Japanese cuisine is short-grain.

Rye

Although rye is known most for its flour, you can buy whole rye berries that can be cooked in liquid into a hot cereal or side dish. Rye flakes, the equivalent of rolled oats, are also available and can be used as a hot cereal or side dish. They have a tangy taste.

Wheat

Wheat, the most important food grown in the world, is a rich source of nourishment. It is, of course, used to make flours, breads, cereals, and pastas.

Whole-wheat grains that have been steamed, dried, and ground into small pieces are called *bulgur*. Depending on how it is processed, some or all of the bran may be removed. Check the bulgur you want to purchase to see if the dark brown bran is still on. Bulgar has a nutty flavor that is excellent by itself or mixed with rice. Its uses are numerous—from salads to soups, from breads to desserts. It is also a nutritious extender and thickener for meat dishes and soups.

Wheat bran is available either processed or unprocessed and is used as an ingredient in cooking or baking. It makes a high-fiber addition to baked goods, such as breads and muffins, and can be substituted for bread crumbs in most recipes.

Wheat germ is separated from the wheat grain and can be purchased at the supermarket either toasted or raw. Wheat germ has a nutty, crunchy texture and can be added to cereal, pancakes, baked goods, casseroles, salads, and breading.

Wheat berries, the actual whole-wheat kernels, are also available cracked, as cracked wheat, in coarse, medium, or fine qualities. Cracked wheat is particularly popular in breads.

Amaranth and Quinoa

Amaranth is one of the newer grains to arrive on the market, yet it has been around for at least 5000 years! An important part of the Aztec diet, it contains a high-quality protein and is rich in calcium. A spicy grain with a slightly peppery taste, amaranth seeds can be cooked to make hot cereal, pilaf, or popped to make a snack or cold cereal. It can also be added to pancake, muffin, and quick-bread batters.

Quinoa is a pale yellow seed that is technically not a cereal grain but a dried fruit. Whereas amaranth was popular with the Aztecs, quinoa was a staple of the Incas in Peru. Like amaranth, quinoa is rich in complete protein (unlike other plant foods) and calcium. Also quinoa, unlike grains in general, contains an appreciable amount of oil (7 grams per 8 ounces). The best-quality quinoa is altiplano quinoa from Bolivia or Peru.

The introduction of diet soft drinks in the 1950s sparked the widespread use of nonnutritive sweeteners. **Nonnutritive sweeteners** contain either no or very few calories. Four different ones will be discussed here: saccharin, cyclamate, aspartame, and acesulfame-K.

Saccharin

Saccharin, discovered in 1879, has been consumed by Americans for more than 100 years. Its use in foods increased slowly until the two world wars, when its use increased dramatically due to sugar shortages. Saccharin is 300 times sweeter than sucrose and is excreted unchanged directly into the urine. It is used in a number of foods and beverages, and when combined with aspartame, its sweetness is intensified. Saccharin by itself has a bitter aftertaste. It is sold in liquid, tablet, packet, and bulk form.

In 1977, the Food and Drug Administration (FDA), which regulates the use of food additives, proposed a ban on its use in foods and allowed its sale as a tabletop sweetener only as an over-the-counter drug. This proposal was based on studies that showed the development of urinary bladder cancer in second-generation rats fed the equivalent of 800 cans of diet soft drinks a day. The surge of public protest against this proposal (there were no other alternative sweeteners available at that time) led Congress to postpone the ban, and the postponement is now extended to 1997. Products containing saccharin must have a warning label that states, "Use of this product may be hazardous to your health. This product contains saccharin, which has been determined to cause cancer in laboratory animals."

Human studies conducted since the FDA ban have not shown an association between saccharin and bladder cancer (Morrison and Buring, 1980; Morgan and Wong, 1985).

Cyclamate

Discovered accidentally in 1937, cyclamate was introduced into beverages and foods in the early 1950s. By the 1960s it dominated the noncaloric sweetener market. It is 30 times sweeter than sucrose and is not metabolized by most people. Cyclamate was banned in 1970 after studies showed that large doses of it, given with saccharin, were associated with increased risk of bladder cancer. Cyclamate is still banned in the United States but is approved and used in more than 40 other countries worldwide. Cyclamate is again under consideration for use in specific products, such as tabletop sweeteners and nonalcoholic beverages. It is stable at hot and cold temperatures and has no aftertaste.

Aspartame

In 1965, aspartame, a low-calorie sweetener, was also discovered accidentally. After being tested in more than 100 scientific studies in animals and humans, it was approved by the FDA in 1981. Aspartame is marketed in the United States under the brand name NutraSweet and as Equal tabletop sweetener. It is 200 times sweeter than sucrose and has an acceptable flavor with no bitter aftertaste.

Aspartame is made by joining two protein components, aspartic acid and phenylalanine, and a small amount of methanol. Aspartic acid and phenylalanine are building blocks of protein. Methanol is found naturally in the body and in many foods, such as fruit and vegetable juices. In the intestinal tract, aspartame is broken down into its three components, which are metabolized in the same way as if they had come from food. Aspartame contains 4 calories per gram, but so little of it is needed that the calorie content is negligible.

Aspartame is used as a tabletop sweetener, to sweeten many prepared foods, and in simple recipes that do not require lengthy heating or baking. Aspartame's components separate when heated over time, resulting in a loss of sweetness. It is best used at the end of the cooking cycle. Aspartame can be found in diet soft drinks, powdered drink mixes, cocoa mixes, pudding and gelatin mixes, frozen desserts, and fruit spreads and toppings. If you drink canned diet soft drinks, chances are they are sweetened with aspartame. Fountain-made diet soft drinks are more commonly sweetened with a blend of aspartame and saccharin, because saccharin helps maintain the right amount of sweetness (Powers, 1994).

The stability of aspartame in liquid in storage, the safety of the products of its metabolism, and symptoms possibly related to its use have provoked concerns and much research. Available evidence suggests that aspartame consumption is safe over the long term and is not associated with serious health effects (Butcho and Kotsonis, 1989; Leon, Hunninghake, Bell, Rassin, and Tephly, 1989).

The FDA uses the concept of an Acceptable Daily Intake (ADI) for many food additives, including aspartame. The ADI represents an intake level that, if maintained each day throughout a person's lifetime, would be considered safe by a wide margin. The ADI for aspartame has been set at 50 milligrams per kilogram of body weight. To take in the ADI for a 150-pound adult, someone would have to drink twenty 12-ounce cans of diet soft drinks.

The only individuals for whom aspartame is a known health hazard are those who have the disease phenylketonuria (PKU), because they are unable to metabolize phenylalanine. For this reason, any product containing aspartame carries a warning label. Some other people may also be sensitive to aspartame and need to limit their intake.

Acesulfame–K

In 1988, the Food and Drug Administration approved a new noncaloric sweetener, acesulfame potassium, or acesulfame–K, for use in dry food products and as a powder or tablet to be used as a tabletop sweetener. It is marketed under the brand names Sunette and Sweet One tabletop sweetener. It is about as sweet as aspartame but is more stable and can be used in baking. Acesulfame–K is approved for use in chewing gums, dry beverage mixes, gelatins, puddings, and nondairy creamers. It may be approved for soft drinks and baked goods. Its taste is reportedly clean and sweet, with no aftertaste in most products.

Acesulfame–K passes through the digestive tract unchanged. The sweetener is used in twenty other countries, including France, Britain, and the Soviet Union. As with aspartame, Sunette is under attack from consumer groups as a possible health risk.

It is important to have a variety of nonnutritive sweeteners in the marketplace, especially for diabetics. Moderation in their use, as well as in the use of caloric sweeteners, seems to be the most prudent advice at this time.

Label Reading Questions and Answers: Carbohydrates

What does "Total Carbohydrate" include?

Total Carbohydrate includes dietary fiber, sugars, and starches (see Figure 2-5).

Nutrition Facts

Serving Size 1 cup (228g)
Servings Per Container 2

Amount Per Serving

Calories 250   Calories from Fat 110

	% Daily Value*
Total Fat 12g	**18%**
Saturated Fat 3g	**15%**
Cholesterol 30mg	**10%**
Sodium 470mg	**20%**
Total Carbohydrate 31g	**10%**
Dietary Fiber 0g	**0%**
Sugars 5g	
Protein 5g	

Vitamin A 4%	•	Vitamin C 2%
Calcium 20%	•	Iron 4%

*Percent Daily Values are based on a 2,000 calorie diet. Your daily values may be higher or lower depending on your calorie needs:

		Calories:	2,000	2,500
Total Fat	Less than		65g	80g
Sat Fat	Less than		20g	25g
Cholesterol	Less than		300mg	300mg
Sodium	Less than		2,400mg	2,400mg
Total Carbohydrate			300g	375g
Dietary Fiber			25g	30g

Calories per gram:
Fat 9   •   Carbohydrate 4   •   Protein 4

FIGURE 2-5.   Nutrition label

What does "Sugars" on the Nutrition Facts label include?

Sugars include those naturally present in the food (for example, lactose in milk and fructose in fruit) as well as those added to the food, such as table sugar, high-fructose corn syrup, and dextrose.

What does "No Added Sugar" mean on a food label?

It means that no sugar or ingredients containing sugars (for example, dried fruit) have been added during processing or packing. However, it doesn't mean that the food is sugar-free. The food can still contain naturally occurring sugar. An example is 100-percent fruit juice, which contains natural sugars but no added sugars. "No added sugar" signals a reduction in calories from sugars only, not from fat, protein, and other carbohydrates.

Why doesn't the nutrition label list a Percent Daily Value for sugars?

There is no Daily Value for sugars because there is not enough scientific evidence to make any recommendations in this area.

Deficiencies of sugar don't exist, and sugar is not associated with any major diseases.

What is the Daily Value for total carbohydrates?

The Daily Value for total carbohydrate is 300 grams, based on a 2000 calorie diet that has about 60 percent of calories from carbohydrates. Use the following chart to check your Daily Value for carbohydrates based on the appropriate calorie level.

Calorie needs/day	Daily Value for Carbohydrates
1600	240 grams or more
1800	270
2000	300
2200	330
2500	375
2800	420
3200	480

What is the Daily Value for dietary fiber? The Daily Value for dietary fiber is 25 grams, which is compatible with current recommendations. For a 1600-calorie diet, your dietary fiber needs are 20 grams. For a 2500-calorie diet, the number of grams increases to 30. The National Cancer Institute recommends that 20 grams is the minimum amount of fiber recommended for all calorie levels below 2000.

What does "Sugar-Free" or "Reduced Sugar" mean on a label?
Sugar-free foods must contain less than 0.5 grams of sugar per serving.
Reduced sugar foods must contain at least 25 percent less sugar than the reference food.

What do "High Fiber," "Good Source of Fiber," and "More or Added Fiber" mean?
High fiber indicates that the food provides 5 grams or more per serving.
Good source of fiber indicates that the food provides from 2.5 to 4.9 grams of fiber per serving.
More or added fiber means that the food provides at least 2.5 grams more fiber per serving than the reference food. Foods making claims about increased fiber content also must meet the definition for "low-fat," or the amount of total fat per serving must appear next to the claim.

CHAPTER

3

Lipids:
Fats and Oils

**KEY
QUESTIONS**

1. What is the difference between fats and oils, and in which foods are each found?
2. What are saturated and unsaturated fats, and in which foods are each found?
3. What is cholesterol, and in which foods is it found?
4. How are lipids digested, absorbed, and metabolized?
5. What functions do fats, cholesterol, and lecithin have in the body and in food?
6. How do lipids impact our health?
7. What can you do to eat less fat, saturated fat, and cholesterol?

QUIZ

Directions: In the following columns, check off each food that is a significant source of fat and/or cholesterol.

Food	Fat	Cholesterol
1. Butter	_____	_____
2. Margarine	_____	_____
3. Split peas	_____	_____
4. Peanut butter	_____	_____
5. Porterhouse steak	_____	_____
6. Flounder	_____	_____
7. Skim milk	_____	_____
8. Cheddar cheese	_____	_____
9. Chocolate chip cookie made with vegetable shortening	_____	_____
10. Green beans	_____	_____

INTRODUCTION

Lipids include fats, oils, cholesterol, and lecithin.

The word *fat* is truly an all-purpose word. We use it to refer to the excess pounds we carry, the blood component that seems to cause heart disease, and the greasy foods in our diet that we feel we ought to cut out. To be more precise about the nature of fat, we need to look at fat in more depth.

To begin, **lipid** is the chemical name for a group of compounds that includes fats, oils, cholesterol, and lecithin. Fats and oils are the most abundant lipids found in nature and are in both plant and animal tissues. A lipid is customarily called a **fat** if it is a solid at room temperature, and it is called an **oil** if it is a liquid at the same temperature. Lipids obtained from animal sources are usually solids, such as butter, whereas oils are generally of plant origin. Therefore, we commonly speak of animal fats and vegetable oils, but we also use the word fat to refer to both fats and oils.

Like carbohydrates, lipids are also composed of carbon, hydrogen, and oxygen. Unlike most carbohydrates, lipids are not long chains of repeating units. Most of the lipids in foods (over 90 percent), and also in the human body, are in the form of triglycerides. Therefore, when we talk about fat in food or in the body, we are really talking about **triglycerides**. The first section in this chapter will explain what triglycerides are.

TRIGLYCERIDES

A triglyceride (Figure 3-1) is made of three **fatty acids** (*tri-* means three) attached to **glycerol**, a derivative of carbohydrate. Glycerol contains three carbon atoms, each attached to one fatty acid. You can think of glycerol as the backbone of the triglyceride.

Fatty acids in triglycerides are made of carbon atoms joined like links in a straight chain. Interestingly, the number of carbons is always an even number. Fatty acids differ from one another in two respects: the length of the carbon chain and the degree of saturation. The length of the chain may be categorized as short chain (6 carbons or less), medium chain (8 to 12 carbons), or long chain (14 to 20 carbons). Most food lipids contain long-chain fatty acids. The length of the chain influences the fat's ability to dissolve in water. Generally, triglycerides do not dissolve in water, but the short- and medium-chain fatty acids have some solubility in water, which will have implications later in our discussion on their digestion, absorption, and metabolism.

Fatty acids are referred to as **saturated** or **unsaturated**. To understand this concept, think of each carbon atom in the fatty-acid chain as having hydrogen atoms attached like charms on a bracelet, as you can see in Figure 3-2. Each "C" represents a carbon atom, each "H" represents a hydrogen atom, and each "O" represents an oxygen atom. Each carbon atom can have a maximum of four bonds, so it can attach to four other atoms. Typically a carbon atom has one bond each to the two carbon atoms on its sides and one bond each to two hydrogens. If each carbon atom in the chain is filled to capacity with hydrogens, it is considered a saturated fatty acid. That's how saturated fatty acid got its name: It is saturated with hydrogen atoms. When a hydrogen is missing from two neighboring carbons, a double bond forms between the carbon atoms, and this type of fatty acid is considered unsaturated.

If you look at Figure 3-2, the top fatty acid in the illustration is saturated: It is filled to capacity with hydrogens. By comparison, the middle and lower fatty acids are unsaturated. This is evident because there are empty spaces without hydrogens in the picture. Wherever hydrogens are

FIGURE 3-1.
A triglyceride

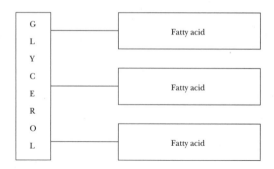

FIGURE 3-2.
Types of
fatty acids

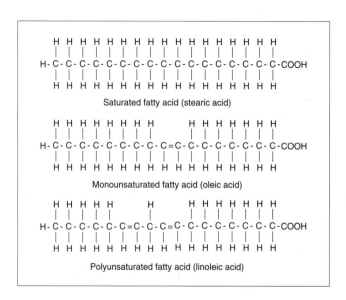

Fatty acids can be
short-, medium-, or
long-chain. They
can also be
saturated,
monounsaturated,
or polyunsaturated.

missing, the carbons are joined by two lines, indicating a double bond. The spot where the double bond is located is called the **point of unsaturation**.

Now that you know what saturated and unsaturated fatty acids are, we need to look at the two types of unsaturated fatty acids. Unsaturated fatty acids are either **monounsaturated** or **polyunsaturated**. A fatty acid that contains only one (*mono-* means one) double bond in the chain is called monounsaturated; if the chain has two or more double bonds, the fatty acid is called polyunsaturated. Figure 3-2 gives examples of monounsaturated and polyunsaturated fatty acids. The monounsaturated fatty acid is missing one pair of hydrogen atoms in the middle of the molecule. The polyunsaturated fatty acid is missing two pairs of hydrogen atoms.

Now that you know about the different types of fatty acids, it's time to get back to the concept of triglycerides. From the three types of fatty acids, we get three types of triglycerides, commonly called fats.

1. A saturated triglycercide, also called a **saturated** fat, is made of three saturated fatty acids.
2. A monounsaturated triglyceride, also called a **monounsaturated** fat, is made of at least one monounsaturated fatty acid.
3. A polyunsaturated triglyercide, also called a **polyunsaturated** fat, is made of at least one polyunsaturated fatty acid.

Now we are ready to see which types of foods the three different fats appear in.

Triglycerides in Food

All food fats, animal or vegetable, contain a mixture of saturated and unsaturated fats. However, saturated fats are mostly found in foods of animal origin and monounsaturated and polyunsaturated fats are mostly found in foods of plant origin and some seafoods. Foods of animal origin include meat, poultry, seafood, milk and dairy products such as butter, and eggs. Foods of plant origin include fruits, vegetables, dried beans and peas, grains, foods made with grains such as breads and cereals, nuts, seeds, and vegetable oils such as corn oil.

Before going into more detail on foods that contain the three types of fats, let's see what each food group contributes in terms of overall fat.

1. Fruits and Vegetables. Whether fresh, canned, or frozen, most fruits and vegetables are practically fat free. The only exceptions are avocados, olives, and coconuts, which contain significant amounts of fat. Also, frozen vegetables that have butter, margarine, or sauces added are probably high in fat. Last, fried vegetables, such as French fried potatoes, are high in fat.
2. Breads, Cereals, Rice, Pasta, and Grains. Most foods in this group are low in fat. Exceptions include most chips, doughnuts, croissants, and many baked goods such as cakes, pies, cookies, biscuits, and muffins. Crackers are also often high in fat.
3. Dry Beans and Peas, Nuts and Seeds. Dry beans and peas are very low in fat. Most nuts and seeds, however, such as peanuts and peanut butter, are quite high in fat.
4. Meat, Poultry, and Seafood. Meat and poultry, and to some extent seafood, contain a bit of fat. The fat content of meat tends to be higher than poultry, and poultry tends to have more fat than seafood. Of course, within each group there are choices that are quite high in fat

Saturated triglycerides = saturated fats. Monounsaturated triglycerides = monounsaturated fats. Polyunsaturated triglycerides = polyunsaturated fats.

Saturated fats are mostly found in animal foods. Unsaturated fats are mostly found in plant foods.

Excellent low-fat or no-fat foods include fruits, vegetables, most breads and cereals, rice, pasta, whole grains, dry beans and peas, and nonfat milk products.

TABLE 3-1.   Total calories and fat in selected fats and oils.

Fat or oil	Calories/Tablespoon	Grams Fat/Tablespoon	Grams Saturated Fat/Tablespoon
Coconut oil	120	13	12
Palm kernel oil	120	13	11
Palm oil	120	13	7
Butter, stick	108	12	7
Lard	115	13	5
Cottonseed oil	120	13	3
Olive oil	119	13	1
Canola oil	120	13	1
Peanut oil	119	13	2
Safflower oil	120	13	1
Corn oil	120	13	2
Soybean oil	120	13	2
Sunflower oil	120	13	1
Shortening	106	12	3
Margarine, stick	100	11	1–3
Margarine, soft tub	100	11	1–2
Margarine, liquid	90	10	1–2
Margarine, whipped	70	8	1–2
Margarine, spread	60	7	1–2
Margarine, diet	50	6	1

Source: U.S. Department of Agriculture.

and choices that are much more moderate in fat. For example, chicken without the skin is low in fat because most of its fat is just under the skin.

5.   Dairy Foods.   Most regular dairy foods are high in fat. Luckily, there are plenty of low-fat alternatives, such as skim milk, nonfat yogurt, and some special low-fat cheeses.

6.   Fats, Oils, Sauces, and Condiments.   Fats, such as vegetable shortening, and oils are almost pure fat. Table 3-1 lists the total calories and fat in selected fats and oils. Sauces often rely on fats and oils for flavor, although many more flavorful sauces are now being made with little or no fat. Condiments such as regular mayonnaise and salad dressings also contain much fat.

As you can see from this discussion, the main contributors to fat in your diet are probably coming from meat, poultry, regular dairy products, regular baked goods, fried foods, oils, and fats. You can't see most of the fat you

TABLE 3-2. Food sources of saturated fat, monounsaturated fat, polyunsaturated fat, and cholesterol.

	Food Sources
Saturated fat	Meat, poultry, dairy products (except nonfat), butter, lard, palm oil, palm kernel oil, and coconut oil
Monounsaturated fat	Olive, canola, peanut, and nut oils
Polyunsaturated fat	Safflower, sunflower, soybean, corn, cottonseed, sesame, and fish oils
Cholesterol	Egg yolk, liver and other organ meats, whole milk and whole-milk cheeses, cream, ice cream, butter, meat, poultry, and seafood

get in the foods you eat, except of course when you add oils and fats. The fatty streaks in meat, under the skin of poultry, in milk and cheese, and in fried foods are not as obvious as the margarine you spread on bread.

In addition to seeing which foods are high in fat, let's look at the saturated fat, monounsaturated fat, and polyunsaturated fat content of foods.

1. Saturated fat is found in fatty cuts of meat, skin-on poultry, whole-milk dairy products such as whole milk and butter, lard, eggs, and in some vegetable oils such as coconut, palm kernel, and palm oils. These vegetable oils are unusual because almost all vegetable oils are rich in unsaturated fats.
2. Polyunsaturated fats are found in greatest amounts in safflower, corn, soybean, cottonseed, sesame, and sunflower oils. These oils are commonly used in salad dressings and as cooking oils. Nuts and seeds also contain polyunsaturated fats, enough to make nuts and seeds a rather high-calorie snack food depending on serving size. Polyunsaturated fats are also found in fish and shellfish.
3. Monounsaturated fats include olive oil, peanut oil, and canola oil. Like other vegetable oils, these are used in salad dressings and for cooking.

The most popular monounsaturated fat is olive oil.

Table 3-2 summarizes the food sources of saturated, monounsaturated, and polyunsaturated fats.

When looking at fat in foods, it is important to distinguish between two different concepts: the percentage of fat by weight and the percentage of calories from fat. To explain these two concepts, let's look at an example. Sliced turkey breast is advertised as being 96 percent fat free.

What this means is that if you weighed out a 3-ounce serving, 96 percent of the weight is not fat. In other words, only 4 percent of its weight is actually fat. It says nothing about how many calories come from fat.

Now if you look on the nutrition label, you will read that a 3-ounce serving contains 3 grams of fat, 27 calories from fat, and 140 total calories. The label also states that the percentage of calories from fat in a serving is 19 percent. To find out the percentage of calories from fat in any serving of food, simply divide the number of calories from fat by the number of total calories, then multiply the answer by 100 as follows.

$$\frac{Calories\ from\ fat\ \text{x}\ 100}{Total\ calories} = \text{Percent of calories from fat}$$

$$\frac{27\ calories\ from\ fat\ \text{x}\ 100}{140\ calories} = 19\%\ \text{fat}$$

This percentage has become more important as recommendations on fat consumption have targeted 30 percent or less of total calories as a desirable daily total from fat. This does not mean, however, that every food you eat needs to derive only 30 percent of its calories from fat. If this were the case, you could not even have a teaspoon of margarine because *all* of its calories come from fat. It is your total fat intake over a few days that is important, not the percentage of fat in just one food or just one meal.

Rancidity

Rancidity is the deterioration of fat, resulting in undesirable flavors and odors. In the presence of air, fat can lose a hydrogen at the point of unsaturation and take on an oxygen atom. This change creates unstable compounds that start a chain reaction, quickly turning a fat rancid. You can tell whether a fat is rancid by its odd odor and taste. The greater the number of points of unsaturation, the greater the possibility that rancidity will develop. This explains why saturated fats are more resistant to rancidity than unsaturated fats.

Vitamin E helps prevent rancidity.

Rancidity is also quickened by heat and ultraviolet light rays. Luckily, vitamin E is present in plant oils and it naturally resists deterioration of the oil. Quite often the food additives butylated hydroxyanisole (BHA) and butylated hydroxytolulene (BHT) are added to some packaged foods such as salad dressings to maintain freshness.

To prevent rancidity, store fat and oils tightly sealed in cool, dark places. For butter and margarine, check dating on the packaging. When oils are refrigerated, they sometimes become cloudy and thicker. This usually clears up after they are left at room temperature again for a few minutes or are put under warm water.

MINI-SUMMARY Most of the lipids in foods, and also in the human body, are in the form of triglycerides. A triglyceride is composed of three fatty acids attached to glycerol. Fatty acids may be saturated or unsaturated. Unsaturated fatty acids are either monounsaturated or polyunsaturated. Fat is found mostly in meat, poultry, regular dairy products, regular baked goods, fried foods, oils and fats. Fat in your diet is both visible, as in margarine or oil, and invisible, as in the fat in whole milk or cheese. Saturated fats are found mostly in animal foods. Monounsaturated and polyunsaturated fats are found mostly in plant foods. Unsaturated fats are more likely to become rancid than saturated fats.

CHOLESTEROL

Cholesterol is the most abundant sterol, a category of lipids. Pure cholesterol is an odorless, white, waxy, powdery substance. You cannot taste it or see it in the foods you eat.

Your body needs cholesterol to function normally. It is present in every cell in your body, including the brain and nervous system, muscle, skin, liver, intestines, heart, and skeleton. The body uses cholesterol to make **bile acids**, which allow us to digest fat, and to make cell membranes, many hormones, and vitamin D. Unfortunately, high blood cholesterol is a risk factor for heart disease and is found in the walls of clogged arteries. This will be discussed in more detail later on.

So which foods contain cholesterol? Cholesterol is found only in foods of animal origin: egg yolks (it's not in the whites), meat, poultry, fish, milk, and milk products (Table 3-3). It is not found in foods of plant origin. Egg yolk and organ meats (liver, kidney, sweetbreads, brain) contain the most cholesterol—one egg yolk contains 213 milligrams of cholesterol. About four ounces of meat, poultry, or fish (trimmed or untrimmed) contain 100 milligrams of cholesterol with the exception of shrimp, which is still higher in cholesterol.

There is no cholesterol in plant foods, such as fruits, vegetables, cereals, grains, and nuts.

In milk products, cholesterol is mostly in the fat, so lower-fat products contain less cholesterol. For example, 1 cup of whole milk contains 33 milligrams of cholesterol, whereas a cup of skim milk contains only 4 milligrams (Table 3-4).

Egg whites and foods that come from plants, such as fruits, nuts, vegetables, grains, cereals, and seeds, have no cholesterol.

We take in about 400 to 500 milligrams of cholesterol daily and the

TABLE 3-3. Cholesterol in foods.

Food and Portion	Cholesterol (milligrams)
Liver, braised, 3 ounces	333
Egg, whole, 1	213
Beef, short ribs, braised, 3 ounces	80
Beef ground, lean, broiled medium, 3 ounces	74
Beef, top round, broiled, 3 ounces	73
Chicken, roasted, without skin, light meat, 3½ ounces	75
Shrimp, moist heat cooked, 3 ounces	167
Scallops, broiled, 3 ounces	47
Lobster, moist heat cooked, 3 ounces	61
Haddock, baked, 3 ounces	63
Mackerel, baked, 3 ounces	64
Swordfish, baked, 3 ounces	43
Milk, whole, 8 ounces	33
Milk, 2% fat, 8 ounces	18
Milk, 1% fat, 8 ounces	10
Skim milk, 8 ounces	4
Cheddar cheese, 1 ounce	30
American processed cheese, 1 ounce	27
Cottage cheese, low-fat, 1%, 1/2 cup	5

Source: National Institutes of Health. 1994. *Step by Step: Eating to Lower Your High Blood Cholesterol.* NIH Publication No. 94-2920.

liver also makes a significant amount of cholesterol. Because the body produces cholesterol, it is not considered an essential nutrient.

MINI-SUMMARY   Cholesterol is present in every cell and is used by the body to make bile acids, which allow us to digest fats, and to make cell membranes, many hormones, and vitamin D. Cholesterol is found only in foods of animal origin, such as egg yolks, meat, poultry, fish, milk, and milk products. It is not found in foods of plant origin. The liver produces cholesterol, so it is not an essential nutrient.

LECITHIN

Lecithin is used to make ready-to-eat baked foods because it is an excellent emulsifier.

Lecithin is considered a phospholipid, a class of lipids that are like triglycerides except that one fatty acid is replaced by a phosphorus-containing substance. Lecithin functions as a vital component of cell membranes. It also acts as an emulsifier. As you know, fats and water do not normally stay

TABLE 3-4. **Nutrition information for milk.**			
Nutrition per 1 cup	*Whole Milk*	*2% Milk*	*Skim Milk*
Calories	150	121	86
Polyunsaturated fat (grams)	less than 1	less than 1	0
Saturated fat (grams)	5	3	less than 1
Cholesterol (milligrams)	33	18	4

Source: National Institutes of Health. 1994. *Step by Step: Eating to Lower Your High Blood Cholesterol.* NIH Publication No. 94-2920.

mixed together but separate into layers. An emulsifier is capable of breaking up the fat globules into small droplets, resulting in a uniform mixture that won't separate. Lecithin keeps fats in solution in the blood, and elsewhere in the body, a most important function. Lecithin is used commercially as an emulsifier in foods such as salad dressings and bakery products.

Although the media have featured lecithin as a wonder nutrient that can burn fat, improve memory, and other similar feats, none of these is true. Enough lecithin is made in the liver that it is not considered an essential nutrient.

MINI-SUMMARY Lecithin, a phospholipid, is a vital component of cell membranes and acts as an emulsifier (keeps fats in solution). It is not an essential nutrient.

DIGESTION, ABSORPTION, AND METABOLISM

Fats are difficult for the body to digest, absorb, and metabolize. The problem is simple. Fat and water do not mix. Minimal digestion of fats occurs before reaching the upper part of the small intestine. Once they reach this area, the gallbladder is stimulated to release **bile** into the intestine. Bile is made by the liver, stored in the gallbladder, and squirted into the intestinal tract when fat is present. Bile contains bile acids that emulsify fat, meaning that they split fats into small globules or pieces. In this manner, fat-splitting enzymes (such as pancreatic lipase) can then do their work. The enzymes break down the triglycerides in food to their component parts—fatty acids and glycerol—so they can be absorbed across the intestinal wall. **Monoglycerides**, triglycerides with only one fatty acid, are also produced.

Once absorbed into the cells of the small intestine, triglycerides are reformed. Now it is time for them to travel in the blood. Both shorter-chain fatty acids and glycerol can travel freely in the blood because they are water soluble. However, triglycerides, monoglycerides, cholesterol, and longer-chain fatty acids would float in clumps and wreak havoc in either the blood or lymph. Because of this, the body wraps them with protein to make them water soluble. The resulting substance is called a **lipoprotein**, a combination of fat *(lipo-)* and protein. Lipoproteins contain triglycerides, protein, cholesterol, and phospholipid, another type of lipid. There are four types of lipoproteins.

Chylomicron is the name of the lipoprotein responsible for carrying mostly triglycerides, and some cholesterol, from the intestines through the lymph system to the bloodstream. In the bloodstream, an enzyme—**lipoprotein lipase**—breaks down the triglycerides into fatty acids and glycerol so they can be absorbed into the body's cells. Once the triglycerides are disposed of, most of what remains of the chylomicron is some protein and cholesterol that is metabolized by the liver.

The primary sites of lipid metabolism are the liver and the fat cells. The liver manufactures triglycerides and cholesterol too. Triglycerides, and some cholesterol, are carried through the body by the liver's version of chylomicrons: **very low density lipoproteins (VLDLs)**. The VLDLs release triglycerides, with the help of lipoprotein lipase, throughout the body. Once the majority of triglycerides are removed, VLDLs are converted in the blood into another type of lipoprotein called **low density lipoprotein (LDL)**.

There are four types of lipoproteins: chylomicrons, VLDL, LDL, and HDL. Each has a special job in the body.

The LDLs, mostly made of cholesterol, transport much of the cholesterol found in the blood to the body's cells. Certain cells (especially in the liver) have the ability to absorb the entire LDL particle. The LDLs not absorbed by cells are somehow involved in depositing cholesterol on the inner blood vessel wall, causing hardening and narrowing of the arteries.

A last type of lipoprotein, **high density lipoprotein (HDL)**, contains much protein and travels throughout the body picking up cholesterol. It is thought that the HDLs carry cholesterol back to the liver for disposal. Thus HDLs help remove cholesterol from the blood, preventing the buildup of cholesterol in the arterial walls.

Most body cells can store only small amounts of fat, but fat cells, can become greatly enlarged with fat. The fat cells of obese people may be many times larger than those of a normal-weight or underweight individual. However, if not enough calories are being consumed to meet the body's needs, the fat cells release fat and start to shrink.

MINI-SUMMARY With the help of bile and various enzymes, fats are broken down into monoglycerides, fatty acids, and glycerol so they can be absorbed across the intestinal wall. Once absorbed into the cells of the small intestine, triglycerides are reformed. Chylomicrons, a type of lipoprotein, carry triglycerides and cholesterol from the intestines through the lymph system to the bloodstream. In the bloodstream, the enzyme lipoprotein lipase breaks down the triglycerides into fatty acids and glycerol so they can be absorbed into the body's cells. Very low density lipoproteins are the liver's equivalent of chylomicrons.

Low-density lipoproteins are mostly made of cholesterol and transport much of the cholesterol found in the blood. High-density lipoprotein travels throughout the body picking up cholesterol.

FUNCTIONS OF LIPIDS

Fats have many vital purposes in the body, where they account for 15 to 25 percent of your weight. At least 50 percent of your fat stores are located under the skin, where fat provides insulation, a cushion around critical organs (like shock absorbers), and optimum body temperature in the cold.

Fats perform many functions both in the body and in food.

Most cells store only small amounts of fat, but specific cells, called adipose (fat) cells, can store loads of fat and actually increase 50 times in weight! If your fat cells are completely filled with fat and you need to store more fat, your body can even produce new fat cells. Dietary fat can be stored in fat cells much quicker and more easily than glucose. Fat stores are a compact way to store lots of energy. Remember that one gram of fat yields 9 calories (carbohydrate and protein yield only 4). Fats provide most of the fuel supply for the muscles.

Fat is an important part of all cell membranes. Fat also transports the fat-soluble vitamins (A, D, E, and K) through the body.

In foods, fats enhance taste, flavor, aroma, crispness (especially in fried foods), juiciness (especially of meat), and tenderness (especially in baked goods). Fat provides a smooth texture and a creamy feeling in the mouth. The love of fatty foods cuts across all ages (just watch a preschooler devour French fries or an elderly adult eat a piece of chocolate cake) and cultures (where fatty foods are available). Eating a meal with fat makes people feel full because fat delays the emptying of the stomach. Fats are therefore said to have **satiety value.** Last, the fat-soluble vitamins and essential fatty acids are found in fatty foods.

Two fatty acids in food are considered to be **essential fatty acids (EFAs)** because the body can't make them. They are essential to our health, and deficiencies in these acids can produce symptoms (although this rarely occurs in the United States). This is why there is presently no RDA for EFAs, although this may change. The two essential fatty acids are called **linoleic acid** and **linolenic acid**. Linoleic acid is called an omega-6 fatty acid because its double bonds appear after the sixth carbon in the chain (see Figure 3-2). Linoleic acid is polyunsaturated and is found in corn, cottonseed, soybean, and safflower oil. It is also found in nuts, seeds, and whole-grain products.

Linolenic acid is the leading omega-3 fatty acid found in food, and, as expected, its double bonds appear after the third carbon in the chain. It appears in some vegetable oils such as canola, walnut, and soybean oils, as well as in margarines made from these oils (Nettleton, 1991). Some leafy vegetables contain linolenic acid, but only in small amounts.

MINI-SUMMARY Many fat cells are located just under the skin where fat provides insulation for the body, a cushion around critical organs, and optimum body temperature in the cold. Fat stores are a compact way to store lots of energy (9 calories per gram). Fat is also present in all cell membranes and transports the fat-soluble vitamins through the body. In foods, fats enhance taste, flavor, aroma, crispness, juiciness, tenderness, and texture. Fats also have satiety value. Linoleic acid (an omega-6 fatty acid) and linolenic acid (an omega-3 fatty acid) are the essential fatty acids. Deficiencies of them are rare.

LIPIDS AND HEALTH

Lipids have been associated with two health problems: heart disease and cancer. First, let's look at heart disease. The higher your blood cholesterol level, the greater your risk or chance of developing coronary heart disease—the most common form of heart disease. Anyone can develop high blood cholesterol, regardless of age, gender, race, or ethnic background. In fact, 52 million American adults now have a high blood cholesterol level.

When there is too much cholesterol in your blood, the excess can become trapped in arterial walls. By building up there, the cholesterol helps to cause hardening of the arteries, called **atherosclerosis**. Atherosclerosis causes most heart attacks. How? The cholesterol buildup narrows the arteries that supply blood to the heart, slowing or even blocking blood flow to the heart. As a result, the heart gets less oxygen than it needs. This weakens the heart muscle, and chest pain (called **angina**) may occur. If a blood clot forms in the narrowed artery, a heart attack or even death can result.

Cholesterol buildup happens slowly—you are not even aware of it. If you lower your high blood cholesterol level, you can slow, stop, or even reverse the buildup—and lower your risk of illness or death from heart disease.

Two types of lipoproteins affect your risk of heart disease.

1. The cholesterol and fat from LDLs, the "bad" cholesterol, are the main sources of dangerous buildup and blockage in the arteries. Thus, the more LDLs you have in your blood, the greater your risk of heart disease.
2. HDLs, the "good" cholesterol, help keep cholesterol from building up in the arterial walls. If your HDL level is low, your risk of heart disease is greater.

A diet with a moderate amount of fat and low amounts of saturated fat and cholesterol can help maintain normal blood cholesterol levels. Since fat, saturated fat, and cholesterol tend to go together in the same foods, lowering your intake of these nutrients is not too confusing.

You may wonder at this point why people with elevated blood cholesterol levels shouldn't just watch how much cholesterol they eat; after all it is the cholesterol that's high. The reason is that high blood cholesterol is in part due to too much saturated fat. Where dietary fat consists mostly of monounsatuated fats, such as olive oil, blood cholesterol levels are lower than when dietary fat is mostly saturated. Heart disease will be discussed in more detail in Chapter 11.

Cancer is the second leading cause of death in the United States following heart disease. Research suggests that the amount and type of fat you eat may play a role in the cause of certain cancers such as breast cancer. This topic is discussed more in Chapter 11.

A diet low in fat, saturated fat, and cholesterol is helpful in preventing heart disease and probably cancer as well.

The omega-3 fatty acids have received much attention because the longer-chain ones, **eicosapentaenoic acid (EPA)** and **docosahexaenoic acid (DHA)**, may reduce the risk of heart disease by lowering the level of fat and LDLs in the blood and also by lessening the chance of blood clots. When blood clots in narrowed arteries, it can cause a heart attack or stroke. EPA and DHA play other important roles as well, such as in growth and development throughout the life cycle and as components in almost all cell membranes (Simpoulos, 1991).

Although the body can convert linolenic acid into EPA and DHA, you can get more EPA and DHA in the body by eating seafood (Nettleton, 1991). Seafood is the only good source of these two omega-3 fatty acids, in particular the fatty fish, such as herring, Pacific oysters, mackerel, and salmon. Other good sources are sea bass, whiting, trout, bluefish, white albacore or bluefin tuna, and Atlantic mackerel. Even fish with less fat contain some omega-3s. But don't expect to find omega-3s in fish sticks or similar products—the omega-3s are lost in processing. Studies have shown that people who eat fish two or three times a week are less likely to die prematurely of heart disease. Although fish-oil supplements are available, their long-term safety and effectiveness is not known, so it is preferable to eat fish twice a week.

MINI-SUMMARY The higher your blood cholesterol level, the greater your risk or chance of developing coronary heart disease—the most common form of heart disease. With a diet moderate in fat and low in saturated fat and cholesterol, you can help maintain normal blood cholesterol levels. Research suggests that the amount and type of fat you eat may play a role in causing certain cancers, such as breast cancer. Certain omega-3 fatty acids found in seafood may help prevent heart disease and play other important roles in the body.

RECOMMENDATIONS AND TIPS FOR NUTRITIOUS FOOD SELECTION

The Dietary Guidelines for Americans recommends a diet low in fat, saturated fat, and cholesterol. In 1990, an important report, *Healthy People 2000: National Health Promotion and Disease Prevention Objectives* was released by the Public Health Service/Department of Health and Human Services. The purpose of the report was to improve health promotion and disease prevention. One often-cited goal of this report is for Americans to reduce dietary fat intake to an average of 30 percent of calories or less, and average saturated fat intake to less than 10 percent of calories among people age 2 and older (U.S. Department of Health and Human Services, 1991) [See Table 3-5]. Dietary recommendations also suggest lowering cholesterol intake to 300 milligrams daily.

According to the most recent National Health and Examination Survey (1988–1991), Americans have been eating less fat (from 36 to 34 percent of calories) and saturated fat (from 13 to 12 percent of calories). However, the drop in percentage of fat calories occurred because we are eating more! In other words, average fat intake did not actually decrease but increased from 81 to 83 grams per day. Because the total number of calories eaten increased, too, the percent of calories from fat went down from 36 to 34 percent. Cholesterol intake is high, about 220 to 360 mil-

TABLE 3-5. Recommended fat and saturated fat intake.		
If Your Total Daily Calories Are	*Total Fat* (grams)*	*Saturated Fat* (grams)*
1,200	40	13
1,500	50	17
1,800	60	20
2,000	67	22
2,200	73	24
2,400	80	27
2,600	86	29
2,800	93	31
3,000	100	33

*Total fat is 30 percent of total calories. Saturated fat is 10 percent of total calories.

ligrams daily (National Cholesterol Education Program Expert Panel, 1993).

The following tips will help guide you in making food choices that are lower in fat, saturated fat, and/or cholesterol.

Meat

1. You can still eat red meat as long as you choose lean cuts (See Table 12-2). Choosing lean red meat gives you all the benefits of meat's protein and iron. Premenopausal women especially need the iron in lean meat. Lean beef cuts include top round and eye of round. Lean veal cuts include shoulder, sirloin, ground veal, and veal cutlets. Lean pork cuts include tenderloin, sirloin, and top loin.

2. Limit high-fat processed meats such as bacon, bologna, salami, hot dogs, and sausage. They are high in saturated fat and total fat. Look for low-fat processed meats.

3. Limit organ meats, such as liver, sweetbreads, and kidneys. Organ meats are high in cholesterol, even though they are fairly low in fat.

Poultry

4. You can buy chicken and turkey pieces with the skin already removed, or buy the pieces with the skin on and remove it yourself before eating. Remember, white meat always contains less saturated fat than dark meat. Removing the skin, particularly from the white meat pieces, can help you get rid of almost all of the saturated fat. Removing the skin from the dark meat thighs and drumsticks also helps.

TABLE 3-6. Meat, poultry, and fish: a comparison.

Food Type (3 ounces, cooked)	Saturated Fat (grams)	Dietary Cholesterol (milligrams)	Total Fat (grams)	Calories
Beef, top round, broiled	3	73	8	185
Beef, whole rib, broiled	10	72	26	313
Chicken, light meat without skin, roasted	1	64	4	130
Chicken, light meat with skin, roasted	3	71	19	189
Ground turkey— breast meat only	<1	35	<2	130
Ground turkey (meat and skin), cooked	3	87	11	200
Cod, baked	<1	47	<1	89

Source: National Institutes of Health. 1994. *Step by Step: Eating to Lower Your High Blood Cholesterol.* NIH Publication No. 94-2920.

5. Limit goose and duck. They are high in saturated fat, even with the skin removed.

6. Try fresh ground turkey or chicken made only from breast meat. Types that don't say "white meat" or "breast" on the label may include the skin and dark meat, so they are higher in fat. Substitute ground turkey or chicken for ground beef.

7. Remember that some (but not all) chicken and turkey hot dogs are lower in saturated fat and total fat than pork and beef hot dogs. There are also "lean" beef hot dogs that are low in fat and saturated fat.

Fish and Shellfish

1. Most fish is lower in fat, saturated fat, and cholesterol than meat and poultry (Table 3-6).

2. Shellfish varies in cholesterol content. Some, like shrimp, are fairly high in cholesterol. Others, like scallops, mussels, and clams, are low. Shellfish have little saturated fat and total fat.

Dairy Foods

1. Buy skim and 1 percent milk rather than whole or 2 percent milk. They have just as much or more calcium and other nutrients as whole milk—with much less saturated fat and cholesterol. They also have fewer calories.

2. Because most cheeses are made with whole milk or cream, they are high in saturated fat and cholesterol. Ounce for ounce, meat, poultry, and regular cheeses have about the same amount of cholesterol, but regular cheeses have much more saturated fat. Fortunately, many cheese makers are starting to offer low-fat versions of cheese favorites such as Cheddar, Swiss, and mozzarella. They use skim milk and vegetable oils to replace some of the cream and other fat. The result is more reduced-fat and fat-free cheeses to choose from. When looking for hard cheeses, go for versions that are "fat-free," "reduced-fat," "low-fat," "light," or "part-skim." When looking for soft cheeses, choose low-fat (1 percent) or nonfat cottage cheese, farmer cheese, or part-skim or light ricotta. Ideally, try to pick a cheese with 3 grams of fat or less per ounce (see Table 13-2).

3. Because ice cream is made from whole milk and cream, it is fairly high in saturated fat and cholesterol. Instead, buy other frozen desserts that are low in saturated fat such as ice milk, low-fat frozen yogurt, low-fat frozen dairy desserts, fruit ices, sorbet, and popsicles.

4. Buy low-fat or nonfat yogurt. Use it as a topping or in recipes.

5. Try low-fat or nonfat sour cream or creamy cheese blends. Many taste as rich as the real thing but have less fat and fewer calories.

Eggs

1. Limit how many egg yolks you eat, preferably to four a week, including the egg yolks in baked goods and processed foods.

2. Substitute two egg whites for each whole egg in recipes. For cakes or cookies, this substitution is acceptable for one or two eggs in most recipes and for three or four in some others. For scrambled eggs and omelets, you can use one whole egg and two egg whites or a commercial egg substitute that contains virtually no cholesterol.

Fat and Oils

1. Choose liquid vegetable oils that are high in unsaturated fats: canola, corn, olive, peanut, safflower, sesame, soybean, and sunflower oils.

2. Buy margarine made with unsaturated liquid vegetable oils as the first ingredient. Choose tub or liquid margarine or vegetable oil spreads. The softer the margarine, the more unsaturated it is.

3. Limit butter, lard, and solid shortenings. They are high in saturated fat.

4. Buy light or nonfat mayonnaise and salad dressings instead of the regular high-fat kinds.

Fruits and Vegetables

1. Buy fruits and vegetables to eat as snacks, desserts, salads, side dishes, and in main dishes. Season with herbs, spices, lemon juice, or fat-free or low-fat mayonnaise. Limit the use of regular mayonnaise or other fatty sauces.

Breads, Cereals, Pasta, Rice and Other Grains, and Dry Peas and Beans

1. Choose whole-grain breads and rolls often.
2. Buy dry cereals; most are low in fat. Limit the high-fat granola, muesli, and oat bran types that are made with coconut or coconut oil. Granola and muesli often have nuts as well, which increases total fat and calories.
3. Buy pasta, rice, and dry peas and beans to use as entrees or in casseroles or soups. Hold the high-fat sauces.
4. Limit baked goods made with lots of saturated fat, such as croissants, muffins, biscuits, butter rolls, doughnuts, and brioche.

Sweets and Snacks

1. For a delicious cake with no fat, try angel food cake and top it with fruit puree or fresh fruit slices.
2. Try fat-free or low-fat cakes, cupcakes, brownies, and pastries.
3. Try cookies lower in fat such as animal crackers, fig and other fruit bars, ginger snaps, graham crackers, and vanilla or lemon wafers.
4. Avoid baked goods, cookies, and crackers with the fats listed in Table 3-7.
5. Bake your own sweets and snacks at home using recipes that contain moderate amounts of fat, preferably high in polyunsaturated fat.
6. Gelatin desserts contain no fat. Make puddings with 1 percent or skim milk.
7. Instead of chips, pick pretzels or air-popped popcorn.

In addition, limit fats by choosing cooking methods such as broiling, roasting, poaching, stir-frying, or baking rather than frying. When roasting, place the meat on a rack so that the fat can drip away. For basting, substitute wine or tomato or lemon juice for fat. Limit the amount of fat used in cooking and, if need be, use vegetable oil or margarine rather than butter, shortening, or lard. Use nonstick cooking equipment. When sautéing, substitute vegetable juice, wine, or defatted stock for the fat, or use vegetable-oil cooking spray. Vegetables can be steamed or microwaved for best appearance, flavor, texture, and nutrient retention.

TABLE 3-7. Sources of saturated fat and cholesterol.

Animal fat	Cream	Meat fat
Bacon fat	Egg and egg-yolk solids	Palm kernel oil
Beef fat	Ham fat	Palm oil
Butter	Hardened fat or oil	Pork fat
Chicken fat	Hydrogenated	Turkey fat
Cocoa butter	vegetable oil	Vegetable oil*
Coconut	Lamb fat	Vegetable shortening
Coconut oil	Lard	Whole-milk solids

*Could be coconut or palm oil.

TABLE 3-8. Fat-saving recipe substitutions.

Instead of	*Use*
Whole milk	Skim or 1 percent milk
Evaporated milk	Evaporated skim milk
Light cream	Equal amounts 1 percent milk and evaporated skim milk
1 cup butter	1 cup margarine or 2/3 cup vegetable oil*
Shortening	Margarine*
Mayonnaise or salad dressing	Nonfat or light mayonnaise or salad dressing
1 whole egg	1/4 cup egg substitute or 2 egg whites
Cheese	Low-fat cheese
Sour cream	Nonfat or low-fat sour cream or yogurt
Fat for "greasing" pan	Nonstick cooking spray

*Note: The texture of baked goods may be different when you use these substitutions. Experiment to find out what works best for you.

Table 3-8 lists fat-saving recipe substitutions, and Table 3-9 gives an example of how to make meals lower in fat.

MINI-SUMMARY Dietary recommendations suggest 30 percent of calories as fat, less than 10 percent from saturated fats, and a maximum of 300 milligrams of cholesterol daily. Tips are outlined to decrease the amount of fat, saturated fat, and cholesterol in your diet.

TABLE 3-9. Examples of an average American menu and a low-fat menu.

Average American Diet (37% fat)	*Low-fat Diet (30% fat)*
Breakfast	
1 fried egg	1 cup corn flakes with blueberries
2 slices white toast	1 cup 1% milk
with 1 teaspoon butter	1 slice rye toast with 1 teaspoon margarine
1 cup orange juice	1 cup orange juice
black coffee or tea	black coffee or tea
Snack	
1 doughnut	1 toasted pumpernickel bagel
	with 1 teaspoon margarine
Lunch	
1 grilled cheese sandwich	1 tuna salad (3 ounces) sandwich
on white bread (2 ounces cheese)	with lettuce and tomato
2 oatmeal cookies	1 graham cracker
black coffee or tea	black coffee or tea
Snack	
20 cheese crackers	1 crisp apple
Dinner	
3 ounces fried hamburger	3 ounces broiled lean ground beef
with catsup	with catsup
1 baked potato	1 baked potato with low-fat plain
with sour cream	yogurt and chives
3/4 cup steamed broccoli	3/4 cup steamed broccoli
with 1 teaspoon butter	with 1 teaspoon margarine
1 cup whole milk	1 cup 1% milk
1 piece frosted marble cake	1 small piece homemade gingerbread
Total fat: 37% of calories	30% of calories
Saturated fat: 19% of calories	10% of calories
Cholesterol: 505 milligrams	186 milligrams

Source: National Cholesterol Education Program. 1987. *Eating to Lower Your Blood Cholesterol.*
Bethesda, MD: National Cholesterol Education Program.

Angina
Atherosclerosis
Bile
Bile acids
Cholesterol
Chylomicron
Docosahexaenoic acid (DHA)
Eicosapentaenoic acid (EPA)
Essential fatty acids
Fat
Fat substitutes
Fatty acids
Glycerol
High-density lipoprotein (HDL)
Hydrogenation
Lecithin
Linoleic acid
Linolenic acid
Lipid

Lipoproteins
Lipoprotein lipase
Low-density lipoprotein (LDL)
Monoglycerides
Monounsaturated fat
Monounsaturated fatty acid
Oils
Point of unsaturation
Polyunsaturated fat
Polyunsaturated fatty acid
Rancidity
Satiety value
Saturated fat
Saturated fatty acid
Trans fatty acids
Triglycerides
Unsaturated fatty acid
Very low density lipoprotein (VLDL)

1. Name four compounds that can be classified as lipids.
2. How are lipids like carbohydrates? How are lipids unlike carbohydrates?
3. Why are triglycerides significant?
4. Draw the structure of a triglyceride.
5. How can fatty acids be different?
6. What is meant by point of unsaturation?
7. Describe what makes saturated fats different from monounsaturated and polyunsaturated fats.
8. List five foods that contain saturated fats, five foods that contain polyunsaturated fats, and three foods that contain monounsaturated fats.
9. Which food groups contribute most dietary fat? Give examples from each group.
10. If a serving of food contains 81 calories and 3 grams of fat, what is the percentage of calories from fat?
11. What causes rancidity? How can rancidity be prevented?
12. What important functions does cholesterol perform?
13. List five foods that contain cholesterol and five foods that do not.

14. In what form are triglycerides absorbed in the small intestine?
15. Name the four lipoproteins and the function of each?
16. List five functions of fat in the body.
17. List five functions of fat in food.
18. Are RDAs set for the essential fatty acids? Why or why not?
19. What's the connection between heart disease and lipids?
20. What are the recommendations for fat, saturated fat, and cholesterol intake?

ACTIVITIES AND APPLICATIONS

1. Quiz

Let's go over how you did on the quiz at the beginning of the chapter. Butter, porterhouse steak, and Cheddar cheese are all significant sources of fat and cholesterol. Margarine, peanut butter, and chocolate-chip cookies made with vegetable shortening are all significant sources of fat but contain no cholesterol. Skim milk, split peas, and green beans do not contain significant amounts of fat or cholesterol. Flounder contains just a tiny amount of fat (about 1 gram) but does have 58 grams of cholesterol, which is significant.

2. Self-Assessment

To find out whether your diet is high in fat, saturated fat, and cholesterol, check yes or no to the following questions.

Do You Usually	YES	NO
1. put butter on popcorn?	___	___
2. eat more red meats (beef, pork, lamb) than chicken and fish?	___	___
3. leave the skin on chicken?	___	___
4. eat whole-milk cheeses, such as Cheddar, American, and Swiss more than three times a week?	___	___
5. sauté or fry foods more than once or twice a week?	___	___
6. eat high-fat lunch meats, hot dogs, and bacon more than three times a week?	___	___
7. leave visible fat on meat?	___	___
8. use regular creamy salad dressings such as Russian, blue cheese, thousand island, and creamy French?	___	___
9. eat potato chips, nacho chips, and/or cream dips more than twice a week?	___	___
10. drink whole milk?	___	___

11. eat more than four eggs a week? ___ ___
12. eat organ meats (liver, kidney, and others)
    more than once a week? ___ ___
13. use mayonnaise, margarine, and/or butter
    often on your sandwiches? ___ ___
14. use vegetable shortening in baking or cooking? ___ ___
15. eat commercially baked goods, including cakes,
    pies, and cookies, more than twice a week? ___ ___

RATINGS: If you answered yes to:

1–3 questions, you are probably eating a diet not too high in fat, saturated fat, and cholesterol.

4–7 questions, you could afford to make some food substitutions, such as skim milk for regular milk, to reduce your fat and saturated fat intake.

8–15 questions, your diet is very likely high in fat, saturated fat, and cholesterol.

3. Changing Eating Habits

If you are eating too much fat, you can make changes a little at a time! Check off one of these things to try (if you are not already doing it) or make up your own, and do it today!

- The next time I eat chicken, I will take the skin off.
- I will limit my daily meat and poultry servings to two 3-ounce servings daily. (A 3-ounce serving is about the size of a deck of cards.)
- This week, I will try a new type of fresh or plain frozen fish.
- I will try a low-fat cheese, such as low-fat Swiss.
- I will switch to 1 percent or skim milk.
- I will try sherbet or ice milk for dessert instead of ice cream.
- I will count the number of eggs I eat per week and see whether I meet the recommendations.
- To cut back on fat, I will use a lower-fat margarine, salad dressing, or mayonnaise.
- I will keep more fruit in the refrigerator so it will be handy for a snack instead of cookies or chips.
- I will buy pretzels instead of chips.
- For breakfast, instead of doughnuts, I will try a hot or cold cereal with skim milk and toast with jelly.
- I will top my spaghetti with stir-fried vegetables instead of a creamy sauce.

4. Reading Food Labels

Following are food labels from two different brands of lasagne, one heavy on cheese and ground beef and the other is a vegetable lasagne made with moderate amounts of cheese. Using the Nutrition Facts given, can you tell which is which? How did you tell?

Lasagne #1	*Lasagne #2*
Nutrition Facts	*Nutrition Facts*
Amount per serving	Amount per serving
Calories 230	Calories 140
Calories from fat 140	Calories from fat 20
Total fat 16 g	Total fat 2.5 g
Saturated 6 g	Saturated 0.5 g
Polyunsaturated 1 g	Polyunsaturated 1 g
Monounsaturated 7 g	Monounsaturated 0.5 g
Cholesterol 74 g	Cholesterol 0 g
Sodium 180 mg	Sodium 180 mg
Total carbohydrate 0 g	Total carbohydrate 21 g
Dietary fiber 0 g	Dietary fiber 5 g
Sugar 0 g	Sugar 0 g
Protein 21 g	Protein 8 g

5. Meat, Poultry, and Seafood Comparison

Using Appendix A, Nutritive Value of Foods, pick out three meat items you eat, three poultry items you eat, and three fish/shellfish items you eat. Make a chart listing the calories, fat, saturated fat, and cholesterol of all these foods. Once the chart is done, ask yourself the following questions.

- Which food has the least/most amount of fat?
- Which food has the least/most amount of saturated fat?
- Which food has the least/most amount of cholesterol?

6. Name That Fat Substitute!

Following are ingredient listings from four different products made with fat substitutes. Using "Food Facts: Everything You Always Wanted to Know About Fat Substitutes" (p. 101) as a guide, identify the fat substitutes in these foods.

Creme-Filled Chocolate Cupcakes: 0 grams of fat per cupcake
Sugar, water, corn syrup, bleached flour, egg whites, nonfat milk, defatted cocoa, invert sugar, modified food starch (corn, tapioca), glycerine, fruc-

tose, calcium carbonate, natural and artificial flavors, leavening, salt, dextrose, calcium sulfate, oat fiber, soy fiber, preservatives, agar, sorbitan monostearate, mono- and diglycerides, carob bean gum, polysorbate 60, sodium stearoyl lactylate, xanthan gum, sodium phosphate, maltodextrin, guar gum, pectin, cream of tartar, sodium aluminum sulfate, artificial color.

Low-Fat Mayonnaise Dressing: 1 gram of fat per tablespoon
Water, corn syrup, liquid soybean oil, modified food starch, egg whites, vinegar, maltodextrin, salt, natural flavors, gums (cellulose gel and gum, xanthan), artificial colors, sodium benzoate and calcium disodium EDTA

Lite Italian Dressing: 0.5 grams of fat per 2 tablespoons
Water, distilled vinegar, salt, sugar, contains less than 2% of garlic, onion, red bell pepper, spice, natural flavors, soybean oil, xanthan gum, sodium benzoate, potassium sorbate and calcium disodium EDTA, yellow #5 and red #40.

Light Cream Cheese: 5 grams fat per 2 tablespoons
Pasteurized skim milk, milk, cream, contains less than 2% of cheese culture, sodium citrate, lactic acid, salt, stabilizers (xanthan and/or carob bean and/or guar gums), sorbic acid, natural flavor, vitamin A palmitate.

American Dietetic Association. 1991. Position of the American Dietetic Association: Fat replacements. *Journal of The American Dietetic Association* 91(10): 1285–88.

Beaudette, T. 1990. The new fat substitutes: Nutritional implications. *Seminars in Nutrition* 10: 1–16.

Blumenthal, D. 1990. Making sense of the cholesterol controversy. *FDA Consumer* 24(5): 12.

Caputo, F. A., and R. D. Mattes. 1992. Human dietary responses to covert manipulations of energy, fat, and carbohydrate in a midday meal. *American Journal of Clinical Nutrition* 56: 36–43.

Fisher, K. D. 1991. Evaluation of the health aspects of caprenin (caprocarpylobehenin). Bethesda, MD: Life Sciences Research Office Federation of American Societies for Experimental Biology.

Foltin, R. W., M. W. Fischman, T. H. Moran, B. J. Rolls, and T. H. Kelly. 1990. Caloric compensation for lunches varying in fat and carbohydrate content by humans in a residential laboratory. *American Journal of Clinical Nutrition* 52: 969–980.

Foltin, R. W., B. J. Rolls, T. H. Moran, T. H. Kelly, A.L. McNelis, and M. W. Fischman. 1992. Caloric, but not macronutrient, compensation by humans for required-eating occasions with meals and snack varying in fat and carbohydrate. *American Journal of Clinical Nutrition* 55: 331–342.

Grundy, S. M. 1990. Cholesterol and coronary heart disease: Future directions. *Journal of the American Medical Association* 264: 3053.

Judd, J. T., B. A. Clevidence, R. A. Muesing, J. Wittes, M. E. Sunkin, and J. J. Podczasy. 1994. Dietary trans fatty acids: effects on plasma lipids and lipoproteins of healthy men and women. *American Journal of Clinical Nutrition* 59: 861–868.

Kalab, M., N. Singer, G. Arille, and V. Young. 1990. Nutritional and functional qualities of microparticulated protein. Symposium Summary.

Kris-Etherton, P. M., Debra Krummel, Mary E. Russell, Darlene Dreon, Sally Mackey, Jane Borchers, and Peter D. Wood. 1988. The effect of diet on plasma lipids, lipoproteins, and coronary heart disease. *Journal of The American Dietetic Association* 88(11): 1373-1400.

Kristal, Alan R., Emily White, Ann L. Shattuck, Susan Curry, Garnet L. Anderson, Ann Fowler, and Nicole Urban. 1992. Long-term maintenance of a low-fat diet: Durability of fat-related dietary habits in the Women's Health Trial. *Journal of The American Dietetic Association* 92(5): 553–559.

Lichtenstein, Alice, 1993. Trans fatty acids, blood lipids, and cardiovascular risk: Where do we stand? *Nutrition Review* 51(11): 340–343.

Lyle, B. J., K. E. McMahon, and P. A. Kreutler. 1992. Assessing the potential dietary impact of replacing dietary fat with other macronutrients. *The Journal of Nutrition* 122: 211–216.

Mann, G. V. 1994. Metabolic consequences of dietary trans fatty acids. *Lancet* 343: 1268–1271.

Mattes, R. D., C. B. Pierce, and M. I. Friedman. 1988. Daily caloric intake of normal-weight adults: Response to changes in dietary energy density of a luncheon meal. *American Journal of Clinical Nutrition* 48: 214–219.

Mattson, Fred H. 1989. A changing role for dietary monounsaturated fatty acids. *Journal of The American Dietetic Association* 89(3): 387–391.

Mattson, Fred H., E. J. Hollenbach, and A. M. Kligman. 1975. Effect of hydrogenated fat on the plasma cholesterol and triglyceride levels of man. *The American Journal of Clinical Nutrition* 28: 726–731.

McDowell, M. A., R. R. Briefel, and K. Alaimo. 1994. Energy and macronutrient intakes of persons ages 2 months and over in the United States: Third National Health and Nutrition Examination Survey, Phase 1, 1988-1991. Advance data from vital and health statistics of the Centers for Disease Control and Prevention. No 255. Hyattsville, MD: National Center for Health Statistics.

Mela, David J. 1992. Nutritional implications of fat substitutes. *Journal of The American Dietetic Association* 92: 472–476.

Mensink, R. P., and M. B. Katan. 1990. Effect of dietary trans fatty acids on high-density and low-density lipoprotein cholesterol levels in healthy subjects. *The New England Journal of Medicine* 323: 439–445.

Nabors, Lyn O'Brien. 1992. Fat replacers: Options for controlling fat and calories in the diet. *Food & Nutrition News* 64: 5–6.

National Cholesterol Education Program Expert Panel. 1993. Second report on detection, evaluation, and treatment of high blood cholesterol in adults (Adult Treatment Panel II) *Circulation* 89(3): 1329–1445.

National Institutes of Health. 1994. *Step by Step: Eating to Lower Your High Blood Cholesterol.* NIH Publication No. 94-2920

Nettleton, Joyce A. 1991. Omega-3 fatty acids: comparison of plant and seafood sources in human nutrition. *Journal of the American Dietetic Association.* 91(3): 331–337.

Peters, J. C., B. N. Holcombe, L. K. Hiller, and D. R. Webb. 1991. Caprenin 3. Absorption and caloric value in adult humans. *Journal of the American College of Toxicology* 10: 357–367.

Segal, M. 1990. Fat substitutes: A taste for the future? *FDA Consumer* 24(10): 25–28.

Simopoulos, A. P. 1991. Omega-3 fatty acids in health and disease and in growth and development. *The American Journal of Clinical Nutrition* 54: 438–463.

Stern, J. S., and M. G. Hermann-Zaidins. 1992. Fat replacements: A new strategy for dietary change. *Journal of The American Dietetic Association* 92: 91–93.

U.S. Department of Agriculture and U.S. Department of Health and Human Services. 1990. Nutrition and Your Health: Dietary Guidelines for Americans. *Home and Garden Bulletin* No. 232.

U.S. Department of Health and Human Services, Public Health Service. 1991. Healthy People 2000: National Health Promotion and Disease Prevention Objectives. Washington, DC: U.S. Government Printing Office.

Webb, D. R., J. C. Peters, R. J. Jandacek, and N. E. Fortier. 1991. Caprenin 2. Short-term safety and metabolism in rats and hamsters. *Journal of the American College of Toxicology* 10: 341–355.

Webb, D. R., and R. A. Sanders. 1991. Caprenin 1. Digestion, absorption, and rearrangement in thoracic duct-cannulated rats. *Journal of the American College of Toxicology* 10: 325–339.

Willett, W. C., and A. Ascherio. 1994. Trans fatty acids: Are the effects only marginal? *American Journal of Public Health* 84: 722–724.

Food Facts: Everything You Always Wanted to Know About Fat Substitutes[1]

The number of low-fat, reduced-fat, and fat-free foods on supermarket shelves has exploded over the past couple of years. Check out the cookies and crackers, baked goods, salad dressings, mayonnaise, and butters and margarine, and you will no doubt see many foods labeled "fat free," "low fat," or "reduced fat." You may have wondered how some foods can be made with less fat yet still taste good. This is where fat substitutes come in.

Fat substitutes are ingredients that mimic the functions of fat in foods, and either contain fewer calories than fat or no calories. So what does fat do in foods? Lots! Fat gives ice cream its creaminess, makes cakes moist and tender, gives cheese its rich flavor, and makes salad dressings smooth and creamy. Making foods with less fat that taste great has been challenging, but it can be done with the help of a variety of fat-reduction ingredients and processing techniques. Reduced-fat foods almost always use more than one fat substitute to replace the fat. There are three categories of fat substitutes: carbohdyrate-based, lipid-based, and protein-based (Table 3-10).

Carbohydrate-Based Fat Substitutes

In many food products with lowered fat content, various types and forms of carbohydrates are used to produce the texture that fat normally supplies. In fact, carbohydrates such as starches and gums were commonly used in foods as thickening agents to supply texture long before their use in developing lower-fat and fat-free food products. Today, carbohydrates continue to play key roles as thickeners, bulking agents, moisturizers and stabilizers in foods such as lower-fat and fat-free frozen desserts, baked goods, cheeses, salad dressings, sauces and gravies, sour cream, yogurt, and puddings.

For instance, modified food starches, maltodextrins and dextrins, which are made from starches, absorb water to form gels that mimic the texture and mouth feel of fat. Polydextrose, a bland starch polymer, acts as a bulking agent to replace some of the volume lost when fat and/or sugar are removed from a food. It also helps keep food moist. It has been used as a partial fat substitute in baked goods, cake frostings, puddings, and frozen desserts. Gums provide a creamy mouth feel and help stabilize emulsions in salad dressings. Cellulose gel, a purified form of cellulose ground to microparticles, supplies mouth feel and flow properties for products such as frozen desserts, sauces, and salad dressings. Algins such as sodium alginate and calcium alginate can also be used as part of a fat-reduction process.

Compared with traditional fats, which contain 9 calories per gram, carbohdyrate-based ingredients provide from 0 to 4 calories per gram, depending on the type and concentration of a particular ingredient. For example, dry forms of maltodextrins provide 4 calories per gram. But when hydrated with water, as required for some products, their caloric contribution drops to 1 to 2 calories per gram of finished product. Other carbo-

[1] Portions of this are being used with permission from the "Uses and Nutritional Impact of Fat Reduction Ingredients," International Food Information Council Foundation, 1995.

hydrates, such as cellulose and xanthan gums, are not digested except by bacteria in the lower intestine, and contribute negligible calories.

Carbohydrate-based fat-reduction ingredients do have their limitations. They cannot replace oils and shortenings used to fry foods. Most are not suitable for cooking or frying. Another problem with starches is taste: They do not always mimic the mouth feel of fat at different levels of concentration. The next category of fat substitutes overcomes these problems but also introduces new concerns.

Lipid-Based Fat Substitutes

Some lipid-based ingredients are actually fats tailored to contribute fewer calories and less available fat to foods. Others are structurally modified to provide no calories or fat.

As with other fat-reduction ingredients, fat-based ingredients are versatile and can be used in a variety of foods including chocolate, margarine, spreads, sour cream, and cheese. In addition, some may be used to fry foods. Because these ingredients are made from fats, they have the same physical properties as fats, including taste, texture, and mouth feel.

Olestra, a lipid-based fat substitute made by Procter & Gamble Company, was approved in 1996 for use in certain snack foods such as potato chips, tortilla chips, and crackers. Procter & Gamble developed olestra, which is being marketed under the trade name Olean, for use in hot and cold foods.

The advantages of olestra are that it keeps its fatlike qualities when heated, it has the mouth feel of regular fat (because it has 80 fatty acids attached to a core sugar), and it carries flavors well. Also, olestra has no calories because it can't be digested. Whereas 1 ounce of regular potato chips contains 150 calories and 10 grams of fat, olestra chips have 60 calories and no fat.

Since olestra can't be digested, and has a molecular structure unlike any other molecule, it had to be approved by the Food and Drug Administration (FDA) as a new food additive and studies had to be done to prove its safety.

During the testing of olestra, two safety issues came up. First, clinical testing indicated that olestra reduces the absorption of fat soluble vitamins (vitamins A, D, E, and K) and carotenoids (substances that may be involved in cancer prevention) from foods eaten at the same time as olestra-containing products. Studies undertaken by Procter & Gamble showed that just 16 chips made with olestra lowered blood lutein (a carotenoid) levels by 20 percent and blood lycopene (another carotenoid) levels by 60 percent. The FDA requires Procter & Gamble to add essential vitamins—vitamins A, D, E, and K— to olestra.

Clinical testing also showed that olestra causes abdominal cramping and loose stools in some individuals. About 3 out of every 10 subjects in Procter & Gamble's studies got diarrhea after eating 20 grams of olestra a day. That's about 40 potato chips or a 2-ounce bag. Some subjects got diarrhea after eating only 16 chips a day.

Due to these concerns, the FDA requires the following labeling statement on all products made with olestra: "This product contains olestra. Olestra may cause abdominal cramping and loose stools. Olestra inhibits the absorption of some vitamins and other nutrients. Vitamins A, D, E, and K have been added." The FDA is also requiring Procter & Gamble to conduct studies to monitor consumption as well as studies on olestra's long-term effects. FDA will formally review these studies in a public meeting of the Foods Advisory Committee in 1998.

Protein-Based Fat Substitutes

Some protein-based fat substitutes are processed by microparticulation. For example, Simplesse is made from egg white and milk protein blended and heated using microparticulation. The protein is shaped into microscopic round particles that roll easily over one another. The aim of the process is to create the feel of a creamy liquid and the texture of fat. Simplesse cannot be used to fry foods but can be used in some cooking and baking. It contains 1 to 2 calories per gram.

The Impact of Fat Substitutes on the Quality of Our Diet

The big question with fat substitutes is: Will foods containing them help us reduce fat and calorie intake or will we compensate by increasing our intake of fat from other foods? In other words, will we have premium ice cream with our no-fat cake or a rich dessert after a no-fat entree? We really don't know the answer to these questions right now, but we can look at the impact of sugar substitutes on our eating habits. Although diet soft drinks were thought to be a great way to take in less sugar and fewer calories, our intake of refined sugars has grown, not decreased, since sugar substitutes came into use.

TABLE 3-10. A guide to fat substitutes.

1. Carbohydrate-Based
   (Starches and gums stabilize water in a gel-like structure. They are hydrophilic and add texture and structure.)

Name	*Description*	*Other Functions*	*Cal/Gm.*
Dextrins	Bland, nonsweet Made from hydrolyzed starches	Some thickening ability Stabilizer	1–4 calories (depends on concentration) Fully digestible

Uses: Salad dressings

Maltodextrin	Nonsweet Made from cornstarch	Bulking agent	4 calories Fully digestible

Uses: Baked products, margarines, salad dressings, mayonnaise

Modified food starches (A starch that has been altered by physical or chemical means)	Made from corn, rice, potato, tapioca	Stabilizers Thickeners Texturizers	4 calories Fully digestible

Uses: Baked goods, mayonnaise, sour cream, puddings, pie fillings, gravies, sauces, gum drops

Polydextrose	Randomly cross-linked polymer of glucose Made from dextrose and small amounts of sorbitol and citric acid	Bulking agent	1 calorie Partially absorbable

Uses: Frozen desserts, puddings, cake frostings, candy, baked goods and mixes

Gums*	Made from seeds, seaweed extracts, and plants	Thickening agents Stabilizers Increase fiber Replaces starch and/or fat	1–3 calories Limited digestion and absorption

Some Gums:
   Xanthum gum (1 cal/gm): synthetic, thickener in salad dressings
   Guar gum (1–3 cal/gm): in dressings, soups, baked goods, ice cream
   Alginates: in salad dressings
   Carrageenan (1 cal/gm): in salad dressings, ice cream, milk products, and reduced-fat ground beef
   Cellulose gum: bulking agent in low-cal foods

2. Lipid-Based

Name	Description	Other Functions	Cal/gm
Olestra	Fatty acid esters of sucrose 6–8 fatty acids on a sucrose core Good carrier of flavors	—	0 Not absorbed

Uses: Snack foods such as chips and crackers

Name	Description	Other Functions	Cal/gm
Caprenin	Esterification of glycerol with 3 fatty acids Like cocoa butter	—	5 calories 1 of fatty acids only partially absorbed.

Uses: Candy.

3. Protein-Based

Name	Description	Other Functions	Cal/gm
Simplesse	Microparticulated protein of milk and egg white proteins Retains water within its structure	—	1–2 calories

Uses: Frozen desserts, cheese foods (will denature if heated too much)

Hot Topic: Trans Fatty Acids

At the turn of the century, it was discovered that liquid vegetable oils could be converted into solid fats by the use of heat, hydrogen, and certain metal catalysts. The process is called **hydrogenation**. The partial hydrogenation process was quickly commercialized to make vegetable shortening (containing 30 to 40 percent trans fatty acids), which is cheaper to make than lard or butter and has a long shelf life. Vegetable shortening is simply vegetable oils that have been partially hydrogenated. The use of these partially hydrogenated fats has increased markedly over this century. Most margarines contain partially hydrogenated oils, and many oils used in deep-fat frying are partially hydrogenated. If you look through your food cabinets and refrigerator, you will find partially hydrogenated oils popping up in many cookies, crackers, peanut butter, and salad dressings.

If hydrogenation makes foods cheaper and gives them longer shelf life, then what's the big deal? Concerns about hydrogenation revolve around what happens to some of the unsaturated fatty acids. Some of them become saturated during the process. Other unsaturated fatty acids, called **trans fatty acids**, lose their natural bend or kink and become straight (like saturated fatty acids). Fats with straight chains can fit closer together, which makes them more solid. This explains why vegetable shortening is a solid.

Research on trans fatty acids has looked at its relationship to heart disease. Studies on the effects of hydrogenated fats on blood lipid levels were first done in the 1960s. Recently, much new data on the health effects of trans fatty acids has appeared. In a seminal study, Mensink and Katan (1990) found that trans fatty acids, when substituted for a polyunsaturated fatty acid, increased total cholesterol and LDL cholesterol and decreased HDL cholesterol. These results have been confirmed by other researchers (Judd et al., 1994).

Going one step further, the noted researchers Mann (1994) and Willett and Ascherio (1994) have hypothesized that both metabolic and epidemiological studies give strong evidence that trans fatty acid intake is causally related to risk of coronary heart disease.

There appears to be clear evidence from well-controlled studies that trans fatty acids, at levels consumed by Americans, have significant adverse effects on blood cholesterol levels. Trans fatty acids from all food sources provide about 5 to 8 percent of energy in a Western-style diet (Lichtenstein, 1993). (It is interesting to note that margarines and shortening without trans fatty acids are available in Europe.) Here's how to avoid trans fat.

1. Eat less fat. Eat moderate amounts of cookies, crackers, chips, pastries, and margarines. Buy lower-fat versions.
2. Avoid deep-fried foods.
3. Use olive oil or canola oil instead of butter, margarine, or shortening.
4. Look for foods labeled "saturated fat free."

Label Reading Questions and Answers: Lipids

What does "Total Fat" (see Fig. 3-3) on the Nutrition Facts label include?

Nutrition Facts

Serving Size 1oz
(28g/about 6 chips)
Servings Per Container 9

Amount Per Serving

Calories 130   Calories from Fat 50

	% Daily Value*
Total Fat 6g	9%
Saturated Fat 1g	5%
Cholesterol 0mg	0%
Sodium 80mg	3%
Total Carbohydrate 19g	6%
Dietary Fiber 1g	4%
Sugars 0g	
Protein 2g	

Vitamin A 0%	•	Vitamin C	0%
Calcium 4%	•	Iron	0%

* Percent Daily Values are based on a 2,000
calorie diet. Your daily values may be higher
or lower depending on your calorie needs:

		Calories:	2,000	2,500
Total Fat	Less than		65g	80g
Sat Fat	Less than		20g	25g
Cholesterol	Less than		300mg	300mg
Sodium	Less than		2,400mg	2,400mg
Total Carbohydrate			300g	375g
Dietary Fiber			25g	30g

FIGURE 3-3. Nutrition Label.

Total fat refers to all the fat in the food: saturated, polyunsaturated, and monounsaturated. Only total fat and saturated fat information are required on the label because high intakes of both are linked to high blood cholesterol, which in turn is linked to increased risk of coronary heart disease. Listing the amount of polyunsaturated and monounsaturated fats in the food is voluntary.

What is the Daily Value for fat?
The Daily Value for fat is 65 grams, which represents 30 percent of total calories in a 2000–calorie diet.

Are trans fatty acids included under "Total Fat"?

No, trans fatty acids are not included in the grams of total fat. This is why when you add up the amounts of saturated, polyunsaturated, and monounsaturated fat, they do not always add up to the full amount declared for total fat.

Why is it that when I multiply the number of grams of fat by 9 calories/gram, the calories I calculate do not equal the "Calories from Fat" on the label?

You are correct to multiply the number of grams of fat in a food by 9 to come up with the number of calories from fat. Because numbers on labels are rounded, your calculated number will not always match the number on the label.

Can a product be labeled "Fat Free" or "Cholesterol Free" and still contain those nutrients?
Under label regulations, they can contain minute amounts of these nutrients. For example, a fat-free food is allowed to contain up to 0.5 grams of fat per serving. A cholesterol-free food is allowed to contain up to 2 milligrams of cholesterol.

What other nutrient claims can be made for fat or cholesterol and how is each defined?
Low fat means the food must contain 3 grams or less of fat per serving.
Reduced fat or **less fat** means that food must contain at least 25 percent less fat per serving than the reference food mentioned on the label. For example, the reference food for reduced-fat mayonnaise is regular mayonnaise.

Saturated fat free means that food contains less than 0.5 grams and less than 0.5 grams of trans fatty acids per serving.

Low saturated fat means that food contains 1 gram or less of saturated fat per serving and not more than 15 percent of calories from saturated fatty acids.

Reduced saturated fat or **less saturated fat** means the food contains at least 25% less of saturated fat per serving than the reference food.

Low-cholesterol foods must contain 20 milligrams or less of cholesterol as well as 2 grams or less of saturated fat per serving.

Reduced cholesterol or **less cholesterol** means the food has at least 25% less cholesterol than the reference food and 2 grams or less of saturated fat per serving.

What does it mean if the Percent Daily Value for cholesterol is 10 percent?

It means that one serving will provide 10 percent of the Daily Value for cholesterol, which is set at 300 milligrams or less. Don't confuse Daily Value with RDAs. There is no RDA for cholesterol (because the body makes enough), but dietary recommendations have consistently stated that cholesterol intake should be at or below 300 milligrams daily, so this figure is used for the Daily Value.

What do the terms "Lean" and "Extra Lean" on meat labels mean?

The following claims can be used to describe meat, poultry, seafood, and game meats.

Lean means less than 10 grams of fat, 4.5 grams or less of saturated fat, and less than 95 milligrams of cholesterol per serving and per 100 grams (about 3 1/2 ounces).

Extra lean means less than 5 grams of fat, less than 2 grams of saturated fat, and less than 95 milligrams cholesterol per serving and per 100 grams (about 3 1/2 ounces).

CHAPTER

4

Protein

**KEY
QUESTIONS**

1. What is protein made of?
2. What functions does protein serve in the body?
3. What happens when protein is denatured, and why is this process significant?
4. How is protein digested, absorbed, and metabolized?
5. Are some proteins of higher quality than others or are all proteins created equal?
6. Do Americans tend to eat too much, too little, or just the right amount of protein each day?
7. What can happen if you eat too much or too little protein?

QUIZ

Directions: Circle the foods that contain protein, even in small amounts.

1. Steak	5. Yogurt	9. Nuts
2. Green beans	6. Milk	10. Bread
3. Chicken	7. Split peas	11. Soybeans
4. Peanut butter	8. Cheese	12. Baked beans

INTRODUCTION

Have you ever wondered why meat, poultry, and seafood are often considered entrees, or main dishes, whereas vegetables and potatoes are side dishes? As recently as the 1950s and 1960s, the abundant protein found in meat, poultry, and seafood was considered the mainstay of a nutritious diet. You could say that these foods took center stage, or more accurately, center plate. As a child, I can remember going to visit my grandparents on Sundays and eating a roast beef dinner during our visit. Yes, we had vegetables too, but the big deal at dinner was the roast that was carefully cooked, sliced, and served (with brown gravy, of course).

Today, protein foods continue to be an important component of a nutritious diet; however, we are more likely to see non-meat protein foods, such as lentils or pasta, occupying the center of the plate. For adults who grew up when beef was king (and not nearly as expensive as it is today) and full-fat bologna sandwiches filled many lunchboxes, making spaghetti without meatballs takes a little getting used to, but more and more meatless meals are being served.

So just what are **proteins**? They are an essential part of all living cells found in animals and plants. The protein found in animal and plant foods is such an important substance that the term *protein* is derived from the Greek word meaning "first." About 16 percent of your body weight (if you're not overweight) is protein. Proteins reside in your skin, hair, nails, muscles, and tendons, to name just a few places. It functions in a very broad sense to build and maintain the body. This chapter discusses its structure, functions, metabolism, and relationship to diet.

STRUCTURE OF PROTEIN

Like carbohydrates and fats, proteins contain carbon, hydrogen, and oxygen. Unlike carbohydrates and fats, proteins contain nitrogen and provide much of the body's nitrogen. Nitrogen is necessary for bodily function; life as we know it wouldn't exist without nitrogen.

Proteins are long chains of **amino acids** strung together much like railroad cars. Amino acids are the building blocks of protein. There are 20 different ones each consisting of a backbone to which a side chain is attached (Figure 4-1). The amino acid backbone is the same for all amino acids, but the side chain varies. It is the side chain that makes each amino acid unique.

Amino acids are the building blocks of protein.

Of the 20 amino acids in proteins (see Table 4-1), nine either cannot be made in the body or cannot be made in the quantities needed. They must therefore be obtained in foods for the body to function properly. This is why we call these amino acids **essential** or **indispensable amino acids**. The remaining 11 can be made in the body. However, under certain circumstances, one or more of these amino acids may become essential.

Essential amino acids cannot be made in the body or cannot be made in adequate quantities, so they must be in your diet.

When the amino-acid backbones join end to end, a protein forms (Figure 4-2). The bonds that form between adjoining amino acids are called **peptide bonds**. Proteins often contain from 35 to several hundred or more amino acids. Protein fragments with 10 or more amino acids are called **polypeptides**.

Each of the over 100,000 different proteins in the body contains its own unique number and sequence of amino acids. In other words, each protein differs in terms of what amino acids it contains, how many it contains, and the order in which they are contained. The number and sequence of the amino acids in the protein chain is called the **primary structure**. The number of possible arrangements is as amazing as the fact that all the words in the English language are made of different sequences of 26 letters. Also, some proteins are made of more than one chain of amino acids. For example, hemoglobin contains four chains of linked amino acids.

After a protein chain has been made in the body, it does not remain

TABLE 4-1. Amino acids.	
Essential Amino Acids	*Other Amino Acids*
Histidine	Alanine
Isoleucine	Arginine
Leucine	Asparagine
Lysine	Aspartic acid
Methionine	Cysteine
Phenylalanine	Glutamic acid
Threonine	Glutamine
Tryptophan	Glycine
Valine	Proline
	Serine
	Tyrosine

FIGURE 4-1.
An amino
acid

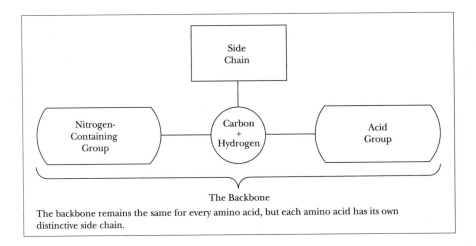

The backbone remains the same for every amino acid, but each amino acid has its own distinctive side chain.

a straight chain. In the instant after a new protein is created, the side chain of each amino acid in the strand either attracts or repels other side chains, resulting in the protein either bending or coiling (Figure 4-3). This bending and coiling is called the protein's **secondary structure**.

One more step must take place before the protein can do any work in the body. Due in part to the interaction of amino acids at some distance from each other in the chain (Figure 4-3), the protein folds and loops. This process of folding results in the protein's **tertiary structure**. In case you are wondering whether a protein's tertiary structure has any real importance, it does! A protein's tertiary structure—how it bends and folds—makes the protein able to perform its functions in the body. Up to

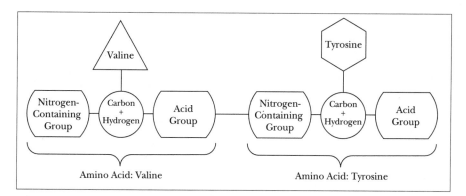

FIGURE 4-2. A part of a protein

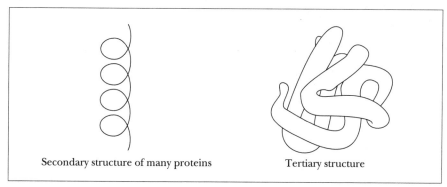

FIGURE 4-3. Primary structure — the number and sequence of amino acids. Secondary structure — bends or coils. Tertiary structure — folds and loops.

this point, the protein wasn't functional. So what exactly does a protein do? That's our next topic.

MINI-SUMMARY   Proteins contain nitrogen. They are long chains of 20 different amino acids, some of which are essential, joined end to end by peptide bonds. Each protein has its own characteristic primary structure (number and sequence of amino acids), secondary structure (bending or coiling), and tertiary structure (folding and looping), which make it functional.

FUNCTIONS OF PROTEIN

After reviewing all of the jobs proteins perform, you will have a greater appreciation of this nutrient. In brief, protein is part of most body structures; builds and maintains the body; is a part of many enzymes, hormones, and antibodies; transports substances around the body; maintains fluid and acid-base balance, and can provide energy for the body (Table 4-2). Now let's take a look at each function separately.

Proteins function as part of the body's structure. For example, protein

TABLE 4-2. Functions of protein.

- Acts as a structural component of the body
- Builds and maintains the body
- Found in many enzymes, hormones, and antibodies
- Transports iron, fats, minerals, and oxygen
- Maintains fluid and acid-base balance
- Provides energy as last resort

can be found in skin, bones, hair, fingernails, muscles, blood vessels, the digestive tract, and blood. It appears in every cell as part of **deoxyribonucleic acid (DNA)**, which carries the genetic code.

DNA holds the code, or blueprint, for making the proteins you need in your body.

Proteins are used for building and maintaining body tissues. Worn-out cells are replaced throughout the body in regular intervals. For instance, your skin today will not be the same skin in a few months. It is constantly being broken down and rebuilt or remodeled, as are most body cells, including the protein within the cells. The greatest amount of protein is needed when the body is building new tissues rapidly, such as during pregnancy or infancy. Additional protein is also needed when body protein is either lost or destroyed as in burns, surgery, or infections.

Proteins are found in many **enzymes**, hormones, and antibodies. Thousands of enzymes have been identified. Almost all the reactions that occur in the body, such as food digestion, involve enzymes. Enzymes are catalysts, meaning that they increase the rate of these reactions, sometimes more than a million times. They do this without being changed in the overall process. Enzymes contain a special pocket called the *active site*. You can think of the active site as a lock into which only the correct key will fit. Various substances will fit into the pocket, undergo a chemical reaction, and then exit the enzyme in a new form, leaving the enzyme to speed up other reactions.

Hormones are chemical messengers secreted into the bloodstream by various organs, such as the liver, to regulate certain body activities so a constant internal environment (called **homeostasis**) is maintained. For example, the hormone **insulin** is released from the pancreas when your blood sugar level goes up, such as after eating lunch. Insulin pushes sugar from the blood into your cells, resulting in lower, more normal blood sugar levels.

Antibodies are blood proteins whose job is to bind with foreign bodies or invaders (scientific name is **antigens**) that do not belong in the body. Invaders could be a viruses, bacteria, or toxins. Each antibody fights a specific invader. For example, there are many different viruses that cause the common cold. An antibody that binds with a certain cold virus is of no use to you if you have a different strain of the cold virus. However, exposure to a cold virus results in increased amounts of the specific type of antibody that can attack it. Next time that particular cold virus comes around, your body remembers and makes the right antibodies. This time the virus is destroyed faster, and your body's response (called the **immune response**) is enough to combat the disease.

Enzymes — catalysts. Hormones — chemical messengers. Antibodies — immune response.

Proteins also act as taxicabs in the body, transporting iron, fats, minerals, and oxygen, quite often through the blood.

Protein also plays a role in body fluid balance (discussed in chapter 6), and the **acid-base balance** of the blood. Normal bodily processes produce acids and bases that can cause major problems, even death, if not buffered or neutralized. The blood must remain neutral; otherwise, dangerous conditions known as **acidosis** (above normal acidity) and alkalosis (above normal alkalinity) can occur. Some blood proteins have the chemical ability to buffer, or neutralize, both acids and bases.

Acid-base balance is the process in which your body buffers the acids and bases normally produced in the body.

In addition, amino acids can be burned to supply energy (4 calories/gram) if absolutely needed. Of course, burning takes them away from their vital functions, but some amino acids can be converted to glucose and burned.

MINI-SUMMARY Protein is part of most body structures; builds and maintains the body; is a part of many enzymes, hormones, and antibodies; transports substances around the body; maintains fluid and acid-base balance; and provides energy for the body.

DENATURATION

Under certain circumstances, a protein's shape is distorted, causing it to lose its ability to function. This process is called **denaturation**. In most cases, the damage cannot be reversed. Denaturation can occur both to proteins in food and to proteins in our bodies.

Denaturation can be caused by high temperatures (as in cooking), ultraviolet radiation, acids and bases, agitation or whipping, high salt concentration, and the salts of mercury, silver, and lead. For example, when you fry an egg, the proteins in the egg white become denatured and turn from clear to white. Denaturation of protein can also occur in the body whenever the blood becomes too acidic or too basic.

Gluten, the protein in flour, denatures during baking to give bread and other baked goods their structure.

MINI-SUMMARY When a protein is denatured, its shape gets distorted so it can no longer function. Protein foods denature during cooking, and proteins in the body can denature if the blood becomes too acidic or basic.

DIGESTION, ABSORPTION, AND METABOLISM

Like lipids, proteins cannot be absorbed across the intestinal membranes until they are broken down into their amino-acid units. Protein digestion starts in the stomach, where stomach acid uncoils the proteins (denaturation) enough to allow enzymes to enter them to do their work. One stomach enzyme, **pepsin**, is the principal digestive enzyme. It splits peptide bonds, making proteins shorter in length.

Digestion is then completed in the small intestine, where pancreatic and intestinal enzymes work on releasing amino acids to be absorbed across the intestinal wall. Because they are water-soluble, amino acids easily travel in the blood to the liver and cells that require them.

An **amino acid pool** in the body provides the cells with a supply of amino acids for making protein. The amino acid pool refers to the overall amount of amino acids distributed in the blood, the organs (such as the liver), and the body's cells. Amino acids from foods, as well as amino acids from body proteins that have been dismantled stock these pools. In this manner, the body recycles its own proteins. If the body is making a protein and can't find an essential amino acid for it, the protein can't be completed and the partially completed protein is disassembled or taken apart. This is important to consider for the next section on protein quality.

MINI-SUMMARY Protein digestion takes place in the stomach and small intestines, where stomach acid and enzymes help break up food proteins into amino acids to be absorbed across the wall of the small intestine. Because they are water-soluble, amino acids easily travel in the blood (as part of the amino acid pool) to the liver and cells that require them.

PROTEIN IN FOOD AND PROTEIN QUALITY

Protein is found in animal and plant foods (Table 4-3). Protein is highest in animal foods, such as beef, chicken, and fish. The amount of protein in one serving of many milk and dairy products is about the same as in one serving of many grains and legumes (dried beans and peas). Of the plant foods, grains, legumes, and nuts usually contribute more protein than vegetables and fruits. Protein-rich foods are usually higher in fat and saturated fat, and always higher in cholesterol, than plant foods (plant foods have no cholesterol). Protein-rich foods also tend to be the most expensive foods to buy when you go to the supermarket or are buying for a foodservice operation.

To understand the concept of protein quality, you need to recall that nine of the 20 amino acids either can't be made in the body or can't be made in sufficient quantity. Food proteins that provide all of the essential amino acids in the proportions needed are called complete proteins. Examples of complete proteins include the animal proteins, such as meats, poultry, fish, eggs, milk, and other dairy products.

An essential amino acid in lowest concentration in a protein is referred to as a **limiting amino acid** because it limits the protein's usefulness unless another food in the diet contains it. **Incomplete protein** contains at least one limiting amino acid. Plant proteins, including dried beans and peas, grains, vegetables, nuts, and seeds, are incomplete. When certain plant foods, such as peanut butter and whole-wheat bread, are eaten over the course of a day, the limiting amino acid in each of these groups is supplied by the other group. Such combinations are called **complementary proteins**.

Complete protein contains all of the essential amino acids in the proportions needed. Incomplete protein has at least one limiting amino acid.

Although plant proteins are incomplete and score lower than animal proteins, they are not low quality. When plant proteins are eaten with other foods, the food combinations usually result in complete protein. In fact, some plant proteins, such as the grains amaranth and quinoa and protein made from soybeans (called "isolated soy protein"), are complete proteins. In adequate amounts and combinations, plant foods can supply the essential nutrients needed for growth and development and overall health. Many cultures around the world use plant proteins extensively. Plant protein foods contribute 65 percent of the protein for each person in the world. For North America alone, plant protein foods only contribute about 32 percent of the protein for each person (Young and Pellett, 1994).

Researchers have developed various ways to score the quality of food proteins. They judge them on how much of their nitrogen the body retains or how well the proteins support growth or maintenance of body tissue. Animal proteins tend to score higher than vegetable proteins, and animal protein is also more digestible. Protein scores have little use in countries where protein consumption is adequate but are useful to scientists working in countries where protein intakes are low.

Food Facts: Meatless Meals in Restaurants and Institutions

The interest in serving meatless meals in restaurants and institutions has grown during the 1990s. Meatless meals make ample use of grains (such as wheat, oats, rice, and barley), beans, peas, lentils, nuts, and seeds. Here are some interesting ways that meatless dishes are being featured on menus in restaurants and institutions.

- All-vegetable combinations are used as fillings for pita pocket sandwiches, soft tortillas, or crepes, and as toppings for pasta and baked potatoes. The fillings may be bound together with sauces using cheese or yogurt.
- Stir-fry dishes omit meat, poultry, and fish. Instead they emphasize fresh vegetables, often with other foods, such as tofu (soybean curd) or even peanuts.
- Vegetables, such as tomatoes, cabbage leaves, and small eggplants are stuffed and baked with many different fillings.

- Vegetarian bars feature assorted grains, beans, pasta, sauces, chopped nuts, and seeds.
- Vegetables, beans, peas, and lentils can be pureed to make dips that can double as sandwich spreads. Examples include black-bean spread and hummus (made from chickpeas).
- Vegetable burgers can be dressed up with almost any traditional burger topping, such as lettuce, tomatoes, salsa, sautéed mushrooms, or grilled pineapple.
- One-dish meals like vegetarian chili, ratatouille, or red beans and rice are flavorful ways to combine plant-based proteins. Main-dish soups are also popular.
- Many excellent international recipes, such as spinach pie from Greece or polenta (cornmeal pudding) are meatless.

MINI-SUMMARY Animal proteins are examples of complete proteins, and most plant proteins are examples of incomplete proteins. By eating complementary plant proteins, you can overcome the problem presented by limiting amino acids and eat a nutritionally adequate diet. Incomplete proteins are not low in quality. In the right amounts and combinations, plant proteins can support growth and maintenance.

PROTEIN AND HEALTH

If you eat too much or too little protein, your health may be affected. First let's look at a high-protein diet. Eating too much protein has no benefits. It will not result in bigger muscles, stronger bones, or increased immunity. In fact, eating more protein than you need may add excessive calories beyond what you require. Extra protein is not stored as protein but is stored as fat if too many calories are being taken in.

Diets high in protein can also be a concern if you are eating a lot of high-fat animal proteins, such as bacon and hamburger, and few vegetable proteins. Comparison of the fat and fiber content of animal and vegetable proteins (Table 4-3) makes clear that plant sources of protein contain less fat and more fiber. They also contain no cholesterol and are rich in vitamins and minerals. Eating too much high-fat animal protein can raise your blood cholesterol levels, which in turn increases your risk of cardiovascular disease. By eating fewer plant proteins, you are also missing out on good sources of fiber and antioxidant nutrients (see Chapter 5), which may protect against cancer.

Published studies show that increased protein intake leads to increased calcium loss (Heany, 1993). This does not necessarily mean that everyone who takes in too much protein is calcium deficient, since the body will make up for this loss by absorbing more calcium in the intestine. However, if an individual has a high protein intake and a low calcium intake, the increased calcium absorption won't compensate enough for its loss. Published studies also show that high protein intakes can worsen kidney problems in patients with renal (kidney) disease (Ahmed, 1991).

On the other hand, eating too little protein can cause problems too, such as slowing down the protein rebuilding and repairing process and weakening the immune system. Developing countries have the most problems with **protein-energy malnutrition (PEM)**. PEM refers to a broad spectrum of malnutrition from mild to serious cases. PEM can occur in infants, children, adolescents, and adults, although it is seen most often in infants and children. PEM develops gradually over weeks or months. In mild cases of PEM, there is weight loss, stunted or slowed growth, and more sedentary behavior.

PEM is prevalent in parts of Central America, South America, Asia, and Africa.

In severe cases of PEM, physicians often see the clinical syndromes called kwashiorkor and marasmus. **Kwashiorkor** is characterized by retarded growth and development, a protruding abdomen due to *edema* (swelling), peeling skin, a loss of normal hair color, irritability, and sadness. **Marasmus** is characterized by gross underweight, no fat stores, and wasting away of muscles. There is no edema, but patients are apathetic. Whereas marasmus is usually associated with severe food shortage, prolonged semistarvation, or early weaning, kwashiorkor is associated with poor protein intake and late weaning (Torun and Chew, 1994).

Mini-Summary There is no benefit to eating too much protein. Eating too much high-fat animal protein can increase your blood cholesterol levels, increase calcium loss from the body (a concern when calcium

TABLE 4-3. Fat, saturated fat, protein, cholesterol and fiber in animal and plant foods.

Animal Foods	Fat (grams)	Saturated Fat (grams)	Protein (grams)	Cholesterol (milligrams)	Fiber (grams)
Beef, ground broiled, 3 oz.	16	6	21	74	0
Chicken breast, roasted, 3 oz.	3	1	27	73	0
Cod, baked, 3 oz.	1	0	19	47	0
Milk, 2%, 8 fl. oz.	5	3	8	18	0
Cheese, American, 1 oz.	9	6	6	27	0
Egg, 1	6	2	6	274	0
Plant Foods					
Lentils, cooked, 1/2 cup	0	0	8	0	5
Peanut butter, 2 tablespoons	16	3	10	0	2
Brown rice, cooked, 1/2 cup	1	0	2	0	1
Spaghetti, whole wheat, 1 cup	1	0	7	0	3
Whole-wheat bread, 2 slices	2	0	6	0	3
Broccoli, chopped 1 cup	0	0	6	0	3
Apple, 1 medium	0.5	0	0.3	0	3

Sources: United States Department of Agriculture Handbook Number 72, 8-1, 8-5, 8-13, 8-15, 8-20.

intake is low), and worsen kidney problems in people with renal disease. Eating too little protein is associated with protein-energy malnutrition.

THE RDA FOR PROTEIN

The RDA for protein for a 174-pound man is 63 grams. For a 138-pound woman, the RDA is 50 grams. For healthy adults, the RDA works out to be 0.36 grams of protein per pound of body weight. This allows for adequate protein to make up for daily losses in urine, feces, hair, and so on. In other words, taking in enough protein each day to balance losses results in a state of protein balance, called nitrogen balance. The RDA for protein is generous and is based on the recommendation that proteins come from both animal and plant foods.

The amount of protein needed daily is proportionally higher during periods of growth, such as during pregnancy and infancy. During these periods, a person needs to eat more protein than is lost, a condition known as **positive nitrogen balance**. **Negative nitrogen balance** occurs during starvation and some illnesses when the body excretes more protein than is taken in.

In the United States, meeting the RDA for protein is rarely a problem. According to U.S. Department of Agriculture (USDA) surveys, 14 to 18 percent of calories in the American diet come from protein, with animal proteins contributing about 65 percent (USDA, 1983, 1986, and 1987). Using the RDA for protein and energy as a guide, the percent of calories from protein should be lower, from 10 to 12 percent.

Positive nitrogen balance occurs during growth and pregnancy. Negative nitrogen balance occurs during starvation and certain illnesses.

MINI-SUMMARY   Most Americans eat more than the RDA for protein. More protein is needed during periods of growth and positive nitrogen balance. Negative nitrogen balance occurs during starvation and some illnesses.

RECOMMENDATIONS AND TIPS FOR NUTRITIOUS FOOD SELECTION

The following tips for nutritious food selection center on the quantity, quality, and variety of protein we eat.

1. **Pick a variety of protein foods to meet your needs.**
2. **Eat enough, but not too much, protein.** Table 4-4 shows the average number of grams of protein in foods. Let us assume you need 50 grams of protein daily, and you normally eat 3 ounces of meat, poultry, fish, or cheese for lunch and supper, 1 cup of milk, 2 serving of vegetables, and 4 servings of bread daily. You are already consuming 66 grams of protein, which would increase to 74 if you add 1 more cup of milk. To cut down on your protein, you could switch from eating 3 ounces of animal protein at lunch or supper to a pasta meal, for example, or eat smaller portions of animal protein.
3. **Balance your consumption of plant and animal sources of protein.** Whereas meats supply important nutrients such as iron, plant sources generally supply starch, fiber, vitamins, and minerals, without much fat or any cholesterol. Plant proteins, which provide less than one-third of protein for Americans, are getting a lot more attention from Americans these days. In more homes and restaurants, plant proteins have acquired new status as entrees (such as vegetarian chili) instead of appearing mostly as side dishes.

TABLE 4-4. Average protein in food groups.	
Food and Serving Size	*Protein (grams)*
Meat, poultry, fish—3 ounces	21
Milk—1 cup	8
Most cheeses—1 ounce	7
Bread—1 slice	3
Ready-to-eat cereals—3/4 cup	3
Starchy vegetables—1/2 cup	2
Vegetables—1/2 cup	2
Fruits—1 piece fresh or 1/2 cup	0
Fat—1 teaspoon	0

4. **When choosing animal proteins, choose those with less fat.** For example, choose lean cuts of beef such as top round or eye of round; white, skinless turkey and chicken; fish; skim milk; and cheeses with 3 grams of fat or less per ounce. Chapter 12 gives more information on choosing low-fat proteins.

MINI-SUMMARY   Pick a variety of protein foods to meet your needs. Eat enough, but not too much, protein. Balance your consumption of plant and animal sources of protein. When choosing animal proteins, choose those with less fat.

KEY TERMS

Acid-base balance
Acidosis
Alkalosis
Amino acid pool
Amino acids
Antibodies
Antigens
Complementary proteins
Complete proteins
Denaturation
Deoxyribonucleic acid (DNA)
Edema
Enzymes
Essential(indispensable)
   amino acid
Homeostasis

Hormones
Immune response
Incomplete proteins
Insulin
Kwashiorkor
Limiting amino acid
Marasmus
Negative nitrogen balance
Pepsin
Peptide bonds
Polypeptides
Positive nitrogen balance
Primary structure
Protein-energy malnutrition
Proteins
Secondary structure
Tertiary structure

In your own words, answer the following questions.

1. How is protein like carbohydrates and fats? How is protein different from carbohydrates and fats?
2. Describe the structure of an amino acid.
3. How is each amino acid different from the others?
4. How many amino acids are considered indispensable? Why are they essential?
5. Describe a protein's primary, secondary, and tertiary structures. What happens when any of these structures are improperly formed?
6. Describe protein's functions.
7. When an egg white cooks, explain what happens to its protein.
8. What can cause denaturation?
9. Describe how protein is digested and absorbed.
10. How are complete proteins different from incomplete proteins?
11. What is meant by complementary proteins?
12. Describe problems that can be caused by consuming too much or too little protein.
13. Why does the RDA for protein increase during pregnancy and infancy?
14. Name two circumstances when an individual might experience negative nitrogen balance.
15. List four considerations to keep in mind when selecting protein foods.

1. Quiz

All the foods listed in the quiz at the beginning of the chapter contain at least some protein.

2. Self-Assessment

In the space provided, write the number of times per week that you eat the foods listed. Does your protein come mostly from animal or plant sources or is it somewhat evenly balanced between the two? Think about the serving sizes of the animal proteins versus the plant proteins. Are the meats, poultry, and fish usually the entrees, and the pasta, rice, vegetables, and dried beans or peas served as side dishes in smaller quantities? What can you do to better balance the two sides if needed?

Animal Protein Sources		Plant Protein Sources	
Red meats	_____	Dried beans	_____
Poultry	_____	Dried peas	_____
Fish	_____	Bread	_____
Milk	_____	Cereals	_____
Cheese	_____	Pasta	_____
Yogurt	_____	Rice	_____
Eggs	_____	Nuts and Seeds	_____
		Vegetables	_____
		(including potatoes)	

**Total Number
  of Servings**   _____

**Total Number
  of Servings**   _____

3. Reading Food Labels

Following are food labels from a beef burger and a vegetable burger. Compare and contrast their nutritional content.

Beef Burger (3 oz.)	**Vegetable Burger** (2.5 oz.)
Nutrition Facts	*Nutrition Facts*
Amount per serving	*Amount per serving*
Calories 230	Calories 140
Calories from fat 140	Calories from fat 20
Total fat 16 g	Total fat 2.5 g
Saturated 6 g	Saturated 0.5 g
Polyunsaturated 1 g	Polyunsaturated 1 g
Monounsaturated 7 g	Monounsaturated 0.5 g
Cholesterol 74 g	Cholesterol 0 g
Sodium 180 mg	Sodium 180 mg
Total carbohydrate 0 g	Total carbohydrate 21 g
Dietary fiber 0 g	Dietary fiber 5 g
Sugar 0 g	Sugar 0 g
Protein 21 g	Protein 8 g

4. How Much Protein Do You Eat?

First, calculate how many grams of protein you need by multiplying your weight (in pounds) by 0.36.

Next, write down everything you ate yesterday, including approximate portion sizes. If yesterday was not a typical day, write down what you normally eat during the course of a day. Using the tables in this chapter and/or Appendix A, find the amount of protein in each food and total your protein intake for the day.

Now you can compare your daily protein intake to the RDA. Do you consume too much, too little, or just about the right amount of protein daily? If you are eating too much, what foods would you cut down on and what foods would you replace them with?

5. *Meat Diet versus Mostly Plant Diet*

Using the tables in this chapter and/or Appendix A, find the amount of protein in each food listed below and total up each list.
Each list represents one day's intake.

Meat-Based Diet		*Plant-Based Diet with Dairy*	
2 eggs	_____	1 cup oatmeal	_____
2 slices white toast	_____	1/2 cup raisins	_____
1/2 cup orange juice	_____	1 corn muffin	_____
1/2 cup milk	_____	1 cup milk	_____
1 doughnut	_____	1 apple	_____
3 ounces roast beef	_____	2 tablespoons peanut butter	_____
1 ounce American cheese	_____	2 tablespoons fruit jam	_____
2 slices white bread	_____	2 slices whole-wheat bread	_____
1 tablespoon mayonnaise	_____	1 banana	_____
1 ounce corn chips	_____	1/2 cup milk	_____
2 cupcakes	_____	4 graham crackers	_____
2 slices pizza	_____	1 cup vegetable soup	_____
1 cup vegetable salad	_____	2 tacos	_____
1 tablespoon dressing	_____	1 cup vegetable salad	_____
12 ounce soft drink	_____	1 tablespoon dressing	_____
1 cup vanilla ice cream	_____	1/2 cup milk	_____
		1 cup vanilla ice milk	_____
Total Protein:	_____	**Total Protein:**	_____

Which diet contains more protein? Do either or both of these diets meet your protein RDA? Is it possible for you to get the protein you need without eating meat, poultry, or seafood?

REFERENCES Ahmed, F. 1991. Effect of diet on progression of chronic renal disease. *Journal of the American Dietetic Association* 91(10): 1266–1267.

Bhattacharyya, A. K. 1986. Protein-energy malnutrition (kwashiorkor-marasmus syndrome): Terminology, classification and evolution. *World Review of Nutrition and Dietetics* 47: 80–133.

Chopra, Joginder G., Allan L. Forbes, and Jean-Pierre Habicht. 1978. Protein in the U.S. diet. *Journal of the American Dietetic Association* 72(3): 253–258.

Hautvast, J. G. A. J. 1987. Panel summary statements: proteins and selected vitamins. American Journal of Clinical Nutrition 45(5): 1044–1046.

Heaney, R. 1993. Protein intake and the calcium economy. *Journal of the American Dietetic Association* 93(11): 1260–1261.

Olowookere, Julius O. 1987. The bioenergetics of protein-energy malnutrition syndrome. *World Review of Nutrition and Dietetics* 54: 1–25.

Olson, R. E. 1989. World food production and problems in human nutrition. *Nutrition Today* (January/February): 15–18.

Sampson, H. A., L. Mendelson, and J. P. Rosen. 1992. Fatal and near-fatal anaphylactic reactions to food in children and adolescents. *New England Journal of Medecine* 327(6): 380–384.

Scrimshaw, Nevin S. 1969. Nature of protein requirements. *Journal of the American Dietetic Association* 54(2): 94–102.

Torun, B., and F. Chew. 1994. Protein-energy malnutrition in M. E. Shils, J. A. Olson, and M. Shike, eds., *Modern Nutrition in Health and Disease.* Philadelphia: Lea & Febiger.

USDA (U.S. Department of Agriculture). 1983. Nationwide Food Consumption Survey 1977–1978. Food Intakes: Individuals in 48 States, Year 1977–78. Report No. I-1. Hyattsville, MD: Consumer Nutrition Division, Human Nutrition Information Service, USDA.

USDA (U.S. Department of Agriculture). 1986. Nationwide Food Consumption Survey. Continuing Survey of Food Intakes by Individuals. Men 19–50 Years, 1 Day, 1985. Report No. 8503. Hyattsville, MD: Consumer Nutrition Division, Human Nutrition Information Service, USDA.

USDA (U. S. Department of Agriculture). 1987. Nationwide Food Consumption Survey. Continuing Survey of Food Intakes by Individuals: Women 19–50 Years and Their Children 1–5 Years, 4 Days, 1985. Report No. 85-4. Hyattsville, MD: Consumer Nutrition Division, Human Nutrition Information Service, USDA.

Young, Vernon R., and Peter L. Pellett. 1994. Plant proteins in relation to human protein and amino acid nutrition. *American Journal of Clinical Nutrition* 59(Suppl.): 1203S–1212S.

Yunginger, J. W., K. G. Sweeney, W. Q. Sturner, L. A. Giannandrea, J. D. Teigland, M. Bray, P. A. Benson, J. A. York, L. Biedrzycki, D. L. Squillace, and R. M. Helm. 1988. Fatal food-induced anaphylaxis. *Journal of the American Medical Association* 260(10): 1450–1451.

Hot Topic: Food Allergies

Do you start itching whenever you eat peanuts? Does seafood cause your stomach to churn? Symptoms like these cause millions of Americans to suspect they have a **food allergy**, when indeed most probably have a **food intolerance**. True food allergies affect a relatively small percentage of people. Experts estimate that only 2 percent of adults, and from 4 to 8 percent of children, are truly allergic to certain foods (Anderson, 1994). So what's the difference between a food intolerance and a food allergy? A food allergy involves an abnormal immune system response. If the response doesn't involve the immune system, it is called a food intolerance. Symptoms of food intolerance may include gas, bloating, constipation, dizziness, or difficulty sleeping.

Food allergy symptoms are quite specific. **Food allergens**, the food components that cause allergic reactions, are usually proteins. When the allergen passes from the mouth into the stomach, the body recognizes it as a foreign substance and produces antibodies to halt the invasion. As the body fights off the invasion, symptoms begin to appear throughout the body. The most common sites (Figure 4-4) are the mouth (swelling of the lips or tongue, itching lips), digestive tract (stomach cramps, vomiting, diarrhea), the skin (hives, rashes, or eczema), and the airways (wheezing or breathing problems). Allergic reactions to foods usually begin within minutes to a few hours after eating.

Food intolerance may produce symptoms similar to those of food allergies, such as

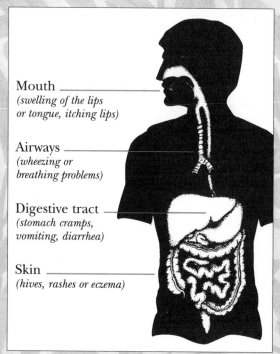

Mouth _____
(swelling of the lips or tongue, itching lips)

Airways _____
(wheezing or breathing problems)

Digestive tract _____
(stomach cramps, vomiting, diarrhea)

Skin _____
(hives, rashes or eczema)

Figure 4-4. Common sites for allergic reactions.

abdominal cramping. But whereas people with true food allergies must avoid offending foods altogether, people with food intolerance can often eat small amounts of the offending food without experiencing symptoms.

Food allergies are much more common in infants and young children, who often outgrow them later. Increased susceptibility of young infants to food allergic reactions is believed to be the result of immunologic immaturity and, to some extent, intestinal immaturity. Older children and adults may lose their sensitivity to certain foods if the responsible food allergen can be identified and completely eliminated from the diet, although some food allergies, such as those to peanuts and nuts, can last a lifetime.

Cow's milk, peanuts, eggs, wheat, and soy are the most common food allergies in children. In many cases, children outgrow these allergies later on in childhood. In general, the more severe the first allergic reaction, the longer it takes to outgrow. Adults are usually most affected by nuts, fish, shellfish, and peanuts.

Most cases of allergic reactions to foods are mild, but some are violent and life-threatening. The greatest danger in food allergy comes from **anaphylaxis**, a rare allergic reaction involving a number of body parts simultaneously. Anaphylaxis is also known as **anaphylactic shock**. Like less serious allergic reactions, anaphylaxis usually occurs after a person is exposed to an allergen to which he or she was sensitized by previous exposure. That is, it does not usually occur the first time a person eats a particular food. Anaphylaxis can produce severe symptoms in as little as 5 to 15 minutes. Signs of such a reaction include difficulty breathing, swelling of the mouth and throat, drop in blood pressure, and loss of consciousness. The sooner anaphylaxis is treated, the greater the person's chance of surviving.

Although any food can trigger anaphylaxis, peanuts, nuts, shellfish, milk, eggs, and fish are the most common culprits (Sampson, Mendelson, and Rosen, 1992; Yunginger, Sweeney, Sturner, et al., 1988). Peanuts are the leading cause of death from food allergies. As little as 1/5 to 1/5000 of a teaspoon of the offending food has caused death.

There is no specific test to predict the likelihood of anaphylaxis, although allergy testing may help determine which foods a person may be allergic to and provide some guidance as to the severity of the allergy. Experts advise people who are prone to anaphylaxis to carry medication—usually injectable epinephrine—with them at all times and to check the medicine's expiration date regularly.

Diagnosing a food allergy begins with a thorough medical history to identify the suspected food, the amount that must be eaten to cause a reaction, the amount of time between food consumption and development of symptoms, how often the reaction occurs, and other detailed information. A complete physical examination and selected laboratory tests are conducted to rule out underlying medical conditions not related to food allergy. Several tests, such as skin-testing and blood tests, are available to determine whether a person's immune system is sensitized to a specific food. In prick-skin testing, a diluted extract of the suspected food is placed on the skin, which is then scratched or punctured. If no reaction at the site occurs, then the skin test is negative and allergy to the food is unlikely. If a bump surrounded by redness (similar to a mosquito bite) forms within 15 minutes, then the skin test is positive and the person may be allergic to the tested food.

Once diagnosed, most food allergies are

treated by avoidance of the food allergen. Newer approaches, such as drugs, are being explored. Avoiding allergens is relatively easy to do at home where you can read food labels and call food manufacturers, but this task becomes harder when you go out to eat. As a food-service professional, you can do the following to help customers with food allergies.

1. Have recipe/ingredient information available for customers with food allergies. Some restaurants designate a person on each shift, who knows this information the best, to be in charge of discussing allergy concerns with customers. To be useful, this information must be accurate and updated regularly. A manufacturer may change the ingredients in salsa, for example, and these changes are important to note.

2. If you are not sure what is in a menu item, don't give the customer false reassurances. It's better to say "I don't know—why not pick something else" than to give false information that could result in the customer's death and hundreds of thousands of dollars in fines and lawsuits.

3. Staff need training in the nature of food allergies, the foods commonly involved in anaphylactic shock, the restaurant's procedure on identifying and handling customers with food allergies, and emergency procedures.

4. Kitchen staff need training in avoiding ingredient substitutions. They also need to be trained to prepare and serve foods without contacting the foods most likely to cause anaphylactic shock: nuts, peanuts, fish, and shellfish. This means that all preparation and cooking equipment should be thoroughly cleaned after working with these foods. Remember that even minute amounts of the offending food, sometimes even a strong smell of the food, can cause anaphylactic reactions.

In short, take it seriously when a customer asks whether there are walnuts in your Waldorf salad. Some customers who ask such questions are probably just trying to avoid an upset stomach, but for some it's a much more serious, and possibly life-threatening, matter. Since you don't know which customer really suffers from food allergies, take every customer seriously.

Table 4-5 lists foods to omit for specific allergies.

	TABLE 4-5. Foods to omit for specific allergies.	
Food Allergen	*Foods to Omit*	*Check Food Labels for*
Milk	All fluid milk including buttermilk, evaporated or condensed milk, nonfat dry milk, all cheeses, all yogurts, ice cream and ice milk, butter, many margarines, most nondairy creamers and whipped toppings, hot cocoa mixes, creamed soups, many breads, crackers and cereals, pancakes, waffles, many baked goods such as cakes and cookies (check the label), fudge, instant potatoes, custards, puddings, some hot dogs and luncheon meats	Instant nonfat dry milk, nonfat milk, milk solids, whey, curds, casein, caseinate, milk, lactose-free milk, lactalbumin, lactoglobulin, sour cream, butter, cheese, cheese food, butter, milk chocolate, buttermilk
Eggs	All forms of eggs, most egg substitutes, eggnog, any baked goods made with eggs such as muffins and cookies or glazed with eggs such as sweet rolls, ice cream, sherbet, custards, meringues, cream pies, puddings, French toast, pancakes, waffles, some candies, some salad dressings and sandwich spreads such as mayonnaise, any sauce made with egg such as hollandaise, souffles, any meat or potato made with egg, all pastas unless egg-free, soups made with eggs or noodles, soups made with stocks that were cleared with eggs, marshmallows	Eggs, albumin, globulin, livetin, ovalbumin, ovomucin, ovomucoid, ovoglobulin egg albumin, ovovitellin, vitellin

Food Allergen	Foods to Omit	Check Food Labels for
Gluten	All foods containing wheat, oats, barley or rye as flour or in any other form, salad dressings, gravies, malted beverages, postum, soy sauce, instant puddings, distilled vinegar, beer, ale, some wines, gin, whiskey, vodka	Flour* (unless from sources noted below), modified food starch, monosodium glutamate, hydrolyzed vegetable protein, cereals, malt or cereal extracts, food starch, vegetable starch, vegetable gum, wheat germ, wheat bran, bran, semolina, malt flavoring, distilled vinegar, emulsifiers, stabilizers.

*Corn, rice, soy, arrowroot, tapioca, and potato do not contain gluten, so they are safe to use.

Label Reading Questions and Answers: Protein

Why is no Percent Daily Value for protein included on food labels (Figure 4-5)?

Nutrition Facts

Serving Size 3 oz cooked fish
(84g/about 1½ fillets)
Servings Per Container about 4

Amount Per Serving

Calories 100   Calories from Fat 10

	% Daily Value*
Total Fat 1g	**2%**
Saturated Fat 0g	**0%**
Cholesterol 80mg	**27%**
Sodium 85mg	**4%**
Total Carbohydrate 0g	**0%**
Dietary Fiber 0g	**0%**
Sugars 0g	
Protein 21g	

Vitamin A 0%	•	Vitamin C 0%
Calcium 2%	•	Iron 6%

* Percent Daily Values are based on a 2,000 calorie diet. Your daily values may be higher or lower depending on your calorie needs:

		Calories:	2,000	2,500
Total Fat	Less than		65g	80g
Sat Fat	Less than		20g	25g
Cholesterol	Less than		300mg	300mg
Sodium	Less than		2,400mg	2,400mg
Total Carbohydrate			300g	375g
Dietary Fiber			25g	30g

Figure 4-5. Nutrition label

Because most Americans get more than enough protein, no Daily Value is necessary. Your daily needs are 0.36 grams of protein per pound of body weight.

If a food is labeled "high in protein" or "good source of protein," what exactly does that mean?

A food labeled "high in protein" must provide at least 10 grams of high-quality protein per serving. A food labeled "good source of protein" must contain at least 5 grams of high-quality protein per serving.

A food I bought yesterday says "more protein" on the label. What can I expect?

A food labeled "more protein" must have at least 5 grams more of high-quality protein per serving than the reference food. Some foods are made with additional protein, and the label can include this information when the product has at least 5 grams more of high-quality protein than the regular product.

CHAPTER

5

Vitamins

**KEY
QUESTIONS**

1. What are the general characteristics of vitamins?
2. What are the functions and food sources of each of the 13 vitamins?
3. At what level, as compared to the RDA, are vitamins toxic?
4. Which vitamins are more likely to be deficient in the American diet?
5. Which vitamins are the most toxic in high doses?
6. How can you conserve vitamins when handling and cooking foods?

QUIZ

1. Which of the following vitamins is most likely to be deficient in the American diet?
   (a) Vitamin E
   (b) Folate
   (c) Thiamin
   (d) Pantothenic acid
2. Which of the following classes of vitamins are more likely to be toxic if taken in excess?
   (a) Water-soluble vitamins
   (b) Fat-soluble vitamins
   (c) A and B
   (d) None of the above
3. A food rich in vitamin C needs to be eaten
   (a) daily
   (b) every other day
   (c) two times each week
   (d) once each week
4. A folate deficiency causes a form of
   (a) osteoporosis
   (b) scurvy
   (c) anemia
   (d) skin inflammation
5. Nutrients can be destroyed due to
   (a) poor receiving practices
   (b) poor storage practices
   (c) overcooking
   (d) all of the above

INTRODUCTION

Vitamins are organic food nutrients that are essential in small quantities for growth and good health. Vitamins are similar because they are made of the same elements: carbon, hydrogen, oxygen, and sometimes nitrogen or cobalt. They differ in the arrangement of their elements and the functions they perform in the body. In the early 1900s, scientists thought they had found the compounds needed to prevent two diseases caused by vitamin deficiencies: scurvy and pellagra. These compounds originally were believed to belong to a class of chemical compounds called amines and were named from the Latin *vita*, or life, plus *amine—vitamine*. Later, the "e" was dropped when it was found that not all of the substances were amines. At first, no one knew what they were chemically so vitamins were identified by letters. Later, what was thought to be one vitamin turned out to be many, and numbers were added, such as the vitamin B complex (for example, vitamin B_1 and vitamin B_6).

Later on, some vitamins were found unnecessary for human needs and were removed from the list, which accounts for some of the numbering gaps. For example, vitamin B_8, adenylic acid, was later found not to be a vitamin. Others, originally given different designations, were found to be the same. For example, vitamins H, M, S, W, and X were all shown to be biotin.

As the number of vitamins being discovered increased, scientists began naming them by their structure or function. Scientists also worked on reproducing the vitamins' structures in the laboratory. Eventually, companies started producing synthetic vitamin supplements with the identical chemical structure as those found in food. The body can't detect whether a vitamin is synthetic or natural—the only thing that matters is that the structure is accurate.

Let's start with some basic facts about vitamins.

1. Very small amounts of vitamins are needed by the human body and very small amounts are present in foods. Some vitamins are measured in IU's (international units), a measure of biological activity; others are measured by weight, in micrograms or milligrams. To illustrate how small these amounts are, remember that 1 ounce is 28.3 grams. A milligram is 1/100 of a gram, and a microgram is 1/1000 of a milligram.
2. Although vitamins are needed in small quantities, the roles they play in the body are enormously important, as you will see in a moment.

3. Most vitamins are obtained through food. Some are also produced by bacteria in the intestine (and are absorbed into the body), and one (vitamin D) can be produced by the skin when it is exposed to sunlight.

4. There is no perfect food that contains all the vitamins in just the right amounts. The best way to assure an adequate vitamin intake is to eat a varied and balanced diet.

5. Vitamins do not contain calories, so they do not directly provide energy to the body. Vitamins provide energy indirectly because they are involved in energy metabolism.

6. Some vitamins in foods are not the actual vitamin but are **precursors**. The body chemically changes the precursor to the active form of the vitamin.

7. A **megadose** of a vitamin is defined as more than 10 times the RDA. It often has toxic effects. Vitamin D, for example, can be toxic when taken at only 5 to 10 times the RDA.

Vitamins are classified according to how soluble they are in either fat or water. **Fat-soluble vitamins** (A, D, E, and K) generally occur in foods containing fat, and they can be stored in the body. **Water-soluble vitamins** (vitamin C and the B-complex vitamins) are not stored appreciably in the body. Now let's take a closer look at the 13 different vitamins.

MINI-SUMMARY Very small amounts of vitamins are needed by the human body, and very small amounts are present in foods. Although vitamins are needed in small quantities, the roles they play in the body are enormously important. Vitamins must be obtained through foods, because vitamins are either not made in the body or not made in sufficient quantities. There is no perfect food that contains all the vitamins in just the right amounts. The best way to assure an adequate intake of vitamins is to eat a varied and balanced diet. Vitamins have no calories so they do not directly provide energy to the body. Some vitamins in foods are not the actual vitamin but rather are precursors. The body chemically changes the precursor to the active form of the vitamin. Megadoses are often toxic. Vitamins are classified according to how soluble they are in either fat or water.

FAT-SOLUBLE VITAMINS

Fat-soluble vitamins include vitamins A, D, E, and K. They generally occur in foods containing fats and are stored in the body either in the liver or in adipose (fatty) tissue until they are needed. Fat-soluble vitamins are absorbed and transported around the body like other fats. If anything interferes with normal fat digestion and absorption, these vitamins may not be absorbed. For instance, people who use mineral oil (as a laxative) at mealtimes will not absorb the fat-soluble vitamins at that meal because they will be excreted with the mineral oil in the feces.

Although it is convenient to be able to store these vitamins so you can survive periods of poor intake, excessive vitamin intake (such as if you are taking large doses of vitamin pills), causes large amounts of vitamins A, D, and K to be stored and may lead to undesirable symptoms.

Fat-soluble vitamins:
Vitamin A.
Vitamin D.
Vitamin E.
Vitamin K.

Vitamin A

During World War I, many children in Denmark developed eye problems. Their eyes became dry, eyelids became swollen, and eventually blindness resulted. A Danish physician read that an American scientist gave milkfat to laboratory animals to cure similar eye problems in animals. At the time Danish children were drinking skim milk because all the milkfat was being made into butter and sold to England. When the Danish doctor gave whole milk and butter to the children, they got better. The Danish government later restricted the amount of exported dairy foods. Dr. E. V. McCollum, the American scientist, eventually found vitamin A (the first vitamin to be discovered) to be the curative substance in milkfat.

Vitamin A has two roles involving the eyes. First, it is essential for the health of the cornea, the clear membrane covering your eye. Without enough vitamin A, the cornea becomes cloudy. Eventually it dries (called **xerosis**) and thickens and can result in permanent blindness (**xerophthalmia**).

Vitamin A is well known for its role in night vision. When there is insufficient vitamin A, you may experience symptoms of night blindness. In **night blindness**, it takes longer to adjust to dim lights after seeing a bright flash of light (such as oncoming car headlights) at night. This is an early sign of vitamin A deficiency. If the deficiency continues, xerosis and xerophthalmia can occur.

Vitamin A is involved in many other functions. It plays a role in cell growth and development, healthy skin and hair, as well as proper bone growth and tooth development in children. Vitamin A is also needed for proper immune system functioning (so you can fight infections) and to maintain the protective linings of your lungs, intestines, urinary tract, and other organs (this also helps to fight infection and disease). Vitamin A is essential for normal reproduction.

Vitamin A:
Night vision.
Healthy cornea
of eye.
Cell growth and
development.
Healthy skin and
hair.
Bone and tooth
development.
Maintenance of
protective linings.
Immune system.
Normal
reproduction.

Vitamin A is found in foods in two forms: **preformed vitamin A** or **retinol** and **provitamin A**. Provitamin A refers to certain members of a class of pigments called carotenoids that contribute red, orange, or yellow color to fruits and vegetables. Provitamin A is converted to vitamin A in the body.

Beta-carotene, the most abundant carotenoid, is an **antioxidant**. Antioxidants combine with oxygen so oxygen is not available to oxidize, or destroy, important substances. Antioxidants prevent the oxidation of unsaturated fatty acids in the cell membrane, DNA (the genetic code), and other cell parts that substances called **free radicals** destroy. In the absence of antioxidants, free radicals destroy cells (possibly accelerating the aging process) and alter DNA (possibly increasing the risk for cancerous cells to develop). Free radicals may also contribute to the development of cardiovascular disease. In the process of functioning as an antioxidant, beta-carotene is itself oxidized or destroyed. The role of beta-carotene as an anticancer agent is being studied.

Vitamin A:
Fortified milk and
cereals.
Dark green
vegetables.
Deep orange fruits
and vegetables.

Certain plant foods are excellent sources of carotenoids. These include dark green vegetables, such as spinach, and deep orange fruits and vegetables, such as apricots, carrots, and sweet potatoes. Beta-carotene has an orange color seen in many vitamin-A-rich fruits and vegetables, but in some cases its orange color is masked by dark green chlorophyll found in vegetables such as broccoli.

Sources of preformed vitamin A include animal products such as liver (a very rich source), vitamin-A-fortified milk, fortified butter and margarine, and fortified cereals. Most ready-to-eat and instant cereals are also fortified with vitamin A. Fortified ready-to-eat cereals usually contain at least 25 percent of the U.S. RDA for vitamin A. Retinol, the active form of vitamin A found in animal foods, is used in fortification. Preformed retinol makes up about two-thirds of our total vitamin A intake.

The RDA for vitamin A is expressed in **retinol equivalents**. Retinol equivalents measure the amount of retinol derived from eating foods that contain preformed vitamin A or provitamin A. To get enough vitamin A, it is recommended that you eat a dark green vegetable or deep orange fruit or vegetable at least every other day. Because the body stores vitamin A in the liver, it is not absolutely necessary to eat a good source every day.

Prolonged use of high doses of vitamin A (usually about 10 times one's RDA) may cause hair loss, bone pain and damage, soreness, liver damage, nausea, and diarrhea. Megadoses are particularly dangerous for pregnant women (it may cause birth defects) and children (it can stunt growth). Only preformed vitamin A, not carotenoids such as beta-carotene, has such effects. When supplements of beta-carotene are taken, the beta-carotene can't be converted fast enough to be toxic.

Vitamin D

Vitamin D differs from all the other nutrients in that it can be made in the body. When ultraviolet rays shine on your skin, a cholesterol-like compound is converted into a precursor of vitamin D and absorbed into the blood. Of course, if you are not in the sun much or if the ultraviolet rays are cut off by heavy clothing, clouds, smog, fog, sunblock, and window glass, there will be less vitamin D produced. On the positive side, a light-skinned person needs only about 15 minutes of sun on the face, hands, and arms two to three times per week to make enough vitamin D (a dark-skinned person needs several hours). Several months' supply of vitamin D can be stored in the body.

Vitamin D is a member of a team of nutrients and hormones that maintain blood calcium levels and ensure an adequate supply of calcium (and phosphorus) for building bones and teeth. Calcium is also used to contract muscles and transmit nerve impulses, so vitamin D ensures that calcium is available for these functions. Vitamin D increases blood calcium levels in any of three ways: it increases calcium absorption in the intestine, decreases the amount of calcium excreted by the kidney, and pulls calcium out of the bones.

Vitamin D: Maintenance of blood calcium levels.

Significant food sources of vitamin D include liver, egg yolks, and fish liver oils. Except for these few foods, only small amounts of vitamin D are found in food. For this reason, milk is normally fortified with vitamin D. Some breakfast cereals and margarines are also fortified with vitamin D. If you drink two cups of milk each day, you will get about half the RDA of vitamin D (the rest comes from other foods and sun exposure). There is no vitamin D added to milk products such as yogurt or cheese.

Vitamin D: Sunshine. Fortified milk. Liver. Egg yolk.

Vitamin D deficiency in children causes **rickets**, a disease in which bones do not grow normally, resulting in bowed legs and knock knees. Vitamin D deficiency in adults causes **osteomalacia**, a disease in which leg and spinal bones soften and may bend. Rickets is rarely seen, but osteomalacia may be seen in elderly individuals with poor milk intake and little sun exposure.

Vitamin D, when taken in excess of the RDA, is the most toxic of all the vitamins. All you need is about 4 to 5 times the RDA to start feeling symptoms of nausea, vomiting, diarrhea, fatigue, confusion, and thirst. It can lead to calcium deposits in the heart and kidneys that can cause severe health problems and even death. Young children and infants are especially susceptible to the toxic effects of too much vitamin D, and megadoses can cause growth failure.

Vitamin E

When you talk about vitamin E, you are actually referring to its four different forms, named after the first four letters of the Greek alphabet: alpha, beta, gamma, and delta. Vitamin E has an important function in the body as an antioxidant, especially to red blood cells in the lungs that pick up oxygen and white blood cells that defend the body from disease. Vitamin E plays a role in iron metabolism and develops and maintains nervous tissues. Vitamin E's role in preventing cardiovascular disease and cancer and delaying aging is still very much in the research stages.

Vitamin E is widely distributed in plant foods. Rich sources include vegetable oils, margarine and shortening made from vegetable oils, and wheat germ (which contains much oil). In oils, vitamin E acts like an antioxidant, thereby preventing the oil from going rancid or bad. Other good sources include whole-grain and fortified breads and cereals, legumes, nuts, seeds, and green leafy vegetables. Except for liver and egg yolks, animal foods are poor sources for vitamin E.

Deficiency is rare, except in infants born prematurely (meaning very early), in part because of vitamin E's wide distribution in plant foods and because the body has significant storage capacity.

Vitamin K

Vitamin K has an essential role in the production of several chemicals (such as prothrombin) involved in blood clotting. Blood clotting is vital in the prevention of excessive blood loss when the skin is broken.

Vitamin K appears in certain foods and is also produced in the body. There are billions of bacteria that normally live in your intestines, and some of them make a form of vitamin K. It is thought that the amount of vitamin K produced by the bacteria is significant and may meet about half of your needs. (An infant is normally given this vitamin after birth to prevent bleeding because the intestine does not yet have the bacteria to produce vitamin K.) Food sources of vitamin K provide the balance needed. Excellent sources of vitamin K include liver and dark green leafy vegetables such as broccoli, collard greens, lettuce, spinach, and cabbage. Other sources include cheese, egg yolk, and soybean oil.

Vitamin K deficiency is rare. Excessive supplementation of a synthetic version of vitamin K can be toxic, so supplements of just vitamin K are not available unless prescribed by a physician.

TABLE 5-1. Vitamins.

Vitamin	*RDA[1] or ESADDI[2]*	*Functions*	*Sources*
Fat-Soluble Vitamins			
Vitamin A	Males: 1,000 Retinol Equivalents Females: 800 Retinol Equivalents	Cell growth and development Healthy skin and hair Bone and tooth development Maintenance of protective linings of lungs, etc. Proper functioning of immune system Normal reproduction Night vision; healthy cornea	Preformed: Liver, fortified milk, fortified cereals Provitamin: Dark green vegetables, deep orange fruits and vegetables
Vitamin D	5 micrograms	Maintenance of blood calcium levels	Fortified milk, liver egg yolk, fortified breakfast cereals, sunshine
Vitamin E	Males: 10 milligrams Females: 8 milligrams	Antioxidant Iron metabolism Maintenance of nervous tissue Protects red and white blood cells	Vegetable oils, margarine, shortening, wheat germ, whole-grain and fortified breads and cereals, legumes, nuts, seeds, green leafy vegetables
Vitamin K	Males: 80 micrograms Females: 65 micrograms	Blood clotting	Dark green leafy vegetables, cheese, soybean oil, Intestinal bacteria
Water Soluble Vitamins			
Vitamin C	60 milligrams	Antioxidant Formation of collagen Wound healing Iron absorption Functioning of immune system Synthesis of some hormones and neurotransmitters	Citrus fruits, tomatoes potatoes, broccoli, cantaloupe, strawberries, fortified juices and cereals

Vitamin	RDA[1] or ESADDI[2]	Functions	Sources
Thiamin	Males: 1.5 milligrams Females: 1.1 milligrams	Coenzyme in energy metabolism Functioning of nervous system Normal growth	Pork, liver, dry beans, peanuts, peanut butter, seeds, whole-grain and enriched breads and cereals
Riboflavin	Males: 1.7 milligrams Females: 1.3 milligrams	Coenzyme in energy metabolism Healthy skin Normal vision	Milk and milk products, organ meats, whole-grain and enriched breads and cereals, some meats
Niacin	Males: 19 milligrams equivalent Females: 15 milligrams equivalent	Coenzyme in energy metabolism Healthy skin Normal functioning of nervous system Normal functioning of digestive tract	Organ meats, meat, poultry, fish, whole-grain and enriched breads and cereals, milk, eggs
Vitamin B$_6$	Males: 2.0 milligrams Females: 1.6 milligrams	Coenzyme in carbohydrate, fat, and protein metabolism Synthesis of red blood cells	Organ meats, meat, poultry, fish, whole grains, fortified cereals, leafy green vegetables, potatoes, bananas, cantaloupe
Folate	Males: 200 micrograms Females: 180 micrograms	Formation of DNA Formation of new cells Iron metabolism	Green leafy vegetables, organ meats, legumes, orange juice
Vitamin B$_{12}$	2.0 micrograms	Activation of folate Normal functioning of the nervous system	Animal foods only: meat, poultry, seafood, eggs, dairy products
Pantothenic Acid	4–7 milligrams	Energy metabolism	Widespread
Biotin	30–100 micrograms	Energy metabolism	Widespread

[1]RDA is for ages 25–50.
[2]Estimated Safe and Adequate Daily Dietary Intakes for adults.

MINI-SUMMARY Table 5-1 summarizes the functions and sources of the fat-soluble vitamins: A, D, E, and K.

WATER-SOLUBLE VITAMINS

Water-soluble vitamins include vitamin C and the B-complex vitamins. The B vitamins work in every body cell, where they function as coenzymes. A coenzyme combines with an enzyme to make it active. The body stores only limited amounts of water-soluble vitamins (except vitamin B_{12}— several years' supply can be stored in the liver); excesses are excreted in the urine. Even though excesses are excreted, excessive supplementation of water-soluble vitamins can cause toxic side effects.

Vitamin C

Scurvy, the name for vitamin C deficiency disease, has been known since biblical times. It was most common on ships where sailors developed bleeding gums, weakness, loose teeth, broken capillaries (small blood vessels) under the skin, and eventually death. Because sailors' diets included fresh fruits and vegetables only for the first part of a voyage, longer voyages resulted in more cases of scurvy. Once it was discovered that citrus fruits prevented scurvy, British sailors were given daily portions of lemon juice. In those days, lemons were called limes, hence British sailors got the nickname "Limeys."

Vitamin C (its chemical name is ascorbic acid, meaning "no-scurvy acid") is important in forming **collagen**, a protein substance that provides strength and support to bones, teeth, skin, cartilage, and blood vessels. It has been said that vitamin C acts like cement, holding together our cells and tissues. It is also important in healing wounds, absorbing iron into the body, fighting infection, and making certain hormones and **neurotransmitters** (chemical substances released by nerve cells that stimulate or inhibit other cells).

Vitamin C:
Antioxidant.
Formation of
collagen.
Wound healing.
Iron absorption.
Functioning of
immune system.

Like beta-carotene and vitamin E, vitamin C is an important antioxidant; it prevents the oxidation of vitamin A and polyunsaturated fatty acids in the intestine. Its antioxidant properties have made vitamin C widely used as a food additive. It may appear on food labels as sodium ascorbate, calcium ascorbate, or simply ascorbic acid.

Foods rich in vitamin C include citrus fruits (oranges, grapefruits, limes, and lemons) and tomatoes. Good sources include white potatoes, sweet potatoes, broccoli, and other green and yellow vegetables, as well as cantaloupe and strawberries. Only foods from the fruit and vegetable groups contribute vitamin C. There is little or no vitamin C in the meat

Vitamin C:
Citrus fruits.
Tomatoes.
Potatoes.
Broccoli.
Cantaloupe.
Strawberries.

TABLE 5-2. Vitamin C in foods.	
Food	*Milligrams Vitamin C*
Fruits	
Orange, 1	80
Kiwi, 1 medium	75
Cranberry juice cocktail, 6 ounces	67
Orange juice, from concentrate, 1/2 cup	48
Papaya, 1/2 cup cubes	43
Strawberries, 1/2 cup	42
Grapefruit, 1/2	41
Grapefruit juice, canned, 1/2 cup	36
Cantaloupe, 1/2 cup cubes	34
Tangerine, 1	26
Mango, 1/2 cup, slices	23
Honeydew melon, 1/2 cup cubes	21
Banana, 1	10
Apple, 1	8
Nectarine, 1	7
Vegetables	
Broccoli, chopped, cooked, 1/2 cup	49
Brussel sprouts, cooked, 1/2 cup	48
Cauliflower, cooked, 1/2 cup	34
Sweet potato, baked, 1	28
Kale, cooked, chopped, 1/2 cup	27
White potato, baked, 1	26
Tomato, 1 fresh	22
Tomato juice, 1/2 cup	22
Cereals	
Cornflakes, 1 cup	15

Source: U.S. Department of Agriculture.

group (except in liver, of course) or the dairy group. Some juices are fortified with vitamin C (if not already rich in vitamin C), as are most ready-to-eat cereals. Many people meet their daily RDA for vitamin C simply by drinking 1/2 cup (4 fluid ounces) of orange juice. This is a good choice because vitamin C is easily destroyed in food preparation and cooking. Table 5-2 lists the vitamin C content of selected foods.

Certain situations require additional vitamin C. These include pregnancy and nursing, growth, fevers and infections, burns, fractures, surgery, cancer, and cigarette smoking. Smoking interferes with the use of vitamin C. In some cases, you can still get all the extra needed by doubling your intake of foods rich in vitamin C.

Deficiencies resulting in scurvy are rare. Scurvy might occur, however, in infants who are fed cow's milk instead of breast milk or formula (they both contain vitamin C), in elderly people with poor intake of fruits and vegetables, and in alcoholics.

The RDA for vitamin C, which was designed to prevent scurvy, may be increased in the next edition of the RDAs. Some research is showing that intake recommendations should not be based simply on preventing scurvy, but rather on what is best for the population. One study found that the optimal daily intake of vitamin C was more like 200 milligrams rather than the 60 milligrams recommended for adults (Levine, 1996). At the 200 milligram level, vitamin C was best absorbed and used by the body's tissues. Unfortunately, this dose of vitamin C causes problems for individuals with certain conditions. More research will give better guidance on what an optimal RDA is for vitamin C.

At doses over 400 milligrams, the body's ability to absorb vitamin C greatly declines and excess vitamin is excreted. Doses over 1000 milligrams (1 gram) daily may be hazardous, and diarrhea and stomach inflammation may occur. If supplements are suddenly stopped, a condition called **rebound scurvy** in which deficiency symptoms appear, may occur.

Thiamin, Riboflavin, and Niacin

Thiamin, riboflavin, and niacin all play key roles as part of coenzymes in energy metabolism. They are essential in the release of energy from carbohydrates, fats, and proteins. They are also needed for normal growth.

Thiamin, riboflavin, and niacin are all coenzymes in energy metabolism.

Thiamin also plays a vital role in the normal functioning of the nerves and muscles, since the nerves send messages to the muscles to contract and relax. Riboflavin is important for healthy skin and normal vision. Niacin is needed for the maintenance of healthy skin and the normal functioning of the nervous system and digestive tract.

Because thiamin, riboflavin, and niacin all help release food energy, the needs for these vitamins increase as calorie needs increase.

Thiamin is widely distributed in foods but mostly in moderate amounts. Pork is an excellent source of thiamin. Other sources include liver, dry beans, peanuts, peanut butter, seeds, wheat germ and whole-grain and enriched breads and cereals.

Thiamin:
Pork.
Legumes.
Peanuts.
Breads and cereals.

Milk and milk products are the major source of riboflavin in the American diet. Other sources include organ meats such as liver (very high

Riboflavin:
Milk and milk
products.
Breads and cereals.

Niacin:
Meat, poultry, fish.
Breads and cereals.

in riboflavin), whole-grain and enriched breads and cereals, chicken and some meats. Because riboflavin breaks down when exposed to light, avoid buying milk in clear glass containers.

The main sources of niacin are meat, poultry, and fish. Organ meats, again, are quite high in niacin. Whole-grain and enriched breads and cereals are also important sources of niacin. All foods containing complete protein, such as those just mentioned and also milk and eggs, are good sources of the precursor of niacin, tryptophan. **Tryptophan**, an amino acid present in some of these foods, is converted to niacin. About half the niacin we use is made from tryptophan.

Deficiencies in thiamin, riboflavin, and niacin are rare, in part because foods such as enriched breads contain all three nutrients. General symptoms for B vitamin deficiencies include fatigue, decreased appetite, and depression.

Toxicity is not a problem except in the case of niacin. Nicotinic acid, a form of niacin, has been prescribed by physicians to lower elevated blood cholesterol levels. Unfortunately it has some undesirable side effects. Starting at doses of 100 milligrams, typical symptoms include flushing, rashes, tingling, itching, hives, nausea, diarrhea, and abdominal discomfort. Flushing of the face, neck, and chest lasts for about 20 minutes after taking a large dose. More serious side effects of large doses include liver malfunction, high blood sugar levels, and abnormal heart rhythm.

Vitamin B₆

Vitamin B$_6$:
Synthesis of red
blood cells.
Coenzyme in
metabolism of
energy nutrients.

Vitamin B_6 is actually three different compounds that can each be changed to the active coenzyme form. Vitamin B_6 plays an important role as part of a coenzyme involved in carbohydrate, fat, and protein metabolism. It is particularly important in protein metabolism, specifically in making and breaking down amino acids. It is also used to make red blood cells (which transport oxygen around the body).

The need for vitamin B_6 is directly related to protein intake. As the intake of protein increases, the need for vitamin B_6 increases.

Vitamin B$_6$:
Meat, poultry, fish.
Whole grains.
Fortified cereals.
Leafy green
vegetables.
Potatoes.·
Bananas and
cantaloupe.

Good sources for vitamin B_6 include organ meats, meat, poultry, and fish. Vitamin B_6 also appears in plant foods; however, it is not as well absorbed from these sources. Good plant sources include whole grains (refined grains are not enriched with this vitamin), potatoes, and some fruits (such as bananas and cantaloupe), and some leafy green vegetables (such as broccoli and spinach). Fortified ready-to-eat cereals are also good sources of vitamin B_6.

Deficiency of vitamin B_6 causes muscle twitching, a type of anemia,

TABLE 5-3. Food sources of folate.

Food	Micrograms per 100g of food—3.5 oz
Dark-green leafy vegetables	120–160
Other vegetables	40–100
Fruits (particularly citrus)	50–100
Beans (legumes)	50–300
Whole grains	60–120
Breakfast cereals	100 or 400

and rashes. Excessive use of vitamin B_6 (more than 2 grams daily for 2 months or more) can cause irreversible nerve damage and symptoms such as numbness in hands and feet and difficulty walking. Doses as low as 50 milligrams may even be toxic. Unfortunately vitamin B_6 supplementation became popular when it appeared that the vitamin may relieve some of the symptoms of premenstrual syndrome and carpal tunnel syndrome, a condition in which a compressed nerve in the wrist causes much pain.

Folate and Vitamin B_{12}

Folate and vitamin B_{12} often work together in the body. Folate is a component of the enzymes required to form DNA, the genetic material contained in every body cell. Folate is therefore needed to make all new cells. Much folate is used to produce adequate numbers of red blood cells, white blood cells, and digestive tract cells.

Excellent sources of folate include green leafy vegetables (the word folate comes from the word *foliage*, meaning leafy), organ meats such as liver and kidney, legumes, orange juice, and brewers' yeast (Table 5-3). Good sources include beef, whole-grain breads and cereals, and fortified ready-to-eat cereals. Much folate is lost during food preparation and cooking, so fresh and lightly cooked foods are more likely to contain more folate.

Vitamin B_{12}, a group of related compounds that contain the mineral cobalt, is present in all body cells. Its most important function is to convert folate into its active forms so that it can make DNA. It also helps in the normal functioning of the nervous system by maintaining the protective cover around nerve fibers.

Folate: Formation of DNA and new cells. In oranges, green leafy vegetables, legumes.

*Vitamin B$_{12}$:
Activates folate.
Normal
functioning of the
nervous system.
Found only in
animal foods.*

Vitamin B$_{12}$ also differs from other vitamins in that it is found only in animal foods such as meat, poultry, fish, shellfish, eggs, milk, and milk products. Plant foods do not contain any vitamin B$_{12}$. Vegetarians who do not eat any animal products need to include vitamin-B$_{12}$-fortified soy milk (or other fortified foods) in their diet or supplements.

Vitamin B$_{12}$ also differs from other vitamins in that it requires two compounds—**R-protein** (produced in most body fluids) and **intrinsic factor** (produced in the stomach)—to be absorbed. Vitamin B$_{12}$ attaches to the R-protein in the stomach and is then released in the small intestine, where it complexes with the intrinsic factor. Vitamin B$_{12}$ is then carried to the ileum (the last segment of the small intestine), where it is absorbed. Vitamin B$_{12}$ is stored in the liver.

A folate deficiency can cause **megaloblastic anemia**, a condition in which the red blood cells are larger than normal and function poorly. Other symptoms may include digestive tract problems such as diarrhea, and mental depression. Groups particularly at risk for folate deficiency are pregnant women, low-birthweight infants, and the elderly.

A folate deficiency may have especially serious consequences during the first few weeks of pregnancy when it may cause neural tube defects. The neural tube is the tissue in the embryo that develops into the brain and spinal cord. Neural tube defects are diseases in which the brain and spinal cord form improperly in early pregnancy. They affect 1 to 2 of every 1000 babies born each year. Neural tube defects include anencephaly, in which most of the brain is missing, and spina bifida. In one form of spina bifida, a piece of the spinal cord protrudes from the spinal column, causing paralysis of parts of the lower body.

The need for folate is critical during the earliest weeks of pregnancy—when most women don't know they are pregnant. However, consuming enough folate during the entire pregnancy is also important. A study of pregnant women showed that those women consuming less than 240 micrograms per day of folic acid had about a two to threefold greater risk of preterm delivery and low birth weight (Scholl et al., 1996).

Because of the importance of folate during pregnancy and the difficulty most women encounter trying to get double the RDA for folate in the diet, the Food and Drug Administration has required manufacturers of certain foods to fortify them with folate. By January 1, 1998, manufacturers of enriched breads, flour, pasta, cornmeals, rice, and other foods must fortify their foods so that one serving provides 40 micrograms of folate, or 10 percent of the daily recommended amount. Women eating folate-fortified foods should not assume that these foods will meet all their folate needs. They should still seek out folate-rich foods.

A vitamin B_{12} deficiency in the body is usually not due to poor intake but rather to a problem with absorption. When vitamin B_{12} is not properly absorbed, **pernicious anemia** develops. Pernicious means ruinous or harmful, and this type of anemia is marked by a megaloblastic anemia (as with folate deficiency) in which there are too many large, immature red blood cells. Symptoms include extreme weakness and fatigue. Nervous system problems also erupt. The cover surrounding the nerves in the body becomes damaged, making it difficult for impulses to travel along them. This causes a poor sense of balance, numbness and tingling sensations in the arms and legs, and mental confusion.

Because deficiencies in folate or vitamin B_{12} cause macrocytic anemia, a physician may mistakenly administer folate when the problem is really a vitamin B_{12} deficiency. The folate would treat the anemia, but not the deterioriation of the nervous system due to a lack of vitamin B_{12}. If untreated, this damage can be significant and sometimes irreversible. When vitamin B_{12} is deficient due to an absorption problem, injections of the vitamin must be given.

Pantothenic Acid and Biotin

Both pantothenic acid and biotin are involved in energy metabolism. Pantothenic acid is needed to release energy from carbohydrates, fats, and protein. Biotin is involved in the metabolism of carbohydrates, fats, and proteins. There is no RDA for either vitamin because the specific requirement has not yet been established; instead, an estimated safe and adequate daily dietary intake has been established.

Both pantothenic acid and biotin are widespread in foods. Good sources of pantothenic acid include meat, eggs, milk, some vegetables, and legumes. Good sources of biotin include liver, egg yolks, cheese, and peanuts. Intestinal bacteria make considerable amounts of biotin. Deficiency and toxicity concerns are not known.

MINI-SUMMARY Table 5-1 summarizes the functions and sources of the water-soluble vitamins.

KEY TERMS

Antioxidant	Preformed vitamin A (retinol)
Beta-carotene	Provitamin A
Carotenoids	R-protein
Collagen	Rebound scurvy
Fat-soluble vitamins	Retinoids
Free radicals	Retinol
Intrinsic factor	Retinol equivalents
Megadose	Rickets
Megaloblastic anemia	Scurvy
Neurotransmitters	Tryptophan
Night blindness	Vitamins
Osteomalacia	Water-soluble vitamins
Pernicious anemia	Xerophthalmia
Precursors	Xerosis

REVIEW QUESTIONS AND EXERCISES

1. List five basic facts about vitamins.
2. Describe two differences between water-soluble and fat-soluble vitamins.
3. Name the vitamins described in the following.
   A. Which vitamin(s) is only present in animal foods?
   B. Which vitamin(s) is found in high amounts in pork and ham?
   C. Which vitamin(s) is found mostly in fruits and vegetables?
   D. Which vitamin(s) needs a compound made in the stomach in order to be absorbed?
   E. Which vitamin deficiency causes osteomalacia?
   F. Which vitamin is made from tryptophan?
   G. Which vitamin(s) is made by intestinal bacteria?
   H. Which vitamin(s) do you need more of if you eat more protein?
   I. Which vitamin(s) is needed for clotting?
   J. Which vitamin(s) is increased during pregnancy?
   K. Which vitamin(s) is known for forming a cellular cement?
   L. Which vitamin has a precursor called beta-carotene?
   M. Which vitamin is made in the skin?
   N. Which vitamin(s) is an antioxidant?
   O. Which vitamin(s) is needed for bone growth and maintenance?
   P. Which vitamin(s), when deficient, causes night blindness?
   Q. Which vitamin(s) is purposely added to milk because no other good sources of it are available?

1. Quiz

Check your answers with these.

1. b
2. b
3. a
4. c
5. d

2. Your Eating Style

Using Table 5-3, circle any food sources that you do not eat at all, or eat infrequently, such as dairy products or green vegetables. Do you eat most of the foods containing vitamins, or do you hate vegetables and maybe fruits too? How often do you eat vitamin-rich foods? The answers to these questions should help you assess whether your diet is adequately balanced and varied, which is necessary to ensure adequate vitamin intake.

3. Supermarket Sleuth

Check the selection of supplements available at your local pharmacy or supermarket. How many supply only 100 percent of the RDA? How many supply 500 percent or more of the RDA? Are any "nonvitamins" being sold?

4. Vitamin Salad Bar

Set up a salad bar using Figure 5-1. You may use any foods you like in your salad bar, as long as you have a good source of each of the 13 vitamins and you fill each of the circles. In each circle, write down the name of the food and which vitamin(s) it is rich in.

FIGURE 5-1.
Vitamin salad bar

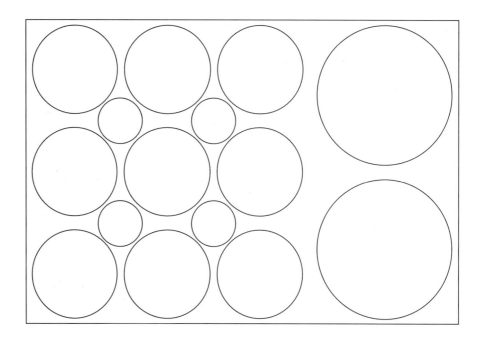

REFERENCES   American Medical Association. 1987. Vitamin preparations as dietary supplements and as therapeutic agents. *Journal of the American Medical Association* 257 (14): 1929–1936.

Bailey, Lynn B. 1992. Evaluation of a new Recommended Dietary Allowance for folate. *Journal of The American Dietetic Association* 92(4): 463–471.

Barness, Lewis A. 1986. Adverse effects of overdosage of vitamins and minerals. *Pediatrics in Review* 8(1): 20–24.

Bell, Linda Schaffer, and Michele Fairchild. 1987. Evaluation of commercial multivitamin supplements. *Journal of The American Dietetic Association* 87(3): 341–345.

Booth, Sarah L., Jean A.T. Pennington, and James Sadowski. 1996. Food sources and dietary intakes of vitamin K-1 (phylloquinone) in the American diet: Data from the FDA Total Diet Study. *Journal of The American Dietetic Association* 96(2): 149–154.

Callaway, C. W. 1987. Statement of vitamin and mineral supplements. *Journal of Nutrition* 117: 1649.

Dairy Council. 1987. Food versus pills versus fortified foods. *Dairy Council Digest* 58(2): 7–12.

Levy, Alan S., and Raymond E. Schucker. 1987. Patterns of nutrient intake among dietary supplement users: Attitudinal and behavioral correlates. *Journal of The American Dietetic Association* 87(6): 754–760.

Manore, Melinda M., Linda A. Vaughan, and William R. Lehman. 1990. Contribution of various food groups to dietary vitamin B_6 intake in free-living, low-income elderly persons. *Journal of The American Dietetic Association* 90(6): 830–834.

Mertz, Walter. 1994. A balanced approach to nutrition for health: The need for biologically essential minerals and vitamins. *Journal of The American Dietetic Association* 94(11): 1259–1262.

Reynolds, Robert D. 1990. Determination of dietary vitamin B_6 intake: Is it accurate? *Journal of The American Dietetic Association* 90(6): 799–801.

Ross, A. Catharine, and Maureen E. Ternus. 1993. Vitamin A as a hormone: Recent advances in understanding the actions of retinol, retinoic acid, and beta carotene. *Journal of The American Dietetic Association* 93(11): 1285–1290.

Scholl, T. O., M. L. Hediger, J. I. Scholl, Chor-San Khoo, and R. L. Fischer. 1996. Dietary and serum folate: Their influence on the outcome of pregnancy. *American Journal of Clinical Nutrition* 63: 520–525.

Slater, T. F., and G. Block. 1991. Antioxidant vitamins and beta-carotene in disease prevention. (Proceedings of a conference held in London, U.K.) *The American Journal of Clinical Nutrition* 53 (Suppl.): 189S–396S.

Stewart, Michael L., Janet T. McDonald, Alan S. Levy, Raymond E. Schucker, and Douglas P. Henderson. 1985. Vitamin/mineral supplement use: A telephone survey of adults in the United States. *Journal of The American Dietetic Association* 85(12): 1585–1590.

Suttie, J.W. 1992. Vitamin K and human nutrition. *Journal of The American Dietetic Association* 92(5): 585–590.

Truswell, A. Stewart. 1985. Vitamins I. *British Medical Journal* 291(6501): 1033–1035.

Truswell, A. Stewart. 1985. Vitamins II. *British Medical Journal* 291(6502): 1103–1106.

Food Facts: How Food Processing, Storage, Preparation, and Cooking Affect Vitamin and Mineral Content

Five factors are responsible for most nutrient loss: heat, exposure to air and light, cooking in water, and baking soda. Because the fat-soluble vitamins are insoluble in water, they are fairly stable in cooking. Water-soluble vitamins easily leach out of foods during washing or cooking. Of all the vitamins, vitamin C is the most fragile and the most easily destroyed during preparation, cooking, or storage. Oxygen and high temperatures readily oxidize or destroy vitamin C. Thiamin and folate are also fragile. Here are some tips for retaining food nutrients.

1. Buy fresh, high-quality food.
2. Examine fresh fruits and vegetables thoroughly for appropriate color, size, and shape.
3. Store fruits and vegetables in the refrigerator (except green bananas, potatoes, and onions) to inhibit enzymes that make fruits and vegetables age and lose nutrients. The enzymes are more active at warm temperatures.
4. Foods should not be stored for too long as lengthy storage causes nutrient loss. Store canned goods in a cool place. Refrigerated goods should be maintained at a temperature of 45 degrees F. or lower, freezer goods at 0 degrees F. or lower. Thermometers should be kept in the refrigerator and freezer to monitor temperatures.
5. When storing food, close up tightly to decrease exposure to the air.
6. Wash vegetables quickly and avoid soaking them.
7. Potatoes and other vegetables that are boiled or baked without being peeled retain many more nutrients than peeled and cut vegetables. In general, the smaller you cut vegetables before cooking, the higher the vitamin loss because leaching and oxidation are increased with increased surface area. Cut vegetables no more than necessary.
8. Keep skins on fruits as much as possible, because more vitamins and minerals reside under the skin than in the center of the fruit.
9. Steaming, microwaving, and stir-frying are good choices to retain nutrients when cooking. Each method is fast and uses little or no water. For boiled vegetables, the longer the cooking time and the more water used, the higher the nutrient loss. Cook quickly and use as little water as possible.
10. Frying temperatures can destroy vitamins in vegetables. For instance, French-fried potatoes lose much of their vitamin C.
11. Never use baking soda with green vegetables to improve appearance—as it causes nutrient loss.
12. Broiled or roasted meats retain more B vitamins than meats that are braised or stewed.
13. Use the cooking water from vegetables and the drippings from meats (after skimming off the fat) to prepare soup and gravy.
14. Prepare foods close to the time they will be served.
15. Don't keep milk in clear glass containers, as light destroys the riboflavin. Factors that destroy vitamins often spoil the color, flavor, and texture of food as well.

Hot Topic: Healthy Cultural Foods

Just as American cuisine has its healthy and not-so-healthy dishes, so do other cuisines from around the world. Here are some tips on healthier menu choices from other countries.

Mexico

Healthy Mexican foods include bean soups and salads, tomatoes, rice, salsa (a spicy tomato-based sauce), soft tortillas filled with chicken and vegetables (as in burritos), fajitas (tortillas wrapped around pieces of grilled meat or poultry and vegetables), salads, and fruit for dessert. Ceviche (marinated seafood in lime juice) and gazpacho (a cold vegetable soup) are also good choices. Refried beans, guacamole (avocado dip), fried foods such as fried tortillas or chicken, and higher-fat ground-beef–filled burritos and tacos, are high in fat.

France

Main dishes with a wine sauce, such as coq au vin (chicken in wine), are a better choice than sauces made with egg yolks and butter, such as hollandaise. Poached fish or entrées steamed "en papillote" are also good choices. The French traditions of serving fresh salad after the entrée and fruit as dessert are healthful.

Italy

Italians in Northern Italy raise beef cattle and dairy cows. In their cooking, they use much beef, cream, and butter, all of which are high in fat. Pasta in northern Italy usually uses eggs. In contrast, in southern Italy where wheat is harvested and olive trees grow, wheat pasta and olive oil, as well as beans and seafood, are popular. Healthy Italian choices include bean and vegetable soups, wheat pasta, tossed salads, wine or tomato sauces, lowfat cheeses, and frozen fruit desserts like ices.

Greece

Healthy Greek foods include appetizers such as tzatziki (yogurt and cucumbers) and spinach with lentil soup, broiled entrées such as fish and shish kabob (with lean meat) and plaki (fish cooked with tomatoes, onions, and garlic), pita bread, and dried figs for dessert. Moussaka, a traditional dish of eggplant and lamb, and desserts made with phyllo tend to be high in fat.

India

Staples of the Indian diet are healthy foods such as rice, beans, lentils, vegetables, and bread. Indian breads include chapatis, a round flatbread made of whole-wheat flour, and naan, a bread that uses yeast to make it rise. Healthy menu choices are dal (lentil) soup, chapati, tandoori chicken (marinated and then roasted in a clay pot or stove), basmati rice, tomato chutney, and fresh mango for dessert. Chutney is a relish made from fruits, vegetables, and herbs that accompanies Indian main dishes. Indian cooking uses many strong spices.

China

There is no single Chinese cooking style. Instead there are a number of regional styles. Vegetables, rice and other grains, and foods made from soybeans are staples in the Chinese diet where meat is served only in small portions. Plain rice is served at all meals. Stir-frying is the most common method of cooking Chinese food. Stir-frying involves cooking bite-sized pieces of food over medium-high heat in a small amount of oil while stirring constantly. Appetizers and entrées that are stir-fried, steamed, or broiled are healthy choices. Steamed brown rice is a good side dish and dessert is often fruit such as pineapple and oranges. Fried foods such as fried rice, egg rolls, and fried noodles are higher in fat. Other fatty foods include duck, goose, and spare ribs. Soy sauce, a popular condiment that is high in sodium, should be served on the side. A low-sodium soy sauce is available.

Japan

Most Japanese cooking is quite healthy, with its emphasis on fresh fish and vegetables prepared with little fat. While Chinese foods are often stir-fried, the Japanese like to simmer, boil, steam, or broil their foods. These are all healthy methods used to prepare their rice, vegetable, and soy dishes. An entrée such as chicken teriyaki (broiled with a sauce) is a better choice than chicken tempura which is deep fried. As in Chinese cooking, soy sauce is popular and it should be served on the side.

Label Reading Questions and Answers: Vitamins

What vitamins are listed on food labels?

Two vitamins, vitamin A and vitamin C, are required on food labels (Figure 5-2). Food manufacturers may list any other vitamins.

Nutrition Facts
Serving Size 1 pizza (184g)
Servings Per Container 1

Amount Per Serving

Calories 560 Calories from Fat 230

	% Daily Value*
Total Fat 25g	**38%**
Saturated Fat 13g	**65%**
Cholesterol 45mg	**16%**
Sodium 1,090mg	**45%**
Total Carbohydrate 60g	**20%**
Dietary Fiber 4g	**16%**
Sugars 7g	
Protein 23g	

Vitamin A 45%	•	Vitamin C 0%
Calcium 50%	•	Iron 8%

* Percent Daily Values are based on a 2,000 calorie diet. Your daily values may be higher or lower depending on your calorie needs:

	Calories:	2,000	2,500
Total Fat	Less than	65g	80g
Sat Fat	Less than	20g	25g
Cholesterol	Less than	300mg	300mg
Sodium	Less than	2,400mg	2,400mg
Total Carbohydrate		300g	375g
Dietary Fiber		25g	30g

Calories per gram:
Fat 9 • Carbohydrate 4 • Protein 4

FIGURE 5-2. Nutrition label.

What information do I get about these vitamins?

The amounts of vitamins A and C are listed as a Percent Daily Value in Nutrition Facts. Daily Values are a guide to the total daily nutrient amount you need based on a 2000-calorie diet. Therefore, the Daily Value may be a little high, a little low, or right on target for you. Percent Daily Values show you how much of the Daily Value is in one serving.

What is the daily value for vitamins A and C?

The Daily Value for vitamin A is 5000 IU, and the Daily Value for vitamin C is 60 mg.

How can I use the Percent Daily Values?

Use the Percent Daily Values to give you a general idea of the nutrient content—whereas a food contains a lot or a little of specific nutrients. You can also use Percent Daily Values to see how foods fit into your overall daily diet and to make comparisons among products.

If the labels claim "good sources of folate," will the Nutrition Facts include more information?

Yes. If a label makes a nutrient claim, that nutrient must be listed on the nutrition label so you will be able to see what the Percent Daily Value is for one serving.

What other nutrient claims can be made for vitamins?

Here are some other claims you may find on food labels, and the definitions set by the government for their use.

Nutrient Claims	*Definition*
High, Rich in, Excellent source of	20 percent or more of the Daily Value
Good Source, Contains, Provides	10 to 19 percent of the Daily Value
More, Enriched, Added	Contains at least 10 percent more of the Daily Value as compared to the reference food

CHAPTER 6

Water and Minerals

1. Why is water an important nutrient?
2. What are the functions and food sources of the 17 minerals?
3. Which minerals are more likely to be deficient in the diet?
4. Are excessive mineral supplements toxic, and if so, which ones?

QUIZ

1. Which of the following minerals is most likely to be deficient in the American diet?
    (a) Phosphorus
    (b) Calcium
    (c) Sulfur
    (d) Cobalt
2. Which of the following classes of minerals are more likely to be toxic if taken in excess?
    (a) Major minerals
    (b) Trace minerals
    (c) Some major and some trace minerals
    (d) None of the above
3. Which of the following foods is an excellent source of iron?
    (a) Fresh pears
    (b) Tomatoes
    (c) Hamburger
    (d) Cake
4. What percentage of the body is water?
    (a) 15 percent
    (b) 35 percent
    (c) 55 percent
    (d) 75 percent
5. Which of the following foods is low in sodium?
    (a) Hot dog
    (b) Canned tomato juice
    (c) Fresh apple
    (d) American cheese

TABLE 6-1 **Major and trace minerals.**	
Major Minerals	*Trace Minerals*
Calcium	Chromium
Chloride	Cobalt
Magnesium	Copper
Phosphorus	Fluoride
Potassium	Iodine
Sodium	Iron
Sulfur	Manganese
	Molybdenum
	Selenium
	Zinc

INTRODUCTION

If you were to weigh all the minerals in your body, they would amount to only 4 or 5 pounds. You need only small amounts of minerals in your diet, but they perform enormously important jobs in your body—building bones and teeth, regulating your heartbeat, and transporting oxygen from the lungs to tissues, to name a few.

Some minerals are needed in relatively large amounts in the diet—over 100 milligrams daily. These minerals, called **major minerals**, include calcium, chloride, magnesium, phosphorus, potassium, sodium, and sulfur. Other minerals, called **trace minerals** or trace elements, are needed in smaller amounts—less than 100 milligrams daily. Iron, fluoride, and zinc are examples of trace minerals. Table 6-1 lists all the major and trace minerals.

Minerals have some distinctive properties not shared by other nutrients. For example, whereas over 90 percent of dietary carbohydrates, fats, and proteins are absorbed into the body, the percentage of minerals that are absorbed varies tremendously. For example, only 5 to 10 percent of the iron in your diet is normally absorbed, about 30 percent of calcium is absorbed, and almost all the sodium you eat is absorbed. Minerals in animal foods tend to be absorbed better than those in plant foods. Unlike vitamins, minerals are not destroyed in food storage or preparation. They are, however, water-soluble, so there is some loss in cooking liquids. Like vitamins, minerals can be toxic when consumed in excessive amounts and may interfere with the absorption and metabolism of other minerals.

Minerals are divided into two categories: major minerals and trace minerals.

MINI-SUMMARY Some minerals are needed in relatively large amounts in the diet—over 100 milligrams daily. These minerals are called major minerals and include calcium, chloride, magnesium, phosphorus, potassium, sodium, and sulfur. Other minerals, called trace minerals or trace elements, are needed in smaller amounts—less than 100 milligrams daily. Minerals are absorbed to varying degrees and are not destroyed in food storage or preparation. Minerals can be toxic when consumed in excessive amounts.

WATER

Deny someone food and he or she can still live for weeks. But death comes quickly, in a matter of a few days, if you deprive a person of water. Nothing survives without water, and virtually nothing takes place in the body without water playing a vital role.

Although variations may be great, the average adult's body weight is generally 50 to 60 percent water—enough, if it were bottled, to fill 40 to 50 quarts. For example, in a 150-pound man, water accounts for about 90 pounds, fat about 30 pounds, with protein, carbohydrates, vitamins, and minerals making up the balance. Men generally have more water than women, a lean person more than an obese person. Some parts of the body have more water than others. Human blood is about 92 percent water, muscle and brain about 75 percent, and bone 22 percent.

The body uses water for virtually all its functions: for digestion, absorption, circulation, excretion, transporting nutrients, building tissue, and maintaining temperature. Almost all body cells need and depend on water to perform their functions. Water carries nutrients to the cells and carries away waste materials to the kidneys.

Water is needed in each step of the process of converting food into energy and tissue. Water in the digestive secretions softens, dilutes, and liquifies the food to facilitate digestion. It also helps move food along the gastrointestinal tract. Differences in the fluid concentration on either side of the intestinal wall enhance the absorption process.

Water serves as an important part of body lubricants, helping to cushion the joints and internal organs, keeping tissues in the eyes, lungs, and air passages moist, and surrounding and protecting the fetus during pregnancy.

Many adults take in and excrete between 8 and 10 cups of fluid daily. Nearly all foods have some water. Milk, for example, is about 87 percent water, eggs about 75 percent, meat between 40 and 75 percent, vegetables from 70 to 95 percent, cereals from 8 to 20 percent, and bread around 35 percent.

The body gets rid of the water it doesn't need through the kidneys and skin and, to a lesser degree, from the lungs and gastrointestinal tract. Water is also excreted as urine by the kidneys along with waste materials carried from the cells. About 4 to 6 cups a day are excreted as urine. The amount of urine reflects, to some extent, the amount of an individual's fluid intake, although despite the amount consumed, the kidneys will always excrete a certain amount each day to eliminate waste products generated by the body's metabolic actions. In addition to the urine, air released from the lungs contains some water, and evaporation that occurs on the skin (when sweating or not sweating) contains water as well.

If normal and healthy, the body maintains water at a constant level. A number of mechanisms, including the sensation of thirst, operate to keep body-water content within narrow limits. You feel thirsty when the blood starts to become too concentrated. Unfortunately, by the time you feel thirsty, you are already much in need of extra fluid, but this can be easily remedied by drinking promptly. It is therefore very important not to ignore feelings of thirst, a concern that is particularly appropriate for the elderly. For healthy individuals, it is not possible to drink too much water—it will simply be excreted.

By the time you feel thirst, you are already a little dehydrated.

There are, of course, conditions in which the various body mechanisms for regulating water balance do not work, such as severe vomiting, diarrhea, excessive bleeding, high fever, burns, and excessive perspiration. In these situations, large amounts of fluids and minerals are lost. The treatment of these conditions are medical problems to be managed by a physician.

MINI-SUMMARY   The average adult's body weight is generally 50 to 60 percent water. The body uses water for virtually all its functions: for digestion, absorption, circulation, excretion, transporting nutrients, building tissue, and maintaining temperature. Almost all body cells need and depend on water to perform their functions. Water carries nutrients to the cells and carries away waste materials to the kidneys. A number of mechanisms, including the sensation of thirst, operate to keep body-water content within narrow limits. You feel thirsty when the blood starts to become too concentrated.

MAJOR MINERALS

Calcium and Phosphorus

Calcium and phosphorus are used for building bones and teeth. Most of the body's calcium and phosphorus is found in the bones and teeth, where they give rigidity to the structures. Bone is being rebuilt every day, with new bone being formed and old bone being taken apart. There is little turnover of calcium in teeth.

Calcium also circulates in the blood, where a constant level is maintained so it is always available for use. Calcium helps blood to clot, muscles to contract (including the heart muscle), nerves to transmit impulses, and also helps maintain normal blood pressure.

Calcium:
Formation of bones
and teeth.
Blood clotting.
Muscle contraction.
Transmission of
nerve impulses.

Like calcium, phosphorus circulates in the blood and is involved in the metabolic release of energy from fat, protein, and carbohydrates. It is also a part of DNA (genetic material) and many enzymes. Normal body processes produce acids and bases that can cause major blood and body problems, such as coma and death, if not buffered (or neutralized) somehow. Phosphorus has the ability to buffer both acids and bases.

The major sources of calcium are milk and milk products. Not all milk products are as rich in calcium as milk (see Table 6-2). As a matter of fact, butter, cream, cottage cheese, and cream cheese contain little calcium. One glass of milk or yogurt or 1½ ounces of cheese each have a little less than half of the RDA for most adults.

Phosphorus:
Formation of bones
and teeth.
Energy metabolism.
Formation of DNA
and many enzymes.
Buffer.

Without milk or milk products in your diet, it may be difficult to get enough calcium. Other good sources of calcium include canned salmon and sardines (as long as the bones are eaten), oysters, calcium-fortified foods such as orange juice, and several greens such as broccoli, collards, kale, mustard greens, and turnip greens. Other greens such as spinach, beet greens, Swiss chard, sorrel, and parsley are calcium-rich but also contain a binder (**oxalic acid**) that seems to prevent some of calcium from being absorbed. Dried beans and peas and certain shellfish contain moderate amounts of calcium but are usually not eaten in sufficient quantities to make a significant contribution. Meats and grains are poor sources.

Calcium and
phosphorus are
both rich in milk
and milk products.

About 30 percent of the calcium you eat is absorbed. The body absorbs more calcium (up to 60 percent) during growth and pregnancy when additional calcium is needed. Absorption is higher for younger people than for older people. Postmenopausal women, who are at high risk of developing osteoporosis—to be discussed later—often absorb the least calcium. Vitamin D helps calcium absorption and is added to milk. Certain substances interfere with calcium absorption, such as the tannins in tea and large amounts of phytic acid, a binder found in wheat bran and whole grains.

Phosphorus is widely distributed in foods and is not likely to be lacking in the diet. Milk and milk products are excellent sources of phosphorus, as they are for calcium. Good sources of phosphorus are meat, poultry, fish, eggs, legumes, and whole-grain foods. Fruits and

TABLE 6-2. **Calcium in selected foods.**

Food	Calcium Content
Milk, skim, 8 ounces	302
Milk, 2%, 8 ounces	297
Milk, whole, 8 ounces	291
Yogurt, low-fat, 8 ounces	415
Yogurt, low-fat with fruit, 8 ounces	345
Yogurt, frozen, 1 cup	200
Ice cream, vanilla, 1 cup lowfat	176
Cottage cheese, lowfat, 1 cup	155
Swiss cheese, 1 ounces	272
Parmesan, grated, 2 tablespoons	138
Cheddar, 1 ounce	204
Mozzarella, 1 ounce	147
American cheese, 1 ounce	174
Cheese pizza, ¼ of 14-inch pie	332
Macaroni and cheese, ½ cup	181
Orange juice, calcium fortified, 8 ounces	330
Sardines, drained, 2 ounces	175
Oysters, cooked, 3 ounces	76
Shrimp, cooked, 3 ounces	33
Tofu, calcium set, 3½ ounces	128
Dried navy beans, cooked, 1 cup	95
Turnip greens, frozen and cooked, 1 cup	249
Kale, frozen and cooked, 1 cup	179
Mustard greens, 1 cup	104
Broccoli, cooked, ½ cup	35
Oatmeal, instant, fortified, 1 packet	160
Pancakes, from mix, one 4-inch pancake	30
Wheat bread, 2 slices	40

Source: U.S. Department of Agriculture Handbook 8, and Home and Garden Bulletin Number 72, and manufacturers.

vegetables are generally low in this mineral. Compounds made with phosphorus are used in processed foods, especially soft drinks (phosphoric acid).

Magnesium

Magnesium is found in all body tissues, with about 60 percent in the bones and the remainder in the soft tissues, such as muscles, and in the blood. It is essential to many enzyme systems responsible for energy conversions in the body and other functions. Magnesium is used in building bones and teeth and relaxes the heart and smooth muscles after contraction. Magnesium also has a role in making protein.

Magnesium is a part of the green pigment **chlorophyll** found in plants, so good sources include green leafy vegetables, potatoes, nuts (especially almonds and cashews), seeds, whole-grain cereals, and legumes such as soybeans. Seafood is also a good source. Meat and dairy products supply small amounts.

We probably take in less than the RDA, but deficiency symptoms are rare.

Sodium

Sodium, potassium, and chloride are collectively referred to as **electrolytes** because, when dissolved in body fluids, they separate into positively or negatively charged particles called **ions**. Potassium, which is positively charged, is found mainly within the cells. Sodium (positively charged) and chloride (negatively charged) are found mostly in the fluid outside the cells.

The electrolytes maintain two critical balancing acts in the body: **water balance** and **acid-base balance**. Water balance means maintaining the proper amount of water in each of the body's three "compartments": inside the cells, outside the cells, and in the blood vessels. Electrolytes maintain the water balance by moving the water around in the body. Electrolytes are also able to buffer, or neutralize, various acids and bases in the body. In addition to its roles in water and acid-base balance, sodium is needed for muscle contraction and transmission of nerve impulses.

The major source of sodium in the diet is salt—a compound made of sodium and chlorine. Salt by weight is 39 percent sodium, and 1 teaspoon contains 2300 milligrams (a little more than 2 grams) of sodium. Many processed foods have high amounts of sodium added during processing and manufacturing, and it is estimated that these foods provide fully 75 percent of the sodium in most people's diets. The following is a list of processed foods high in sodium:

Canned, cured, and/or smoked meats and fish, such as bacon, salt pork, sausage, scrapple, ham, bologna, corned beef, frankfurters, luncheon meats, canned tuna fish and salmon, and smoked salmon.

Many cheeses, especially processed cheeses such as processed American cheese

Salted snack foods, such as potato chips, pretzels, popcorn, nuts, and crackers

Food prepared in brine, such as pickles, olives, and sauerkraut

Canned vegetables, tomato products, soups, and vegetable juices

Prepared mixes for stuffings, rice dishes, and breading

Dried soup mixes and bouillon cubes

Food Groups	Sodium, mg	Food Group	Sodium, mg
TABLE 6-3. **Where's the salt?**			
Bread, Cereal, Rice, and Pasta		Natural cheeses, 1½ oz.	110-450
Cooked cereal, rice, pasta, unsalted, ½ cup	Trace	Process cheeses, 2 oz.	800
Ready-to-eat cereal, 1 oz.	100-360		
Bread, 1 slice	110-175	*Meat, Poultry, Fish, Dry Beans, Eggs, and Nuts*	
		Fresh meat, poultry, fish, 3 oz.	Less than 90
Vegetable		Tuna, canned, water pack, 3 oz.	300
Vegetables, fresh or frozen, cooked		Bologna, 2 oz.	580
without salt, ½ cup	Less than 70	Ham, lean, roasted, 3 oz.	1,020
Vegetables, canned or frozen			
with sauce, ½ cup	140-460	*Other*	
Tomato juice, canned, ¾ cup	660	Salad dressing, 1 tbsp.	75-220
Vegetable soup, canned, 1 cup	820	Ketchup, mustard, steak sauce, 1 tbsp.	130-230
		Soy sauce, 1 tbsp.	1,030
Fruit		Salt, 1 tsp.	2,000
Fruit, fresh, frozen, canned ½ cup	Trace	Dill pickle, 1 medium	930
		Potato chips, salted, 1 oz.	130
Milk, Yogurt, and Cheese		Corn chips, salted, 1 oz.	235
Milk, 1 cup	120	Peanuts, roasted in oil, salted, 1 oz.	120
Yogurt, 8 oz.	160		

Source: U.S. Department of Agriculture

Certain seasonings such as salt, sea salt, garlic salt, onion salt, celery salt, seasoned salt, soy sauce, Worcestershire sauce, horseradish, catsup, and mustard

Table 6-3 illustrates the salt content of food in the various food groups. Salt is also used in food preparation and at the table for seasoning.

In addition to the sodium in salt, sodium appears in monosodium glutamate (MSG), baking powder, and baking soda. Other possible sources of dietary sodium include the sodium found in some local water systems and in medications, such as some antacids. Unprocessed foods also contain natural sodium, but in small amounts (with the exception of milk and some milk products).

There is no RDA for sodium. Instead, there is an estimated minimum requirement: 500 milligrams. The sodium intake of Americans is easily 6 times this amount—varying from 3 to 8 grams daily. The Nutrition Facts Label lists a Daily Value of 2400 mg per day for sodium.

Overconsumption of sodium, particularly as salt, is a concern because many studies have shown that a high sodium intake is associated with higher blood pressure. Most evidence suggests that many people at risk for high blood pressure reduce their chances of developing this condition by consuming less salt or sodium. Some questions remain, partly because other factors may interact with sodium to affect blood pressure.

Potassium is found in many fruits and vegetables, milk and yogurt.

Potassium

Potassium, an electrolyte found mainly in the fluid inside the individual body cells, helps maintain water balance and acid-base balance along with sodium. In the blood, potassium assists in muscle contraction, including maintaining a normal heartbeat, and sending nerve impulses.

Potassium is distributed widely in foods, both plant and animal. Unprocessed, whole foods such as fruits and vegetables (especially winter squash, potatoes, oranges, and grapefruits), milk, and yogurt are excellent sources of potassium.

A potassium deficiency is uncommon in healthy people but may result from dehydration or from using a certain class of blood pressure medications called **diuretics**. Diuretics cause increased urine output and some cause an increased excretion of potassium as well. Symptoms of a deficiency include muscle cramps, weakness, nausea, and abnormal heart rhythms that can be very dangerous, even fatal.

Chloride is in salt.

Chloride

Chloride, another important electrolyte, helps maintain water balance and acid-base balance. It is also a part of hydrochloric acid, which is quite highly concentrated in the stomach juices. Hydrochloric acid aids in protein digestion, destroys harmful bacteria, and increases the absorption of calcium and iron. The most important source of dietary chloride is sodium chloride, or salt. If sodium intake is adequate, there will be ample chloride as well.

Other Major Minerals

The body doesn't use the mineral sulfur by itself, but uses the nutrients it is found in, such as protein and thiamin. The protein in hair, skin, and nails is particularly rich in sulfur. There is no RDA for sulfur. Protein foods supply plentiful amounts of sulfur and deficiencies are unknown.

MINI-SUMMARY   The functions and sources of the major minerals are listed in Table 6-4.

TABLE 6-4. **Minerals.**

Minerals	RDA[1] or ESADD[2]	Functions	Sources
Major Minerals			
Calcium	800 milligrams	Formation of bones and teeth Blood clotting Muscle contraction Transmission of nerve impulses	Milk and milk products, canned salmon and sardines (with bones), oysters, calcium-fortified foods, broccoli, collards, kale, mustard greens, turnip greens
Phosphorus	800 milligrams	Formation of bones and teeth Energy metabolism Formation of DNA and many enzymes Buffer	Milk and milk products, meat, poultry, fish, eggs, legumes, whole grains
Magnesium	Males: 350 milligrams Females: 280 milligrams	Energy metabolism Formation of bones and teeth Muscle contraction protein synthesis	Green leafy vegetables, potatoes, nuts, seeds, whole-grain cereals, legumes
Sodium	500 milligrams[3]	Water balance Acid-base balance Buffer Muscle contraction Transmission of nerve impulses	Salt, processed foods, MSG
Potassium	2,000 milligrams[3]	Water balance Acid-base balance Buffer Muscle contraction Transmission of nerve impulses	Many fruits and vegetables (potatoes, oranges, grapefruit), milk, and yogurt
Chloride	750 milligrams[3]	Water balance Acid-base balance Part of hydrochloric acid in stomach	Salt
Sulfur	No RDA	Part of some amino acids Part of thiamin	Protein foods

TABLE 6-4.   Minerals.

Minerals	RDA[1] or ESADDI[2]	Functions	Sources
Trace Minerals			
Copper	1.5–3.0 milligrams	Iron metabolism Formation of hemoglobin Collagen formation energy release	Organ meats, shellfish whole-grain breads and cereals legumes, nuts, dried fruits
Fluoride	1.5–4.0 milligrams	Strengthening of developing teeth	Water
Iodine	150 micrograms	Normal functioning of thyroid gland Normal metabolic rate	Iodized salt
Iron	Males: 10 milligrams Females: 15 milligrams	Part of hemoglobin and myoglobin Part of some enzymes Energy metabolism Needed to make new cells	Liver, meats, shellfish, enriched breads and cereals, green leafy vegetables, legumes, dried fruit, egg yolk
Selenium	Males: 70 micrograms Females: 55 micrograms	Activation of an antioxidant	Seafood, meat, liver, eggs, whole grains and vegetables (if soil is rich in selenium)
Zinc	Males: 15 milligrams Females: 12 milligrams	Part of many enzymes Wound healing Bone formation Development of sexual organs General growth and maintenance Taste perception and appetite	Protein foods, whole grain fortified cereals, some legumes, dairy products
Chromium	50–200 micrograms	Works with insulin	Liver, meat, whole grains, nuts

[1]RDA is for ages 25–50.

[2]Estimated Safe and Adequate Daily Dietary Intakes for adults.

[3]There is no RDA or ESADDI for sodium, potassium, and chloride. These numbers are estimated minimum requirements.

TABLE 6-5.　Iron in foods.	
Foods	Milligrams Iron
Meat and Poultry	
Beef liver, 3 ounces	5.3
Sirloin steak, 3 ounces	2.6
Hamburger, 3 ounces, lean	1.8
Chicken breast, 3 ounces	0.9
Shellfish	
Oysters, breaded, fried, 1	3.0
Clams, raw, 3 ounces	2.6
Vegetables	
Spinach, 1 cup, frozen, cooked	2.9
Legumes	
Great Northern beans, 1 cup	4.9
Black beans, 1 cup	2.9
Tofu, 2½ inch x 2¾ inch x 1 inch cube	2.3
Eggs	
Egg yolk, 1	0.9
Dried Fruits	
Apricots, ¼ cup	1.5
Raisins, ¼ cup	0.7
Breads and Cereals	
Corn flakes cereal, 1 ounce	1.8
Whole-wheat bread, 1 slice	1.0
White bread, 1 slice	0.7

Source: Nutritive Value of Foods, U.S. Department of Agriculture Home and Garden Bulletin Number 72.

TRACE MINERALS

Trace minerals (Table 6-1) represent an exciting area for research, because our understanding of many trace minerals is just now emerging. Like vitamins, minerals can be toxic at high doses. Unlike vitamins, many trace minerals are toxic at levels only several times higher than recommendations. Also, trace minerals are highly interactive with each other. For example, taking extra zinc can cause a copper deficiency. For this reason, it is advisable to consult a physician for supplementation exceeding one and one-half times the recommended levels.

Iron

Iron is part of hemoglobin, myoglobin, and some enzymes.

Iron, one of the most abundant metals in the universe and one of the most important in the body, is a key component of **hemoglobin**, a part of red blood cells that carries oxygen to body cells. Cells require oxygen to break down glucose and produce energy. Iron is also part of **myoglobin**, a muscle protein that stores and carries oxygen. Iron works with many enzymes in energy metabolism and is needed to make new cells as well as certain hormones and neurotransmitters.

Meat is a particularly rich source of iron. To increase iron absorption, eat a vitamin C-rich food at the same meal.

About one-third of iron in the American diet comes from beef and enriched breads, rolls, and crackers. Other sources include liver, poultry, shellfish, fortified cereals, legumes, green leafy vegetables, egg yolks, and dried fruits (see Table 6-5).

The ability of the body to absorb and use iron from different foods varies from 3 percent for some vegetables to 35 percent from red meat. The average is about 15 percent. The predominant form of iron in animal foods, called **heme iron**, is absorbed and used twice as readily as iron in plant foods, called **nonheme iron**. Animal foods also contain some nonheme iron. The presence of vitamin C in a meal increases nonheme iron absorption, as does consuming meat, poultry, and fish. Some foods actually decrease iron consumption: coffee, tea, phytic acid in whole grains, oxalic acid in some vegetables, and calcium supplements. The body increases or decreases iron absorption as needed, but it absorbs iron more efficiently when iron stores are low and during growth spurts or pregnancy. Some iron is stored in the bone marrow and in the liver.

Iron deficiency is the most common nutritional deficiency. If severe enough, it results in **iron-deficiency anemia**, a condition in which the size and number of red blood cells are reduced. This condition may result from inadequate intake of iron or from blood loss. Symptoms of iron-deficiency anemia include fatigue, pallor, irritability, and lethargy. Iron-deficiency anemia is a real concern in the United States, more so for

Lead has no known functions or health benefits for humans. In fact, it is a highly toxic metal that can damage the nervous, cardiovascular, renal, immune, and gastrointestinal systems and is particularly dangerous for children. In children, lead has a particularly damaging effect on intellectual development. In addition, lead interferes with the manufacture of heme, the oxygen-carrying part of hemoglobin in red blood cells. Lead consumption in childhood can mean stunted growth and a lower IQ. Damage to the child's nervous system is permanent.

New research on lead shows that it may be dangerous at low levels in adults. Low levels of lead may contribute to hypertension and harm the kidneys. Significant sources of lead include lead-based paint, the overwhelming source, and also drinking water carried in lead pipes, lead-soldered cans, and some ceramic dishes covered with lead glaze. Lead can be in any home's water, so it is advisable to have your water tested—especially in high-risk households where women are pregnant or there are children under six years of age. In addition to the problem with lead pipes, some faucets contain lead and leach lead into the water.

Although the number of cans produced in the United States that use lead solder has decreased to under 4 percent, the number of imported cans with lead solder is unknown. The only way to make sure that a can is not soldered with lead is to choose one-piece aluminum cans (like those for soft drinks) or cans with welded seams that have shiny metal around the seam. Cans that are soldered are not so shiny around the seam because some solder is usually obvious.

Most ceramic glaze contains lead, which, if properly fired and sealed, does not cause any concern. However, some ceramic cookware (and dishware), from both outside and inside the United States, has been found to leach lead in dangerous amounts into food. Ceramic items in your home may include fine china, stoneware, earthenware, and ironstone. Unfortunately, there is no way of telling whether a ceramic piece has an unsafe amount of lead unless you do a test using a lead-testing kit. Lead also leaches from lead crystal, and it can leach into any liquid, not just alcohol. Here are precautions to follow to lessen your chances of lead poisoning.

1. Don't store foods in ceramic cookware or dishes unless you are sure they are lead-free.
2. Avoid using ceramic dishes to serve acidic foods and beverages, which cause more lead to be leached out. Examples of acidic foods include citrus juices, apple juice, tomato products, cola-flavored soft drinks, coffee, or tea.
3. Heat also causes more lead to be leached out, so avoid cooking and microwaving with ceramic cookware or dishes that you are not sure of.
4. Do not use, and perhaps dispose of, any china on which the glaze is corroded or has a chalky gray residue when dry.
5. Be cautious about using very old china and highly decorated handcrafted china.
6. If buying new ceramic cookware or dishes, select a manufacturer, such as Corning, that produces lead-free glazes.
7. Do not use lead crystal every day, and never use it to store food or beverages. Also, never let children use it.
8. If in doubt, check it out: buy a lead-testing kit. They cost from $20 and up in hardware stores.

women than men. It is also a concern for infants and children. Children with this condition show symptoms of behavioral problems (short attention span, restlessness) when in reality they need more dietary iron. The RDA for iron is higher for women of childbearing age than for men because women have to replace menstrual blood losses. It is not unusual for menstruating women to regularly consume less than the iron RDA. Iron supplementation authorized by a physician may be helpful.

Although the body generally avoids absorbing huge amounts of iron, some people can absorb large amounts. The problem with iron is that once it is in the body, it is hard to get rid of. For individuals who can absorb much iron, large doses of iron supplements can damage the liver and do other damage, a condition called **iron overload**. It is especially important to keep iron supplements away from children, because they are so toxic they can kill. Children under age 3 are at particular risk.

Zinc

*Zinc:
Part of many enzymes.
Wound healing.
Bone formation.
Development of sexual organs.
General growth and maintenance.
Taste perception and appetite.*

Zinc is involved in enzymes that catalyze at least 50 different metabolically important bodily reactions. Zinc assists in wound healing, bone formation, cell reproduction, development of sexual organs, and general tissue growth and maintenance. Zinc is also important for taste perception and appetite.

Protein-containing foods are all good sources of zinc, particularly meat, poultry, and shellfish. Only about 40 percent of the zinc we eat is absorbed into the body. Whole grains, fortified cereals, some legumes, and dairy products are good sources as well. Zinc is much more readily available, or absorbed better, from animal foods. Iron and zinc are often found in the same foods. Like iron, zinc is more likely to be absorbed when animal sources are eaten and when the body needs it more.

*Zinc:
Protein foods.
Whole grain breads and cereals.
Some legumes.*

Deficiencies are more likely to show up in pregnant women, the young, and the elderly. Signs of severe deficiency include growth retardation, delayed sexual maturation, decreased sense of taste, poor appetite, delayed wound healing, and immune deficiencies. Marginal deficiencies do occur in the United States. When overdoses of zinc (only a few milligrams above the RDA) are taken, it causes a copper deficiency and less iron is absorbed. Since zinc supplements can be fatal at lower levels than many of the other trace minerals, zinc supplements should be avoided unless a physician prescribes them.

Iodine

Iodide, the form in which iodine is found in food, is required in extremely small amounts for normal **thyroid gland** functioning. The thyroid gland, located in the neck, is responsible for producing two important hormones that maintain a normal level of metabolism and that are essential for normal growth and development and bone and protein synthesis. Iodine is necessary for these hormones to be produced.

Iodine is not found in many foods: mostly saltwater fish and grains grown in iodine-rich soil (once covered by the oceans, soil in the central states contains little iodine). Iodized salt was introduced in 1924 to combat iodine deficiencies. Iodine also finds its way accidentally into milk (cows receive iodine-containing drugs, and dairy equipment is sterilized with iodine-containing compounds), into baked goods through iodine-containing compounds used in processing, and foods that have certain food colorings. Because iodine can be toxic at high levels, some industries are trying to cut back on its use.

Selenium

Until 1979, it was not known that selenium is an essential mineral. The first RDA for selenium was announced in 1989. Selenium is a component of enzymes that act like antioxidants along with vitamin E to prevent oxidative tissue damage. Excellent sources include seafood, meat, and liver. Because selenium is found in the soil, vegetables and whole grains may be a good source of selenium as well if the soil is selenium-rich. Selenium deficiency can cause a type of heart disease, but this is rare in the United States. When megadoses of selenium are taken over a long time span, diarrhea, nausea, vomiting, hair loss, and malaise can result.

Selenium activates an antioxidant. It is found in seafood, meat, liver, eggs, and foods grown in selenium-rich soils.

Fluoride

Fluoride is the term used for the form of fluorine that appears in drinking water and in the body. The terms **fluoride** and **fluorine** are used interchangeably. In children, fluoride strengthens the mineral composition of the developing teeth so they resist the formation of dental caries, or cavities. The American Dental Association estimates that for every dollar spent on fluoridation, about $50 are saved in subsequent dental costs.

The major source of fluoride is drinking water. Some water supplies are naturally fluoridated, and many supplies have fluoride added, usually at a concentration of 1 part fluoride to a million parts water. Fluoride levels in water are stated in concentrations of parts per million (ppm). About 1 ppm is ideal. Less than 0.7 ppm isn't adequate to protect developing teeth. More than about 1.5 to 2.0 ppm can lead to **mild fluorosis,** a condition that causes small, white, virtually invisible opaque areas on teeth. In its most severe form, fluorosis causes a distinct brownish

Fluoride strengthens developing teeth and is found in fluoridated water.

mottling or discoloring. Artificial fluoridation of water uses an optimum standard set by the Environmental Protect Agency of 0.7 to 1.2 ppm, depending on locality (a lower amount is needed in warmer parts of the country, where people drink more water).

Only fluoride taken internally, whether in drinking water or dietary supplements, can strengthen babies' and children's developing teeth to resist decay. Once the teeth have erupted, they are beyond help from ingested fluoride. Supplements are important for the approximately 40 percent of Americans who do not have adequately fluoridated water supplies.

For both children and adults, fluoride applied to the surface of the teeth can nonetheless add protection, at least to the outer layer of enamel, where it plays a role in reducing decay. The most familiar form, of course, is fluoride-containing toothpaste, introduced in the early 1960s. Fluoride rinses are also available, as are applications by dental professionals. All such products are regulated by the Food and Drug Administration (FDA). They are considered effective adjuncts to ingested fluoride, and are the only useful sources of tooth-strengthening fluoride for teenagers and adults.

Some health groups have been concerned that fluoride is a cancer risk. In 1991, based on a review of 50 human studies, scientists from the Public Health Service (which includes the National Institutes of Health, the Center for Disease Control, and the FDA) reported that optimal fluoridation of drinking water does not pose a detectable cancer risk. The report did observe, however, that there are multiple sources of fluoride and commented that, "In accordance with the prudent health practice of using no more than the amount necessary to achieve a desired effect, health professionals and the public should avoid excessive and inappropriate fluoride exposure."

Chromium works with insulin. It is found in brewer's yeast, lean beef, and some fruits and vegetables.

Chromium

Chromium works with insulin to transfer glucose and other nutrients from the bloodstream into the body's cells. Chromium deficiency results in a condition much like diabetes in which the blood glucose level is abnormally high. Chromium also plays an important role in the body's use of fats and proteins. Although advertised as helping you lose weight and put on muscle, well-designed research studies have not shown these effects. The role of chromium in possibly lowering blood cholesterol levels is still under investigation. Good sources of chromium are whole, unprocessed foods, such as whole grains and breads and cereals made with whole grains, wheat germ, lean beef, and some fruits and vegetables, such as corn on the cob, tomatoes, sweet potatoes, and apples. The richest source is brewer's (nutritional) yeast. Although chromium supplements are safer than zinc or iron, megadoses are not advised.

Copper

Copper works with iron to form hemoglobin. It also aids in forming collagen, a protein that gives strength and support to bones, teeth, muscle, cartilage, and blood vessels. Copper is a part of many important enzymes, such as those involved in the nervous system and energy release.

Copper occurs mostly in unprocessed foods. Organ meats, shellfish, legumes, nuts, dried fruits, and whole-grain breads and cereals are rich sources.

Copper-deficient diets are linked to heart disease, causing cholesterol and blood pressure to go up. Copper deficiency is rare, but marginal deficiencies do occur. Single doses of copper only 4 times the recommended level can cause vomiting and nervous-system disorders.

Copper:
Iron metabolism.
Formation of hemoglobin.
Collagen formation.
Energy release.

Copper:
Organ meats.
Shellfish.
Whole grain breads and cereals.
Legumes.
Nuts.
Dried fruits.

Other Trace Minerals

Cobalt is a part of vitamin B_{12} and is therefore needed to form red blood cells. The dietary source of cobalt is vitamin B_{12}, which is found in animal foods.

Manganese is needed for bone formation and as part of many enzymes involved in energy metabolism and the metabolism of carbohydrate, fats, and protein. It is found in many foods, especially whole grains, dried beans, nuts, and leafy vegetables. A deficiency is unknown.

Molybdenum is a part of a number of enzymes. It appears in legumes, whole grains, nuts, and organ meats. Deficiency does not seem to be a problem.

As time goes on, more trace minerals will be recognized as essential to human health. There are currently several trace minerals essential to animals that are likely to be essential to humans as well. Possible candidates for nutrient status include arsenic, boron, cadmium, lithium, nickel, silicon, tin, and vanadium.

MINI-SUMMARY The functions and sources of the trace minerals are listed in Table 6-4.

OSTEOPOROSIS

Osteoporosis is the most common bone disease. Characterized by loss of bone density and strength, osteoporosis is associated with debilitating fractures, especially in people age 45 and older. Bone loss develops over a span of many years and is largely symptomless, although some women may experience chronic spinal pain or muscle spasms in the back. Often, the first sign of osteoporosis is a wrist or hip fracture or a compression fracture that causes the vertebrae in the upper back to collapse, curving the spine into the "dowager's hump" that has come to symbolize osteoporosis.

As many as 8 million Americans, 80 percent of them women, now suffer from the condition, with more than 1.5 million osteoporosis-related fractures occurring annually. A little less than half of women over 50 will experience an osteoporosis-related fracture in their lifetime. Another 17 million women are at risk.

Luckily, osteoporosis can be prevented, detected, and treated, and it is never too late to do something about it.

Although bones seem to be as lifeless as rocks, they are in fact composed of living tissue that is continually being broken down and rebuilt in a process called *remodeling*. It takes about 90 days for old bone to be broken down and replaced by new bone; then the cycle begins anew. Bones continue to grow in strength and size until a person's early thirties, when peak bone mass is attained. Men achieve more peak bone mass than women. Optimal bone mass and size will only be attained if there has been enough calcium in the diet. After that, bone is broken down faster than it is deposited, resulting in decreased bone mass (about 1 percent per year). In men, bone loss is slow but constant. For women, bone loss speeds up during the five years following menopause due to decreased production of estrogen, and then slows to about the same rate as before menopause.

Besides being influenced by age, sex, and estrogen levels, bone health is also influenced by diet and exercise. For maximum bone health, adequate amounts of calcium and vitamin D need to be taken in. Unfortunately, most women (especially teenagers) do not consume the RDA for calcium (McBean, Forgac, and Finn, 1994). During the five to ten years after the beginning of menopause, optimal calcium, intake is important. Although some bone loss in inevitable, it can be kept to its programmed minimum with adequate calcium from the diet. The National Institutes of Health has recommended 1500 milligrams of calcium for postmenopausal women and 1000 milligrams of calcium for women aged 25 to 49 and women who are getting estrogen replacement therapy. The recommendation for both men and women over 65 is 1500 milligrams of calcium daily, almost double the current RDA. The RDA for calcium will likely be increased in the next edition. The National Institutes of Health has already recommended calcium in larger amounts

TABLE 6-6. 1994 recommendations for calcium intake by the National Institutes of Health, Consensus Development Panel on Optimal Calcium Intake.

Age/Gender	NIH Recommendations	Current RDAs
Birth–1 yr	400–600 mg	400–600 mg
1–5 yrs	800 mg	800 mg
6–10 yrs	800–1200 mg	1200 mg
11–24 yrs	1200–1500 mg	1200 mg
Females, 25–49 yrs	1000 mg	800 mg
Females, pregnant/nursing	1200–1500 mg	1200 mg
Females, postmenopausal, 50–64 yrs:		
On estrogen replacement therapy	1000 mg	800 mg
Not on estrogen replacement therapy	1500 mg	800 mg
Males, 25–64 yrs	1000 mg	800 mg
Males/females, 65 yrs+	1500 mg	800 mg

than in the RDA (Table 6-6) (NIH Consensus Development Panel on Optimal Calcium Intake, 1994).

Exercise also influences bone health, and participation in sports and exercise increases bone density in children. For older adults, exercise helps improve strength and balance, making it less likely for them to have a fall. To benefit bone health, exercise must be weight bearing or strength training. Also, exercise benefits only the bones used, such as the leg bones when biking or walking.

The best approach to osteoporosis is prevention—the reason why calcium intake is so important. Starting in childhood through young adulthood (when bones are forming), adequate calcium intake is vital to having more bone mass at maturity. Adequate intake of calcium is also important after early adulthood.

Individuals who are aware of the problems of osteoporosis sometimes take calcium supplements. Many calcium supplements provide mixtures of calcium with other compounds such as calcium carbonate, a good source of calcium. There are also powdered forms of calcium-rich substances, such as bonemeal and dolomite (a rock mineral). These are dangerous because they may contain lead and other elements in amounts that constitute a risk. Excessive intake of calcium can cause problems such as possible urinary stone formation, constipation, and decreased absorption of iron and other nutrients.

Other ways to prevent osteoporosis include regular weight-bearing or strength-training exercise (as already mentioned), consumption of adequate milk for vitamin D, exposure to the sun (for more vitamin D), estrogen therapy for women, moderate consumption of alcohol and caffeine, and avoiding smoking.

It has been known for some time that estrogen therapy at and after menopause prevents osteoporosis-related fractures. Conjugated estrogens—a mixture of estrogens from natural sources—received FDA approval as a treatment for osteoporosis in 1988. Although the hormone decreases the risk of osteoporosis and heart disease, with long-term use it may increase the risk of breast and endometrial cancers. Estrogen therapy (which is also helpful in treating menopause symptoms) is a poor choice for some groups of women, such as those who have estrogen-sensitive breast cancer.

MINI-SUMMARY The best approach to osteoporosis is prevention—taking in the RDA for calcium, regular exercise, consuming milk for adequate vitamin D, consuming moderate amounts of alcohol, and avoiding smoking. Estrogen therapy may be advised for some menopausal women.

RECOMMENDATIONS AND TIPS FOR NUTRITIOUS FOOD SELECTION

The rules that apply to vitamins also apply to minerals. For example, a balanced and varied diet in which no foods are overemphasized or omitted is essential to adequate mineral consumption. Following are some tips to assure yourself an adequate and varied diet.

1. Select foods daily from each of these groups: fruits; vegetables; whole-grain breads and cereals and other grain products; milk and dairy foods; meats, poultry, fish, eggs, and legumes.
2. Select and make one new recipe each week that uses one or more foods that you do not normally eat.
3. Buy a recipe book emphasizing foods lacking in your diet, such as vegetables or grains.
4. When food shopping, make it a point to buy one new nutritious food each time you shop.
5. When eating out, avoid your old standby; order something different.

Following are some tips to ensure adequate fluid intake.

1. When you are thirsty, drink beyond the point when you think you have had enough fluid.
2. Keep a pitcher of water and a glass close to you during the day so that you are reminded to take a drink and can easily do so.
3. Drink at least 1 cup of fluid with each meal and snack.
4. Stop every time you pass a water fountain and have a drink.
5. Be sure the beverages you like to drink are available.
6. Make water in a glass appear more appealing by adding ice and a twist of lemon, lime, or orange. Use a fancy glass.

The trick to drinking enough fluids daily is to make it a habit to drink more frequently.

KEY TERMS

Acid-base balance	Iron-deficiency	Osteoporosis
Chlorophyll	anemia	Oxalic acid
Diuretic	Iron overload	Thyroid gland
Electrolytes	Major minerals	Trace minerals
Hemoglobin	Mild fluorosis	Water balance
Heme iron	Myoglobin	
Ions	Nonheme iron	

REVIEW QUESTIONS AND EXERCISES

1. List four basic facts about minerals.
2. Describe the difference between major minerals and trace minerals.
3. How much of your actual weight is water?
4. List six functions of water.
5. What is one concern with the thirst mechanism?
6. Name the mineral(s)
   a. involved in bone formation.
   b. found mostly in milk and milk products.
   c. that help maintain water and acid-base balance.
   d. depleted by some diuretics.
   e. found in the stomach juices.
   f. important for a healthy heart.
   g. found in certain water supplies.
   h. found in salt.
   i. found in heme.
   j. that causes a form of anemia.
   k. that occur in the soil.
   l. that are part of vitamin B_{12}.
7. Name five factors that enhance the development of osteoporosis.

**ACTIVITIES
AND
APPLICATIONS**

1. Quiz
Check your answers with these.
   a. b
   2. b
   e. c
   4. c
   5. c

FIGURE 6-1.
Mineral salad bar

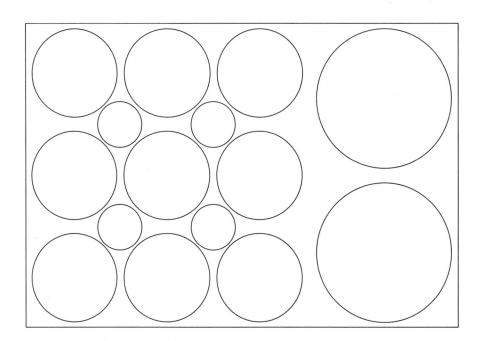

2. Your Eating Style
   Using Table 6-4, circle any food sources of minerals that you do not eat at all, or eat infrequently, such as dairy products or green vegetables. Do you eat many of the foods containing minerals, or only a moderate amount of them? How often do you eat mineral-rich foods? The answers to these questions should help you assess whether your diet is adequately balanced and varied to ensure adequate mineral intake.

3. *How Much Do You Drink?*

Keep a diary of how many fluid ounces you drink in one day, including beverages such as coffee and soft drinks but excluding alcoholic beverages. Convert the number of fluid ounces to the number of cups by dividing the total ounces by 8. Then compare this number to the 8 to 10 cups you need daily. Did you drink enough fluid? When might you need over 10 cups daily?

4. *Mineral Salad Bar*

Set up a salad bar using Figure 6-1. You may use any foods you like in your salad bar as long as you have a good source of each of the minerals listed in Table 6-4 and you fill each of the circles. In each circle, write the name of the food and which mineral(s) it is rich in.

5. *Sodium Countdown*

Using Appendix A, "Nutritive Value of Foods," list the sodium content of ten of your favorite foods. How much would each contribute to the daily maximum recommendation of 1800 to 2400 milligrams of sodium?

REFERENCES

American Dietetic Association. 1994. Position of the American Dietetic Association: The impact of fluoride on dental health. *Journal of The American Dietetic Association* 94(11): 1428–1431.

American Dietetic Association. 1996. Position of The American Dietetic Association: Vitamin and mineral supplementation. *Journal of The American Dietetic Association* 96(1): 73–77.

American Medical Association. 1983. Sodium in processed foods. *Journal of The American Medical Association* 249(6): 784–798.

Anderson, Richard A., and Adriane S. Kozlovsky. 1985. Chromium intake, absorption, and excretion of subjects consuming self-selected diets. *American Journal of Clinical Nutrition* 41(6): 1177–1183.

Black, M. R., D. M. Medeiros, E. Brunett, and R. Welke. 1988. Zinc supplements and serum lipids in young adult white males. *American Journal of Clinical Nutrition* 47: 970.

Bronner, Felix. 1994. Calcium and osteoporosis. *American Journal of Clinical Nutrition* 60: 831–836.

Dietary Supplement Health and Education Act of 1994. Public Law 103-417, 108 STAT: 4325–4335.

Food and Nutrition Board, National Academy of Sciences—National Research Council. 1989. Recommended Dietary Allowances. Washington, DC: National Academy Press.

Harland, Barbara, and Barbara Harden-Williams. 1994. Is vanadium of human nutritional importance yet? *Journal of The American Dietetic Association* 94(8): 891–894.

Hecht, Annabel. 1986. Electrolytes, the charge in the body's power system. *FDA Consumer* 20(6): 25–27.

Hertzler, Ann A., and Thomas R. McAnge. 1986. Development of an iron checklist to guide food intake. *Journal of The American Dietetic Association* 86(6): 782–786.

Johnson, M. A., and S. E. Kays. 1990. Copper: Its role in human nutrition. *Nutrition Today* (January/February): 6–9.

Lever, A. F. 1986. Should recommendations be made to reduce dietary sodium intake? *Proceedings of the Nutrition Society* 45(3): 259–262.

McBean, Lois D., Tab Forgac, and Susan Calvert Finn. 1994. Osteoporosis: Visions for care and prevention–A conference report. *Journal of The American Dietetic Association* 94(6): 668–671.

Mertz, Walter. 1994. A balanced approach to nutrition for health: The need for biologically essential minerals and vitamins. *Journal of The American Dietetic Association* 94(11): 1259–1262.

Mertz, Walter. 1983. The significance of trace elements for health. *Nutrition Today* (September/October 1983): 26–31.

Mertz, Walter. 1981. The essential trace elements. *Science* 213(4514): 1332–1338.

Monsen, Elaine R. 1988. Iron nutrition and absorption: Dietary factors which impact iron bioavailability. *Journal of The American Dietetic Association* 88(7): 786–790.

NIH Consensus Development Panel on Optimal Calcium Intake. 1994. *Journal of The American Dietetic Association* 272(24): 1942–1947.

Pennington, Jean A. T. 1990. A review of iodine toxicity reports. *Journal of The American Dietetic Association* 90(11): 1571–1581.

Pennington, Jean A. T., and Barbara E. Young. 1991. Total Diet Study of nutritional elements, 1982-1989. *Journal of The American Dietetic Association* 91(2): 179–183.

Pennington, Jean A. T., Barbara E. Young, and Dennis B. Wilson. 1989. Nutritional elements in U.S. diets: Results from the Total Diet Study, 1982 to 1986. *Journal of The American Dietetic Association* 89(5):659–664.

Pennington, Jean A. T., and John W. Jones. 1987. Molybdenum, nickel, cobalt, vanadium, and strontium in total diets. *Journal of The American Dietetic Association* 87(12): 1644–1650.

Pennington, Jean A. T., Barbara E. Young, Dennis B. Wilson, Roger D. Johnson, and John E. Vanderveen. 1986. Mineral content of foods and total diets: The Selected Minerals in Foods Survey, 1982 to 1984. *Journal of The American Dietetic Association* 86(7): 876–891.

Turnlund, Judith R. 1988. Copper nutriture, bioavailability, and the influence of dietary factors. *Journal of The American Dietetic Association* 88(3): 303–308.

Vokes, T. 1987. Water homeostasis. *Annual Review of Nutrition* 7: 383–406.

Wardlaw, Gordon M. 1993. Putting osteoporosis in perspective. *Journal of The American Dietetic Association* 93(9): 1000-1006.

Hot Topic: Are Dietary Supplements Necessary?

About 40 percent of Americans use dietary supplements on a regular basis. The supplement industry is huge: It's worth over $4 billion per year and provides over 3000 products. Dietary supplements in the marketplace include vitamins; essential minerals; protein; amino acids; botanicals such as ginseng and yohimbe; extracts from animal glands; garlic extract; fish oils; fibers such as acacia and guar gum; compounds not generally recognized as foods or nutrients, such as bioflavonoids, enzymes, germanium, nucleic acids, and paraaminobenzoic acid; and mixtures of these ingredients.

The reasons people take supplements are quite diverse. Various explanations include assurance of adequate nutrient intake, increased vitality, improved athletic performance, enhanced resistance to illness, and general well-being. There is little evidence to suggest that supplement users take in fewer nutrients from foods than non-supplement users. Unfortunately, many people take supplements without any guidance. Very few—under 10 percent—of Americans who regularly take vitamins do so under the guidance of their physician.

Obtaining nutrients through eating a variety of foods is the best way to get essential nutrients for a couple of reasons. First, there are probably substances in food that we have not yet realized are essential to the body or are helpful in preventing disease. For example, a chemical found in broccoli (and also in cauliflower, kale, carrots, and brussel sprouts) seems to block tumor formation in animals and may do the same in humans. Second, problems with nutrient overdoses or imbalances are less likely to occur from eating foods than from taking pills. Although most Americans can get needed vitamins and minerals through food, situations do occur when supplements may be necessary, as follows:

Pregnant or lactating women may need iron and folate.

Strict vegetarians may need vitamin B_{12}, calcium, iron, and zinc—nutrients that may be hard to get enough of when eating only plant foods.

People eating less than 1200 calories a day—such as dieters and some elderly who get little exercise—may need vitamin and mineral supplements because it is hard to get enough nutrients in such low-calorie diets.

Premenopausal women sometimes develop iron-deficiency anemia and may require iron supplements.

People on certain medications that interact with nutrients, or people with certain illnesses, may require supplements.

If you really feel you need additional nutrients, your best bet is to buy a multivitamin and mineral supplement that supplies 100 percent of the RDA for 10 or so essential nutrients. It can't hurt and may act as a safety net for individuals who eat haphazardly. But no such supplement can adequately take the place of food and serve as a permanent substitute for improving a poorly constructed diet. In other words, use vitamin and mineral supplements to "supplement" a good diet, not substitute for a poor diet.

When buying supplements, be sure to read the label carefully. The Food and Drug Administration (FDA) oversees labeling of supplements and regulates supplements as foods, as long as no drug claims are made for them. The FDA does not require safety testing of any supplements. If a supplement is unsafe or has misleading label information, it is up to the FDA, not the manufacturer, to provide that this is so. The Dietary Supplement Health and Education Act of 1994 has a different set of regulations for health claims on supplements than those allowed for foods. A statement for a dietary supplement may be made on its label if it meets these 3 criteria.

1. The statement claims a benefit related to a classical nutrient deficiency disease and discloses the prevalence of such disease in the United States, describes the role of a nutrient or dietary ingredient intended to affect the structure or function in humans, characterizes the documented mechanism by which a nutrient or dietary ingredient acts to maintain such structure or function, or describes general well-being from consumption of a nutrient or dietary ingredient.
2. The manufacturer of the dietary supplement has substantiation that such statement is truthful and not misleading.
3. The statement contains, prominently displayed and in boldface type, the following: This statement has not been evaluated by the Food and Drug Administration. This product is not intended to diagnose, treat, cure, or prevent any disease.

Other precautions for buying and using supplements include these:

- Be sure to tell health-care providers about all supplements you take, including concentrations and amounts.
- Children, adolescents, older or chronically ill people, and women who are pregnant or are breast-feeding should not use high-potency supplements or those used for medicinal purposes unless they are under supervision of a physician.
- Keep supplements far away from children, preferably locked away in a cabinet. Although you might not think of supplements as a poison, iron-containing supplements are the leading cause of pediatric poisoning death for children under 6 in the United States. Some supplements can be fatal depending on the vitamin or mineral, the dosage, and the child's size.

Label Reading Questions and Answers: Minerals

What minerals are listed on food labels?

Three minerals are required on food labels: sodium, calcium, and iron (Figure 6-2). Food manufacturers may list any other minerals.

Nutrition Facts

Serving Size 3 oz
(84g/about ½ stalk)
Servings Per Container about 2.5

Amount Per Serving

Calories 30	Calories from Fat 0

	% Daily Value*
Total Fat 0g	**0%**
Saturated Fat 0g	**0%**
Cholesterol 0mg	**0%**
Sodium 20mg	**1%**
Total Carbohydrate 5g	**2%**
Dietary Fiber 3g	**11%**
Soluble Fiber 1g	
Sugars 0g	
Protein 3g	

Vitamin A 25%	•	Vitamin C 110%
Calcium 4%	•	Iron 4%

* Percent Daily Values are based on a 2,000 calorie diet. Your daily values may be higher or lower depending on your calorie needs:

	Calories:	2,000	2,500
Total Fat	Less than	65g	80g
Sat Fat	Less than	20g	25g
Cholesterol	Less than	300mg	300mg
Sodium	Less than	2,400mg	2,400mg
Total Carbohydrate		300g	375g
Dietary Fiber		25g	30g

FIGURE 6-2. Nutrition Facts.

What information do I get about these minerals?

For sodium, the number of milligrams in one serving is given, as well as the Percent Daily Value. The amounts of calcium and iron are listed as a Percent Daily Value. Daily Values are a guide to the total daily nutrient amount you need based on a 2000-calorie diet. Therefore, the Daily Value may be a little high, a little low, or right on target for you. Percent Daily Values show how much of the Daily Value is in one serving.

What is the daily value for sodium, calcium, and iron?

The Daily Value for: sodium is 2400 milligrams, for calcium is 1000 milligrams, and for iron is 18 milligrams.

How can I use the Percent Daily Values?

Use the Percent Daily Values to provide a general idea of the nutrient content— whether a food contains a lot or a little of specific nutrients. You can also use Percent Daily Values to see how foods can fit into your overall daily diet and to make comparisons among products.

If a label claims to be a "good source of iron," will the Nutrition Facts include more information?

Yes. If a label makes a nutrient claim, that nutrient must be listed on the nutrition label so you see what the Percent Daily Value is for one serving.

What other nutrient claims can be made with vitamins, and what do they mean?

Here are some other claims you may find on food labels, and the definitions set by the government for their use.

Nutrient Claims	Definition
High, Rich In, Excellent Source of	20 percent or more of the Daily Value
Good Source, Contains, Provides	10 to 19 percent of the Daily Value
More, Enriched, Fortified, Added	Contains at least 10 percent more of the Daily Value when compared to the reference food

What nutrient claims are allowed for sodium, and what do they mean?

Sodium-free: less than 5 milligrams of sodium

Very low sodium: 35 milligrams or less of sodium

Low sodium: 140 milligrams or less of sodium

Reduced or less sodium: at least 25 percent less sodium than the reference food

Light in sodium: at least 50 percent less sodium than the reference food

CHAPTER

7

Putting It All Together

1. What are the seven U.S. dietary guidelines?
2. How can you use the Food Guide Pyramid and the exchange lists in planning meals?
3. How can you use food labeling to help plan meals?

QUIZ

Directions: Answer the following question by filling in the blanks. How many minimum servings per day do you need of the following foods?

1. Breads, cereals, and other grain products   ____ servings
2. Fruits   ____ servings
3. Vegetables   ____ servings
4. Meat, poultry, fish, and alternates   ____ servings
5. Milk, cheese, and yogurt   ____ servings

DIETARY RECOMMENDATIONS

Dietary recommendations have been published for the healthy American public for almost 100 years. Early recommendations centered on encouraging intake of certain foods to prevent deficiencies, fight disease, and enhance growth. Although deficiency diseases have been virtually eliminated, they have been replaced by diseases of dietary excess and imbalance—problems that now rank among the leading causes of illness and death in the United States. Diseases such as heart disease and cancer touch the lives of most Americans and generate substantial health-care costs. More recent dietary guidelines have therefore centered on modifying the diet, in most cases cutting back on certain foods, to prevent lasting degenerative diseases such as heart disease.

Dietary recommendations are quite different from the RDAs. Whereas the RDAs deal with specific nutrients, dietary recommendations discuss specific foods and food groups that will help individuals meet the RDA. The RDAs also tend to be written in a technical style. Dietary recommendations are usually written in easy-to-understand terms.

The most recent set of U.S. dietary recommendations are the **Dietary Guidelines for Americans** (fourth edition), published in 1995. These guidelines are for healthy Americans age 2 years and over—not for younger children and infants, whose dietary needs differ. Dietary Guidelines for Americans reflect recommendations of nutrition authorities who agree that enough is known about diet's affect on health to encourage certain dietary practices. They should be applied to diets consumed over several days and not to single meals or foods.

The first two guidelines form the framework for the diet: "Eat a variety of foods" for the nutrients and calories you need, and "Balance the food you eat with physical activity—maintain or improve your weight." The next two guidelines stress the need for many Americans to change their diets to be lower in fat, saturated fat, and cholesterol, and higher in grain products, vegetables, and fruits. Other guidelines suggest moderate use of sugars, salt and sodium, and alcoholic beverages. These guidelines call for avoiding extremes in diet; both eating too much and eating too little can be harmful.

The Dietary Guidelines refer to the **Food Guide Pyramid** (discussed next) and nutrition information found on food labels. The following is a summary of the Dietary Guidelines for Americans.[1]

1. **Eat a variety of foods.**

To obtain the nutrients and other substances needed for good health, vary the foods you eat. Foods contain combinations of nutrients and other healthful substances. No single food can supply all nutrients in the amounts you need. To make sure you get all the nutrients and other substances needed for health, choose the recommended number of daily servings from each of the five major food groups displayed in the Food Guide Pyramid (Figure 7-1).

The 1995 Dietary Guidelines for Americans try to state goals in a positive, rather than negative, manner.

Foods vary in their amounts of calories and nutrients. Some foods such as grain products, vegetables, and fruits have many nutrients and other healthful substances but are relatively low in calories. Fat and alcohol are high in calories. Foods high in both sugars and fat contain many calories but often are low in vitamins, minerals, or fiber.

Growing children, teenage girls, and women have higher needs for some nutrients such as calcium and iron.

Where do vitamin, mineral, and fiber supplements fit in? Supplements may help to meet special nutritional needs. However, supplements do not supply all of the nutrients and other substances present in foods that are important to health. Supplements of some nutrients taken regularly in large amounts are harmful. Daily vitamin and mineral supplements at or below the Recommended Dietary Allowances are considered safe but are usually unnecessary for people who eat the variety of foods in the Food Guide Pyramid.

For the first time in 1995, the Dietary Guidelines addressed the topic of vegetarian diets, stating that they can be nutritionally adequate when planned properly.

Supplements are sometimes needed to meet specific nutrient requirements. For example, older women and others with little exposure to sunlight may need a vitamin D supplement.

Enjoy eating a variety of foods. Get the many nutrients your body

[1]Adapted from *Nutrition and Your Health: Dietary Guidelines for Americans,* Fourth Edition, 1995, U. S. Department of Agriculture and U. S. Department of Health and Human Services.

FIGURE 7-1

The food guide pyramid—
a guide to daily food choices

> **Key**
>
> ◊ Fat (naturally occurring and added)
> □ Sugars (added)
>
> The symbols show fat and added sugars in foods.
> They come mostly from the fats, oils, and sweets group.
> But foods in other groups—such as cheese or ice cream
> from the milk group or french fries in the vegetable
> group—can also provide fat and added sugars.

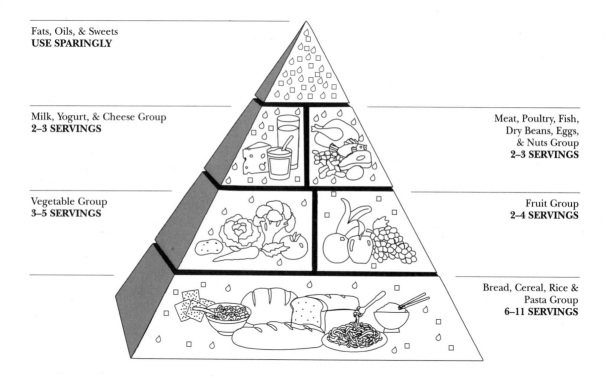

Fats, Oils, & Sweets
USE SPARINGLY

Milk, Yogurt, & Cheese Group
2–3 SERVINGS

Meat, Poultry, Fish,
Dry Beans, Eggs,
& Nuts Group
2–3 SERVINGS

Vegetable Group
3–5 SERVINGS

Fruit Group
2–4 SERVINGS

Bread, Cereal, Rice &
Pasta Group
6–11 SERVINGS

Looking at the Pieces of the Pyramid

The Food Guide Pyramid emphasizes foods from the five major food
groups shown in the three lower sections of the Pyramid. Each of these
food groups provides some, but not all, of the nutrients you need.
Foods in one group can't replace those in another. No one of these
major food groups is more important than another—for good health,
you need them all.

Source: U.S. Department of Agriculture and the U.S. Department of Health and Human Services.

TABLE 7-1. To decrease calorie intake.

- eat a variety of foods that are low in calories and high in nutrients—check the Nutrition Facts Label.
- eat less fat and fewer high-fat foods.
- eat smaller portions and limit second helpings of foods high in fat and calories.
- eat more vegetables and fruits without fats and sugars added in preparation or at the table.
- eat pasta, rice, breads, and cereals without fats and sugars added in preparation or at the table.
- eat less sugars and fewer sweets (like candy, cookies, cakes, soda).
- drink less or no alcohol.

needs by choosing among the varied foods you enjoy from these groups: grain products, vegetables, fruits, milk and milk products, protein-rich plant foods (beans, nuts), and protein-rich animal foods (lean meat, poultry, fish, and eggs). Remember to choose lean and low-fat foods and beverages most often. Many foods you eat contain servings from more than one food group. For example, soups and stews may contain meat, beans, noodles, and vegetables.

2. **Balance the food you eat with physical activity—maintain or improve your weight.**

   Many Americans gain weight in adulthood, increasing their risk for high blood pressure, heart disease, stroke, diabetes, certain types of cancer, arthritis, breathing problems, and other illness. Therefore, most adults should not gain weight. If you are overweight and have one of these problems, you should try to lose weight, or at the very least, not gain additional weight.

   Healthy diets and exercise can help people maintain a healthy weight, and may also help them lose weight. It is important to recognize that overweight is a chronic condition that can be controlled only with long-term changes. To reduce caloric intake, eat less fat and control portion sizes (see Table 7-1). If you are not physically active, spend less time in sedentary activities, such as watching television, and be more active throughout the day. As people lose weight, the body becomes more efficient at using energy and the rate of weight loss may decrease. Increased physical activity will help you continue losing weight and avoid gaining it back (see Table 7-2).

TABLE 7-2. **To increase calorie expenditure by physical activity.**

Remember to accumulate 30 minutes or more of moderate physical activity on most—preferably all—days of the week.

Examples of moderate physical activitites for healthy U.S. adults

- walking briskly (3–4 miles per hour)
- conditioning or general calisthenics
- home care, general cleaning
- racket sports such as table tennis
- mowing lawn, power mower
- golf—pulling cart or carrying clubs
- home repair, painting
- fishing, standing/casting
- jogging
- swimming (moderate effort)
- cycling, moderate speed (<10 miles per hour)
- gardening
- canoeing leisurely (2.0–3.9 miles per hour)
- dancing

Source: Adapted from Pate, et al., *Journal of the American Medical Association*, 1995, Vol. 273, p.404.

3. **Choose a diet with plenty of grain products, vegetables, and fruits.**

Grain products, vegetables, and fruits are key parts of a varied diet. They are emphasized in this guideline because they provide vitamins, minerals, complex carbohydrates (starch and dietary fiber), and other substances important for good health. They are also generally low in fat, depending on how they are prepared and what is added to them at the table. Most Americans of all ages eat fewer than the recommended number of servings of grain products, vegetables, and fruits, even though consumption of these foods is associated with a substantially lower risk for many chronic diseases, including certain types of cancer (Table 7-3).

Most of the calories in your diet should come from grain products, vegetables, and fruits. These include grain products high in complex carbohydrates—breads, cereals, pasta, rice—found at the base of the Food Guide Pyramid, as well as vegetables such as potatoes and corn. Dry beans (like pinto, navy, kidney, and black beans) are included in the meat and beans group of the Pyramid, but they can count as servings of vegetables instead of meat alternatives.

Plant foods provide fiber. Fiber is found only in plant foods such as

TABLE 7-3. **For a diet with plenty of grain products, vegetables, and fruits, eat daily:**

6–11 servings of grain products (breads, cereals, pasta, and rice).
- Eat products made from a variety of whole grains, such as wheat, rice, oats, corn, and barley.
- Eat several servings of whole-grain breads and cereals daily.
- Prepare and serve grain products with little or no fats and sugars.

3–5 servings of various vegetables and vegetable juices.
- Choose dark-green leafy and deep yellow vegetables often.
- Eat dry beans, peas, and lentils often.
- Eat starchy vegetables, such as potatoes and corn.
- Prepare and serve vegetables with little or no fats.

2–4 servings of various fruits and fruit juices.
- Choose citrus fruits or juices, melons, or berries regularly.
- Eat fruits as desserts or snacks.
- Drink fruit juices.
- Prepare and serve fruits with little or no added sugars.

whole-grain breads and cereals, beans and peas, and other vegetables and fruits. Because there are different types of food fibers, choose a variety of foods daily. Eating a variety of fiber-containing plant foods is important for proper bowel function, can reduce symptoms of chronic constipation, diverticular disease, and hemorrhoids; and may lower the risk for heart disease and some cancers. However, some of the health benefits associated with a high-fiber diet may come from other components present in these foods, not from fiber alone.

Plant foods provide a variety of vitamins and minerals essential for health, such as vitamin C, vitamin B_6, carotenoids, and folate. The antioxidant nutrients found in plant foods (for example, vitamin C, carotenoids, vitamin E, and certain minerals) are presently of great interest to scientists and the public because of their potentially beneficial role in reducing the risk of cancer and certain other chronic diseases.

4. **Choose a diet low in fat, saturated fat, and cholesterol.**

Some dietary fat is needed for good health. Fats supply energy and essential fatty acids and promote absorption of the fat-soluble vitamins A, D, E, and K. Most people are aware that high levels of saturated fat and cholesterol in the diet are linked to increased blood cholesterol levels and a greater risk for heart disease. More Americans are now eating less fat,

> **TABLE 7-4. For a diet low in fat, saturated fat, and cholesterol, eat daily:**

Fats and Oils
- Use fats and oils sparingly in cooking and at the table.
- Use small amounts of salad dressings and spreads such as butter, margarine, and mayonnaise. Consider using lowfat or fat-free dressings for salads.
- Choose vegetable oils and soft margarines most often because they are lower in saturated fat than solid shortenings and animal fats, even though their caloric content is the same.
- Check the Nutrition Facts Label to see how much fat and saturated fat are in a serving; choose foods lower in fat and saturated fat.

Grain Products, Vegetables, and Fruits
- Choose lowfat sauces with pasta, rice and potatoes.
- Use as little fat as possible to cook vegetables and grain products.
- Season with herbs, spices, lemon juice, and fat-free or lowfat salad dressings.

Meat, Poultry, Fish, Eggs, Beans and Nuts
- Choose two to three servings of lean fish, poultry, meats, or other protein-rich foods, such as beans, daily. Use meats labeled "lean" or "extra lean." Trim fat from meat; take skin off poultry. (Three ounces of cooked lean beef or chicken without skin—a piece the size of a deck of cards—provides about 6 grams of fat; a piece of chicken with skin or untrimmed meat of that size may have as much as twice this amount of fat.) Most beans and bean products are almost fat-free and are a good source of protein and fiber.
- Limit intake of high-fat processed meats such as sausages, salami, and other cold cuts; choose lower fat varieties by reading the Nutrition Facts Label.
- Limit the intake of organ meats (three ounces of cooked chicken liver have about 540 mg of cholesterol); use egg yolks in moderation (one egg yolk has about 215 mg of cholesterol). Egg whites contain no cholesterol and can be used freely.

Milk and Milk Products
- Choose skim or lowfat milk, fat-free or lowfat yogurt, and lowfat cheese.
- Have two to three lowfat servings daily. Add extra calcium to your diet without added fat by choosing fat-free yogurt and lowfat milk more often. (One cup of skim milk has almost no fat, 1 cup of 1 percent milk has 2.5 grams of fat, 1 cup of 2 percent milk has 5 grams [one teaspoon] of fat, and 1 cup of whole milk has 8 grams of fat.) If you do not consume foods from this group, eat other calcium-rich foods.

saturated fat, and cholesterol-rich foods than in the recent past, and fewer people are dying from the most common form of heart disease. Still, many people continue to eat high-fat diets, the number of overweight people has increased, and the risk of heart disease and certain cancers (also linked to fat intake) remains high. This guideline emphasizes the continued importance of choosing a diet with less total fat, saturated fat, and cholesterol (Table 7-4).

Choose a diet that provides no more than 30 percent of total calories from fat. The upper limit on the grams of fat in your diet depends on the calories you need. Mono- and polyunsaturated fat sources should replace saturated fats within this 30 percent limit. Partially hydrogenated vegetable oils, such as those used in many margarines and shortenings, contain a particular form of unsaturated fat, known as trans fatty acids, that may raise blood cholesterol levels, although not as much as saturated fat.

Advice in the previous sections does not apply to infants and toddlers under age 2. After that age, children should gradually adopt a diet that, by age 5, contains no more than 30 percent of calories from fat.

Children by the age of 5 should be getting only 30% of their calories from fat, just like their parents.

5. **Choose a diet moderate in sugars.**

Sugars which are carbohydrates, come in many forms. Dietary carbohydrates also include the complex carbohydrates starch and fiber. During digestion, all carbohydrates except fiber break down into sugars. Sugars and starches occur naturally in many foods that also supply other nutrients. Examples of these foods include milk, fruits, some vegetables, breads, cereals, and grains. Americans eat sugars in many forms, and most people like their taste. Some sugars are used as natural preservatives, thickeners, and baking aids in foods; they are often added to foods during processing and preparation or when they are eaten. The body cannot tell the difference between naturally occurring and added sugars because they are chemically identical.

Scientific evidence indicates that high-sugar diets do not cause hyperactivity or diabetes. If you wish to maintain your weight while eating less fat, replace the lost fat calories with an equal number of calories from fruits, vegetables, and grain products, found in the lower half of the Food Guide Pyramid. Some foods that contain a lot of sugars supply calories but few or no nutrients. These foods are located at the top of the Pyramid. For very active people with high calorie needs, sugars can be an additional source of energy.

Sugar substitutes such as sorbitol, saccharin, and aspartame are added to many foods. Most sugar substitutes do not provide significant calories and therefore may be useful in the diets of people concerned about

TABLE 7-5.   **For healthier teeth and gums:**

- eat fewer foods containing sugars and starches between meals.
- brush and floss teeth regularly.
- use a flouride toothpaste.
- ask your dentist or doctor about the need for supplemental fluoride, especially for children.

calorie intake. Foods containing sugar substitutes, however, may not always be lower in calories than similar products that contain sugars.

Both sugar and starches can promote tooth decay (Table 7-5).

6.   **Choose a diet moderate in salt and sodium.**

Sodium and salt are found mainly in processed and prepared foods. Sodium and sodium chloride—known commonly as salt—occur naturally in foods, usually in small amounts. Salt and other sodium-containing ingredients are often used in food processing. Some people add salt and salty sauces, such as soy sauce, to their food at the table, but most dietary sodium or salt comes from foods to which salt has already been added during processing or preparation. Although many people add salt to enhance the taste of foods, their preference may weaken with eating less salt.

Sodium is associated with high blood pressure. In the body, sodium plays an essential role in regulating fluids and blood pressure. Many studies in diverse populations have shown that a high sodium intake is associated with higher blood pressure. Most evidence suggests that many people at risk for high blood pressure reduce their chances of developing this condition by consuming less salt or sodium. Some questions remain, partly because other factors may interact with sodium to affect blood pressure.

Following other guidelines in the *Dietary Guidelines for Americans* may also help prevent high blood pressure. An important example is the guideline on weight and physical activity. The role of body weight in blood pressure control is well documented. Blood pressure increases with weight and decreases when weight is reduced. The guideline to consume a diet with plenty of fruits and vegetables is relevant because fruits and vegetables are naturally lower in sodium and fat and may help with weight reduction and control. Consuming more fruits and vegetables also increases potassium intake, which may help to reduce blood pressure (Table 7-6). Increased physical activity helps lower blood pressure and control weight.

TABLE 7-6. Some good sources of potassium.

- Vegetables and fruits in general, especially
  - potatoes and sweet potatoes
  - spinach, swiss chard, broccoli, winter squashes, and parsnips
  - dates, bananas, cantaloupes, mangoes, plantains, dried apricots, raisins, prunes, orange juice, and grapefruit juice
  - dry beans, peas, lentils
- Milk and yogurt are good sources of potassium and have less sodium than cheese; cheese has much less potassium and usually has added salt.

TABLE 7-7. To consume less salt and sodium:

- Read the Nutrition Facts Label to determine the amount of sodium in the foods you purchase. The sodium content of processed foods—such as cereals, breads, soups and salad dressings—often varies widely.
- Choose foods lower in sodium and ask you grocer or supermarket to offer more low-sodium foods. Request less salt in your meals when eating out or traveling.
- Add small amounts if you salt foods in cooking or at the table. Learn to use spices and herbs, rather than salt, to enhance the flavor of food.
- When planning meals, consider that fresh and most plain frozen vegetables are low in sodium.
- When selecting canned foods, select those prepared with reduced or no sodium.
- Remember that fresh fish, poultry, and meat are lower in sodium than most canned and processed ones.
- Choose foods lower in sodium content. Many frozen dinners, packaged mixes, canned soups, and salad dressings contain a considerable amount of sodium. Remember that condiments such as soy and many other sauces, pickles, and olives are high in sodium. Ketchup and mustard, when eaten in large amounts, can also contribute significant amounts of sodium to the diet. Choose lower-sodium varieties.
- Choose fresh fruits and vegetables as a lower-sodium alternative to salted snack foods.

Most Americans consume more salt than is needed. The Nutrition Facts Label lists a Daily Value of 2400 mg per day for sodium. One level teaspoon of salt provides about 2300 milligrams of sodium.

Fresh fruits and vegetables have very little sodium. The food groups in the Food Guide Pyramid include some foods that are high in sodium and other foods that have very little sodium, or can be prepared in ways that add flavor without adding salt. Read the Nutrition Facts Label to compare and help identify foods lower in sodium within each group. Use herbs and spices to flavor food. Try to choose forms of foods that you frequently consume that are lower in sodium and salt (Table 7-7).

TABLE 7-8. What is moderation?

Moderation is defined as no more than one drink per day for women and no more than two per day for men.

Count as a drink:
- 12 ounces of regular beer (150 calories)
- 5 ounces of wine (100 calories)
- 1.5 ounces of 80-proof distilled spirits (100 calories)

7. **If you drink alcoholic beverages, do so in moderation.**

Alcoholic beverages have been used to enhance the enjoyment of meals by many societies throughout human history. Unfortunately, they supply calories but few or no nutrients. They also have harmful effects when consumed in excess, including altered judgment, dependency on alcohol, and many other serious health problems. If adults choose to drink alcoholic beverages, they should consume them only in moderation (Table 7-8).

In 1990, an important report, *Healthy People 2000: National Health Promotion and Disease Prevention Objectives,* was released by the Public Health Service/Department of Health and Human Services. The purpose of this report was to improve health promotion and disease prevention. The first national effort to establish a public health agenda for the United States occurred in 1979. Improved nutrition is one of 22 priorities identified in *Healthy People 2000.* Within improved nutrition are 21 subpriorities (Table 7-9). Several objectives aim for specific, measurable changes in what Americans eat, as well as increased accessibility to healthier foods. Throughout, the report emphasizes healthy choices in diet, exercise, weight control, and other risk factors for disease.

MINI-SUMMARY The most recent dietary recommendations, *Dietary Guidelines for Americans* (4th edition), list seven guidelines: eat a variety of foods; balance the food you eat with physical activity—maintain or improve your weight; choose a diet with plenty of grain products, vegetables, and fruits; choose a diet low in fat, saturated fat, and cholesterol; choose a diet moderate in sugars, salt, and sodium, and drink alcoholic beverages in moderation. Included in *Healthy People 2000's* public health agenda are 22 nutrition goals for Americans.

TABLE 7-9. Nutrition Goals from *Healthy People 2000*.

1. Reduce coronary heart disease deaths to no more than 100 per 100,000 people.

2. Reverse the rise in cancer deaths to achieve a rate of no more than 130 per 100,000 people.

3. Reduce overweight to a prevalence of no more than 20 percent among people age 20 and older and no more than 15 percent among adolescents ages 12 through 19.

4. Reduce growth retardation among low-income children ages 5 and younger to less than 10 percent.

5. Reduce dietary fat intake to an average of 30 percent of calories or less and average saturated fat intake to less than 10 percent of calories among people age 2 and older.

6. Increase complex carbohydrates and fiber-containing foods in the diets of adults to 5 or more daily servings for vegetables (including legumes) and fruit, and to 6 or more daily servings for grain products.

7. Increase to at least 50 percent the proportion of overweight people age 12 and older who have adopted sound dietary practices combined with regular physical activity to attain an appropriate body weight.

8. Increase calcium intake so at least 50 percent of youth ages 12 through 24 and 50 percent of pregnant and lactating women consume 3 or more servings daily of foods rich in calcium, and at least 50 percent of people age 24 and older consume 2 or more servings daily.

9. Decrease salt and sodium intake so at least 65 percent of home meal preparers prepare foods without adding salt, at least 80 percent of people avoid using salt at the table, and at least 40 percent of adults regularly purchase foods modified or lower in sodium.

10. Reduce iron deficiency to less than 3 percent among children age 1 through 4 and among women of childbearing age.

11. Increase to at least 75 percent the proportion of mothers who breastfeed their babies in the early postpartum period and to at least 50 percent

the proportion who continue breastfeeding until their babies are 5 to 6 months old.

12. Increase to at least 75 percent the proportion of parents and caregivers who use feeding practices that prevent baby-bottle tooth decay.

13. Increase to at least 85 percent the proportion of people age 18 and older who use food labels to make nutritious food selections.

14. Achieve useful and informative nutrition labeling for virtually all processed foods and at least 40 percent of fresh meats, poultry, fish, fruits, vegetables, baked goods, and ready-to-eat carry-away foods.

15. Increase to at least 5000 brand items the availability of processed food products that are reduced in fat and saturated fat.

16. Increase to at least 90 percent the proportion of restaurants and institutional foodservice operations that offer identifiable low-fat, low-calorie food choices, consistent with the Dietary Guidelines for Americans.

17. Increase to at least 90 percent the proportion of school lunch and breakfast services and childcare foodservices with menus that are consistent with the nutrition principles in the Dietary Guidelines for Americans.

18. Increase to at least 80 percent the receipt of home food services by people age 65 and older who have difficulty in preparing their own meals or are otherwise in need of home-delivered meals.

19. Increase to at least 75 percent the proportion of the nation's schools that provide nutrition education from preschool through grade 12, preferably as part of quality school health education.

20. Increase to at least 50 percent the proportion of worksites with 50 or more employees that offer employee nutrition education and/or weight-management programs.

21. Increase to at least 75 percent the proportion of primary care providers who provide nutrition assessment and counseling and/or referral to qualified nutritionists or dietitians.

MENU PLANNING GUIDES

In this section we discuss two methods for menu planning: food groups and exchange lists.

Food Groups

In 1958 the United States Department of Agriculture published *Food for Fitness—A Daily Food Guide* that included a description of the **basic four food groups**. The four food groups included meats and meat substitutes, milk and milk products, fruits and vegetables, and grains. Each group contained foods of similar origin and nutrient content. For example, the grain group included foods such as breads and cereals made from grains that provide thiamin, niacin, and iron.

According to the basic four food group plan, you should eat at least two servings daily from the meat group, two servings from the milk group, four servings of fruits and vegetables, and four servings of grains. The suggested servings from the four food groups for adults supplies about 1200 calories and provides 80 percent of the 1950s RDAs for protein, vitamins A and C, thiamin, riboflavin, niacin, calcium, and iron. The four food groups were designed to guard against nutrient deficiencies.

The basic four food group concept has also become outdated. When the concept was developed there were RDAs for less than 10 nutrients; in the most recent version (1989) of the RDA, there are requirements for 26 nutrients. Also, the emphasis has switched from eating enough of different foods to prevent deficiencies to balancing your diet to prevent diseases such as heart disease and cancer.

The Food Guide Pyramid is based on consumer research — maybe that's why it's getting more attention than the Basic Four Food Groups.

The Food Guide Pyramid (Figure 7-1), the most recent food guidance system developed by the USDA, is based on USDA's research on what foods Americans eat, what nutrients are in these foods, and how to apply variety, moderation, and balance to your daily meals and snack choices. The Pyramid focuses on fat because most American diets are too high in fat. Following the Pyramid will help you keep your intake of total fat and saturated fat low.

The Pyramid includes foods from the five food groups shown in the three lower sections of the Pyramid.

1. Breads, cereals, rice, and pasta
2. Fruits
3. Vegetables
4. Meat, poultry, fish, dry beans, eggs, and nuts
5. Milk, cheese, and yogurt

TABLE 7-10. What counts as a serving?*

**Grain Products Group
(bread, cereal, rice, and pasta)**
- 1 slice of bread
- 1 ounce of ready-to-eat cereal,
- 1/2 cup of cooked cereal, rice, or pasta

Vegetable Group
- 1 cup of raw leafy vegetables
- 1/2 cup of other vegetables—cooked or chopped raw
- 3/4 cup of vegetable juice

Fruit Group
- 1 medium apple, banana, orange
- 1/2 cup of chopped, cooked, or canned fruit
- 3/4 cup of fruit juice

**Milk Group
(milk, yogurt, and cheese)**
- 1 cup of milk or yogurt
- 1 1/2 ounces of natural cheese
- 2 ounces of processed cheese

**Meat and Beans Group
(meat, poultry, fish, dry beans, eggs, and nuts)**
- 2–3 ounces of cooked lean meat, poultry, or fish
- 1/2 cup of cooked dry beans or 1 egg counts as 1 ounce of lean meat. Two tablespoons of peanut butter or 1/3 cup of nuts count as 1 ounce of meat.

*Some foods fit into more than one group. Dry beans, peas, and lentils can be counted as servings in either the meat and beans group or vegetable group. These "cross over" foods can be counted as servings from either one or the other group, but not both. Serving sizes indicated here are those used in the Food Guide Pyramid and based on both suggested and usually consumed portions necessary to achieve adequate nutrient intake. They differ from serving sizes on the Nutrition Facts Label, which reflect portions usually consumed.

TABLE 7-11. How many servings do you need each day?

	Women & Some Older Adults	Children, Teen Girls Active Women, Most Men	Teen Boys & Active Men
Caloric Level*	About 1600	About 2200	About 2800
Bread group	6	9	11
Vegetable group	3	4	5
Fruit group	2	3	4
Milk group	2–3**	2–3**	2–3**
Meat group	5 ounces	6 ounces	7 ounces
Total fat (grams)	53	73	93

*These are the calorie levels if you choose low-fat, lean foods from the 5 major food groups and use foods from the fats and sweets group sparingly.
**Women who are pregnant or breastfeeding, teenagers, and young adults to age 24 need 3 servings.

Source: U.S. Department of Agriculture and the U.S. Department of Health and Human Services.

Plant foods (grains, vegetables, and fruits) are the foundation of a healthy Pyramid diet.

At the base of the Pyramid are breads, cereals, rice, and pasta—all foods from grains. You need the most servings of these foods each day. Foods from the grain products group, along with vegetables and fruits (the next level), are the basis of healthful diets. Vegetables and fruits are placed on the same level because they both include foods that come from plants. On the next level are two groups of foods that come mostly from animals: milk, yogurt, and cheese; and meats, poultry, fish, dry beans, eggs, and nuts.

The Pyramid shows a range of servings for each major food group. The number of servings that are right for you depends on how many calories you need, which in turn depends on your age, sex, size, and activity level. Almost everyone should have at least the lowest number of servings in the ranges. Serving sizes are listed in Table 7-10, and the suggested number of servings for various individuals are given in Table 7-11. Unfortunately, the Pyramid's serving sizes do not always correspond to the serving sizes on the new food label. This is because the serving sizes on food labels are meant to reflect what people normally eat, whereas the serving sizes for the Pyramid are recommended sizes.

The following suggestions on calorie level are based on recommendations of the National Academy of Sciences and on calorie intakes reported by people in national food-consumption surveys.

1600 calories is about right for many sedentary women and some older adults.

2200 calories is about right for most children, teenage girls, active women, and many sedentary men. Pregnant or breastfeeding women may need somewhat more.

2800 calories is about right for teenage boys, many active men, and some very active women.

The small tip of the Pyramid shows fats, oils, and sweets, such as salad dressings, cream, butter, margarine, sugar, soft drinks, candies, and sweet desserts, but these do not make a food group (there are no pictures at the tip of the Pyramid). These foods supply calories and little else nutritionally; most people should use them sparingly. Some fat symbols (teardrops) or added sugar symbols (rectangles) are shown in the other food groups. That's to remind you that some foods in these groups can also be high in fat and added sugars. Many foods in the milk, meat, and beans groups (which include egg and nuts, as well as meat, poultry, and fish) are also high in fat, as are some processed foods in the grain group. Choosing lower-fat options among these foods allows you to eat the recommended

TABLE 7-12. **Checklist for healthy menus.**

If you write out your menus, select several to help you answer the questions below. Then answer the following questions.

	YES	NO
1. Does a day's menu provide at least the lower number of servings from each of the major food groups?		
6 servings of grain products?	____	____
2 servings of fruit?	____	____
3 servings of vegetables?	____	____
2–3 servings of lean meat or the equivalent (totaling 5 ounces per day)?	____	____
2 servings of milk, yogurt, or cheese?	____	____
2. Do the menus have several servings of whole-grain breads or cereals each day?	____	____
3. Do menus for a week include several servings of:		
Dark-green leafy vegetables, such as spinach, broccoli, romaine lettuce?	____	____
Dry beans or peas, such as kidney beans, split peas, lentils?	____	____
4. Do menus include some vegetables and fruits with skins and seeds (baked potatoes with skin, summer squash, berries, apples, or pears with peels)?	____	____
5. Underline all of the foods in your menus that are high in fat, sugars, or sodium.		
Are other foods that are served with them lower in fat, sugars, or sodium?	____	____
Are other meals on the same day lower in fat, sugar, or sodium, so that total intake is moderate?	____	____
6. Are the menus practical for you in time, cost, and family acceptance?	____	____

Source: Preparing Foods and Planning Menus Using the Dietary Guidelines, U.S. Department of Agriculture, Home and Garden Bulletin No. 232–238, 1990.

servings from these groups and increase the amount and variety of grain products, fruits, and vegetables in your diet without going over your calorie needs. When choosing foods for a healthful diet, consider the fat and added sugars in your choices from all the food groups, not just fats and sweets from the Pyramid tip.

You can achieve a healthful, nutritious eating pattern with many combinations of foods from the five major food groups. Choosing a variety of foods within and across food groups improves dietary patterns because foods within the same group have different combinations of nutrients and other beneficial substances. It also makes meals more interesting. Meals can have rice, pasta, potatoes, or bread at the center of the plate, accompanied by other vegetables and fruit, and lean and low-fat foods from the other groups.

Table 7-12 is a checklist for healthy menus.

TABLE 7-13. Nutrient content of exchange lists.

Groups/Lists	Carbohydrate (grams)	Protein (grams)	Fat (Grams)	Calories
Carbohydrate Group				
Starch	15	3	1 or less	80
Fruit	15	—	—	60
Milk				
Skim	12	8	0-3	90
Low-fat	12	8	5	120
Whole	12	8	8	150
Other carbohydrates	15	varies	varies	varies
Vegetables	5	2	—	25
Meat and Meat Substitute Group				
Very lean	—	7	0-1	35
Lean	—	7	3	55
Medium-fat	—	7	5	75
High-fat	—	7	8	100
Fat Group	—	—	5	45

Source: Exchange Lists for Meal Planning, 1995, American Diabetes Association and American Diabetic Association.

Exchange Lists

Whereas the food group system groups foods by their protein, vitamin, and mineral content, the exchange system groups foods by their calorie, carbohydrate, fat, and protein content. Each food on a list has approximately the same amount of calories, carbohydrate, fat, and protein as another in the portions listed, so that any listed food can be exchanged for any other food on the same list.

The **Exchange Lists for Meal Planning** have been developed by the American Diabetes and American Dietetic Association for use primarily by diabetics who need to regulate what and how much they eat (see Appendix D). They are also often used in weight control because they are relatively easy to learn and master, and they afford a good deal of control over calorie intake. There are seven exchange lists of like foods. Each food on a list has approximately the same amount of calories, carbohydrate, fat, and protein as another in the portions listed, so that any food on a list can be exchanged, or traded, for any other food on the same list (see Table 7-13). The seven exchange lists are starch, fruit, milk, other carbohydrates,

Exchange lists have also been developed for diabetics and individuals with renal disease.

vegetables, meat and meat substitutes, and fat. Diabetics can exchange starch, fruit, or milk choices within their meal plans because they all have about the same amount of carbohydrate per serving. Chapter 11 goes into more detail about diabetics and the diabetic diet.

Each exchange list has a typical member with an easy-to-remember portion size:

Starch—1 slice bread, 80 calories
Meat—1 ounce lean meat, 55 calories
Vegetable—1/2 cup cooked vegetable, 25 calories
Fruit—1 small apple, 60 calories
Milk—1 cup skim milk, 90 calories
Fat—1 teaspoon margarine, 45 calories

The meat exchange is broken down into very lean, lean, medium-fat, and high-fat meat and meat alternates. Very lean and lean meats are encouraged. The milk exchange contains skim, low-fat, and whole-milk exchanges. Fats are divided into three groups, based on the main type of fat they contain: monounsaturated, polyunsaturated, or saturated. There is also a listing of free foods that contain negligible calories.

Both systems have their good and bad points. Whereas the Food Guide Pyramid plan encourages variety, nutrient adequacy, and balance—no group of foods is overemphasized—the Exchange Lists also promote moderation and variety. The Food Guide Pyramid is easier to use, but the Exchange Lists are more accurate in terms of calories and nutrients consumed.

MINI-SUMMARY Both food groups and exchange lists can assist in menu planning. The newest food group concept is the Food Guide Pyramid, which includes five food groups and displays plant foods (grains, vegetables, and fruits) as the foundation of a healthy diet. The most popular set of exchange lists were designed for diabetics. The exchange system groups foods by their calorie, carbohydrate, fat, and protein content. Each food on a list can be traded for any other food on that list.

USING THE NEW FOOD LABELS

Food labels have become scorecards for millions of health-conscious Americans. Facts found on labels tell not only what the product is but what ingredients are in it, manufacturer information, nutrition information, and frequently sell-by or use-by dates.

Figure 7-2.
Food label

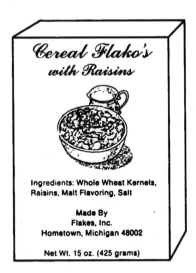

Since 1938 the federal government has required basic information on food labels. The Food and Drug Administration (FDA) regulates labels on all packaged foods except for meat, poultry, and egg products—foods regulated by the U.S. Department of Agriculture (USDA). The amount of information on food labels varies, but all food labels must contain at least:

Read the food label and set a better table!

The name of the food

The net contents or net weight—the quantity of the food itself without the packaging (in English and metric units)

The name and place of business of the manufacturer, packer, or distributor

A list of ingredients.

Nutrition information is also required for most foods, our next topic.

For most foods, all ingredients must be listed on the label and must be identified by their common names to help consumers identify ingredients that they are allergic to or want to avoid for other reasons. The ingredient that is present in the largest amount, by weight, must be listed first. Other ingredients follow in descending order according to weight (Figure 7-2). This gives consumers an idea of an ingredient's proportion of in a food.

The FDA has always required that the ingredients of packaged foods be listed on the labels. But certain common foods, such as mayonnaise,

TABLE 7-14. Product dates.

Pull Date. This is the last day that the manufacturer recommends that the product remain on sale. This date takes into consideration additional time for storage and use at home, so if the food is bought on the pull date, it still can be eaten at a later date. How long the product should be offered for sale and how much home storage is allowed are determined by the manufacturer, based on knowledge of the product and the product's shelf life.

Quality assurance or freshness date. This date shows how long the manufacturer thinks a food will be of optimal quality. The label, may read: "Best if used by October 1996." This doesn't mean, however, that the product shouldn't be used after the suggested date.

Pack date. This is the date the food was packaged or processed.

Expiration date. This is the last day on which a product should be eaten. State governments regulate these dates for perishable items, such as milk and eggs.

---

macaroni, and bread, made according to "standard" recipes set by the FDA, were exempt from this requirement. The FDA now considers listing all ingredients necessary even for standardized foods, mainly because many of today's consumers, unlike their parents or grandparents, don't know what these foods are made of. The FDA now requires the following:

- The listing of all FDA-certified color additives by name.
- Identification of caseinate as a milk derivative when used in foods that claim to be nondairy, such as coffee whiteners, because some people with milk allergies use nondairy products.
- Declaration of sulfites used in standardized foods because some people are allergic to these preservatives.
- Declaration of protein hydrolysates, used in many foods as flavors and flavor enhancers. Most important, for consumers with religious or cultural dietary requirements, the food source of the additive must be identified.
- Declaration of monosodium glutamate (MSG), a flavor enhancer, whether added as a separate ingredient or as a component of protein hydrolysates.
- Declaration of the percentage of actual fruit or vegetable juice on the label of all juice beverages, whether full strength or diluted. Juice blends that identify individual juices on the labels must declare the percentage of each identified juice.

FIGURE 7-3.

Location of
nutrition facts

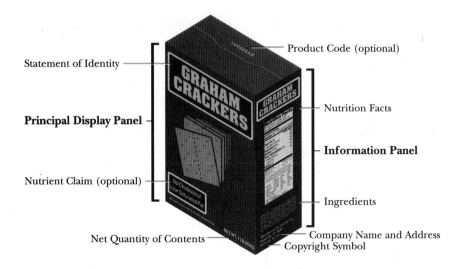

FIGURE 7-3.

Location of nutrition facts

Statement of Identity

Product Code (optional)

Principal Display Panel

Nutrition Facts

Information Panel

Nutrient Claim (optional)

Ingredients

Net Quantity of Contents

Company Name and Address
Copyright Symbol

Labels also often contain product dates. Table 7-14 explains the different types of product dates on food packages.

Nutrition Facts

Under the Nutrition Labeling and Education Act of 1990 and regulations from the Food and Drug Administration and the U.S. Department of Agriculture, virtually all food labels must now give information about a food's nutritional content. Nutrition information is mandatory on processed foods that are meaningful sources of nutrients—that is, on about 90 percent of processed foods. Excluded are plain coffee and tea, most spices, small packages (generally those no larger than a package of Life Savers), and foods produced by small businesses (those with food sales of less than $50,000 a year or total sales of less than $500,000 a year).

The basics on how to read "Nutrition Facts" (see Figure 7-3 and 6-2) are covered in the last section of Chapter 1. In addition, "Label Reading Questions and Answers" (Chapters 1 through 6) explain how to read labels specifically for information on calorie, carbohydrates, fat, protein, vitamins, and minerals.

For raw fruits and vegetables, grocery stores are asked to provide nutrition information on the 20 most frequently consumed items in each category. This program is voluntary, and if at least 60 percent of stores display the information, the guidelines will continue to be voluntary. Nutrition information for fresh meat, poultry, and seafood is probably also available in appropriate sections of the supermarket.

A modified form of nutrition labeling is required for vitamin and mineral supplements. The label will show the amount and percent of the Daily Value of all vitamins and minerals, and the amount of calories and food components—such as fat, carbohydrates, or fiber—present in more than insignificant amounts. (Daily Values are a guide to the total nutrient amount you need for a day based on a 2000-calorie diet.)

Nutrient Claims

The FDA now has a dictionary that food producers, marketers, and consumers can consult for consistent and uniform definitions on an expanded list of nutrient content claims. Phrases such as "high in calcium," "low fat," "sugar free"—describe the amount of a nutrient in a food but don't tell exactly how much. These **nutrient content claims** differ from Nutrition Facts, which do list specific nutrient amounts. You need to read them both. Together, nutrient content claims and Nutrition Facts help you compare one food with another and choose foods for a healthful diet.

Consider a package of macaroni and cheese. The claim might say "rich in calcium." The Nutrition Facts panel shows that one serving supplies 20 percent of the Daily Value for calcium. Macaroni and cheese really is an excellent calcium source. Of course, when you use nutrient content claims in choosing foods, always check the other nutrients on the Nutrition Facts panel to see how the food fits into your overall diet.

Products must meet strict nutrition requirements before they can carry these claims. Daily Values help define nutrient content claims. For example, to say "high in fiber," a food must provide at least 20 percent of the Daily Value for fiber—that is, 5 grams of fiber per serving. The government strictly defines terms such as: *free, low, high, reduced, less, light, fewer, more* and *good source.* Table 7-15 gives more information on each descriptor.

If a food label contains a descriptor for a certain nutrient but the food contains other nutrients at levels known to be less healthy, the label would have to bring that to consumers' attention. For example, if a food making a low-sodium claim is also high in fat, the label must state "see back panel for information about fat and other nutrients."

Health Claims

The Nutrition Labeling and Education Act of 1990 provided, for the first time, the specific statutory authority to allow food labels to carry claims about the relationship between the food and specific diseases or health conditions. This was a major shift in labeling philosophy. Until 1984, a food product making such a claim on its label was treated as a

TABLE 7-15.   Food and Drug Administration label dictionary.

Just like the Nutrition Facts, nutrient content claims are defined for one serving. For example, that means that a high-fiber cereal has 5 or more grams of fiber *per serving*.

Nutrient (Content Claim)	**Definition** (per serving)
CALORIES	
Calorie free	less than 5 calories
Low calorie	40 calories or less
Reduced or fewer calories	at least 25% fewer calories*
Light or lite	one-third fewer calories or 50% less fat*
SUGAR	
Sugar free	less than 0.5 gram sugars
Reduced sugar or less sugar	at least 25% less sugars*
No added sugar	no sugars added during processing or packing, including ingredients that contain sugars, such as juice or dry fruit
FAT	
Fat free	less than 0.5 gram fat
Low fat	3 grams or less of fat
Reduced or less fat	at least 25% less fat*
Light	one-third fewer calories of 50% less fat*
SATURATED FAT	
Saturated fat free	less than 0.5 gram saturated fat
Low saturated fat	1 gram or less saturated fat and no more than 15% of calories from saturated fat
Reduced or less saturated fat	at least 25% less saturated fat*
CHOLESTEROL	
Cholesterol free	less than 2 milligrams cholesterol and 2 grams or less of saturated fat
Low cholesterol	20 milligrams or less cholesterol and 2 grams or less of saturated fat
Reduced or less cholesterol	at least 25% less cholesterol* and 2 grams or less saturated fat
SODIUM	
Sodium free	less than 5 milligrams sodium
Very low sodium	35 milligrams or less sodium
Low sodium	140 milligrams or less sodium
Reduced or less sodium	at least 25% less sodium*
Light in sodium	50% less*
FIBER	
High fiber	5 grams or more
Good source of fiber	2.5 to 4.9 grams
More or added fiber	at least 2.5 grams more*
OTHER CLAIMS	
High, rich in, excellent source of	20% or more of Daily Value*
Good source, contains, provides	10% to 19% of Daily Value*
More, enriched, fortified, added	10% or more of Daily Value*
Lean**	less than 10 grams fat, 4.5 grams or less saturated fat, and 95 milligrams cholesterol
Extra lean**	less than 5 grams fat, 2 grams saturated fat, and 95 milligrams cholesterol

*as compared with a standard serving size of the traditional food
**on meat, poultry, seafood, and game meats

drug and considered misbranded unless the claim was backed up by an approved new drug application.

The FDA has examined the scientific evidence on relationships between ten nutrients and the risks of certain diseases, and has authorized eight such claims—the only ones that can be used in a label. The claims may show a link between the following.

- Calcium and osteoporosis. A calcium-rich diet is linked to a reduced risk of osteoporosis, a condition in which the bones become soft or brittle.
- Fat and cancer. A diet low in total fat is linked to a reduced risk of some cancers.
- Saturated fat and cholesterol and heart disease. A diet low in saturated fat and cholesterol can help reduce the risk of heart disease.
- Fiber-containing grain products, fruits, and vegetables and cancer. A diet rich in high-fiber grain products, fruits, and vegetables can reduce the risk of some cancers.
- Fruits, vegetables, and grain products that contain fiber and heart disease. A diet rich in fruits, vegetables, and grain products that contain fiber can help reduce the risk of heart disease.
- Sodium and high blood pressure. A low-sodium diet may help reduce the risk of heart disease.
- Fruits and vegetables and some cancers. A low-fat diet rich in fruits and vegetables (foods that are low in fat and may contain dietary fiber, vitamin A, or vitamin C) is linked to a reduced risk of some cancers.
- Folic acid and neural tube birth defects. Women who consume 0.4 mg of folic acid daily reduce their risk of giving birth to a child affected with a neural tube defect.

The wording on health claims may differ. For example, a claim on a macaroni and cheese package linking calcium and osteoporosis reads:

> Regular exercise and a healthy diet with enough calcium helps teen and young adult white and Asian women maintain good bone health and may reduce their risk of osteoporosis later in life.

Regulations for the general requirements for health claims set forth a number of definitions to clarify their meanings. One of the most significant defines certain nutrient levels that would disqualify a health claim. Disqualified are those foods that contain more than 13 grams of fat, 4 grams of saturated fat, 60 milligrams of cholesterol, or 480 milligrams of sodium per amount commonly consumed, per labeled serving size, and per 100 grams (about 3 ounces).

MINI-SUMMARY All food labels must contain the name of the product; the net contents or net weight; the name and place of business of the manufacturer, packer, or distributor; a list of ingredients in order of predominance by weight; and nutrition information. Figure 7-3 explains how to read "Nutrition Facts." Any nutrient or health claims on food labels must comply with Food and Drug Administration regulations and definitions.

KEY TERMS

Basic four food groups
Dietary Guidelines for Americans
Dietary recommendations
Exchange Lists for Meal Planning
Food Guide Pyramid
Healthy People 2000: National Health Promotion
    and Disease Prevention Objectives
Nutrient content claims

REVIEW QUESTIONS

In your own words, answer the following questions.

1. What is the name of the most recent set of U.S. dietary recommendations? List the seven recommendations made and give a tip for implementing each one.
2. Should the Food Pyramid or other U.S. dietary recommendations be applied to diets consumed over several days and or to single meals or foods?
3. What was the purpose of the *Healthy People 2000* report? Give five examples of nutrition objectives given in this report.
4. Draw the Food Guide Pyramid and include five examples of each group, their serving sizes, and recommended number of servings per day from each group.
5. Where do fats, oils, and sweets fit into the Food Guide Pyramid?
6. What do the teardrops and inverted rectangles stand for on the Pyramid?
7. Why are the foods in the base of the Pyramid so important?
8. Describe how the exchange lists work. For which group were they originally designed?
9. Name each exchange list and give an example of a food from it and the food's calorie content.
10. What mandatory information is on food labels?
11. What is a nutrient claim? Give an example. How are nutrient claims regulated?
12. What is a health claim? Give an example. How are health claims regulated?

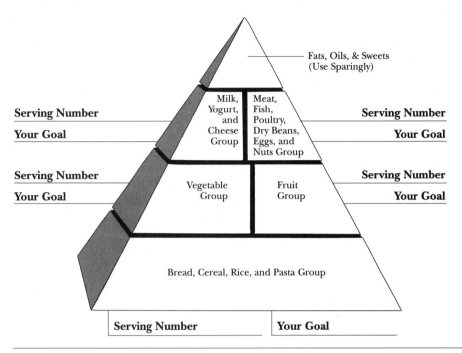

FIGURE 7-4.
Pyramid check-up

---

1. Quiz

Check your answers.

1. Breads, cereals, and other grain products   6 servings
2. Fruits   2 servings
3. Vegetables   3 servings
4. Meat, poultry, fish, and alternates   2 servings
5. Milk, cheese, and yogurt   2 to 3 servings
   (3 servings of the dairy group are needed by breastfeeding or pregnant women, teenagers, and young adults up to age 24.)

2. Pyramid Check-Up

Using Table 7-11 as a guide, estimate the minimum number of servings you need from each group in the Pyramid. Enter those numbers on the lines on the Pyramid that read "Your Goal" (Figure 7-4).

Next, record the foods and serving sizes (estimate as best you can) of what you ate yesterday. Using Table 7-10, determine how many Pyramid servings you had and write your totals on the Pyramid labeled "Serving Number." How does your intake compare to the recommended intake? Do you consume at least the minimum number of servings from each group? If not, identify three ways you can better balance your diet.

3. Supermarket Sleuth

Examine foods from each of the following supermarket sections, and write down nutrient claims (such as "low fat") given on at least two different foods from each section. (Don't forget—fresh fruits and vegetables, meat, poultry, and seafood don't have labels—look for nutrition information nearby.) Also look at the label to see what nutrition facts support this claim.

Produce
Frozen foods
Fresh meats, poultry, and fish dairy
Cereals
Cookies

During your search, find one food item with a health claim and write it down.

4. Label Reading at Breakfast

Look closely at the "Nutrition Facts" for each food you normally eat for breakfast, such as cereal, milk, and juice. Add up the Percent Daily Values for fat, saturated fat, cholesterol, sodium, total carbohydrate, protein, vitamin A, vitamin C, calcium, and iron. How nutritious is your breakfast?

5. Label Comparison

Here are labels from regular mayonnaise and low-fat mayonnaise dressing. Which is which? Compare and contrast the labels.

Nutrition Facts	*Nutrition Facts*
(Serving size: 1 tablespoon)	(Serving size: 1 tablespoon)
Amount per serving	Amount per serving
Calories 25	Calories 100
Calories from fat 10	Calories from fat 99
Total fat 1 g	Total fat 11 g
Saturated 0 g	Saturated 2 g
Polyunsaturated 0.5 g	Polyunsaturated 6 g
Monounsaturated 0 g	Monounsaturated 3 g
Cholesterol 0 mg	Cholesterol 5 mg
Sodium 140 mg	Sodium 180 mg
Total carbohydrate 4 g	Total carbohydrate 0 g
Sugars 3 g	Sugars 0 g
Protein 0 g	Protein 0 g

Not a significant source of dietary fiber, vitamin A, vitamin C, calcium, and iron.

6. Exchange Lists

Using the Exchange Lists for Meal Planning, write a lunch menu using the following exchanges.

2 starches
2 meats/meat substitutes
1 vegetable
1 fruit
1 milk
1 fat
Any free foods

7. Menu Evaluation

This is one day's menu for an adult woman. Suggest some changes to increase nutrients, starch, and fiber and to moderate fat, sugars, and sodium?

Breakfast
1 grapefruit with 1 teaspoon sugar
1 slice white toast with 1 teaspoon margarine and 1 teaspoon jam
1 cup coffee with 1 tablespoon nondairy creamer

Lunch
1 hot-dog bun
1 hot dog with mustard
Coleslaw (1/2 cup cabbage with 2 tablespoons carrot and 2 tablespoons mayonnaise)
1 dill pickle strip
1 can of cola

Snack
4 vanilla sandwich cookies

Dinner
3 ounces roast beef with 2 tablespoons gravy
1/2 cup canned corn
Salad (1 cup iceberg lettuce, 1/2 tomato, 2 tablespoons Italian dressing)
1 slice apple pie
1 cup 2 percent milk

Snack
1/2 cup ice cream

REFERENCES   Achterberg, Cheryl, Elaine McDonnell, and Robin Bagby. 1994. How to put the Food Guide Pyramid into practice. *Journal of tthe American Dietetic Association* 94(9): 1030–1035.

American Diabetes Association and American Dietetic Association. 1995. *Exchange Lists for Meal Planning.* Alexandria, VA: American Diabetes Association.

American Dietetic Association. 1995. Position of the American Dietetic Association: Food and nutrition misinformation. *Journal of the American Dietetic Association* 95(6): 705–707.

Barrett, Steven. 1990. *Health Schemes, Scams, and Frauds.* Mt. Vernon, NY: Consumer Reports Books.

Committee on Diet and Health, Food and Nutrition Board, National Research Council. 1989. *Diet and Health: Implications for Reducing Chronic Disease Risk.* Washington, DC: National Academy Press.

Danford, Darla E., and Marilyn G. Stephenson. 1991. Healthy People 2000: Development of nutrition objectives. *Journal of the American Dietetic Association* 91(12): 1517–1519.

Department of Health and Human Services, Public Health Service, U.S. Food and Drug Administration, and International Food Information Council Foundation. 1994. *The New Food Label: There's Something in It for Everybody.* Rockville, MD: Food and Drug Administration.

Haughton, Betsy, Joan Dye Gussow, and Janice M. Dodds. 1987. An historical study of the underlying assumptions for United States food guides from 1917 through the Basic Four Food Group Guide. *Journal of Nutrition Education* 19(4): 169–176.

Havas, S., J. Heimendinger, K. Reynolds, R. Baranowski, T. A. Nicklas, D. Bishop, D. Buller, G. Sorensen, S. A. A. Beresford, A. Cowan, and D. Damron, 1995. 5 a day for better health: A new research initiative. *Journal of the American Dietetic Association* 94(1): 32–36.

Jarvis, William T. 1980. Food quackery is dangerous business. *Nutrition News* 43(1): 1–2.

Kurtzweil, Paula. 1994. Food label close-up. *FDA Consumer*

Short, Sarah. 1994. Health quackery: Our role as professionals. *Journal of the American Dietetic Association* 94(6): 607–611.

Truswell, A. Stewart. 1987. Evolution of dietary recommendations, goals, and guidelines. *American Journal of Clinical Nutrition* 45(5): 1060–1072.

U.S. Department of Agriculture. 1994. *The Food Label, the Pyramid, and You.* Home and Garden Bulletin Number 266.

U.S. Department of Agriculture and Human Nutrition Information Service. 1992. *The Food Guide Pyramid.* Home and Garden Bulletin No. 252.

U.S. Department of Agriculture and Human Nutrition Information Service. *Preparing Foods & Planning Menus Using the Dietary Guidelines.* Home and Garden Bulletin No. 232-8.

U.S. Department of Agriculture and Human Nutrition Information Service. *Shopping for Food & Making Meals in Minutes Using the Dietary Guidelines.* Home and Garden Bulletin No. 232-10.

U.S. Department of Agriculture and U.S. Department of Health and Human Services. 1995. *Nutrition and Your Health: Dietary Guidelines for Americans,* 4th ed. Home and Garden Bulletin.

U.S. Department of Health and Human Services, Public Health Service. 1988. *The Surgeon General's Report on Nutrition and Health: Summary and Recommendations.* Washington, DC: U.S. Government Printing Office.

U.S. Department of Health and Human Services, Public Health Service. 1991. *Healthy People 2000: National Health Promotion and Disease Prevention Objectives.* Washington, DC: U.S. Government Printing Office.

U.S. Department of Health and Human Services, Public Health Service, and National Institutes of Health. 1992. *Fast & Easy: Fruits and Vegetables for Busy People.* NIH Publication No. 93-3247.

Food Facts: 5 a Day For Better Health!

In 1991 the National Cancer Institute introduced its 5 a Day for Better Health Program to encourage Americans to eat 5 or more servings of fruits and vegetables every day (the Food Guide Pyramid recommends at least 3 servings of vegetables and 2 servings of fruits). Overall Americans eat about 2.5 servings of fruits and vegetables daily. The program is a joint venture of the National Cancer Institute and the Produce for Better Health Foundation, a nonprofit foundation representing the fruit and vegetable industry.

Many fruits and vegetables are rich sources of vitamins and other nutrients and most contain dietary fiber. They have no cholesterol and almost all are naturally low in calories, fat, and sodium (see Table 7-16). One serving is 1/2 cup of fruit, 3/4 cup juice, 1/2 cup cooked vegetable, 1 cup leafy vegetable (such as leaf lettuce), or 1/4 cup dried fruit. It is recommended that you eat at least 1 vitamin-A-rich selection (such as apricots, cantaloupe, papaya, broccoli, carrots, spinach, sweet potatoes, or tomatoes) and one vitamin-C-rich selection (such as citrus fruits, cantaloupe, honeydew, strawberries, watermelon, broccoli, or tomatoes) every day.

Fruits and vegetables may lower your risk of cancer. It is estimated that 35 percent of all cancer deaths are related to what we eat—a diet high in fat and low in fiber. Fruits and vegetables help reduce your risk of cancer because they are low in fat and are rich sources of vitamin A, vitamin C, and fiber. A low-fat diet that is low in saturated fat and cholesterol and includes plenty of high-fiber foods also decreases the risk of heart disease.

How close are you to eating 5 fruits and vegetables a day? How many servings of fruits or vegetables did you eat yesterday?

At breakfast   _____
At lunch   _____
At dinner   _____
For a snack   _____
For dessert   _____
Total   _____

To work more fruits and vegetables into your diet, try one or more of the following tips.

FOR BREAKFAST:

Drink a glass of juice.

Add sliced bananas or fruit to your cereal.

Have a bowl of fruit such as melon or peaches.

Top your pancakes with fruit instead of syrup.

FOR LUNCH:

Have a salad or soup that contains vegetables.

Add zucchini, carrot, or celery sticks to your brown bag lunch.

Eat a piece of fresh fruit, such as an apple or orange, or a couple of plums or kiwis.

Add greens, sprouts, and tomatoes to your sandwich.

FOR A SNACK:

Nibble on some grapes or a banana.

Take along some dried fruit, such as raisins, apricots, prunes, or figs. Keep assorted dried fruits in the glove compartment of your car for a quick snack anytime.

Have a glass of juice.

Keep cut raw vegetables in the refrigerator.

FOR DINNER:

Add vegetables to your main dishes, such as broccoli to your pasta or casserole.

Add raw vegetables or fruit to your green salad.

Use fruits as a garnish on main dishes.

Serve two vegetables.

FOR DESSERT:

Liven up a plain dessert with fresh fruit.

Top your frozen yogurt with pineapple or papaya.

Add chopped fruit or berries to muffins, cakes, or cookies.

If you don't like peeling and chopping fruits and vegetables, select ones that require little peeling and chopping, such as baby carrots, cherry tomatoes, grapes, apples, or broccoli spears. Also, supermarkets are now doing the slicing and dicing, so you can buy ready-to-eat fruit and vegetables.

TABLE 7-16. **Nutritional content of fresh produce.**

	Household Serving Sizes	Serving Size (g)	Serving Size (oz)	Calories (Kcal)	Fat (g)	Sodium (mg)	Dietary Fiber (g)	(% of U.S. RDA) Vit. A	Vit. C	Calcium	Iron
Apple	1 med. apple	154	5.5	80	1	0	5	*	6	*	*
Asparagus	5 spears	93	3.5	18	0	0	2	10	10	*	*
Avocado	1/3 med. avocado	55	2	120	12	5	2	*	5	*	*
Banana	1 med. banana	126	4.5	120	1	0	3	*	15	*	2
Bell pepper	1 med. pepper	148	5.5	25	1	0	2	2	130	*	*
Broccoli	1 med. stalk	148	5.5	40	1	75	5	10	240	6	4
Cabbage	1/12 med. head	84	3	18	0	30	2	*	70	4	*
Cantaloupe	1/4 med. melon	134	5	50	0	35	0	80	90	2	2
Carrot	1 med. 7" long 1 1/4" diameter	78	3	40	1	40	1	330	8	2	*
Cauliflower	1/6 med. head	99	3	18	0	45	2	*	110	2	2
Celery	2 med. stalks	110	4	20	0	140	2	*	15	4	*
Cherry	21 cherries; 1 cup	140	5	90	1	0	3	*	10	2	*
Cucumber	1/3 med. cucumber	99	3.5	18	0	0	0	4	6	2	2
Grape	1½ cups grapes	138	5	85	0	3	2	3	9	2	2
Grapefruit	1/2 med. grapefruit	154	5.5	50	0	0	6	6	90	4	*
Green bean	3/4 cup cut beans	83	3	14	0	0	3	2	8	4	*
Green onion	1/4 cup chopped	25	1	7	0	0	0	3	20	*	5
Honeydew	1/10 med. melon	134	5	50	0	50	1	*	40	*	2
Iceberg lettuce	1/6 med. head	89	3	20	0	10	1	2	4	*	*
Kiwifruit	2 med. kiwifruit	148	5.5	90	1	0	4	2	230	4	4
Leaf lettuce	1 1/2 cups shredded	85	3	12	0	40	1	20	4	4	*
Lemon	1 med. lemon	58	2	18	0	10	0	*	35	2	*
Lime	1 med. lime	67	2.5	20	0	1	3	*	35	2	2
Mushrooms	5 med. mushrooms	84	3	25	0	0	0	*	2	*	*
Nectarine	1 med. nectarine	140	5	70	1	0	3	20	10	*	*
Onion	1 med. onion	148	5.5	60	0	10	3	*	20	4	*
Oranges	1 med. orange	154	5.5	50	0	0	6	*	120	4	*
Peach	2 med. peaches	174	6	70	0	0	1	20	20	*	*
Pear	1 med. pear	166	6	100	1	1	4	*	10	2	2
Pineapple	2 slices, 3" diameter 3/4" thick	112	4	90	1	10	2	*	35	*	*
Plum	2 med. plums	132	4.5	70	1	0	1	9	20	*	*
Potato	1 med. potato	148	5.5	110	0	10	3	*	50	*	8
Radishes	7 radishes	85	3	20	0	35	0	*	30	*	*
Strawberries	8 med. berries	147	5.5	50	0	0	3	*	140	2	2
Summer squash	1/2 med. squash	98	3.5	20	0	0	1	4	25	2	2
Sweet corn	kernels from 1 med. ear	90	3	75	1	15	1	5	10	*	3
Sweet potato	1 med. 5" long, 2" diameter	130	4.5	140	0	15	3	520	50	3	4
Tangerine	2 med., 2 3/8" diameter	168	6	70	0	2	2	30	85	2	*
Tomato	1 med. tomato	148	5.5	35	1	10	1	20	40	*	2
Watermelon	1/18 med. melon; 2 cups diced	280	10	80	0	10	1	8	25	*	2

*Contains less than 2% of the U.S. RDA of this nutrient.
Source: U.S. Food and Drug Administration.

The *U.S. Surgeon General's Report on Nutrition and Health* defines food quackery as "the promotion for profit of special foods, products, processes, or appliances with false or misleading health or therapeutic claims." Have you ever seen advertisements for supplements that are guaranteed to help you lose weight or herbal remedies to prevent serious disease? If a product claim seems just too good to be true, it probably is too good to be true. The problem with quackery is not just loss of money—you can be harmed as well. When you listen to a quack, you usually stop your regular medical treatment and don't receive, or even seek, further care from a legitimate medical professional.

Nutrition is brimming with quackery, in part because different cultures attribute health-promoting characteristics to certain foods and also because nutrition is such a young science. Research on many fundamental nutrition issues, such as the relationship between sodium and hypertension, is far from being resolved, yet research scientists publicize their results long before the results can be said to really prove a scientific theory. Unfortunately, because much research is only in its early stages, the public has been bombarded with conflicting ideas about issues that relate directly to two very important parts of their lives: their health and their eating habits. This conflict leaves the public confused about the truth, and vulnerable to dubious health products (most often nutrition products) and practices—on which people spend between $10 to $30 billion annually.

Misinformation proliferates because in many states anyone can call him or herself a dietitian or nutritionist. Only about half the states require a license to use the title "dietitian." In addition, one may even buy mail-order B.S., M.S., or Ph.D. degrees in nutrition from "schools" in the United States. In all states, nutrition books that are entirely bogus can be published and sold. Unfortunately, they should be sold in the fiction section but wind up looking just like legitimate health books.

A quack is someone who makes excessive promises and guarantees that a nutrition product or practice will enhance your physical and mental health by, for example, preventing or curing a disease, extending your life, or improving some facet of your performance. Here's how to recognize a quack:

1. Their promises are too good to be true. For example, lecithin pills will burn fat, or a certain nutrition product is a miracle cure for a disease.
2. They use dubious diagnostic tests, such as hair analysis, to detect supposed nutritional deficiencies and illnesses. Then they offer a variety of nutritional supplements such as bee pollen, coenzyme Q, or spirulina as remedies against deficiencies and disease.
3. They rely on testimonials as proof of effectiveness.
4. They place too much importance on diet and its connection to disease. Some use food essentially as medicine.
5. They often lack any valid medical or health care credentials.
6. They come across more as salespeople than as medical professionals.
7. They offer simple answers to complex problems.

8. They claim to be persecuted and sabotaged by governmental and medical institutions.
9. Their theories and promises are not written in medical journals using a peer review process but appear in books written only for the lay public.

But where can you find accurate nutritional information? In the United States the largest and most visible group of professionals in the nutrition field are the over 50,000 registered dietitians (RDs). Registered dietitians are recognized by the medical profession as the legitimate providers of nutrition care. They have specialized education in human anatomy and physiology, diet therapy, foods and food science, the behavioral sciences, and foodservice management. Registered dietitians must complete at least a bachelor's degree, an internship or equivalent experience, and a qualifying examination. Continuing education is required to maintain RD status. Registered dietitians work in private practice, hospitals, nursing homes, wellness centers, business and industry, and many other settings. Most are members of the American Dietetic Association.

For answers to your nutrition questions, try the following sources:

National Center for Nutrition and Dietetics (the public education initiative of the American Dietetic Association and its Foundation)—Consumer Nutrition Hot Line: 1(800)366-1655

Your county's Cooperative Extension service

County or state health departments

University nutrition or home economics departments

Hospital food and nutrition departments.

Local or state offices of the American Dietetic Association, American Home Economics Association, American Medical Association, or American Heart Association.

National Cancer Institute—call 1(800)4-CANCER. Hours: Monday through Friday, 9 am to 10 pm Eastern time. Closed on holidays.

In addition to using the expertise of an RD, you can ask some simple questions that will help you judge the validity of nutrition information seen in the media or heard from friends.

1. What are the credentials of the source? Does the person have academic degrees in a scientific or nutrition-related field?
2. Does the source rely on emotions rather than scientific evidence or use sensationalism to get a message across?
3. Are the promises of results for a certain dietary program reasonable or exaggerated? Is the program based on hard scientific information?
4. Is the nutrition information presented in a reliable magazine or newspaper, or is the information published in an advertisement or a well-known publication of questionable reputation?
5. Is the information someone's opinion or the result of years of valid scientific research, with possible practical nutrition implications?

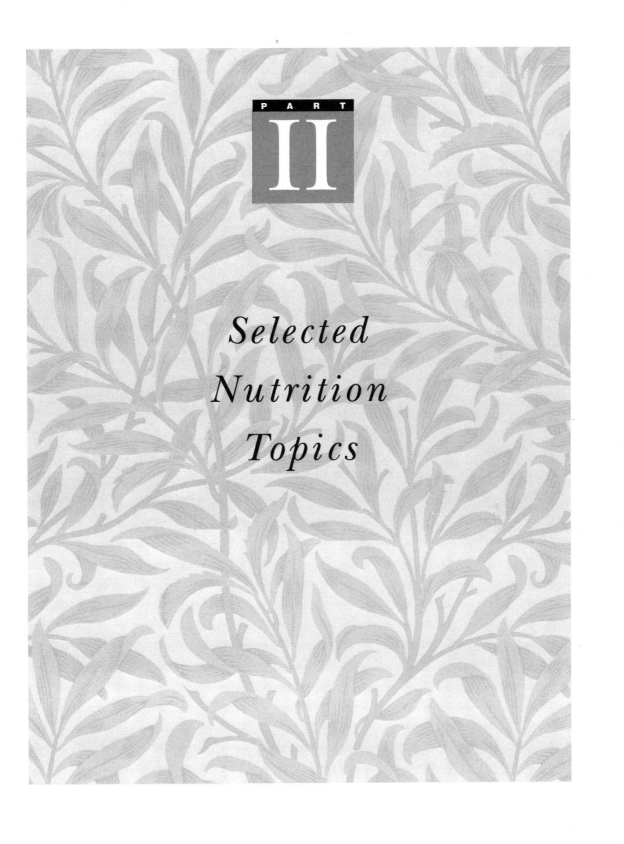

PART

II

*Selected
Nutrition
Topics*

CHAPTER 8

Nutrition Over the Life Cycle

KEY QUESTIONS

1. Can diet provide all the nutrients needed to meet the special needs of pregnancy and lactation?
2. Why is good nutrition important during pregnancy and lactation?
3. From which food groups do pregnant or lactating women need more servings?
4. How much does an infant grow during the first year?
5. Why is breastfeeding recommended over formula feeding?
6. What is the progression of foods for an infant during the first year of life?
7. What special nutrient needs do growing children and adolescents have?
8. What influences nutrient intakes of children and adolescents?
9. How should you plan menus for children and adolescents?
10. Which factors influence the nutrition status of adults and older adults (persons over 65)?
11. How do you plan menus for healthy adults and older adults?

QUIZ

QUIZ

1. Following are the requirements of the Food Guide Pyramid for healthy adults. Fill in the number of servings from each group needed for pregnant and lactating women

Food Group	Minimum Number of Servings	Servings Needed Pregnancy	During Lactation
Meat, poultry, fish, and alternates	2	_____	_____
Milk and dairy products	2	_____	_____
Fruits	2	_____	_____
Vegetables	3	_____	_____
Breads, cereals, grains	6	_____	_____

2. In which order are the following solid foods introduced to infants?
   Whole egg
   Vegetable
   Cereal
   Meat

3. After the age of one, a child's rate of growth decreases.
   True   False

4. Preschoolers commonly have favorite foods that they eat frequently.
   True   False

5. The baby's first teeth cut through the gums
   (a) right after birth.
   (b) between 2 to 6 months.
   (c) between 6 to 10 months.
   (d) after the first birthday.
6. School lunch programs are intended to provide at least what proportion of a child's Recommended Dietary Allowance for calories, protein, iron, calcium, vitamin A, and vitamin C?
   (a) one-fourth
   (b) one-third
   (c) one-half
   (d) no minimum is set
7. Children and adolescent's eating behaviors are affected by
   (a) parents.
   (b) siblings.
   (c) peers.
   (d) school.
   (e) all of the above.
8. Binge eating and then purging is a hallmark of which disease?
   (a) anorexia nervosa
   (b) bulimia nervosa
   (c) binge eating disorder
   (d) all eating disorders
9. Iron is often a problem nutrient for children and adolescents.
   True   False
10. During adolescence, boys put on twice as much muscle as girls, and girls lay down fat stores under the skin.
    True   False
11. There is less room for empty calories in the diet of an elderly person.
    True   False
12. The most prevalent nutrition-related problems of the elderly are chronic conditions that require modified diets.
    True   False

INTRODUCTION

Although much nutrition advice we hear on television or read about in magazines is for adults—and indeed the first part of this book is mostly for adults—other groups have their own special nutrition needs and concerns too. What do pregnant women, babies, children, and even teenagers have in common? They are all growing, and growth demands more nutrients. Did you know that a one-month-old baby, as compared to an adult, needs twice the amount, proportionally, of many vitamins and minerals? At the other end of the age spectrum, the fastest-growing age group in the United States is the over-85 group. As people age, many new factors affect their nutrition status: the aging process, onset of chronic diseases such as heart disease, living alone, inability to get out to food shop, dentures, and so on.

This chapter takes you from pregnancy through infancy, childhood, and adolescence and on to the golden years. Along the way, we will explore the nutritional needs and factors affecting nutrition status for each group, along with menu-planning guides.

PREGNANCY

From a modest one-cell beginning, an actual living and breathing baby is born after 40 weeks. From 8 weeks after conception until birth, the infant in the mother's uterus is called a **fetus.** At 8 weeks the fetus is about 1 inch long and has a beating heart and gastrointestinal and nervous systems. To cushion and protect the **fetus,** it floats in a protected bag, or sac, called the **amniotic sac.** From the second to eighth week after conception, the infant is called an **embryo.**

During the first month of pregnancy, an organ called the **placenta** develops to provide an exchange of nutrients and wastes between fetus and mother and to secrete the hormones necessary to maintain pregnancy. If a mother is not sufficiently nourished during early pregnancy (when she probably doesn't even know she's pregnant), the placenta will not perform properly and the fetus will not get optimal nourishment.

Nutrition During Pregnancy

The nutritional status of women before and during pregnancy influences both the mother's and the baby's health. Factors that place a woman at nutritional risk during pregnancy include an inadequate diet, smoking, and other influences described in Table 8-1.

TABLE 8-1   Nutrition risk factors for pregnant women.

- Pregnancy during adolescence.
- Inadequate diets.
- Multiple birth (twins, triplets, and so on)
- Use of cigarettes, alcohol, or illicit drugs
- Lactose intolerance
- Underweight or overweight at time of conception
- Gaining too few or too many pounds during pregnancy

TABLE 8-2.   Optimum weight gain in pregnancy.

Weight at Conception	*Optimum Weight Gain*
Normal weight	25–35 pounds
Underweight	28–40 pounds
Overweight	15–25 pounds

Components of Weight Gain	*Pounds*
Fetus	8 pounds
Placenta	1.5 pounds
Amniotic fluid	2.0 pounds
Increase in size of uterus, breast, fluid and blood volume	12 pounds
Fat	2.0 to 8.0 pounds

Table 8-2 shows optimum weight gain during pregnancy. Underweight women (10 percent or more below their desirable weight) must either gain weight before or gain more weight during pregnancy. Overweight women need to lose weight before or gain less weight during pregnancy, otherwise they are at greater risk of developing gestational diabetes and hypertension, both of which can cause complications. Table 8-2 also shows that of the weight gained, about 8 pounds is actually baby, with the rest serving to support the baby's growth.

Both prepregnancy weight and weight gain during pregnancy directly influence infant birth weight. The newborn's weight is the number-one indicator of his or her future health status. A newborn who weighs less than 5 1/2 pounds is referred to as a **low birth weight baby.** These babies are at higher risk for disease and experience more difficulties surviving the first year. Often the mother of a low birth weight baby has a history of poor nutrition status before and/or during pregnancy. Other factors associated with low birth weight are smoking, alcohol use, drug use, and certain disease conditions.

For healthy babies, pregnant women need to eat more calories, but not a whole lot more. If a pregnant woman "eats for two" during pregnancy, she is probably asking for trouble! Pregnancy does increase calorie needs, but only about 300 calories. Within that measly 300 calories, however, the pregnant woman must pack more protein and more of 13 different vitamins and minerals! See Table 8-3 for a comparison of RDA for nonpregnant and pregnant women.

Although pregnancy is not a time to diet, it is fine to exercise and appropriate types of exercise are encouraged.

During the first 13 weeks of pregnancy (referred to as the **first trimester**), the total weight gain is between 2 and 4 pounds. Thereafter, about 1 pound per week is normal. Corresponding with the timing of weight gain, it makes sense that the greatest need for calories begins around the tenth week of pregnancy and continues until birth. The two major factors influencing calorie requirements during pregnancy are the woman's activity level and basal metabolic rate (BMR). The BMR increases to support the growth of the fetus. Pregnancy is no time to diet or follow a fad diet, which could have dangerous implications for the fetus.

Protein needs increase from 45 to 50 grams for nonpregnant women to 60 grams for pregnant women. The RDAs for protein are generous during pregnancy and probably high for some women. Meeting protein needs is rarely a problem.

During pregnancy, calcium, phosphorus, and magnesium are necessary for the proper development of the skeleton and teeth. In adequate amounts, calcium may help reduce high blood pressure and the incidence of pre-eclampsia, a sometimes deadly disorder marked by high blood pressure after the sixth month of pregnancy. On the positive side, much more calcium (about double) is absorbed through the intestine. On the negative side, many women do not eat enough calcium-rich foods during pregnancy or lactation. The need for calcium and phosphorus is moderately high (1200 milligrams) but can be met by having at least three servings from the dairy group each day. Magnesium is found in green leafy vegetables, nuts, seeds, legumes, and whole grains.

The need for folate more than doubles during pregnancy. This makes perfect sense when you realize that folate is needed to sustain the growth of new cells and the increased blood volume that occur during pregnancy. Folate is critical in the first four to six weeks of pregnancy (when most women don't even know they are pregnant) because this is when the **neural tube,** the tissue that develops into the brain and spinal cord, forms. Without enough folate, birth defects of the brain and spinal cord, such as **spina bifida,** can occur. In spina bifida, parts of the spinal cord are not

TABLE 8-3. Recommended Dietary Allowances for nonpregnant adult women compared to pregnant and lactating women.

Nutrient	Nonpregnant Women 15–25+ Years	Pregnancy (2nd & 3rd trimesters)	Lactation 1st 6 months	Lactation 2nd 6 months
Energy (kcal)	2200	+300	+500	+500
Protein (g)	44–50	60	65	62
Vitamin A (μg RE)	800	800	1300	1200
Vitamin D (μg)	5–10	10	10	10
Vitamin E (mg *a*-TE)	8	10	12	11
Vitamin K (μg)	55–65	65	65	65
Vitamin C (mg)	60	70	95	90
Thiamin (mg)	1.1	1.5	1.6	1.6
Riboflavin (mg)	1.3	1.6	1.8	1.7
Niacin (mg NE)	15	17	20	20
Vitamin B_6 (mg)	1.5–1.6	2.2	2.1	2.1
Folate (μg)	180	400	280	260
Vitamin B_{12} (μg)	2.0	2.2	2.6	2.6
Calcium (mg)	800–1200	1200	1200	1200
Phosphorous (mg)	800–1200	1200	1200	1200
Magnesium (mg)	280–300	320	355	340
Iron (mg)	15	30	15	15
Zinc (mg)	12	15	19	16
Iodine (μg)	150	175	200	200
Selenium (μg)	50–55	65	75	75

Source: *Recommended Dietary Allowances.* ©1989 by the National Academy of Sciences, National Academy Press, Washington, DC.

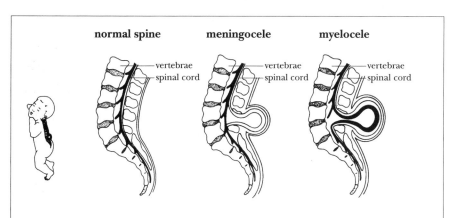

FIGURE 8-1.

Spina bifida aperta

Compared to the normal spine (left), the spine of a baby with spina bifida aperta has a noticeable sac. When the sac is small (center), it can be repaired and there will be no muscle paralysis. But in 90 percent of cases, a portion of the undeveloped spinal cord protrudes through the spine and into the sac (right), causing paralysis and incontinence.

TABLE 8-4.	**Current supplementation recommendations: National Academy of Sciences (1990).**	
Nutrient	*Candidates for Supplementation*	*Level of Nutrient Supplementation*
Iron	All pregnant women (2nd and 3rd trimesters)	30 mg ferrous iron daily
Folic acid	Pregnant women with suspected dietary inadequacy of folate	300 µg/day
Vitamin D	Complete vegetarians and others with low intakeof vitamin D-fortified milk	10 µg/day
Calcium	Women under age 25 whose daily dietary calcium intake is less than 600 mg	600 mg/day
Vitamin B_{12}	Complete vegetarians	2 µg/day
Zinc/copper	Women under treatment with iron for iron deficiency anemia	15 mg Zn/day .2 mg Cu/day
Multivitamin-mineral supplements	Pregnant women with poor diets and for thosewho are considered high risk: multiple gestation, heavy smokers, alcohol/drug abusers, other	Preparation containing iron-30 mg zinc-15 mg copper-2 mg calcium-250 mg vitamin B_6-2 mg folate-300 µg vitamin C-50 mg vitamin D-5 µg

Source: Institute of Medicine. 1990. Nutrition During Pregnancy. Washington, DC: National Academy Press.

properly fused, so gaps are present (Figure 8-1). Not every woman who has insufficient folate during early pregnancy will have a child with such a birth defect. However, if all women of childbearing age consumed enough folate, 50 to 70 percent of birth defects of the brain and spinal cord could be prevented, according the the U.S. Centers for Disease Control and Prevention.

Folate is also critical during the entire pregnancy. A study of pregnant women showed that those women consuming less than 240 micrograms per day of folic acid had about a two- to threefold greater risk of preterm delivery and low birth weight (Scholl et al., 1996).

Because of the importance of folate during pregnancy and the difficulty most women encounter trying to get double the RDA for folate through diet, the Food and Drug Administration has required manufacturers of certain foods to fortify them with folate. By January 1, 1998, manufacturers of enriched breads, flour, pasta, corn meals, rice, and other foods must fortify their foods so that one serving provides 40 micrograms of folate, or 10 percent of the daily recommended amount. Women eating folate-fortified foods should not assume that these foods will meet all their folate needs. They should still seek out folate-rich foods.

Since vitamin B_{12} works with folate to make new cells, increased amounts of this vitamin are also needed. As long as animal products, such as meat and milk, are being consumed, vitamin B_{12} deficiency is not a concern.

Along with folate and vitamin B_{12}, iron also helps in the formation of blood—it is necessary for hemoglobin in both maternal and fetal red blood cells. After 34 weeks of pregnancy, a woman's blood volume has increased 50 percent from the time of conception. Although iron absorption does increase during pregnancy, whether the diet can supply enough iron is questionable. The National Academy of Sciences recommends iron supplements daily during pregnancy.

In the past it was thought that sodium restriction was necessary for women with **edema,** or tissue swelling. It is now known that moderate swelling is normal during pregnancy and that sodium restriction is unnecessary and could actually be harmful for a healthy pregnant women.

Table 8-4 lists the current supplementation recommendations for pregnant women. The only nutrient suggested for all pregnant women is iron.

Menu Planning During Pregnancy

To plan menus properly, certain diet-related concerns that occur during pregnancy need to be discussed. These include morning sickness, changes in taste and smell, constipation, heartburn, and the intake of alcohol, saccharin, aspartame, and mercury and polychlorinated biphenyls.

Nausea and vomiting, commonly referred to as morning sickness (although it can occur at any time of day), may be due to an increase in one or more of the 30 hormones that increase during pregnancy. The hallmarks of morning sickness are nausea and vomiting. Aversion to certain odors and fatigue also accompany the nausea and vomiting. Constipation may also be a concern. Each woman experiences it a little bit differently. Morning sickness lasts for an average of 17 weeks, but for some unlucky women it lasts until delivery. From 50 to 90 percent of women experience some gastrointestinal discomfort in early pregnancy

Morning sickness is a misnomer: it can occur any time of the day or night.

(Erick, 1993). A major health concern with morning sickness is that it can cause dehydration, which in turn causes nausea.

Dietary advice in the past concentrated on small, carbohydrate-rich meals and tea and crackers. For many women, this dietary advice doesn't work. Recent advice centers on eating whatever foods you can keep down, even foods that aren't terribly nutritious, such as potato chips. The logic behind this recommendation is that tastes change when you are sick and you often crave something when you feel ready to eat. It's better to eat that food and keep it down than to eat something that is not appealing and throw it up. During pregnancy, women often develop a fine-tuned sense of smell, which often adds to their nausea. The smell of foods and cooking can make them sick.

Pregnant women commonly report changes in taste and smell. They may prefer saltier foods and crave sweets and dairy products such as ice cream. Certain foods they may have aversions to include alcohol, caffeinated drinks, and meats. Their cravings and aversions do not necessarily reflect actual physiological needs.

Constipation is not uncommon, due to the relaxation of gastro-intestinal muscles. It can be counteracted by eating more high-fiber foods, drinking more fluids, and getting additional exercise.

Heartburn is a common complaint toward the end of pregnancy when the growing uterus crowds the stomach. This condition has nothing to do with the heart but is actually a painful burning sensation in the esophagus. It occurs when stomach contents, which are acidic, flow back into the lower esophagus. Possible solutions include eating small and frequent meals, eating slowly and in a relaxed atmosphere, avoiding caffeine, wearing comfortable clothes, and not lying down after eating.

Several food and beverage ingredients may affect the course and outcome of pregnancy, including alcohol, saccharin and aspartame, and mercury and polychlorinated biphenyls (PCBs).

If you look at the label on any bottle of beer, wine, or liquor, you will see the following.

> Government Warning: According to the Surgeon General, women should not drink alcoholic beverages during pregnancy because of the risk of birth defects.

Alcohol and pregnancy don't mix. During pregnancy, alcohol crosses the placenta, and high alcohol levels can build up in the fetus. Alcohol can limit the amount of oxygen delivered to the fetus, oxygen that is vital to its development, as well as slow the growth of cells. It can also produce abnormal cells.

TABLE 8-5.   **Daily food guide for pregnancy and lactation.**

Food Group	Servings	Serving Size
Meat/meat alternative	3—pregnancy to include 1 serving legumes 3—lactation	2 ounces cooked lean meat, poultry, or fish 2 eggs 2 ounces cheese 1/2 cup cottage cheese 1 cup dried beans or peas 4 tablespoons peanut butter
Milk and Dairy	3—pregnancy (4 for teenagers) 4—lactation	1 cup milk, yogurt, pudding or custard 1 1/2 ounces cheese 1 1/2 to 2 cups cottage cheese
Vegetables*	3—5 during pregnancy and lactation	1/2 cup cooked or juice 1 cup raw
Fruits	2—4 during pregnancy and lactation	Portion commonly served, such as a medium apple or banana
Grain	6—11 during pregnancy and lactation	1 slice whole-grain or enriched bread 1 cup ready-to-eat cereal 1/2 cup cooked cereal or pasta 1/2 bagel or hamburger roll 6 crackers 1 small roll 1/2 cup rice or grits
Fats, sweets, and alcohol**		Includes butter, margarine, salad dressings, mayonnaise, oils, candy, sugar, jams, jellies, syrups, soft drinks, beer, wine, liquor, and any other fats, sweets, and alcohol

* A source rich in vitamin C (citrus, strawberries, melons, tomatoes) is needed daily; a source rich in vitamin A (dark green and deep yellow vegetables) is needed every other day.

** In general, the amount of these foods to use depends on the number of calories you require. Get your essential nutrients in the other food groups first before choosing foods from this group.

The heavy consumption of alcohol during pregnancy may cause a variety of symptoms called **fetal alcohol syndrome** (**FAS**). FAS children may show signs of mental retardation, growth retardation, brain damage, and facial deformities. Newborns with FAS are generally small in size and irritable because of alcohol withdrawal. The most serious concern with FAS infants is their impaired physical and mental development. They have problems gaining weight and are frequently mentally retarded.

You don't have to be a chronic alcoholic to have problems with FAS. Even moderate drinkers can have babies that show subtle signs of FAS. These women also have a higher rate of miscarriages and low birth weight

TABLE 8-6.   Sources of problem nutrients during pregnancy.

Nutrient	Food Sources
Fiber	Bran, dried beans and peas, whole-grain breads and cereals, fruits and vegetables, nuts, seeds
Folate	Organ meats, legumes, dark green leafy vegetables, orange juice, whole-wheat breads and cereals,
Vitamin D	Vitamin D fortified milk
Iron	Red meat, liver, shellfish, poultry, dried fruit, beans, nuts, whole-grain and enriched breads and cereals
Calcium	Milk, dairy products, calcium-fortified orange juice
Magnesium	Green leafy vegetables, nuts, seeds, whole grains, and legumes
Zinc	Red meat, liver, poultry, fish, legumes

babies. The American Academy of Pediatrics recommends that women stop drinking alcohol as soon as they plan to become pregnant, because harm can be done during the first six to eight weeks, when a woman doesn't yet know for sure whether she is pregnant.

Studies reveal that neither saccharin nor aspartame are known to cause problems during pregnancy. However, use of both saccharin and aspartame should be moderated in pregnancy.

High levels of mercury have been found in certain large fish, including swordfish, large tuna, shark, halibut, and marlin. According to the Center for Science in the Public Interest, pregnant women should limit their intake of tuna to a half-pound per week and completely avoid the other fish listed. Pregnant women should also avoid eating fish contaminated with PCBs: fresh-water carp, wild catfish, lake trout, whitefish, bluefish, mackerel, and striped bass.

Table 8-5 is a daily food guide for pregnancy. Problems can arise when an individual omits entire or substantial parts of certain groups. For instance, vegetarians, who do not eat any food of animal origin, need varied, adequate diets and supplements to obtain adequate vitamin B$_{12}$, calcium, zinc, and vitamin D (unless getting adequate sunshine). Individuals who avoid the dairy group may need calcium and vitamin D supplements unless they eat foods fortified with these nutrients, such as calcium-fortified orange juice.

The following are some menu-planning guidelines for pregnant and lactating women.

1. Offer a varied and balanced selection of nutrient-dense foods. Because energy needs increase less than nutrient needs, empty calories are rarely an acceptable choice.
2. In addition to traditional meat entrees, choose entrees based on legumes and/or grains and dairy products. Beans, peas, rice, pasta, and cheese can be used in many entrees. Chapter 10 covers vegetarianism and has much information on meatless entrees.
3. Be sure to offer dairy products made with skim or low-fat milk.
4. Use a variety of whole-grain and enriched breads, rolls, cereals, rice, pasta, and other grains.
5. Use assorted fruits and vegetables in all areas of the menu, including appetizers, salads, entrees, side dishes, and desserts.
6. Be sure to have good sources of problem nutrients: fiber, vitamin B_6, folate, vitamin D, iron, calcium, magnesium, and zinc (See Table 8-6.).
7. Be sure to use iodized salt.

MINI-SUMMARY Women's nutritional status before and during pregnancy influences both the mother and baby's health. Both prepregnancy weight and weight gain during pregnancy directly influence infant birth weight, the most important indicator of the baby's future health status. Although a pregnant woman should consume only 300 additional calories, she must take in more nutrients such as iron, folate, zinc, and vitamin B_{12}. Iron supplements will likely be prescribed because diet just isn't enough. When menu planning, keep in mind that pregnant women need nutrient-dense foods, an extra serving from the dairy and meat/meat alternate groups, and plenty of fruits and vegetables. Recent advice for morning sickness is to let women eat whatever foods they feel they can keep down, without worrying excessively about how nutritious they are. Moderate use of saccharin and aspartame are advised during pregnancy but it is probably best to stay away from alcoholic beverages.

NUTRITION AND MENU PLANNING DURING LACTATION

Tables 8-3 and 8-5 show the RDA and daily food guide for breast-feeding mothers. During lactation, the period of milk production, 500 additional calories and more protein are necessary. Actually, more than 500 extra calories are needed daily, but some (about 150 each day) are supplied by extra fat stored during pregnancy. Lactating mothers, who normally produce about 25 ounces of milk a day, also need at least 2 to 3 quarts of water each day to prevent dehydration. Extra cups of coffee contain extra fluid but also contribute excess caffeine, which can cross to the baby and cause irritability.

A poor diet will not affect the quality of the milk as much as it will affect the quantity of milk produced.

A balanced, varied, and adequate diet (at least 1800 calories) is critical to successful breast-feeding and infant health. If the mother is not eating properly, any nutritional deficiencies are more likely to affect the quantity of milk she makes, rather than the quality. Menu-planning guidelines for lactating women follow those for pregnant women, with emphasis on fluids, dairy products, fruits, and vegetables. Occasional consumption of small amounts of alcohol will probably have no consequences. The National Research Council suggests iron supplementation for the mother to replenish stores depleted during pregnancy. Lactating vegetarian mothers who eat no food of animal origin need to pay special attention to getting enough calories, iron, zinc, calcium, vitamin D, and vitamin B_{12} (Specker, 1994).

MINI-SUMMARY During lactation, mothers need 500 extra calories a day, plenty of fluids, two extra servings from the dairy group, one extra serving from the meat/meat alternate group, and a variety of nutrient-dense foods. If the mother is not eating right, the quantity of milk will be adversely affected. Small amounts of alcohol or caffeine are probably okay.

INFANCY: THE FIRST YEAR OF LIFE

The nutrient needs of infants are about double those of an adult when viewed in proportion to their weights. Little wonder, considering that infants generally double their birth weight in the first four to five months and then triple their birth weight by the first birthday. An infant will also grow 50 percent in length by the first birthday. (In other words, a baby who was 20 inches at birth grows to 30 inches in one year.)

Nutrition During Infancy

Newborns need a plentiful supply of all nutrients, and nutrients especially those necessary for growth, such as vitamins C and D, folate, vitamin B_{12}, calcium, and iron. The RDA is set for infants from 0 to 6 months, and then from 7 to 12 months. By 6 months, growth occurs at a slower rate.

"Breast is best."

For the first 4 to 6 months of life, the source of all nutrients is breast milk or formula. In other words, the infant's diet is breast milk or formula. Breast milk is recommended for all infants in the United States under ordinary circumstances from birth to 12 months (Institute of Medicine, 1991). A baby needs breast milk for the first year of life, and as long as desired after that.

The number of women who are choosing to breast-feed is increasing. Current estimates are that more than 50 percent of American mothers breastfeed their babies in the hospital but only 19 percent are still breastfeeding 6 months later. The reasons behind this increase include research findings that show definite health benefits of breast milk, as well as support and information groups that communicate breast-feeding guidelines and advantages. However, too few mothers breast-feed. The goal set by the U.S. Department of Health and Human Services is to have 75 percent of mothers nursing their babies in early infancy and 50 percent continuing to nurse their babies for 5 or 6 months. Unfortunately, women who are young, unemployed, and on low incomes are the least likely to breast-feed. Their babies could greatly benefit from breast-feeding because they typically face the highest risk of health problems.

The following list shows the advantages of breast-feeding as compared to formula feeding.

1. Breast milk is nutritionally superior to any formula or other type of feeding. It provides exactly the right proportion and form of calories and nutrients needed for optimal growth, brain development, and digestion. Cow's milk contains a different type of protein than breast milk and infants can have difficulty digesting it. It also provides the essential fatty acids, which are lacking in formula. The composition of breast milk changes to meet the needs of the growing infant.
2. Newborns are less apt to be allergic to breast milk than to any other food.
3. Suckling promotes the development of the infant's jaw and teeth. It's harder work to get milk out of a breast than a bottle; and the exercise strengthens the jaw and encourages the growth of straight, healthy teeth. The baby at the breast can control the flow of milk by sucking and stopping. With a bottle, the baby must constantly suck or react to the pressure of the nipple in the mouth.
4. Breast-feeding promotes a close relationship—a bonding, between mother and child. At birth, infants see only 12 to 15 inches: the distance between a nursing baby and its mother's face.
5. Breast milk is less likely to be mishandled. Some formulas require accurate dilutions, and all are much more apt to be mishandled, which can result in foodborne illness.

6. Breast milk helps the infant build up immunities to infectious disease because it contains the mother's antibodies to disease. Breast-fed infants are much less likely to develop serious respiratory and gastro-intestinal illnesses.
7. Breast milk also contains growth factors, thought to help in developing body tissues, and hormones and other substances that may subtly shape the newborn's brain and behavior.
8. Breast-feeding may reduce the risk of breast cancer for the mother.
9. Breast-feeding is less expensive.
10. Breast-fed infants have lower rates of hospital admissions, ear infections, diarrhea, rashes, allergies, and other medical problems than bottle-fed babies.

Breast-feeding is not recommended if the mother uses addictive drugs, drinks more than a minimal amount of alcohol, is on certain medications, or is HIV (the virus that causes AIDS) positive.

If the infant or mother is not exposed regularly to sunlight or if the mother's intake of vitamin D is low, the breast-fed infant may need vitamin D. Vitamin D supplements are generally recommended for breast-fed infants.

Formula feeding is an acceptable substitute for breast-feeding and has some advantages. Some women find formula feeding more convenient (others find breast-feeding more convenient). Other family members can take part in formula feeding. For some women who are uncomfortable with breast-feeding, even after education, formula feeding is the method of choice.

All formulas must meet nutrient standards set by the American Academy of Pediatrics. The three forms of formulas on the market are ready-to-feed, liquid concentrate that needs to be mixed with equal amounts of water, and powdered formulas, which also need to be mixed with water. All formulas must be handled in a sanitary manner to prevent contamination and possible food poisoning.

Cow-based formulas are normally used unless the baby is allergic to the protein or sugar in milk. In that case, a soy-based formula is used. For the baby who is allergic to both cow-based and soy-based formulas, predigested formulas are available. Symptoms of allergies usually include diarrhea and/or vomiting. Cow's milk has too much protein and minerals and too little essential fatty acids, vitamin C, and iron. Therefore it is not recommended until 12 months of age, when the baby is less likely to be allergic to it. Babies are normally switched slowly from formula to cow's milk.

TABLE 8-7.   Tips for breast-feeding success.

- *Get an early start:* Nursing should begin within an hour after delivery if possible, when an infant is awake and the suckling instinct is strong. Even though the mother won't be producing milk yet, her breasts contain colostrum, a thin fluid that contains antibodies to disease.

- *Proper positioning:* The baby's mouth should be wide open, with the nipple as far back into his or her mouth as possible. This minimizes soreness for the mother. A nurse, midwife, or other knowledgeable person can help her find a comfortable nursing position.

- *Nurse on demand:* Newborns need to nurse frequently, at least every two hours, and not on any strict schedule. This will stimulate the mother's breasts to produce plenty of milk. Later, the baby can settle into a more predictable routine. But because breast milk is more easily digested than formula, breast-fed babies often eat more frequently than bottle-fed babies.

- *Delay artificial nipples:* It's best to wait a week or two before introducing a pacifier, so that the baby doesn't get confused. Artificial nipples require a different sucking action than real ones. Sucking at a bottle could also confuse some babies in the early days. They, too, are learning how to breast-feed.

- *Air dry:* In the early postpartum period or until her nipples toughen, the mother should air dry them after each nursing to prevent them from cracking, which can lead to infection. If her nipples do crack, the mother can coat them with breast milk or other natural moisturizers to help them heal. Vitamin E oil and lanolin are commonly used, although some babies may have allergic reactions to them. Proper positioning at the breast can help prevent sore nipples. If the mother's very sore, the baby may not have the nipple far enough back in his or her mouth.

- *Watch for infection:* Symptoms of breast infection include fever and painful lumps and redness in the breast. These require immediate medical attention.

- *Expect engorgement:* A new mother usually produces lots of milk, making her breasts big, hard and painful for a few days. To relieve this engorgement, she should feed the baby frequently and on demand until her body adjusts and produces only what the baby needs. In the meantime, the mother can take over-the-counter pain relievers, apply warm, wet compresses to her breasts, and take warm baths to relieve the pain.

- *Eat right, get rest:* To produce plenty of good milk, the nursing mother needs a balanced diet that includes 500 extra calories a day and six to eight glasses of fluid. She should also rest as much as possible to prevent breast infections, which are aggravated by fatigue.

Whether breast-fed or formula fed, the infant's iron stores are relatively depleted by 4 to 6 months, at which time they typically start to eat iron-fortified cereals. Fluoride supplements may also be prescribed for the formula-fed baby unless the formula is made with fluoridated water.

Feeding the Infant

Successful infant feeding requires cooperative functioning between the mother and her baby. Feeding time should be a pleasurable period for both parent and child, so be sure to be comfortable and relaxed to better enjoy the experience. Ideally, the feeding schedule should be based on reasonable self-regulation by the baby. By the end of the first week of life, most infants want 6 to 8 feedings a day. Formula-fed babies are fed about every 4 hours and breast-fed babies about every 2 to 3 hours.

The mother must breast-feed the child as soon as possible after delivery to enhance success. **Colostrum,** a yellowish fluid, is the first secretion to come from the breast a day or so after delivery. It is rich in proteins, antibodies, and other factors that protect against infectious disease. Colostrum changes to **transitional milk** between the third and sixth days, and by the tenth day the major changes are finished.

The breast-feeding process begins with the infant using a sucking action that stimulates hormones to move milk into the ducts of the breast. This process is referred to as milk **letdown** and is hindered if the mother is tired or anxious. A baby will most often empty a breast in about 10 minutes of nearly continuous sucking. The baby should empty at least one breast per feeding in order to stimulate the breast to produce more milk. To assure that the newborn is getting enough milk, newborns need to be nursed frequently. In order to nurse the child successfully, the mother needs adequate rest, nutrition, and fluids, as well as education and support to decrease anxiety. Table 8-7 lists tips for breast-feeding success.

Babies are ready to eat semi-solid foods such as hot cereal when they can sit up and open their mouths. This usually occurs between 5 to 7 months of age. Other signs that babies are ready for spoon feeding are when they:

- have doubled their birth weight.
- drink more than a quart of formula per day.
- seem hungry often.
- opens their mouths in response to seeing food coming.

Although some parents think that feeding of solids will help the baby to sleep through the night, this is not often so. Feeding of solid food before a baby is ready can create problems because the baby's digestive system is not ready for it. Feeding solids early also increases the risk of allergies and the chances of choking, and may encourage overfeeding.

Most babies can digest starchy foods at around 4 months of age. Once a baby starts on solid foods, it is important to make sure the baby gets sufficient fluids. Up to this point, breast milk or formula met the baby's need for fluids. Now, however, drinking water or other fluid is needed to prevent dehydration. Proportionally, babies have more water in their bodies than adults do. They can become dehydrated very quickly due to hot weather, diarrhea, or vomiting, so fluids need to be offered at these times.

Although eating solid food is certainly simple for an adult, it involves a number of difficult steps for the baby. First the infant must have enough muscle control to close his or her mouth over the spoon, scrape the food from the spoon with the lips, and then move the food from the front to the back of the tongue. By about 16 weeks, a baby generally has these skills, but probably no teeth! The baby's first teeth will cut through the gums between 6 to 10 months of age. If a baby can't swallow well enough to get the food from the back of the tongue into the pharynx, the baby will gag. The **gag reflex** prevents choking and sometimes results in vomiting.

Foods are generally introduced as follows. Keep in mind that the order of introducing different types and textures of foods is tied to the baby's developmental stages.

- 4 to 6 months: Iron-fortified baby cereals
- 5 to 7 months: Strained or pureed vegetables and fruits
- 7 to 9 months: Strained or soft protein foods (meat, chicken, fish, cheese, yogurt, beans, egg yolk)
                    Finger foods such as crackers
                    Fruit juice
- 9 to 12 months: Soft, chopped foods (finely chopped at first)
                    Breads and grain products
- 12 months: Cut-up table foods
                    Whole milk
                    Whole eggs

The first solid food is iron-fortified baby cereal mixed with breast milk or formula. Usually, rice cereal is offered first because it is the least likely to cause an allergic reaction. Barley and oatmeal cereals follow. The iron found in these cereals is very important to meet the infant's high iron needs. Avoid putting cereals or any other solids into the infant's bottle.

Once the baby is used to various cereals, pureed or mashed vegetables and fruits can be tried at about 5 to 6 months. It is a good idea to start

TABLE 8-8. Food guide for infants.

Age	Food*	Amount
0–4 months	Breast milk or formula**	21–29 ounces, formula, 5–8 feedings daily. 6–8 nursings.
4–6 months	Breast milk or formula	27–39 ounces formula, 4–6 feedings daily. 4–5 nursings.
	Iron-fortified infant cereal (usually starts at 5 months)	Give 1 tablespoon with mother's milk/ formula to start. Start with rice cereal. Give once to twice daily. Can work up to 1½ tablespoons twice daily.
5–7 months	Strained vegetables and fruits	Give 1–2 teaspoons once to twice daily. First fruits can be applesauce, pears, peaches, and bananas. First vegetables can be carrots, squash, and sweet potatoes. Slowly increase to 2 tablespoons twice daily.
7–9 months	Breast milk or formula	30–32 ounces formula, 3–5 feedings daily. 3–5 nursings.
	Iron-fortified infant cereal	3 tablespoons plus mother's milk/formula twice daily.
	Strained fruits and vegetables	3 tablespoons twice daily.
	Strained plain meats	1 to 2 tablespoons twice daily.
	Crackers, plain toast, or teething biscuit	When baby has teeth, offer these foods after other foods are eat.
	Fruit juice (vitamin C fortified, non-acid) (usually starts at 5 months)	Start with 2 ounces watered down juice, usually apple juice. Limit fruit juice to 1/2 cup daily.
9–12 months	Breast milk or formula (Your physician may suggest switching to whole milk at 10 months or after.)	24–32 ounces formula, 3–4 times daily. 3–4 nursings.
	Fruit juice (vitamin C fortified)	1/2 cup daily.
	Iron-fortified infant cereal	3–4 tablespoons plus mother's milk/formula twice daily.
	Vegetables, cut up	3–4 tablespoons twice daily.
	Fruits, cut up	3–4 tablespoons twice daily.
	Meats, cut up	2–3 tablespoons twice daily.
	Egg (usually at 12 months)	1 egg = 1 serving of meat.
	Bread and grain products	1/2 slice four times daily.

*Avoid the following foods in the first year because of possible allergic reactions: chocolate, nuts, berries, tomatoes, shellfish.
**Physician may request iron-fortified formula by third or fourth month.

with vegetables so that the baby does not become accustomed to the sweet taste of fruits (babies like sweets) and then reject the vegetables. When adding new foods to the infant's diet, always do so one at a time (and in small quantities) so that, if there is an allergic reaction (such as hives or diarrhea), you will know which food caused it. Introduce new vegetables and fruits about 3 or 4 days apart. Babies adjust differently to new tastes and new textures. If the baby does not like a certain food, offer it a few days later. By offering new foods when the baby is hungry, like at the beginning of a meal, he or she is more likely to eat them.

Instead of purchasing jarred baby foods, some mothers make their own with a food processor or blender.

Fruit juice that is fortified with vitamin C can be started about the seventh month. Although some babies get two or more bottles a day of apple juice (or other type of juice), it is a good idea to limit juice to a half-cup, or 4 fluid ounces, daily. Sometimes a baby who drinks too much juice starts drinking less mother's milk or formula. Another problem with fruit juice can occur when you let your baby go to sleep with a bottle in his or her mouth. The natural sugars in the juice can cause serious tooth decay, called **baby bottle tooth decay.** Letting a baby go to bed with a bottle of formula, cow's milk, or breast milk will also cause baby bottle tooth decay.

Never put a baby to bed with a bottle in his mouth.

Before a baby can move on to finger foods, he or she has to be able to grab them. At about 8 months, a baby discovers and starts to use the thumb and forefinger together to pick things up (called the **pincer grasp**). From about 6 months, the baby has been using the palm (called the **palmar grasp**) to do this. Suitable finger foods include chopped ripe bananas, dry cereal, and pieces of cheese. About this time infants can also start eating protein foods. Poultry and fish must be very tender, and meat will have to be chopped or cut very fine and possibly moistened.

Between 10 and 12 months of age, babies may have four to six sharp teeth, and many are eating soft, chopped foods with the family. At this time it is appropriate to let your child begin drinking from a cup. It takes time, but sooner or later your child will get the idea.

By one year of age, infants can enjoy cut-up table foods as well as whole milk. By 12 months, a baby should be almost entirely self-feeding. Children should not be switched to low-fat milk until they are at least 2 years old because they need the fat in whole milk for proper growth and development. Table 8-8 is a food guide for infants from birth to 12 months.

The foods that babies can choke on are generally of just the right size to close off the top of the windpipe, thereby preventing air from entering the lungs.

Several foods should be avoided during the first year. Because honey and liquid corn syrup may be contaminated with botulism, these foods may cause food poisoning or foodborne illness in children younger than 1 year. Certain foods are also more apt than others to cause choking. They include nuts, raisins, hot dogs, popcorn, whole grapes, peanut butter,

Figure 8-2a.
Growth chart
for girls

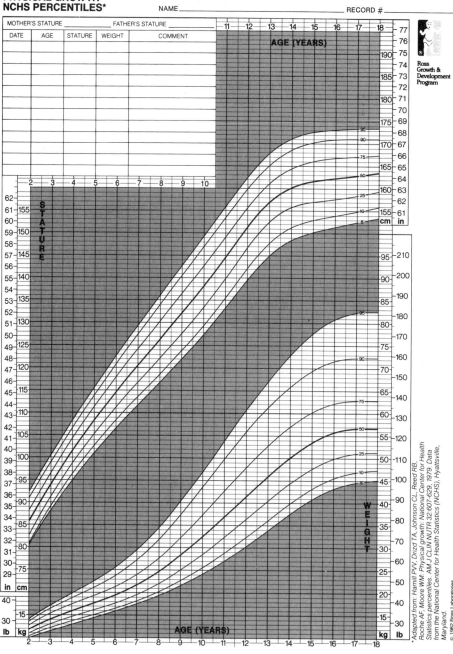

GIRLS: 2 TO 18 YEARS
PHYSICAL GROWTH
NCHS PERCENTILES*

NAME _____   RECORD # _____

Ross
Growth &
Development
Program

*Adapted from: Hamill PVV, Drizd TA, Johnson CL, Reed RB,
Roche AF, Moore WM. Physical growth: National Center for Health
Statistics percentiles. AM J CLIN NUTR 32:607-629, 1979. Data
from the National Center for Health Statistics (NCHS), Hyattsville,
Maryland.

© 1982 Ross Laboratories

**BOYS: 2 TO 18 YEARS
PHYSICAL GROWTH
NCHS PERCENTILES***

NAME _____ RECORD # _____

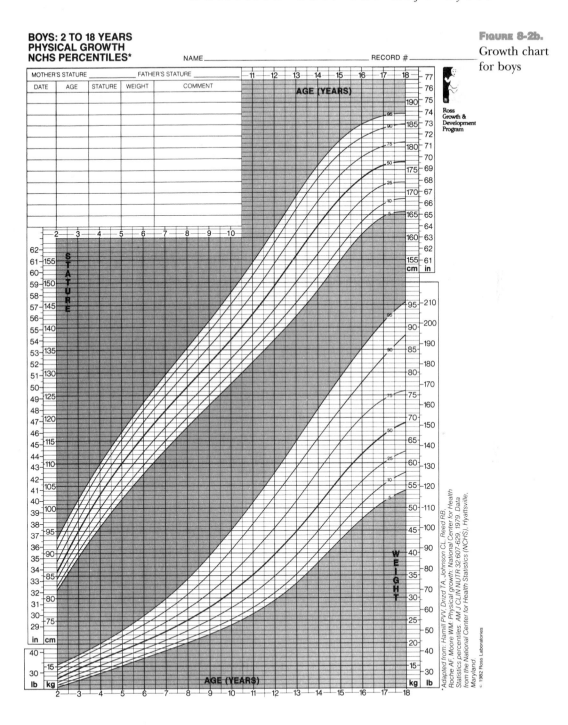

* Adapted from: Hamill PVV, Drizd TA, Johnson CL, Reed RB, Roche AF, Moore WM: Physical growth: National Center for Health Statistics percentiles. AM J CLIN NUTR 32:607-629, 1979. Data from the National Center for Health Statistics (NCHS), Hyattsville, Maryland

© 1982 Ross Laboratories

FIGURE 8-2b.

Growth chart for boys

Ross
Growth &
Development
Program

Age	Weight (lbs.)	Height (in.)	Calories*	Protein(grams)
1–3	29	35	1300	16
4–6	44	44	1800	24
7–10	62	52	2000	28

TABLE 8-9.   Recommended Dietary Allowances for calories and protein for children.

Energy allowances for children are based on median energy intakes of children of these ages followed in longitudinal growth studies.

Source: Recommended Dietary Allowances, 1989 by the National Academy of Sciences, National Academy Press, Washington, DC.

chunks of apple or pear, and cherries with pits. Other foods are also more apt to cause allergies: milk, eggs, wheat, nuts, chocolate, and shellfish. Whole milk and eggs are usually introduced at about 10 to 12 months.

MINI-SUMMARY   The growth rate during the first year will never be duplicated again. The nutrient needs of infants are about double those of an adult when viewed in proportion to their weight. For the first 4 to 6 months, the only food an infant should get is either breast milk or formula. Breast milk is recommended for many reasons. It is nutritionally superior to formula, and newborns are less likely to be allergic to it. Breast milk contains antibodies, to help babies build up immunities, and growth factors, to help babies develop. Breast-fed babies are generally given vitamin D supplements. For formula-fed babies, the formula is generally cow-based. If the baby is allergic to it, then a soy-based formula is used. A baby is generally ready to eat semi-solid foods between 5 to 7 months. The progression of foods starts with iron-fortified baby cereals, strained or pureed vegetables and fruits, strained or soft protein foods, finger foods, fruit juice, to soft chopped foods, and finally cut-up table foods by age one. Whole milk and whole eggs are not recommended until 12 months because of possible allergic reactions. Infants start getting baby teeth after 6 months and many have 4 to 6 teeth by their first birthday. Foods that cause choking, such as nuts and raisins, should be avoided.

CHILDHOOD

Around age one, the growth rate decreases markedly. Yearly weight gain now approximates 4 to 6 pounds per year. Children can expect to grow about 3 inches per year between ages 1 and 7, and then 2 inches per year until the pubertal growth spurt. Until adolescence, growth will come in spurts, during which the child will grow more and eat more.

Figure 8-2 shows growth charts for boys and girls that compare the child's height and weight to national percentiles. For example, if a girl is in the 90th percentile of height for her age, out of 100 girls her age she is taller than 89 and shorter than 10. These growth charts are commonly used by physicians to indicate a child's overall health and adequacy of calorie intake from ages 2 to 18. Growth charts are also available for infants and toddlers up to age 3.

After age 1, children start to lose baby fat and become leaner, with muscle accounting for a larger percentage of body weight. The legs become longer, and the baby now starts to look like a child and walk, run, and jump like a child. By age 2, brain growth is 75 percent complete. A child's head size in relation to body size starts to decrease and look more normal, and by age 6 to 10, the brain becomes adult size.

By about age 1, the child has 6 to 8 teeth, and by age 2 the baby teeth are almost all in. Between ages 6 and 12, these teeth are gradually replaced with permanent teeth. After the first birthday, as children's physical capabilities and desire for independence increase, they are more capable of feeding themselves. By age 18 months, many children can successfully use a spoon without too much spilling, and by 24 months many children can drink properly from a cup.

Nutrition During Childhood

Table 8-9 shows the RDA for calories and protein for children and compares them to the RDA for 25- to 50-year-old males. A one-year-old needs roughly 1000 calories a day, and a three-year-old about 1300. By age 10, a child needs about 2000 calories. Energy needs of children of similar age, sex, and size can vary due to differing BMRs (basal metabolic rates), growth rates, and activity levels. Both energy and protein needs decline gradually per pound of body weight.

During growth spurts, the requirements for calories and nutrients are greatly increased. Appetite fluctuates tremendously, with a good appetite during **growth spurts** (periods of rapid growth), and a seemingly terrible appetite during periods of slow growth. Parents may worry and force a child to eat more than needed at such times, when the child appears to be "living on air." A decreased appetite in childhood is perfectly normal. As long as the child is choosing nutrient-dense calories, nutritional problems are unlikely. In preparation for the adolescent growth spurt, children accumulate stores of nutrients, such as calcium, that will be drawn upon later, as intake cannot meet all the demands of this intensive growth spurt.

TABLE 8-10. Age-appropriate cooking activities.

2 1/2–3 Year Olds
- Wash fruits and vegetables
- Peel bananas
- Stir batters
- Slice soft foods with table knife (cooked potatoes, bananas)
- Pour
- Fetch cans from low cabinets
- Spread with a knife (soft onto firm)
- Use rotary egg beater (for a short time)
- Measure (e.g., chocolate chips into 1 cup measure)

4–5 Year Olds
- Grease pans
- Open packages
- Peel carrots
- Set table (with instruction)
- Shape dough for cookies/hamburger patties*

- Snip fresh herbs for salads or cooking
- Wash and tear lettuce for salad, separate broccoli, cauliflower
- Place toppings on pizza or snacks

6–8 Year Olds
- Take part in planning part of or entire meal
- Set table (with less supervision)
- Make a salad
- Find ingredients in cabinet or spice rack
- Shred cheese or vegetables
- Garnish food
- Use microwave, blender or toaster oven (with previous instruction)
- Measure ingredients
- Present prepared food to family at table
- Roll and shape cookies

9–12 Year Olds
- Depending on previous experience, plan and prepare an entire meal

*Caution children not to put their hands in their mouths while handling raw hamburger meat. It can carry harmful bacteria. They should wash hands after shaping patties.

Although calorie and protein intakes are rarely inadequate in American children, there are concerns about iron intake. Lack of iron can cause decreased energy and affect behavior, mood, and attention span. A balanced diet with adequate consumption of iron-rich foods such as lean meat (ground meat for younger children is easier to chew), enriched breads and cereals, and legumes is important to get enough iron. A source of vitamin C, such as citrus fruits, increases the amount of iron absorbed.

To prevent coronary heart disease early in life, medical authorities generally agree that by age 5 all healthy children should comply with the following guidelines for adults.

1. Reduce total fat intake to 30 percent of calories.
2. Reduce saturated fat intake to less than 10 percent of calories.
3. Consume no more than 300 milligrams of cholesterol daily.

Some parents have overzealously interpreted these guidelines and restricted the fat content of their childrens' diets to the point where the children received inadequate calories, which then interferes with normal growth. After age 2, parents may want to limit fatty meats and cheeses and use 2 percent milk.

Preschoolers exhibit some food-related behaviors that drive their parents crazy, such as **food jags** (eating mostly one food for a period of time). Food jags usually don't last long enough to cause any harm. Preschoolers often pick at foods or refuse to eat vegetables or drink milk. Lack of variety, erratic appetites, and food jags are typical of this age group. Toddlers (ages 1 to 3) tend to be pickier eaters than older preschoolers (ages 4 to 5). Toddlers are just starting to assert their independence and love to say "no" to parental requests. They may wage a control war and parents need to set limits without being too controlling or rigid. Here are several tactics for dealing with preschoolers' (and school-age children's) food habits.

1. Make mealtime as relaxing and enjoyable as possible.
2. Don't nag, bribe, force, or even cajole a child to eat. Stay calm. Pushing or prodding children almost always backfires. Children learn to hate the foods they are encouraged to eat and to desire the foods used as rewards, such as cake and ice cream. Once children know that you won't allow eating to be made into an issue of control, they will eat when they're hungry and stop when they're full. Your child is the best judge of when he or she is full.
3. Allow children to choose what they will eat from two or more healthy choices. You are responsible for choosing which foods are offered, and the child is responsible for deciding how much he or she wants of those foods.
4. Let children participate in food selection and preparation. Table 8-10 lists cooking activities for children of various ages.
5. Respect your child's preferences when planning meals, but don't make your child a quick peanut butter sandwich, for instance, if he or she rejects your dinner.
6. Make sure your child has appropriately sized utensils and can reach the table comfortably.
7. Preschoolers love rituals, so start them early with the habit of eating three meals plus snacks each day at fairly regular times. Also, eat with your preschooler and model good eating habits.
8. Expect preschoolers to reject new foods at least once, if not many times. Simply continue presenting the new food, perhaps prepared

When we force children to clean their plates, we are not letting them determine when they are full, an important skill that can help prevent obesity later in life.

differently, and one day they will try it (usually after 12 to 15 exposures).

9. Let the child serve himself or herself small portions.

10. Do not use desserts as a reward for eating meals. Make dessert a normal part of the meal and make it nutritious.

11. Ask children to try new foods (just a little bite!) and praise them when they try something different. Encourage them by telling them about someone who really likes the food or relating the food to something they think is fun. Realize, though, that some children are less likely to try new things, including new foods.

12. If all else fails, keep in mind that children under six have more taste buds (which may explain why youngsters are such picky eaters) and that this, too, will pass.

Luckily, school-age children are much better eaters. Although they generally have better appetites and will eat from a wider range of foods, they often dislike vegetables and casserole dishes.

Both preschoolers and school-age children learn about eating by watching others: their parents, their siblings, their friends, and their teachers. Parents, siblings, and friends provide role models for children and influence children's developing food patterns. Parents' interactions with their children will also influence what foods they or will not accept.

See the "Hot Topic" later in this chapter for more on the School Lunch and Breakfast Programs.

When children go to school, their peers influence their eating behaviors as well as what they eat for lunch. Lunch for school-age children often consists of the school lunch or a packed lunch from home.

Having breakfast makes a difference in how kids perform at school (Pollitt, 1995). Breakfast also makes a significant contribution to the child's intake of calories and nutrients for the day. Children who skip breakfast usually don't make up for the calories at other meals (Nicklas, Bao, Webber, and Berenson, 1993). If a child gets both breakfast and lunch at school, these meals together typically contribute about 50 percent of the day's calories.

Preschoolers and school-age children also learn about food by watching television. Research shows that children who watch a lot of television are more apt to be overweight. It not only takes them away from more robust activities but exposes them to commercials that are often for sugared cereals, candy, and other empty-calorie foods (Kotz and Story, 1994).

Both obesity and inactivity are currently on the rise in school-age children, especially among adolescents. In a well-known study of children's dietary intakes in a biracial community, ten-year-old children in the late 1980s were found to be 3 pounds heavier than their counterparts 14 years

TABLE 8-11. Daily food guide for children and adolescents.

Food Groups	Average Size Serving	1–3	4–6	7–10	11–14	15–18
High vitamin A vegetables and fruits		1/2–1 1/2	1 1/2–2	2	2–3	2–3**
Broccoli, chicory, brussels sprouts	1/2 cup cooked 1 cup raw					
Greens: beets, collard, dandelion, mustard, kale bok choy, watercress Swiss chard, carrots, pumpkin, sweet potato and yams, winter squash	1/2 medium potato, yam, squash					
Apricots, cantaloupe, mango, papaya	1/2 small cantaloupe, mango or papaya					
Vitamin C rich fruits and vegetables		1	1	1	1	1
Orange and orange juice, grapefruit and grapefruit juice, tomato and tomato juice, tangerines, papaya, cantaloupe, strawberries, acerola cherry, mango, green and red peppers, cauliflower, strawberries, raw cabbage	1 medium fruit 1/2 cup fruit juice 1 cup tomato juice 3/4 cup strawberries 1/2–1 cup raw vegetables					
Other fruits and vegetables		2–2 1/2	2–3	2–3	4–5	4–5**
Asparagus, artichokes, beets, corn, green peas, celery, lettuce, potatoes, string beans, summer squash, turnips, náme, plantain, cucumbers, zucchini, chili pepper	1/2 cup cooked 1 cup raw					
Apple, banana, cherries, pineapple, watermelon	1 medium fruit 1 cup pineapple or watermelon					
Protein foods		1 1/2–2	2–2 1/2	2 1/2–3	3	4–5**
Animal—Fish, chicken, turkey, duck, lean meat (beef, pork, lamb, goat, rabbit), liver, kidney, tongue	1–2 ounces cooked					

Food Groups	Average Size Serving	1–3	4–6	7–10	11–14	15–18
Vegetables—Legumes: dried peas and beans, soybeans, tofu, peanut butter, legumes nuts and seeds	1/2 cup cooked legumes 2 tablespoons peanut butter 3 ounces tofu 1 medium egg					
		3–4 wk	3–4 wk	2–3 wk	2–3 wk	2–3 wk
Milk and milk products		2–3	3	3*	3*	3*
Milk, fluid: whole, low-fat, skim	1 cup fluid milk					
Milk, dry: whole, skim						
Milk, evaporated						
Yogurt—plain, flavored	1 cup					
Cheese—cottage, pot, farmer, American, Cheddar	1 1/2 ounces hard cheese					
Pudding/custard/flan						
Ice cream						
Ice milk						
Sherbert						
Grains: cereals, breads, grain products		3–4	7–8	8–11	8–11	9–10
Bread: whole-wheat, white, rolls	1 slice					
Biscuits, muffins (made with whole grain or enriched white flour)	1 medium					
Pancakes, waffles	2 small					
Cereals	1/2 cup cooked 3/4 cup ready-to-eat					
Rice: white, brown, wild						
Pasta: noodles, macaroni, spaghetti	1/2 cup cooked					
Cornmeal, grits, bulgar, hominy						
Tortillas: flour, corn	6 inches					
Pizza	1/8 slice of 14" pizza					
Fats		2	3	3–5	4–5	4
Salad oil, cooking oil	1 teaspoon					
Margarine						
Mayonnaise						

*Use low-fat milk. **Lower number servings for females.

Source: Reprinted from *Practical Nutrition: A Quick Reference for the Health Care Practitione* by M.D. Simko, C. Cowell, and M. S. Hreha, pp. 302–305, with permission of Aspen Publishers, Inc., ©1989.

previously, yet total calorie intake was about the same and fewer calories came from fat (Nicklas, 1995). The increase in weight was probably related to inactivity. Although the children ate fewer fat calories in the late 1980s, they still ate more fat, saturated fat, and cholesterol than recommended.

So what can parents do to make sure their children eat nutritious diets and get exercise? Be a good role model by eating a well-balanced and varied diet. Have nutritious food choices readily available at home and serve a regular, nutritious breakfast. Maintain regular family meals as much as possible. Family meals are an appropriate time to model healthy eating habits and try out new foods. Also, limit television watching and encourage physical activity.

Menu Planning for Children
Table 8-11 gives a daily food pattern for children from ages 1 to 18.

PRESCHOOLERS

1. Offer simply prepared foods and avoid casseroles or any foods that are mixed together, as children need to identify what they are eating.
2. Offer at least one colorful food, such as carrot sticks.
3. Preschoolers like nutritious foods in all food groups but are often reluctant to eat vegetables. Part of this problem may be due to the difficulty involved in getting them onto a spoon or fork. Vegetables are more likely to be accepted if served raw and cut up as finger foods. However, when serving celery, be sure to take off the strings. Serve cooked vegetables somewhat undercooked, so they are a little crunchy. Brightly colored, mild-flavored vegetables such as peas and corn are more popular with kids.
4. Provide at least one soft or moist food that is easy to chew at each meal. A crisp or chewy food is important, too, to develop chewing skills.
5. Avoid strong-flavored and highly salted foods. Children have more taste buds than adults, so these foods taste too strong to them.
6. Preschoolers love carbohydrate foods, including cereals, breads, and crackers, as they are easy to hold and chew.
7. Smooth-textured foods such as pea soup or mashed potatoes should not have any lumps—children find this unusual.
8. Before age 4, when food-cutting skills start to develop, food needs to be served in bite-size pieces that are either eaten as finger foods or with utensils. For example, cut meat into strips or use ground meat, cut fruit into wedges or slices, and serve pieces of raw vegetables instead of a mixed salad. Other good finger foods include cheese

sticks, wedges of hard-boiled eggs, dry ready-to-eat cereal, fish sticks, arrowroot biscuits, and graham crackers.

9. Serve foods warm, not hot; a child's mouth is more sensitive to hot and cold than an adult's. Also, little children need little plates, utensils, and cups, as well as seats that allow them to reach the table comfortably.

10. Cut-up fruit and vegetables make good snacks. Let preschoolers spread peanut butter on crackers or use a spoon to eat yogurt. Snacks are important to preschoolers because they need to eat more often than adults.

11. To minimize choking hazards for children under 4:

> Slice hotdogs in quarters lengthwise.
> Shred hard raw vegetables and fruits.
> Remove pits from apples, cherries, plums, peaches, and other fruits.
> Cut grapes in half lengthwise.
> Spread peanut butter thin.
> Chop nuts and seeds fine.
> Check to make sure fish is boneless.
> Avoid popcorn and hard candies.

12. Children learn to like new foods by being presented with them repeatedly.

Insist children sit down during mealtime or snacks. Never let them lie down or run around while eating, as this can cause choking.

SCHOOL-AGE CHILDREN

1. Serve a wide variety of foods, including children's favorites: tuna fish, pizza (use vegetable toppings), macaroni and cheese, hamburgers (use lean beef combined with ground turkey breast), hot dogs (use low-fat varieties), and peanut butter.

2. Good snack choices are important, as children do not always have the desire or the time to sit down and eat. Snacks can include fresh fruits and vegetables, dried fruits, fruit juices, breads, cold cereals, popcorn (without excessive fat), pretzels, tortillas, muffins, milk, yogurt, cheese, pudding, sliced lean meats and poultry, and peanut butter.

3. Balance menu items that are higher in fat with those containing less fat.

4. Pay attention to serving sizes (see Table 8-11).

5. Children's most common nutritional problem is iron-deficiency anemia. Offer iron-rich foods such as meat in hamburgers or roast beef sandwiches, peanut butter, baked beans, chili, dried fruits, and fortified dry cereals.

6. As children grow, they need to eat more high-fiber foods, such as fruits, vegetables, beans and peas, and whole-grain foods. Whereas adults need at least 25 grams of fiber daily, children need a daily amount equal to or greater than their age plus 5 grams (Williams, 1995). In other words, a 12-year-old needs 17 grams of fiber daily.

TABLE 8-12.	**Recommended Dietary Allowances for adolescents for calories and protein**			
Age	*Weight*	*Height*	*Calories**	*Protein*
Males				
11–14	99	62	2500	45
15–18	145	69	3000	59
19–24	160	70	2900	58
25–50	174	70	2900	63
Females				
11–14	101	62	2200	46
15–18	120	64	2200	44
19–24	128	65	2200	46
25–50	138	64	2200	50

*Energy allowances are based on median energy intakes of people of those ages followed in longitudinal growth studies.

Source: Recommended Dietary Allowances: ©1989 by the National Academy of Sciences, National Academy Press, Washington, DC.

All children up to age 10 need to eat every 4 to 6 hours to keep their blood glucose at a desirable level; therefore, snacking is necessary between meals. Nutritious snack choices for both preschoolers and school-age children are noted above.

Snacks as well as meals should provide good sources of calcium, such as dairy foods, and iron and zinc, such as meats and legumes. If a child drinks little or no milk, try adding flavorings to milk such as chocolate or strawberry, or make cocoa, milkshakes, puddings, and custards. Milk can be fortified with powdered milk by blending 2 cups of fluid milk with 1/3 cup powdered milk. One cup of fortified milk is equal to 1 1/2 cups of regular milk. Powdered milk can also be added in baking and to casseroles, soups, sauces, gravies, ground meats, mashed potatoes, and scrambled eggs. Cheese and yogurt, of course, are also good sources of calcium.

MINI-SUMMARY By a child's first birthday, the growth rate decreases markedly and yearly weight gain until puberty is about 4 to 6 pounds. By the second birthday, the baby teeth are almost all in. During growth spurts, children's appetites are good, otherwise, their appetites may seem poor. Preschoolers can be fussy eaters, often have food jags, and can take the pleasure out of mealtime. Guidelines for eating with preschoolers and menu planning for them are detailed. Children's eating habits are influenced by family, friends, teachers, availability of school breakfast and lunch programs, and television. Menu-planning guidelines for school-age children are detailed. The most common nutritional problem of children is iron-deficiency anemia.

ADOLESCENCE

Puberty, the process of physically developing from a child to an adult, starts at about age 10 or 11 for girls and 12 or 13 for boys. In girls, it peaks at age 12 and is completed by age 15. In males, it peaks at age 14 and is completed by age 19. The timing of puberty and rates of growth show much individual variation. During the 5 to 7 years of pubertal development, adolescents gain about 20 percent of adult height and 50 percent of adult weight. Most of the body organs double in size, and almost half of total bone growth occurs.

Whereas before puberty the proportion of fat and muscle was similar in males and females, males now put on twice as much muscle as females, and females gain proportionately more fat. In adolescent girls, an increasing amount of fat is being stored under the skin, particularly in the abdominal area. The male also experiences a greater increase in bone mass than females.

Nutrition During Adolescence

Table 8-12 compares the RDA for calories and protein for adolescent males and females to adult needs. A major limitation of the RDAs for adolescents is that they are categorized according to age groups and are not related to stages of physical maturity, which show individual variation. The highest levels of nutrients are for individuals growing at the fastest rate.

Teenagers are not fed. They feed themselves.

Males now need more calories, protein, calcium, iron, and zinc for muscle and bone development than females; however, females need increased iron due to the onset of menstruation. Owing to their big appetites and calorie needs, teenage boys are more likely than girls to get sufficient nutrients. Females have to pack nutrients into fewer calories, which can become difficult if they decrease their food intake in an effort to lose weight.

With their increased independence, adolescents assume responsibility for their own eating habits. Teenagers are not fed; they make most of their own food choices. They eat more meals away from home, such as at fast-food restaurants, and skip more meals than previously. Irregular meals and snacking are common due to busy social lives and after-school activities and jobs. Teenagers will tell you that they lack the time or discipline to eat right, although many are pretty well informed about good nutrition practices. Ready-to-eat foods such as cookies, chips, and soft drinks are readily available, and teenagers pick them up as snack foods. Studies show that snacks contribute one-quarter to one-third of total daily calories and make substantial nutrient contributions except for iron.

Adolescents often have a variety of lunch options when they are at school. These choices may include leaving the school to buy lunch, eating a lunch from the National School Lunch Program, buying à la carte foods in the school cafeteria that do not qualify as a lunch in the National School Lunch Program, or buying food from a school store or vending machines. Although Federal regulations prohibit the sale of carbonated beverages, chewing gum, water ices, and most hard candies in the foodservice area or cafeteria during mealtimes, vending machines with these foods are often found just outside of the cafeteria. State, local, or school rules may close vending machines during mealtime and other times during the school day. Two professional associations, The American Dietetic Association and the American School Food Service Association, have concerns that the foods sold in vending machines, school stores, and à la carte cafeterias, discourage students from eating meals provided by the National School Lunch and Breakfast programs (American Dietetic Association, 1991; American School Food Service Association, 1991).

The media have a powerful influence on adolescents' eating patterns and behaviors. Advertising for not-so-nutritious foods and fast foods permeates television, radio, and billboards. In addition, questionable eating habits are portrayed on television shows. In a study of 12- to 17-year-old adolescents, the prevalence of obesity increased 2 percent for each additional hour of television watched.

A typical meal at a fast-food restaurant—a 4-ounce hamburger, French fries, and a regular soft drink—is high in calories, fat, and sodium. However, more nutritious choices are available at fast-food restaurants. Smaller hamburgers, milk, salads, and grilled chicken sandwiches are examples of more nutritious options.

Parents can positively influence adolescents' eating habits by being good role models and by having dinner and nutritious breakfast and snack foods available at home. Adolescents can become involved in food purchasing and preparation. Parents can also influence their children's fitness level by limiting sedentary activities and encouraging exercise.

Both adolescent boys and girls are influenced by their body image. Adolescent boys may take nutrition supplements and fill up on protein in hopes of becoming more muscular. Adolescent girls who feel they are

For adolescent girls, this is a time when many eating disorders appear. The next section discusses eating disorders in detail.

overweight may skip meals and modify their food choices in hopes of losing weight. Teens who need to lose weight should limit the amount of high-fat food and/or substitute lower-fat choices, such as skim milk for whole milk or nonfat frozen yogurt instead of ice cream. High-fat foods such as French fries and candy bars that have no low-fat substitutes should be eaten only once in a while or in very small amounts. Whether overweight or not, teens need regular exercise.

Menu Planning for Adolescents

Table 8-11 shows a daily food guide for adolescents.

1. Emphasize complex carbohydrates such as assorted breads, rolls, cereals, fruits, vegetables, potatoes, pasta, rice, and dried beans and peas. These foods supply calories along with needed nutrients. Whole-grain products are preferred.
2. Offer well-trimmed lean beef, poultry, and fish. Don't think that just because adolescents need more calories that fatty meats are in order. Their fat calories should be less saturated.
3. Low-fat and skim milk need to be offered at all meals. Girls are more likely to need to select skim milk than males. Other forms of calcium also need to be available, such as pizza, macaroni and cheese and other entrees using cheese, yogurt, frozen yogurt, ice milk, puddings, and custards made with skim milk.
4. Offer margarine; many adolescents are probably used to eating it at home.
5. Have nutritious choices available for hungry on-the-run adolescents looking for a snack. Nutritious snack choices include fresh fruit, muffins and other quick breads, crackers or rolls with low-fat cheese or peanut butter, vegetable-stuffed pita pocket, yogurt or cottage cheese with fruit, or fig bars.
6. Emphasize quick and nutritious breakfasts, such as whole-grain pancakes or waffles with fruit, juices, whole-grain toast or muffin with low-fat cheese, cereal topped with fresh fruits, or a bagel with peanut butter.
7. The nutrients most often lacking in adolescent diets are iron, folate, and calcium. Significant iron sources include meats, poultry, fish, eggs, legumes, and dried fruits. Vitamin C aids the absorption of iron from legumes and dried fruits. Folate is found in leafy green vegetables, orange juice, and beans and peas. Calcium may be lacking for those who have an inadequate intake of milk and other dairy products. If teenagers frequently drink soft drinks instead of milk, they may not have enough calcium in their diets to support bone growth.

MINI-SUMMARY The pubertal growth spurt starts at about age 10 for girls and 12 for boys. During the 5 to 7 years of pubertal development, the adolescent gains about 20 percent of adult height and 50 percent of adult weight. Boys gain twice as much muscle and more bone mass than girls, who gain proportionately more fat. Males now need more calories, protein, calcium, iron, and zinc for muscle and bone development than females, who need increased amounts of iron due to menstruation. Teenagers make most of their own food choices, which are influenced by their body image, peers, and the media. Menu-planning guidelines for adolescents are detailed.

EATING DISORDERS

Each year millions of Americans develop serious and sometimes life-threatening eating disorders. The vast majority—more than 90 percent—of those afflicted with eating disorders are adolescent and young adult women. One reason that women in this age group are particularly vulnerable to eating disorders is their tendency to go on strict diets to achieve an "ideal" figure. Researchers have found that such stringent dieting can play a key role in triggering eating disorders. The actual cause of eating disorders is not entirely understood, but many risk factors have been identified. Risk factors may include a high degree of perfectionism, low self-esteem, genetics, or family preoccupation with dieting and weight.

Eating-disorder patients deal with two sets of issues: those surrounding their eating behaviors and those surrounding their interactions with others and themselves. Eating disorders are considered a mental disorder, and both psychotherapy and medical nutrition therapy are cornerstones of treatment.

Approximately 1 percent of adolescent girls develop **anorexia nervosa,** a dangerous condition in which they can literally starve themselves to death. Another 2 to 3 percent of young women develop **bulimia nervosa,** a destructive pattern of excessive overeating followed by vomiting or other "purging" behaviors to control their weight. The most recently recognized eating disorder, **binge eating disorder,** could turn out to be the most common. With this disorder, binges are not followed by purges, so these individuals often become overweight. Eating disorders also occur in men and older women, but much less frequently.

The consequences of eating disorders can be severe, with one in ten cases leading to death from starvation, cardiac arrest, or suicide over the course of ten years. The outlook is better for bulimia than for anorexia; anorexia patients tend to relapse more. Many patients with anorexia or

There are now three recognized forms of eating disorders: anorexia nervosa, bulimia nervosa, and binge eating disorder. Eating disorders are classified as forms of mental illness.

bulimia also suffer from other psychiatric illnesses such as clinical depression, anxiety, obsessive-compulsive disorder, or substance abuse. Fortunately, increasing awareness of the dangers of eating disorders—sparked by medical studies and extensive media coverage of the illness—has led many people to seek help. Nevertheless, some people with eating disorders refuse to admit that they have a problem and do not get treatment. Family members and friends can help recognize the problem and encourage the person to seek treatment. The earlier treatment is started, the better the chance of a full recovery.

Anorexia Nervosa

People who intentionally starve themselves suffer from anorexia nervosa. This disorder, which usually begins in young people around the time of puberty, involves extreme weight loss—at least 15 percent below the individual's normal body weight. Many people with the disorder look emaciated but are convinced they are overweight. Sometimes they must be hospitalized to prevent starvation. Let's look at a typical case.

Deborah developed anorexia nervosa when she was 16. A rather shy, studious teenager, she tried hard to please everyone. She had an attractive appearance but was slightly overweight. Like many teenage girls, she was interested in boys but concerned that she wasn't pretty enough to get their attention. When her father jokingly remarked that she would never get a date if she didn't take off some weight, she took him seriously and began to diet relentlessly—never believing she was thin enough even when she became extremely underweight.

Soon after the pounds started dropping off, Deborah's menstrual periods stopped. As anorexia tightened its grip, she became obsessed with dieting and food, and developed strange eating rituals. Every day she weighed all the food she would eat on a kitchen scale, cutting solids into minuscule pieces and precisely measuring liquids. She would then put her daily ration in small containers, lining them up in neat rows. She also exercised compulsively, even after she weakened and became faint.

No one could convince Deborah that she was in danger. Finally, her doctor insisted that she be hospitalized and carefully monitored for treatment of her illness. While in the hospital, she secretly continued her exercise regimen in the bathroom. It took several hospitalizations and a good deal of individual and family outpatient therapy for Deborah to face and solve her problems.

One of the most frightening aspects of the disorder is anorexics continue to think they are overweight, even when they are bone-thin.

Food and weight become obsessions. For some, the compulsiveness shows up in strange eating rituals or the refusal to eat in front of others. It is not uncommon for anorexics to collect recipes and prepare gourmet feasts for family and friends but not partake in the meals themselves.

In anorexic patients, starvation can damage vital organs such as the heart and brain. To protect itself, the body shifts into "slow gear": menstrual periods stop and breathing, pulse, and blood pressure rates drop. Nails and hair become brittle. The skin dries, yellows, and becomes covered with soft hair called **lanugo.** Reduced body fat leads to lowered body temperature and the inability to withstand cold.

Mild anemia, swollen joints, reduced muscle mass, and lightheadedness are also common. If the disorder becomes severe, patients may lose calcium from the bones, making them brittle and prone to breakage. They may also experience irregular heart rhythms and heart failure.

Bulimia Nervosa

People with bulimia nervosa consume large amounts of food and then rid their bodies of excess calories by vomiting, abusing laxatives or diuretics, taking enemas, or exercising obsessively. Some use a combination of all these forms of purging. Because many individuals with bulimia "binge and purge" in secret and maintain normal or above-normal body weight, they can often successfully hide their problem for years. Let's take a look at Lisa.

Lisa developed bulimia at age 18. Like Deborah, her strange eating behavior began when she started to diet. She too dieted and exercised to lose weight, but unlike Deborah, she regularly ate huge amounts of food and maintained her normal weight by forcing herself to vomit. Lisa often felt like an emotional powder keg—angry, frightened, and depressed.

Unable to understand her own behavior, she thought no one else would either, so she felt isolated and lonely. Typically, when things were not going well, she would be overcome with an uncontrollable desire for sweets. She would eat pounds of candy and cake at a time and often not stop until she was exhausted or in severe pain. Then, overwhelmed with guilt and disgust, she would make herself vomit.

While recuperating in a hospital from a suicide attempt, she was referred to an eating disorders clinic, where she got into group therapy. She also received medications to treat the illness and the understanding and help she so desperately needed from others who had the same problem.

Individuals with this disorder may binge and purge once or twice a week or as much as several times a day. Dieting heavily between episodes of binging and purging is also common.

As with anorexia, bulimia typically begins during adolescence. The condition occurs most often in women but is also found in men. Many individuals with bulimia, ashamed of their strange habits, do not seek help until they reach their thirties or forties. By this time, their eating behavior is deeply ingrained and more difficult to change.

Bulimic patients—even those of normal weight—can severely damage their bodies by frequent binge eating and purging. Vomiting causes serious problems: The acid in vomit wears down the outer layer of the teeth and can cause scarring on the backs of hands when fingers are pushed down the throat to induce vomiting. Further, the esophagus becomes inflamed and the glands near the cheeks become swollen.

Binge Eating Disorder

Binge eating disorder resembles bulimia in that it is characterized by episodes of uncontrolled eating, or binging. However, binge eating disorder differs from bulimia in that its sufferers do not purge their bodies of excess food. Binge eating was recognized as a mental disorder in 1994. This is not to say that binge eating is a recent development—it's been around for a long time, but only lately has it been categorized as a mental disorder.

Binge eaters feel that they lose control of themselves when eating. They eat large quantities of food and do not stop until they are uncomfortably full. Usually, they have more difficulty losing weight and keeping it off than do people with other serious weight problems. Most people with this disorder are obese and have a history of weight fluctuations. Binge eating disorder is found in about 2 percent of the general population—more often in women than men. Binge eating disorder occurs in about 30 percent of people participating in medically supervised weight control programs.

Treatment

The sooner a disorder is diagnosed, the better the chances that treatment can work. The longer abnormal eating behaviors persist, the more difficult it is to overcome the disorder and its effects on the body. In some cases, long-term treatment is required.

Once an eating disorder is diagnosed, the clinician must determine whether the patient is in immediate medical danger and requires hospitalization. Although most patients can be treated as outpatients, some need hospital care, as in the case of severe purging or risk of suicide.

TABLE 8-13. Do you have an eating disorder?

A positive answer to one or more of these questions may indicate an eating disorder.

1. Do you eat large amounts of food in a very short period while feeling out of control and by yourself?
2. Do you frequently eat a lot of food when you are not hungry and usually when you are alone?
3. Do you feel guilty after overeating?
4. Do you make yourself vomit or use laxatives or diuretics to purge yourself?
5. Do you carefully make sure you eat only a small number of calories each day, such as 500 calories or less, and exercise a lot?
6. Do you avoid going out to maintain your eating and exercise schedule?
7. Do you feel that food controls your life?

TABLE 8-14. Common symptoms of eating disorders.

Symptoms	Anorexia Nervosa*	Bulimia Nervosa*	Binge Eating Disorder
Excessive weight loss in relatively short period of time	X		
Continuation of dieting although bone-thin	X		
Dissatisfaction with appearance; belief that body is fat, even though severely underweight	X		
Loss of monthly menstrual periods	X		
Unusual interest in food and development of strange eating rituals	X		
Eating in secret	X	X	X
Obsession with exercise	X	X	
Serious depression	X	X	X
Binging—consumption of large amounts of food		X	X
Vomiting or use of drugs to stimulate vomiting, bowel movements, and urination		X	
Binging but no noticeable weight gain		X	
Disappearance into bathroom for long periods of time to induce vomiting		X	
Abuse of drugs or alcohol		X	X

*Some individuals suffer from anorexia and bulimia and have symptoms of both disorders.

Eating-disorder patients commonly work with a treatment team that includes an internist, a nutritionist, an individual psychotherapist, and someone who is knowledgeable about psychoactive medications used in treating these disorders. Treatment usually includes individual psychotherapy, family therapy, cognitive-behavioral therapy, medical nutrition therapy, and possibly medications such as antidepressant drugs.

Eating disorders, unfortunately, have a very high death rate; one out of every ten patients will die. With that in mind, prevention of these diseases needs to be seriously examined. Research has identified the community groups most important to reach: junior high school students, coaches, and parents (Whisenant and Smith, 1995).

Table 8-13 lists questions to help individuals determine whether they have an eating disorder.

MINI-SUMMARY As pictured in Table 8-14, there are three different types of eating disorders. Most people afflicted with these problems are adolescent girls and young women. The sooner the disorder is diagnosed, the better the chances for successful treatment. Treatment usually includes individual psychotherapy, family therapy, cognitive-behavior therapy, medical nutrition therapy, and possibly medications. Of all types of mental illness, eating disorders have one of the highest death rates.

THE ELDERLY

By the year 2000, about one in four Americans will be 65 years of age or older. The fastest-growing age group in the United States comprises those over age 85! With the baby boom generation entering their fifties, the graying of America is in full swing. This trend is seen in the growing number of retirement communities and nursing facilities. Not only are there more elderly, but they are living longer. A 65-year-old woman can probably expect to live into her eighties. Her male counterpart still has about 14 more years.

Before looking at nutrition during aging, let's take a look at what happens when we age. Studies suggest that the maximum efficiency of many organ systems occurs between ages 20 and 35. After age 35, the functional capability of almost every organ system declines. Similar changes occur in adults as they age, but the rate of decline shows great individual variation. Both genetics and environmental factors such as nutrition affect the rate of aging. Conversely, changes brought about by the aging process affect nutrition status. Of particular importance are changes that affect digestion, absorption, and metabolism of nutrients.

The basal metabolic rate declines between 8 and 12 percent from age 30 to 70 and is accompanied by a 25 to 30 percent loss in muscle mass. Combined with a general decrease in activity level, these factors clearly indicate a need for decreased calorie intake, which generally does take place during aging. But the elderly need not lose all that muscle mass. Studies have shown that when the elderly do regular weight training exercises, they increase their muscular strength, increase basal metabolism, improve appetite, and improve blood flow to the brain.

Overall, the functioning of the cardiovascular system declines with age. The work load of the heart increases due to atherosclerotic deposits and less elasticity in the arteries. The heart does not pump as hard as before, and cardiac output is reduced in elderly people who do not remain physically active. Blood pressure increases normally with age. Pulmonary capacity decreases by about 40 percent throughout life. This decrease does not restrict the normal activity of healthy older persons but may limit vigorous exercise. Kidney function deteriorates over time, and the aging kidney is less able to excrete waste. Adequate fluid intake is important, as is avoiding megadoses of water-soluble vitamins because they will put a strain on the kidney to excrete them. Last, loss of bone occurs normally during aging and osteoporosis is common (see Chapter 6).

Factors Affecting Nutrition Status

The nutrition status of an elderly person is greatly influenced by many variables, including physiological, psychosocial, and socioeconomic factors.

PHYSIOLOGICAL FACTORS

- **Disease.** The presence of disease, both acute and chronic, and use of modified diets can affect nutrition status. The elderly are major users of modified diets. The most prevalent nutrition-related problems of the elderly are chronic conditions that require modified diets. Certain chronic diseases are associated with **anorexia,** such as gastrointestinal disease, congestive heart failure, renal disease, and cancer (Roe, 1992). Other diseases, such as stroke, are not associated with anorexia but can cause the individual to take in little food.

  Anorexia means lack of appetite.

- **Less muscle mass.** With aging, there is less muscle mass, so the basal metabolic rate decreases. As the basal metabolic rate slows down, the number of calories needed by the elderly decreases.

- **Activity level.** Because active individuals tend to eat more calories than their sedentary counterparts, they are more likely to ingest more nutrients.

TABLE 8-15. Nutrients depleted by selected drugs.

Drug Group	Drug	Nutrients Depleted
Analgesics	Uncoated aspirin	Iron
Antacids	Aluminum or magnesium hydroxide	Phosphate, calcium, and folate
	Sodium bicarbonate	calcium, folate
Antiulcer drugs	Cimetidine	B_{12}
Chemotherapeutic agents	Methotrexate	Folate
Cholesterol-lowering agents	Cholestyramine	Fat, vitamins A and K
Diuretics	Lasix	Potassium
Laxatives	Mineral oil	Vitamins A, D, and K

- **Dentition.** Approximately 50 percent of Americans have lost their teeth by age 65. Despite widespread use of dentures, chewing still presents problems for many elderly.
- **Functional disabilities.** Functional disabilities interfere with the ability of the elderly to perform daily tasks, such as the purchasing and preparation of food and eating. These disabilities may be due to arthritis or rheumatism, stroke, visual impairment, heart trouble, or dementia. One study reported that 39 percent of the elderly subjects needed help food shopping and 26 percent needed help making meals (Ford et al., 1988).
- **Taste and smell.** Sensitivity to taste and smell decline slowly with age (Rolls, 1992). The taste buds become less sensitive and the nasal nerves that register aromas need extra stimulation to detect smells. That's why seniors may find ordinarily seasoned foods too bland. Medications also may alter an individual's ability to taste.
- **Changes in the gastrointestinal tract.** The movement of food through the gastrointestinal tract slows down over time, causing problems such as constipation, a frequent complaint of older people. Constipation may also be related to low fiber and fluid intake, medications, or lack of exercise. Other frequent complaints include nausea, indigestion, and heartburn. (Heartburn, a burning sensation in the area of the throat, has nothing to do with the heart. It occurs when acidic stomach contents are pushed into the lower part of the esophagus or throat.)
- **Medications.** More than half of seniors take at least one medication daily, and many take six or more a day. Medications may alter appetite or the digestion, absorption, and metabolism of nutrients (Table 8-15).

- **Thirst.** Many elderly suffer a diminished perception of thirst—especially problematic when they are not feeling well (Rolls and Phillips, 1990). Because the aging kidney is less able to concentrate urine, more fluid is lost, setting the stage for dehydration.

PSYCHOSOCIAL FACTORS

- **Cognitive functioning.** Poor cognitive functioning may affect nutrition, or perhaps poor nutritional status contributes to poor cognitive functioning (Goodwin, Goodwin, and Garry, 1983).
- **Social support.** An individual's nutritional health results in part from a series of social acts. The purchasing, preparing, and eating of foods are social events for most people. For example, elderly people may rely on one another for rides to the supermarket, cooking, and sharing meals. The benefits of social networks or support are largely due to the companionship and emotional support they provide. It is anticipated that this has a positive effect on appetite and dietary intake.

SOCIOECONOMIC FACTORS

- **Education.** Higher levels of education are positively associated with increased nutrient intakes.
- **Income.** In a large study of older Americans using data from the Nationwide Food Consumption Survey 1977–78, money spent on food was found to be a highly significant predictor of dietary quality (Murphy, Maradee, and Neuhaus, 1990).
- **Living arrangements.** The elderly, particularly women, are more likely to be widowed. The trend has been for widows and widowers in the United States to live alone after the spouse dies. Research focusing on the impact of living arrangements on dietary quality showed that living alone is a risk factor for dietary inadequacy for older men, especially those over age 75 years of age, and for women only in the youngest age group (55 to 64).
- **Availability of federally funded meals.** The availability of nutritious meals through federal programs such as Meals on Wheels, in which meals are delivered to the home, are crucial to the nutritional health of many elderly.

Another popular elderly feeding program is the Congregate Meals Program in which the elderly go to a senior center to eat.

Nutrition for the Later Years

A recent survey completed for the new Nutrition Screening Initiative—targeted at improving the nutritional health status of the aging—shows that, although 85 percent of seniors surveyed believe that nutrition is important for their health and well-being, few act on their beliefs. Further,

30 percent admit to skipping at least one meal a day. These numbers may well soar as America continues to gray at an increasing rate. Studies of the elderly have shown that maintaining adequate calorie intake is vital to good nutrition (Murphy, Davis, Neuhaus, and Lein, 1990).

The daily food guide for an elderly individual is the same as that for a younger adult using the Food Guide Pyramid. Because the elderly consume fewer calories, this means that there is less room in the diet for empty calorie foods such as sweets, alcohol, and fats. At a time when good nutrition is so important to good health, there are many obstacles to eating right, including a basic lack of nutrition knowledge.

Most RDAs for older adults are based on data from younger people because little research has been done on the elderly, although more has been recently undertaken to fill this gap. For most nutrients, the RDAs are the same for older adults as for younger adults (ages 25 to 50). The need for the energy vitamins (thiamin, riboflavin, and niacin) decreases as fewer calories are taken in. There is only one set of RDAs for older adults ages 51 and older.

Nutrients of concern to the elderly include the following.

- **Protein.** Because calorie needs decrease with age but amino acid needs do not decline, the elderly need to eat more calories from protein foods than previously. Approximately 12 to 14 percent of calories should come from protein (Young, 1992). More protein is needed for elderly in poor health.
- **Vitamin B_{12}.** The elderly have a problem with vitamin B_{12} even if they take in enough The stomach of an elderly person secretes less gastric acid and pepsin, both of which are necessary to break vitamin B_{12} from its polypeptide linkages in food. The result is that less vitamin B_{12} is absorbed. Vitamin B_{12} is necessary to convert folate into its active form so that folate can do its job of making new cells, such as new red blood cells. Vitamin B_{12} also maintains the protective cover around nerve fibers. A deficiency in vitamin B_{12} can cause a type of anemia as well as nervous system problems that can cause a poor sense of balance, numbness and tingling in the arms and legs, and mental confusion. If a vitamin B_{12} deficiency is due to problems in absorption, injections are recommended.
- **Vitamin D.** Several factors adversely affect the vitamin D status of the elderly. First, the elderly tend to be outside less so they make less vitamin D from exposure to the sun. Also, they have less of the vitamin D precursor in the skin necessary to make vitamin D, and older women absorb less vitamin D from food. Because milk is the only

dairy product with vitamin D added to it, milk is important to getting enough vitamin D. If milk intake is low, supplements may be recommended.

- **Calcium.** Current intakes for calcium are below the recommendations for individuals over 65 years of age (1500 milligrams) from the National Institutes of Health (Table 6-6). To meet this recommendation, an elderly person would need to eat four servings of dairy products or other calcium-rich foods. Because this can be difficult, supplements may be recommended.
- **Zinc.** Because the elderly take in less than the RDA for zinc, and the importance of zinc in cell production, wound healing, the immune system, and taste, attention needs to be placed on getting enough of this mineral.

Here are some ways the elderly can increase their chances of eating nutritiously.

1. Eat with other people. This usually makes mealtime more enjoyable and stimulates appetite. Taking a walk before eating also stimulates appetite.
2. Prepare larger amounts of food and freeze some for heating up at a later time. This saves cooking time and is helpful if you are reluctant to cook for yourself.
3. If big meals are too much, eat small amounts more frequently during the day. Eat regular meals.
4. If getting to the supermarket is a bother, go at a time when it is not busy or, if you have the money, engage a delivery service .
5. Use unit pricing and sales to cut back on the amount of money you spend on food.
6. Take advantage of community meal programs for the elderly, such as Meals on Wheels.
7. To perk up a sluggish appetite, increase your use of herbs, spices, lemon juice, vinegar, and garlic.

Menu Planning for the Later Years

Basic menu-planning guidelines for older adults are found in the Food Guide Pyramid described in Chapter 7. Guidelines specifically for older adults are listed here.

1. Offer moderately sized meals. Older adults frequently complain when given too much food because they hate to see waste. Restaurants might reduce the size of their entrees by 15 to 25 percent (Schur, 1995).

Hot Topic: Creative Pureed Foods

In the past, pureed foods had the reputation of looking pretty miserable when served in most hospitals and nursing facilities. Pureed meat and vegetables were often scooped into small bowls (which for some reason are called "monkey" dishes), covered with gravy, and sent away to some unfortunate patient as supper.

Pureed diets are often necessary for individuals with chewing or swallowing disorders. But that doesn't mean they need runny, liquid foods. On the contrary, the hardest foods for these individuals to swallow are runny foods. The easiest texture to swallow resembles that of mashed potatoes.

Luckily, times have changed. Many cooks are using thickeners to help shape pureed foods so they look like the original foods (Figure 8-3). Thickeners are often powdered and can be mixed directly with liquids and pureed foods. Although there are several commercial thickeners available, such as Thick & Easy, some cooks use thickeners such as cornstarch or instant mashed potato flakes.

Preparing pureed foods is a challenge not only because the foods must look good and be the right consistency for swallowing, but also because the volume of pureed foods differs from that of regular foods. Fruits and vegetables tend to decrease in volume when pureed so 1/2 cup of pureed peaches, for example, would contain more calories and nutrients than 1/2 cup of regular peaches. On the other hand, meats almost double in volume because of the liquid required to puree them. Using standardized recipes ensures that pureed foods

- are nutritionally adequate.
- are the right consistency.
- look and taste appropriately.
- are not too expensive (recipes cut down on waste).

2. Emphasize complex carbohydrates and high-fiber foods such as fruits, vegetables, grains, and beans. Older people requiring softer diets may have problems chewing some high-fiber foods. High-fiber foods that are soft in texture include cooked beans and peas, bran cereals soaked in milk, canned prunes and pears, and cooked vegetables such as potatoes, corn, green peas, and winter squash.

3. Moderate the use of fat. Many seniors don't like to see their entree swimming in a pool of butter. Use lean meats, poultry, or fish and sauces prepared with vegetable or fruit purees. Have low-fat dairy products available such as skim or 1% milk.

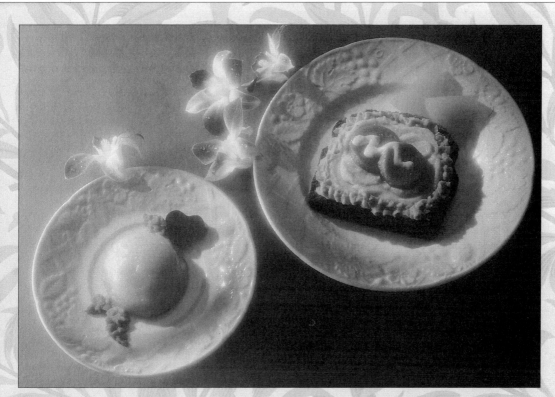

FIGURE 8-3.   Creative and attractive pureed foods using thickeners. Pureed peaches, pureed ham on slurried pumpernickel with pureed lettuce and tomato wedges, garnished with pureed cantaloupe thickened with Menu Magic's Thicken Right.™(Courtesy: Menu Magic, Indianapolis, Indiana)

4. Dairy products are important sources of calcium, vitamin D, protein, potassium, vitamin B_{12} and riboflavin.
5. Offer adequate but not too much protein. Use a variety of both animal and vegetable sources. Providing protein on a budget, as in a nursing home, need not be a problem. Lower-cost protein sources include beans and peas, cottage cheese, macaroni and cheese, eggs, liver, dried skim milk, chicken, and ground beef.

TABLE 8-16   Most and least favorite foods of various age groups.

Age Group	Favorite Foods	Least Favorite Foods
Children (ages 5 to 12)	Sweet foods, fruit flavors, peanut butter and jelly sandwiches, cheese, bananas, grapes, brownies, cookies, ice cream, milk, juice.	Cooked vegetables
Teens (ages 13 to 18)	Burgers, melted cheese toppings, French fries, fried appetizers, sodas, salads and yogurt for health-conscious segment.	Casseroles such as stews and goulash
Young adults (ages 19 to 24)	Sweet, starchy, and fast foods; soup, salads, and vegetables; chocolate; soda and designer beverages including coffees and fruit juices; new ethnic and regional cuisines; vegetarian dishes for health-conscious segment.	
Young adults (ages 25 to 34)	Overstuffed sandwiches, munchies, pasta, grilled chicken, sophisticated comfort foods, fresh breads, creamy and cheesy textures, ethnic and regional dishes, soft drinks, specialty coffees.	
Baby boomers (ages 35 to 54)	Eclectic foods; major fans of Italian, Asian, Mexican, and Southwestern cuisines; soda, fresh juices, and iced tea; healthful options.	
Mature middle-agers (ages 55 to 70)	Personal comfort foods, familiar American foods, fried foods, chocolate desserts, coffee and tea, healthful options.	
Seniors (ages 70 and over)	Familiar foods, sweet foods, soft-textured foods (for breakfast eaters), ethnic and regional dishes, hot coffee and tea, decaffeinated drinks.	Hot foods served lukewarm. Undercooked vegetables.

Sources: Weiss, Steve. 1995 Market driven menus: A coming of age. *Restaurants & Institutions* 105(6): 62–86.
The California Table Grape Commission Survey, 1989.

6. Moderate the use of salt. Many seniors are on low-sodium diets and recognize a salty soup when they taste it. Avoid highly salted soups, sauces, and other dishes. It is better to let them season food to taste.

7. Use herbs and spices to make foods flavorful. Seniors are looking for tasty foods just like anyone else, and they may need them more than ever!

8. Offer a variety of foods, including traditional menu items and cooking from other countries and regions of the United States.

9. Fluid intake is critical, so offer a variety of beverages. Diminished sensitivity to dehydration may cause older adults to drink less fluid than needed. Special attention must be paid to fluids, particularly for those who need assistance with eating and drinking. Beverages such as water, milk, juice, coffee, or tea, and foods such as soup contribute to fluid intake.

10. Intake of the following vitamins and minerals may be inadequate in older adults and needs to be considered when menu planning: vitamin B_{12}, vitamin D, calcium, and zinc. See Tables 5-1 and 6-4 for food sources.

11. If chewing is a problem, softer foods can be chosen to provide a well-balanced diet. Following are some guidelines for soft diets.

- Use tender meats, and if necessary, chop or grind them. Ground meats can be used in soups, stews, and casseroles. Cooked beans and peas, soft cheeses, and eggs are additional softer protein sources.
- Cook vegetables thoroughly and dice or chop by hand if necessary after cooking.
- Serve mashed potatoes or rice, with gravy if desired.
- Serve chopped salads.
- Soft fruits such as fresh or canned bananas, berries, peaches, pears, or melon, as well as applesauce, are some good choices.
- Soft breads and rolls can be made even softer by dipping them briefly in milk.
- Puddings and custard are good dessert choices.
- Many foods that are not soft can be easily chopped by hand or blended in a blender or food processor to provide additional variety.

Table 8-16 lists the most and least favored foods of various age groups.

MINI-SUMMARY The graying of America is in full swing. During aging, the functional capability of almost every organ declines, and muscle tissue and mass decreases. Along with a declining basal metabolic rate, the need for calories decreases. The nutrition status of an elderly person is greatly influenced by many variables: presence of disease, activity level, quality of dentition, functional disabilities, decline in taste and smell acuity, changes in the gastrointestinal tract, use of medications, diminished sense of thirst, level of cognitive functioning, available social support, level of education and income, living arrangements, and availability of federally funded meals. The daily food guide for an elderly individual is the same as that for a younger adult using the Food Guide Pyramid. The nutritional needs of the elderly are being researched, since little has been known in the past. Menu-planning guidelines are listed.

KEY TERMS

Amniotic sac	Heartburn
Anorexia	Lactation
Anorexia nervosa	Lanugo
Baby-bottle tooth decay	Low birth weight baby
Binge eating disorder	Milk letdown
Bulimia nervosa	Morning sickness
Colostrum	Neural tube
Edema	Palmar grasp
Embryo	Pincer grasp
Fetal alcohol syndrome (FAS)	Placenta
Fetus	Puberty
First trimester	Spina bifida
Food jag	Team nutrition
Gag reflex	Transitional milk
Growth spurts	

In your own words, answer each question.

1. What is the difference between an embryo and a fetus?
2. What organ forms during early pregnancy that can be adversely affected by poor nutrition? Describe its role.
3. Why is the nutritional status of women important before and during pregnancy?
4. List five nutritional risk factors for pregnant women.
5. How many more calories a day should a pregnant woman eat? Is it okay for a pregnant woman to get her extra calories from a high-calorie food such as cake? Why or why not?
6. How much weight is normally gained during a 40-week pregnancy? At what rate is the weight gained? How much of the weight gain is attributable to the baby?
7. Which nutrients are particularly important during pregnancy? Why? Which of these nutrients is given in supplement form?
8. What is the dietary advice for morning sickness, constipation, and heartburn?
9. Should sodium be restricted if a pregnant woman has moderate swelling? Why or why not?
10. How many servings from each Food Guide Pyramid group are needed by pregnant and lactating women?
11. Why don't alcohol and pregnancy mix?
12. Are saccharin, aspartame, and caffeine dangerous during pregnancy?
13. List five menu-planning guidelines for pregnant or lactating women.
14. How many extra calories per day should a lactating woman consume? Why are calories increased at this time?
15. Which nutrient is necessary in supplemental form during lactation? Which other nutrient is especially important?
16. Describe an infant's growth pattern for the first year. During which months does the infant need the greatest amount of nutrients?
17. List five advantages of breastfeeding over bottle feeding.
18. Why isn't cow's milk recommended for infants before age 12 months?
19. How often is breast milk or formula given to infants during the first 6 months?
20. In what order are foods introduced and when?
21. Which foods cause baby-bottle tooth decay?
22. Which foods should be avoided during the first year and why?
23. Describe when children start getting their baby teeth and when they are replaced with permanent teeth.
24. List five techniques parents can use to encourage healthy eating and make mealtime fun and relaxing.

25. At what age does puberty start for boys versus girls? How long does it last? How much growth occurs at this time? Who puts on more muscle and bone mass?
26. What influences children's and adolescents' eating habits?
27. List five menu-planning guidelines for children and adolescents.
28. What are the major characteristics of anorexia nervosa, bulimia nervosa, and binge eating disorder? How are eating disorders treated?
29. List ten factors affecting the nutritional status of the elderly.
30. List five menu-planning guidelines for the elderly.

ACTIVITIES AND APPLICATIONS

1. Quiz

Check your answers against the following.

Food Group	Minimum Number of Servings	Servings Needed During Pregnancy	& Lactation
Meat, poultry, fish, and alternates	2	3	3
Milk and dairy products	2	3	4
Fruits	2	2	2
Vegetables	3	3	3
Breads, cereals, grains	6	6	7

2. Cereal, vegetable, meat, whole egg
3. True
4. True
5. c
6. b
7. e
8. b
9. True
10. True
11. True
12. True

2. Television Watch

Watch Saturday morning children's television for at least 1 hour and record the name of each advertiser and what it is advertising. How many of the total number of advertisers advertised food? Were the majority of advertised foods healthy foods or junk foods?

3. *What Influenced Your Childhood Eating Habits?*

Think back to when you were a child and a teenager. What influenced what you put into your mouth? Consider influences such as home, school, friends, and relatives. Which positively influenced your eating style? Which negatively?

4. *Interview*

Interview someone who has direct experience feeding babies and children. Ask him or her about the difficulties and pleasures of feeding young ones. Ask about the children's food preferences and eating habits. Ask how well the young child accepted new foods.

4. *Menu Planning for Preschoolers*

Write a 5-day menu for a day-care center with children ages 1 to 5. Plan a lunch plus morning and afternoon snacks. Allow two menu choices for the lunch entree. Keep in mind eating styles, dietary needs, and general dietary guidelines when planning the menu. If you know someone with young children, ask him or her to look at your menu and tell you whether children will like your choices.

5. *Menu Planning for Children/Adolescents*

Write a 5-day lunch menu for elementary or high school students. The menu must provide an entree, milk, and at least one other food. The average daily menu must provide one-third of the RDA for calories, protein, iron, calcium, vitamin A, and vitamin C. Only 30 percent of total calories can come from fat. Saturated fat can provide no more than 10 percent of total calories.

6. *Eldercare Menu*

Visit or phone the food-service director of a local nursing home, congregate meals feeding center, or continuing care retirement community. Ask about the type of menu being used (restaurant-style or cycle menu) and foods being offered. What are the major meal-planning considerations used in planning meals for the elderly? What special circumstances come up that are unique to them?

REFERENCES   American Academy of Pediatrics, Committee on Nutrition. 1986. Prudent life-style for children: Dietary fat and cholesterol. *Pediatrics* 78(3): 521–25.

American Dietetic Association. 1991. Position of the American Dietetic Association: Competitive foods in schools. *Journal of the American Dietetic Association* 11(9): 1123–1125.

American Dietetic Association. 1993. Position of the American Dietetic Association: Nutrition, aging, and the continuum of health care. *Journal of the American Dietetic Association* 93(1): 80–82.

American Dietetic Association. 1993. Position of the American Dietetic Association: Promotion and support of breast feeding. *Journal of The American Dietetic Association* 93(4): 467–469.

American Dietetic Association. 1994. Position of the American Dietetic Association: Nutrition intervention in the treatment of anorexia nervosa, bulimia nervosa, and binge eating. *Journal of The American Dietetic Association* 94(8): 902–907.

American School Food Service Association. 1991. *Position Statement: Nutrition Policy for Food Available at School (Competitive Foods)*. Alexandria, VA: American School Food Service Association.

Anderson, John A. 1994. Tips when considering the diagnosis of food allergy. *Topics in Clinical Nutrition* 9(3): 11–21.

Barness, Lewis A. 1985. Infant feeding: formula, solids. *Pediatric Clinics of North America* 32(2): 355–362.

Bigler-Doughten, Sharon, and R. Michael Jenkins. 1987. Adolescent snacks: Nutrient density and nutritional contribution to total intake. *Journal of the American Dietetic Association* 87(12): 1678–1679.

Bock, A. A., and F. M. Atkins. 1990. Patterns of food hypersensitivity during sixteen years of double-blind, placebo-controlled food challenges. *Journal of Pediatrics* 117: 561–567.

Brown, Judith E., and M. Story. 1990. "Let them eat cake" or a prescription for improving the outcome of pregnancy?: A response to nutrition during pregnancy, Parts I and II. *Nutrition Today* (6): 18–23.

Davies, Louise. 1988. Practical nutrition for the elderly. *Nutrition Reviews* 46(2): 83–87.

Davis, Maradee A., Suzanne P. Murphy, John M. Neuhaus, and David Lein. 1990. Living arrangements and dietary quality of older U.S. adults. *Journal of The American Dietetic Association* 90(12): 1667–1672.

Dietz, William H. 1987. Childhood obesity. *Annals of the New York Academy of Sciences* 499: 47–54.

Dietz, William H., and Steven L. Gortmaker. 1985. Do we fatten our children at the television set? Obesity and television viewing in children and adolescents. *Pediatrics* 75(5): 807–811.

Epstein, Leonard H., Rena R. Wing, and Alice Valoski. 1985. Childhood obesity. *Pediatric Clinics of North America* 32(2): 363–379.

Erick, Miriam. 1993. *No More Morning Sickness: A Survival Guide for Pregnant Women*. New York: Plume.

Erick, Miriam, and Hahn, Nancy I. 1994. Battling morning (noon and night) sickness: New approaches for treating an age-old problem. *Journal of The American Dietetic Association* 94(2): 147–148.

Ford, A. B., S. J. Folmar, R. B. Salmon, J. H. Medalie, A. W. Roy, and S. S. Galazka. 1988. Health and function in the old and very old. *Journal of the American Geriatrics Society* 36: 187–193.

Goodwin, J. S., J. M. Goodwin, and P. J. Garry. 1983. Association between nutritional status and cognitive functioning in a healthy elderly population. *Journal of the American Medical Association* 249: 2917–2921.

Gordan, Gilbert S., and Cynthia Vaughan. 1986. Calcium and osteoporosis. *Journal of Nutrition* 116(2): 319–322.

Guenther, Patricia M. 1986. Beverages in the diets of American teenagers. *Journal of The American Dietetic Association* 86(4): 493–499.

Harper, Alfred E. 1982. Nutrition, aging, and longevity. *American Journal of Clinical Nutrition* 36(10): 737–749.

Hegsted, D. M. 1986. Calcium and osteoporosis. *Journal of Nutrition* 116(11): 2316–2319.

Institute of Medicine. 1990. *Nutrition During Pregnancy*. Washington, DC: National Academy Press.

Institute of Medicine. 1991. *Nutrition During Lactation*. Washington, DC: National Academy Press.

Jacobson, Michael F., Lisa Y. Lefferts, and Anne Witte Garland. 1991. *Safe Food: Eating Wisely in a Risky World*. Venice, CA: Living Planet Press.

Jones, Kenneth L. 1986. Fetal alcohol syndrome. *Pediatrics in Review* 8(4): 122–126.

Kamath, Savitri. 1982. Taste acuity and aging. *American Journal of Clinical Nutrition* 36(10): 766–775.

Kenney, M. A., J. H. McCoy, A. L. Kirby, E. Carter, A. J. Clark, G. W. Disney, C. D. Floyd, E. E. Glover, M. K. Korslund, H. Lewis, M. Liebman, S. W. Moak, S. J. Ritchey, and S. F. Stallings. 1986. Nutrients supplied by food groups in diets of teenaged girls. *Journal of The American Dietetic Association* 86(11): 1549–1555.

Kotz, Krista, and Mary Story. 1994. Food advertisements during children's Saturday morning television programming: Are they consistent with dietary recommendations? *Journal of The American Dietetic Association* 94(11): 1296–1300.

Kurinij, Natalie, Mark A. Klebanoff, and Barry I. Graubard. 1986. Dietary supplement and food intake in women of childbearing age. *Journal of The American Dietetic Association* 86(11): 1536–1540.

Leaf, Alexander. 1988. The aging process: Lessons from observations in man. *Nutrition Reviews* 46(2): 40–44.

Lecos, Chris W. 1984-85. Diet and the elderly. *FDA Consumer* 18(10): 10–13.

Lynch, Sean R., Clement A. Finch, Elaine R. Monsen, and James D. Cook. 1982. Iron status of elderly Americans. *American Journal of Clinical Nutrition* 36(11): 1032–1045.

McIntosh, W. A., Karen S. Kubena, Juliann Walker, Dana Smith, and Wendall A. Landmann. 1990. The relationship between beliefs about nutrition and dietary practices of the elderly. *Journal of the American Dietetic Association* 90(5): 671–676.

Munro, Hamish N., Paolo M. Suter, and Robert M. Russell. 1987. Nutritional requirements of the elderly. *Annual Review of Nutrition* 7: 23–49.

Murphy, Suzanne P., Maradee A. Davis, John M. Neuhaus, and D. Lein. 1990. Factors influencing the dietary adequacy and energy intake of older Americans. *Journal of Nutrition Education* 22(6): 284–291.

Nicklas, Theresa A. 1995. Dietary studies of children: the Bogalusa Heart Study experience. Journal of The American Dietetic Association 95(10): 1127–1133.

Nicklas, Theresa, Weihang Bao, Larry S. Webber, and Gerald S. Berenson. 1993. Breakfast consumption affects adequacy of total daily intake in children. *Journal of The American Dietetic Association* 93(8): 886–891.

Nutrition Screening Initiative. 1991. *Nutrition Screening Manual for Professionals Caring for Older Americans*. Washington, DC: Nutrition Screening Initiative.

Papa, Anne. 1986. The forgotten generation: Marketing to the over 50 crowd. *Restaurants USA* 6(9): 11–14.

Parker, Sharon L., Magdalena Krondi, and Patricia Coleman. 1993. Food perceived by adults as causing adverse reactions. *Journal of The American Dietetic Association* 93(1): 40–44.

Perkin, Judy E. 1994. Update on food allergy research. *Topics in Clinical Nutrition* 9(3): 22–32.

Pipes, Peggy, and Trahms, Cristine M. 1993. *Nutrition in Infancy and Childhood*, 5th ed. St. Louis, MO: Mosby-Year Book, Inc.

Pollitt, Ernesto. 1995. Does breakfast make a difference in school? *Journal of The American Dietetic Association* 95(10): 1134–1139.

Richman, J. William. 1994. *Pureed Foods with Substance and Style*. Gaithersburg, IL: Aspen Publishers.

Riggs, B. Lawrence, and L. Joseph Melton III. 1986. Involutional osteoporosis. *New England Journal of Medicine* 314(26):1676–1687.

Roe, D. A. 1985. Therapeutic effects of drug-nutrient interactions in the elderly. *Journal of The American Dietetic Association* 85(2): 174–181.

Roe, D. A. 1986. Drug-nutrient interactions in the elderly. *Geriatrics* 41(1): 57–74.

Roe, D. A. 1992. *Geriatric Nutrition*. Englewood Cliffs, NJ: Prentice Hall.

Rolls, B. J. 1992. Aging and apetite. *Nutrition Reviews* 51(12): 422–426.

Rolls, B. J., and M. B. Phillips. 1990. Aging and disturbance of thirst and fluid balance. *Nutrition Reviews* 48: 137–144.

Sampson, Hugh A., L. Mendelson, and J. P. Rosen. 1992. Fat and near fatal anaphylactic reactions to foods in children and adolescents. *New England Journal of Medicine* 327(6): 380–84.

Sampson, Hugh A., and D. D. Metcalfe. 1992. Food allergies. *Journal of the American Medical Association* 268(20): 2840–2844.

Sandstead, Harold H. 1985. Some relations between nutrition and aging. *Journal of The American Dietetic Association* 85(2): 171–172.

Satter, Ellyn. 1991. *Child of Mine: Feeding with Love and Good Sense*. Palo Alto, CA: Bull Publishing.

Schur, S. 1995. Older diner need wiser menu choices. *Restaurants USA* 15(9): 36–38.

Smith, Everett L., Patricia E. Smith, and Gilligan, Catherine. 1988. Diet, exercise and chronic disease patterns in older adults. *Nutrition Reviews* 46(2): 52–61.

Somerville, Sylvia. 1995. Food-allergy awareness: Decreasing the danger in dining out. *Restaurants USA* 15(10): 35–38.

Specker, B. L. 1994. Nutritional concerns of lactating women consuming vegetarian diets. *American Journal of Clinical Nutrition* 59(Suppl.): 11825–11865.

Story, Mary, and Michael D. Resnick. 1986. Adolescents' views on food and nutrition. *Journal of Nutrition Education* 18(4):188–192.

Strain, E. C., G. K. Mumford, K. Silverman, and R. R. Griffiths. 1994. Caffeine dependence syndrome. *Journal of the American Medical Association* 272(13): 1043–1048.

Suitor, Carol W. 1991. Perspectives on nutrition during pregnancy. *Journal of The American Dietetic Association* 91(1): 96–98.

Suter, Paolo M., and Robert M. Russell. 1987. Vitamin requirements of the elderly. *American Journal of Clinical Nutrition* 45(3): 501–512.

U. S. Department of Health and Human Services, Public Health Service. 1991. *Healthy People 2000: National Health Promotion and Disease Prevention Objectives.* Washington, DC: U.S. Government Printing Office.

Walker, Dellmar, and Roy E. Beauchener. 1991. The relationship of loneliness, social isolation, and physical health to dietary adequacy of independently living elderly. *Journal of The American Dietetic Association* 91(3):300–304.

Watkin, Donald M. 1982. The physiology of aging. *American Journal of Clinical Nutrition* 36(10):750–758.

Whisenant, Sheryl, L, and Smith, Barbara A. 1995. Eating disorders: current nutrition therapy and perceived needs in dietetics education and research. *Journal of The American Dietetic Association* 95(10): 1109–1112.

Williams, Christine L. 1995. Importance of dietary fiber in childhood. *Journal of The American Dietetic Association.* 95(10): 1140–1146, 1149.

Williams, Sue Rodwell, and Bonnie S. Worthington-Roberts, eds. 1992. *Nutrition Throughout the Life Cycle,* 2nd ed. St. Louis: Mosby-Year Book.

Worthington-Roberts, Bonnie, and Sue Rodwell Williams. 1993. *Nutrition in Pregnancy and Lactation,* 5th ed. St. Louis: Mosby-Year Book.

Young, V. R. 1992. Macronutrient needs in the elderly. Nutrition Reviews 50(12): 454–462.

Yunginger, J. W., K. G. Sweeney, W. Q. Sturner, L. A. Giannandrea, J. D. Teigland, M. Bray, P. Benson, J. York, L. Biedrzcki, D. Squillace, and R. Helm. 1988. Fatal food-induced anaphylaxis. *Journal of the American Medical Association* 260(10): 1450–1452.

Food Facts: Caffeine

Check out how much you know, or don't know, about caffeine.

True or False?

1. Tea has more caffeine than coffee.
2. Brewed coffee has more caffeine than instant coffee.
3. Some nonprescription drugs contain caffeine.
4. Caffeine is a nervous system stimulant.
5. Withdrawing from regular caffeine use causes physical symptoms.

Check your answers as you read on.

Caffeine, a stimulant, is the most widely used psychoactive substance in the world. Eighty percent of Americans drink at least one caffeine-containing beverage each day, and average caffeine consumption is about 280 milligrams. Caffeine is present in over 60 plant species in various parts of the world, such as the coffee bean in Arabia, the tea leaf in China, the kola nut in West Africa, and the cocoa bean in Mexico.

Coffee, tea, cola, and cocoa are the most common sources of caffeine in the American diet (Table 8-17) with coffee being the chief source. The caffeine content of coffee or tea depends on the variety of coffee bean or tea leaf, the particle size, the brewing method, and the length of brewing or steeping time. Brewed coffee always has more caffeine than instant coffee, and espresso coffee always has more caffeine than brewed coffee. Espresso is made by forcing hot pressurized water through finely ground, dark-roast beans. Because it is brewed with less water, it contains more caffeine than regular coffee.

Table 8-18 defines various specialty coffees.

In soft drinks, caffeine is both a natural and an added ingredient. The Food and Drug Administration requires caffeine as an ingredient in colas and pepper-flavored beverages and allows it to be added to other soft drinks as well. About 5 percent of the caffeine in colas and pepper-flavored soft drinks is obtained naturally from cola nuts; the remaining 95 percent is added. Caffeine-free soft drinks contain virtually no caffeine and make up a small part of the soft drink market.

Numerous prescription and non-prescription drugs also contain caffeine. It is often used in alertness or stay-awake tablets, headache and pain relief remedies, cold products, and diuretics. When caffeine is an ingredient, it must be listed on the product label.

Caffeine is absorbed very well into the body and is rapidly absorbed into the bloodstream. For most people, caffeine increases blood pressure and heart rate, increases attentiveness and performance, and gives relief from fatigue. In high doses it can produce insomnia, nervousness, a racing heart, and other troublesome symptoms. Many people build a tolerance to caffeine's effects that may then lead to increased usage.

It is easy to become dependent on caffeine. When caffeine is withdrawn, symptoms include headache, fatigue, irritability, depression, and poor concentration. The symptoms peak on day 1 or 2 and progressively decrease over the course of a week. It has been shown that even moderate con-

TABLE 8-17.   Caffeine content of beverages, foods, and drugs.

Item	Milligrams Caffeine Average	Range	Item	Milligrams Caffeine Average	Range
Coffee (5-ounce cup)			Cocoa		
Brewed, drip method	115	110–150	Cocoa beverage		
Instant	65	30–120	(5-ounce cup)	4	2–20
Decaffeinated, brewed	3	2–5	Chocolate milk beverage		
Decaffeinated, instant	2	1–5	(8 ounces)	5	2–7
			Milk chocolate (1 ounce)	6	1–15
Tea (5–ounce cup)			Dark chocolate,		
Brewed,			semisweet (1 ounce)	20	5–35
major U.S. brands	40	20–90	Baker's chocolate		
Brewed,			(1 ounce)	26	26
imported brands	60	25–110	Chocolate-flavored syrup		
Instant	30	25–50	(1 ounce)	4	4
Iced (12-ounce glass)	70	67–76			
			Prescription drugs:		
Soft drinks (12-ounce can)			(caffeine per tablet or capsule)		
Cola, pepper		30–46	Cafergot (migraine headaches)		100
Decaffeinated cola, pepper		0–2	Norgesic Forte (muscle relaxant)		60
Cherry cola		36–46	Fiorinal (tension headache)		40
Lemon-lime		0	Darvon (pain relief)		32
Other citrus		0–64	Synalogos-DC (pain relief)		30
Root beer		0	Nonprescription drugs:		
Ginger ale		0	(caffeine per tablet or capsule)		
Tonic water		0	Alertness Tablets		
Other regular soda		0–44	No Doz		100
Juice added		0	Pain Relief		
Diet cola, pepper		0.6	Anacin, Maximum		
Decaffeinated diet cola,			Strength Anacin		32
pepper		0–0.2	Vanquish		33
Diet cherry cola		0–46	Excedrin		65
Diet lemon-lime,			Midol		32
diet root beer		0	Diuretics		
Other diets		0–70	Aqua-Ban		100
Club soda, seltzer,			Cold/Allergy Remedies		
sparkling water		0	Coryban-D capsules		30

Source: Lecos, Chris W. 1987–1988. Caffeine jitters: Some safety questions remain. *FDA Consumer* 21(10): 22–27.

TABLE 8-18. **Specialty coffees.**

Espresso. Strong, concentrated coffee made by forcing hot water under pressure through finely ground, dark-roasted coffee beans. Serving size is small, about $1\frac{1}{2}$ to 4 ounces.

Espresso doppio. A double espresso.

Espresso macchiato. Espresso made with just a touch of foamed milk on top.

Cafe Americano. Espresso diluted with hot water to the strength of regular American coffee. Usually a 6-ounce cup.

Cafe latte. Espresso with 75 percent steamed milk.

Cafe mocha. Espresso with steamed milk and mocha or chocolate syrup and topped with whipped cream. The coffee equivalent of a hot fudge sundae.

Cappuccino. A blend of equal parts espresso, foamed milk, and steamed milk.

---

sumption—about one or two 10-ounce cups of coffee daily (or the equivalent of caffeine from other sources)—often causes people to experience these debilitating symptoms of caffeine withdrawal. To minimize withdrawal symptoms, experts recommend reducing one's caffeine intake by about 20 percent a week over 4 to 5 weeks.

Although caffeine use has stirred fears in the past (it reportedly caused pancreatic cancer and birth defects), moderate use probably confers the benefits of caffeine with few of the risks. There are, however, two groups of individuals who should abstain from caffeine. In some susceptible people with heart disease, caffeine can cause irregular heart beats. Caffeine is also not recommended for individuals with peptic ulcers, because caffeine increases the production of stomach acid. Pregnant and lactating women should consume caffeine in moderation—less than two cups of coffee a day. Studies on caffeine and pregnancy have shown conflicting results, so moderation is recommended.

High intakes of caffeine may be linked to heart attacks and bone loss in women. Once an individual drinks more than two 10-ounce cups of coffee daily, there is added cardiac risk among both smokers and nonsmokers, and especially in people with high blood pressure. Women who consume caffeine and drink little or no milk lose more calcium in their urine and have less dense bones than do women who don't consume any caffeine. For optimum bone density, women should moderate their caffeine intake and get at least two to three servings from the milk group daily.

Hot Topic: School Lunch and Breakfast Programs

TABLE 8-19.   Interesting facts about school lunch and breakfast programs.

- Over 25 million lunches are served through the National School Lunch program every school day. Only McDonald's provides more meals in the U.S.
- Over 93,000 schools participate in the School Lunch program—almost 99 percent of all public schools and 78 percent of all private schools.
- About 40 percent of school lunches are provided free to needy children, and 7 percent are offered at reduced prices. The rest are sold at full price, which averages about $1.15.
- More than half of America's students eat a lunch made by the National School Lunch program, and 18 percent of children bring lunch from home.

Through its National School Meal Programs, the U.S. Department of Agriculture provides breakfasts and lunches to more than 25 million children each school day. Legislation that established the National School Lunch Program was signed by President Harry Truman in 1946. Twenty years later, in 1966, the U.S. Department of Agriculture instituted the School Breakfast Program. About 60 percent of schools that offer the school lunch program also offer the school breakfast program.

The nutrition standards for school meals were never significantly changed until 1994 when Congress passed the Healthy Meals for Healthy Americans Act. By fall of 1996, all meals served through the National School Lunch and School Breakfast programs must comply with the Dietary Guidelines for Americans. The force behind this change was that study after study of school lunch meals found that they were not conforming to the Dietary Guidelines for Americans. In particular, meals were consistently higher than recommended in fat and saturated fat.

The requirements originally set for school lunches stipulated that lunches must provide five items: 2 ounces of meat or alternate, 2 or more servings of fruit and/or vegetables, 1 serving of bread or alternate, and 8 ounces of milk. The new requirements allow schools to move away from this food-based system to what is called a nutrient-analysis system. Using the nutrient-analysis system, school lunch directors look at the nutrients provided in a one-week menu. The highlight of the new regulations is that school lunch menus must provide over the course of a week no more than 30 percent of total calories as fat and no more than 10 percent of total calories as saturated fat. The new regulations do allow a food-based system that follows the old school lunch pattern, but with increased servings of fruits, vegetables, breads and grains. Lunch menus must still provide one-third of the RDA for calories, protein, iron, calcium, vitamin A, and vitamin C, and breakfast menus must provide one-quarter of the same nutrients.

The Healthy Meals for Healthy Americans Act will also introduce new ways to appeal to children's taste; nutrition education for children, parents, and teachers; and changes in program administration to make it work better and more efficiently. Team Nutrition is a project of the U.S. Department of Agriculture to implement the School Meals Initiative for Healthy Children. Team Nutrition is a network of public and private partnerships across the U.S. with the United States Department of Agriculture. USDA's Team Nutrition is designed to help make implementation of the new policy easier and more successful. Team Nutrition will:

- Provide training and technical assistance to schools to ensure that school nutrition and food service personnel have the education, motivation, training, and skills necessary to provide healthy meals that appeal to children.

- Promote food choices for a healthy diet to children by actively involving them in making those food choices, reaching them where they learn, live, eat, and play. Through Team Nutrition, research-based messages have been developed reflecting the Dietary Guidelines for Americans and the Food Guide Pyramid and will help children to expand the variety of foods in their diet, construct a diet lower in fat, and add more fruits, vegetables, and grains to the foods they already eat.

- Provide Team Nutrition In-School curricula for Pre-K to 12th grades. This is a comprehensive activity-based program designed to build skills and motivate children to make food choices for a healthy diet.

- Provide new School Lunch and Breakfast recipes that meet the Dietary Guidelines for Americans, such as Beef Taco Pie made with beef, salsa and low-fat cheddar cheese layered between tortillas.

CHAPTER

9

Weight Management and Exercise

**KEY
QUESTIONS**

1. How is obesity defined?
2. What are the advantages and disadvantages of the three methods of measuring obesity?
3. What are the health implications of obesity?
4. What are possible causes of obesity?
5. What needs to be done in a comprehensive weight-reduction program to maximize weight loss?
6. How can a diet be designed to increase a person's ability to stick to it?
7. What is the relationship between exercise and weight loss?
8. What is behavior and attitude modification theory, and how is it used to help someone lose weight?
9. What are crucial elements of a weight-maintenance program?
10. How can an underweight person gain weight?
11. What are the important elements of nutrition for the athlete?

QUIZ

Quiz
Circle the correct answer.

1. Skipping meals is a good way to lose weight.	*True*	*False*
2. The nondieting approach to weight loss emphasizes exercise and reduced fat intake.	*True*	*False*
3. A diet under 1000 calories is a safe plan for weight loss for most dieters.	*True*	*False*
4. Dieters should not eat snacks between meals.	*True*	*False*
5. The best way to lose weight is to eat less, exercise more, and modify negative eating behaviors and attitudes.	*True*	*False*
6 Dieters should not eat anything after 7 P.M.	*True*	*False*
7. Dieters should weigh in every morning.	*True*	*False*
8. In order to lose weight, dieters need to eliminate high-calorie junk food such as cookies.	*True*	*False*
9. Exercise is crucial for weight loss.	*True*	*False*
10. Athletes need high-fat diets because of their increased calorie needs.	*True*	*False*

INTRODUCTION

Americans trying to lose weight have plenty of company. According to a 1995 report from the Institute of Medicine, tens of millions of Americans are dieting at any given time and spending more than $33 billion yearly on weight-reduction products, such as diet foods and drinks. Yet, studies over the last two decades by the National Center for Health Statistics show that obesity in the United States is actually on the rise. Today, approximately 35 percent of women and 31 percent of men age 20 and older are considered obese, up from about 30 percent and 25 percent, respectively, in 1980. Studies also show that dieters, more often than not, regain most or all of any weight loss.

The words obesity and overweight are generally used interchangeably; however, they have different meanings. Overweight refers to an excess of body weight that includes all tissues, such as fat, bone, and muscle. Obesity refers to an excess of body fat. It is possible to be overweight without being obese, as in the case of a body builder who has a substantial amount of muscle mass. It is possible to be obese without being overweight, as in the case of a very sedentary person who is within the desirable weight range but who nevertheless has an excess of body fat. However, most overweight people are also obese and vice versa.

Obesity is now considered a disease—not a moral failing. Obesity is a disease in which many factors are involved: genetic, environmental, psychological, and others. It occurs when energy intake exceeds the amount of energy expended over time. In a small number of cases obesity is caused by illnesses such as hypothyroidism or the result of taking medications, such as steroids, that can cause weight gain.

Because so many factors affect how much or how little food a person eats and how that food is metabolized by the body, losing weight is not simple. This chapter discusses how obesity impacts on health, theories that try to explain what causes obesity, and treatment to lose and maintain weight loss. Exercise, an important activity for obese and nonobese individuals, is also examined along with nutrition for athletes.

"HOW MUCH SHOULD I WEIGH?"

Overweight is generally defined as body weight between 10 and 19 percent over desirable weight. **Obesity** is 20 percent or more over desirable weight and is classified into three categories: mild, moderate, and severe. **Mild obesity** is 20 to 40 percent, **moderate obesity** is 41 to 91 percent, and **severe obesity** is 100 percent or more over desirable weight.

Overweight: Body weight 10 - 19% over desirable weight.
Obesity: Body weight 20% or more over desirable weight.

Hot Topic: Diet Pills

The 1991/1992 Weight Loss Practices Survey, sponsored by the Food and Drug Administration (FDA) and the National Heart, Lung, and Blood Institute, found that 5 percent of women and 2 percent of men trying to lose weight use diet pills. Products considered by FDA to be over-the-counter weight control drugs are primarily those containing the active ingredient phenylpropanolamine (PPA), such as Dexatrim and Acutrim. PPA is also used as a nasal decongestant in over-the-counter cough and cold products. Consumers need to read the labels of decongestants to see if they contain PPA because it is not advisable to take PPA in 2 products at the same time for different uses. Using diet pills containing PPA generally does not make a big difference in the rate of weight loss, at best one-half pound per week greater weight loss.

In 1996 the FDA approved the first new appetite suppressant drug in 22 years. Although it helps makes people feel full, the new drug, dexfenfluramine, does not eliminate the need to diet or exercise. In studies, the drug has been shown to work with some, but not all, patients. Because of the risk of a rare but dangerous lung disorder, it must be used under the close supervision of a physician. A bigger safety concern with dexfenfluramine, which alters the brain chemical serotonin to make people feel full without eating as much, is whether it causes brain damage. While the FDA works with the drug's manufacturer to do further longer-term studies on its effects on the human brain, the drug is available by prescription under the name Redux and it costs about $2 a day.

There are pros and cons about the use of diet pills. Although they do help some people lose weight initially, what happens when they stop taking the diet pill? After all, you can't take diet pills forever. Most can be used for only a few months or a year. Others will argue that diet pills are needed to obtain that initial weight loss. Whether pro or con, keep in mind that only a small minority of dieters use pills.

To calculate percent of desirable weight, use the following equation.

$$\frac{\text{Actual weight}}{\text{Desirable weight}} \times 100 = \text{Percent of desirable weight}$$

For example, if your actual weight is 120 pounds and your desirable weight is 100 pounds, your percent of desirable weight would be 120 percent.

Over 90 percent of obesity falls into the mild category, which can be treated with diet, exercise, and behavior modification. Moderately obese people are often treated with very-low-calorie liquid diets under medical supervision and behavior therapy. Very-low-calorie diets are usually between 400 and 800 calories per day and contain enough high-quality protein, vitamins, and minerals to meet the RDA. This type of diet is called a liquid diet because it is a powder that mixes with water to make a drink. No other foods are usually allowed. Severely obese people may be treated surgically under certain circumstances. Surgery normally decreases the size of the stomach in hopes of limiting caloric intake in the future.

Obesity can be measured using various methods. **Height-weight tables**, the most widely used weight goals in the United States for the past 40 years, are easy to use and understand. These tables were developed by the Metropolitan Life Insurance Company and represent weight for height associated with the lowest mortality within its insured population. Individuals with significant diseases at the time of policy issue are screened out of the study. Life insurance data have unique value because of the large number of observations, the extensiveness and reliability of the mortality information, and because they are long-term studies. They are not without criticisms, which we discuss later.

The 1959 Metropolitan Life Desirable Weight table had been used for over twenty years when it was replaced in 1983 by a newer table. To use Tables 9-1 and 9-2, you need to calculate your body frame size. Extend your arm and bend it upwards into a 90-degree angle. Keep your fingers straight. Place the thumb and index finger of your other hand on the two bones on either side of your elbow. Measure the space between your fingers with a tape measure or ruler. Compare these measurements with the normal or medium values in the following tables.

	Women		Men	
Height	*Elbow Breadth*	*Height*	*Elbow Breadth*	
4'9"–4'10"	*2¼"–2½"*	*5'1"–5'2"*	*2½"–2⅞"*	
4'11"–5'2"	*2¼"–2½"*	*5'3"–5'6"*	*2⅝"–2⅞"*	
5'3"–5'6"	*2⅜"–2⅝"*	*5'7"–5'10"*	*2¾"–3"*	
5'7"–5'10"	*2⅜"–2⅝"*	*5'11"–6'2"*	*2¾"–3⅛"*	
5'11"	*2½"–2¾"*	*6'3"*	*2⅞"–3¼"*	

If your measurement is less than the normal value for your height and gender, you are considered to have a small frame; if your measurement is greater, you have a large frame.

Note that the 1983 table does not use the term **desirable weight**. Desirable weight is the weight associated with the lowest mortality; it does not imply that disease is minimized at this weight. Because the term **desirable** means different things to different people and has created confusion, Metropolitan decided to label its 1983 tables simply "Height and Weight Tables." The major difference between the 1959 and 1983

There are many height/weight tables, each with its own good points and bad points.

TABLE 9-1. Metropolitan Life Insurance 1959 desirable weights for men and women, ages 25 and over, according to height and frame.

| | Men, Weight in Pounds (indoor clothing) | | | | Women, Weight in Pounds (indoor clothing) | | |
Height (in shoes)*	Small Frame	Medium Frame	Large Frame	Height (in shoes)*	Small Frame	Medium Frame	Large Frame
5'2"	112–120	118–129	126–141	4'10"	92–98	96–107	104–119
5'3"	115–123	121–133	129–144	4'11"	94–101	98–110	106–122
5'4"	118–126	124–136	132–148	5'	96–104	101–113	109–125
5'5"	121–129	127–139	135–152	5'1"	99–107	104–116	112–128
5'6"	124–133	130–143	138–156	5'2"	102–110	107–119	115–131
5'7"	128–137	134–147	142–161	5'3"	105–113	110–122	118–134
5'8"	132–141	138–152	147–166	5'4"	108–116	113–126	121–138
5'9"	136–145	142–156	151–170	5'5"	111–119	116–130	125–142
5'10"	140–150	146–160	155–174	5'6"	114–123	120–135	129–146
5'11"	144–154	150–165	159–179	5'7"	118–127	124–139	133–150
6'	148–158	154–170	164–184	5'8"	122–131	128–143	137–154
6'1"	152–162	158–175	168–189	5'9"	126–135	132–147	141–158
6'2"	156–167	162–180	173–194	5'10"	130–140	136–151	145–163
6'3"	160–171	167–185	178–199	5'11"	134–144	140–155	149–168
6'4"	164–175	172–190	182–204	6'	138–148	144–159	153–173

*Allow 1" heels for men's's shoes and 2" heels for women's shoes.

tables is that the weights are higher on the 1983 tables. The tables indicate an average increase in weight for short men of about 13 pounds, or 10 percent; for medium-height men, about 7 pounds, or 5 percent; and among tall men, 2 pounds, or 1 percent. For short women, the average increase in weight was about 10 pounds, or 9 percent; for medium-height women, 8 pounds, or 6 percent; and among tall women, 3 pounds or 2 percent.

The Metropolitan tables are not without criticism. Frame size was not determined by any objective method in the 1959 tables, and the use of elbow width to determine frame size in 1983 may or may not eliminate this problem. In any case, elbow width was not measured in the insured population, so its accuracy is questionable. Because life insurance holders include disproportionate numbers of white males from upper and middle classes under 60 years old, the tables have been criticized as not being truly representative of the American population, particularly people at lower socioeconomic levels. Also, the insured have been weighed only once, when applying for the insurance. Another criticism of the tables lies in the fact that the weights say nothing about body composition. For instance, a 250-pound linebacker at 6 feet 2 inches would be considered overweight according to the tables, yet his excess pounds are not fat, but muscle. Conversely, a person whose weight is within the appropriate

TABLE 9-2. Metropolitan Life Insurance 1983 height and weight tables.

| | Men, Weight in Pounds (indoor clothing) | | | | Women, Weight in Pounds (indoor clothing) | | |
Height (in shoes)*	Small Frame	Medium Frame	Large Frame	Height (in shoes)*	Small Frame	Medium Frame	Large Frame
5'2"	128–134	131–141	138–150	4'10"	102–111	109–121	118–131
5'3"	130–136	133–143	140–153	4'11"	103–113	111–123	120–134
5'4"	132–138	135–145	142–156	5'	104–115	113–126	122–137
5'5"	134–140	137–148	144–160	5'1"	106–118	115–129	125–140
5'6"	136–142	139–151	146–164	5'2"	108–121	118–132	128–143
5'7"	138–145	142–154	149–168	5'3"	111–124	121–135	131–147
5'8"	140–148	145–157	152–172	5'4"	114–127	124–138	134–151
5'9"	142–151	148–160	155–176	5'5"	117–130	127–141	137–155
5'10"	144–154	151–163	158–180	5'6"	120–133	130–144	140–159
5'11"	146–157	154–166	161–184	5'7"	123–136	133–147	142–163
6'	146–160	157–170	164–188	5'8"	126–139	136–150	146–167
6'1"	152–164	160–174	168–192	5'9"	129–142	139–153	149–170
6'2"	155–168	164–178	172–197	5'10"	132–145	142–156	152–173
6'3"	158–172	167–182	176–202	5'11"	135–148	145–159	155–176
6'4"	162–176	171–187	181–207	6'	138–151	148–162	158–179

*Height for both men and women includes 1" heel. Body weight for women includes 3 pounds for indoor clothing: for men it includes 5 pounds of indoor clothing.

weight range may indeed have excess fat stores.

Table 9-3 shows suggested weights for adults from the 1995 *Dietary Guidelines for Americans*. Although the previous set of these guidelines allowed individuals over 35 to weigh more than shown in this table, the idea of allowing more pounds in middle age and older age does not seem to promote health. Research studies, some of which are very large, have shown that no matter whether you are young or old, as weight goes up so does the incidence of increased LDL cholesterol levels, high blood pressure, and diabetes. The higher weights in Table 9-3 apply to people with relatively large amounts of muscle and bone.

A second method of measuring degree of obesity is **body mass index**, a mathematical formula that correlates weight with body fat. The BMI is calculated as follows:

$$BMI = \frac{body\ weight\ (in\ kilograms)}{height\ (in\ meters)\ 2}$$

The BMI has a direct and continuous relationship to morbidity (incidence of disease) and mortality in studies of large populations; however, it is harder to understand.

The BMI is a more sensitive indicator than height-weight tables and can be easily calculated using a nomogram (Figure 9-1). Each nomogram

Body mass index more accurately tells you about your weight than height/weight tables.

TABLE 9-3. Suggested weights for adults.					
Height*	*Weight in pounds†*	*Height**	*Weight in pounds†*	*Height**	*Weight in pounds†*
4'10"	91–119	5'5"	114–150	6'0"	140–184
4'11"	94–124	5'6"	118–155	6'1"	144–189
5'0"	97–128	5'7"	121–160	6'2"	148–195
5'1"	101–132	5'8"	125–164	6'3"	152–200
5'2"	104–137	5'9"	129–169	6'4"	156–205
5'3"	107–141	5'10"	132–174	6'5"	160–211
5'4"	111–146	5'11"	136–179	6'6"	164–216

*Without shoes
†Without clothes

Source: Dietary Guidelines for Americans (1995)

provides desirable weight and the 20 percent and 40 percent overweight level of men and women of varying heights and weights. These values are read off the central scale after a ruler is placed across the nomogram between the height and weight values. When the BMI exceeds 27.8 for males and 27.2 for females, there are increased obesity-related health risks (National Institutes of Health, 1985).

Another way to measure obesity is to examine the percentage of your body that is fat. For men, a desirable percentage of body fat is 13 to 25 percent, for women, about 17 to 29 percent. When a man's body fat goes over 25 percent fat (or 29 percent for a woman), health risks increase. Body fat is most often measured by using special calipers to measure the skinfold thickness of the triceps and other parts of the body. Because half of all your fat is under the skin, this method is quite accurate when performed by an experienced professional.

Calculate your waist-to-hip ratio.

Recent research suggests that more important than the amount of extra fat a person carries is where it is located. Rather than examining weight for height or other definitions, obesity can be defined in terms of waist-to-hip ratio. Waist-to-hip ratio can be calculated by dividing the number of inches around the waistline by the circumference of the hips. For example, someone who has a 27-inch waist and 38-inch hips would have a ratio of 0.71. A woman whose ratio is 0.8 or higher would be at high risk of weight-related health problems (such as heart disease, hypertension, and diabetes), as would a man whose ratio is 1.0 or above.

Numerous studies show that fat in the hips and thighs is less health-threatening than abdominal fat. Whereas other fat cells empty directly into general circulation, the fatty acid contents of abdominal fat cells go straight to the liver before being circulated to the muscles. This process interferes with the liver's ability to clear insulin from the bloodstream. As

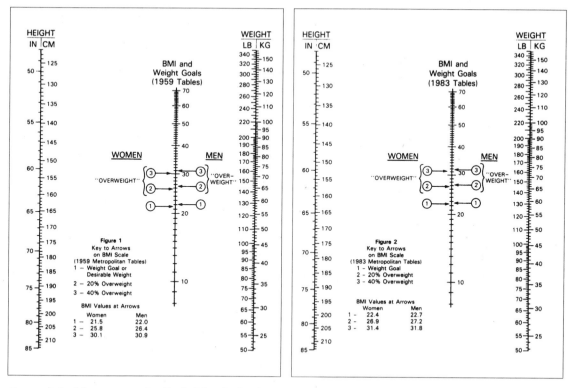

FIGURE 9-1. Nomograms for Body Mass Index based on 1959 and 1983 Metropolitan Life Insurance Company Tables. Weights and heights are without clothing.

blood levels of insulin increase, muscles and other cells become insulin-resistant, and blood glucose levels rise as a result. In response, the pancreas cranks out more insulin, prompting the autonomic nervous system (which controls heart rate, blood pressure, and other vital signs) to produce norepinephrine, an adrenalin-like chemical that raises blood pressure. This sets the stage for the development of diabetes, hypertension, and heart problems.

Obesity can be defined by using height-weight tables, BMI, percentage body fat, and waist-to-hip ratio.

MINI-SUMMARY   Obesity can be defined by using height-weight tables, body mass index (BMI), percentage body fat, and waist-to-hip ratio.

HEALTH IMPLICATIONS OF OBESITY

In general, mortality increases with an increase in relative weight, and this increase is steeper in men and women under age 50 than in older persons. An obese individual is at increased risk for hypertension, high blood cholesterol levels, adult-onset diabetes, and coronary heart disease. Obese people do have more hypertension, diabetes, and high blood cholesterol levels, as well as other cardiovascular problems.

Obese people are also at higher risk for developing certain types of cancer. Obese men are at higher risk for colon, rectal, and prostate cancer. Obese women are at higher risk for breast, uterine, and ovarian cancer.

Conditions aggravated by obesity include breathing problems, abdominal hernia, arthritis, varicose veins, gout, gallbladder disease, and pregnancy. In addition, obese individuals are higher surgical risks.

Obesity creates a psychological burden that, in terms of suffering, may be its greatest adverse effect. Obese people, particularly children, are ridiculed, teased, and excluded by their peers. They are also victims of discrimination. They are self-conscious about their weight and frequently blame themselves.

Weight reduction is recommended for excess body weight of 20 percent or more. Weight reduction is strongly sought when excess fat is combined with any of the following conditions: non-insulin-dependent diabetes, family history of diabetes, high blood pressure, high blood lipid or cholesterol levels, coronary heart disease, or gout. Losing weight often decreases blood pressure and blood cholesterol levels and brings diabetes under better control. Although obesity does not cause these medical conditions, losing weight can help to reduce some of their negative aspects.

MINI-SUMMARY An obese individual is at increased risk for hypertension, high blood cholesterol levels, adult-onset diabetes, cancer (certain types), and coronary heart disease. Conditions aggravated by obesity include abdominal hernia, arthritis, varicose veins, gout, gallbladder disease, and pregnancy. In addition, obese individuals are higher surgical risks.

THEORIES OF OBESITY

As researchers try to figure out why some people get fat and others don't, it is becoming increasingly apparent that obesity has a variety of causes—heredity, environment, metabolism, and level of physical activity—and therefore no single cure.

The body has an almost limitless capacity to store fat. Not only can each fat cell balloon to more than 10 times its original size, but should the available cells get filled to the brim, new ones will propagate. As the body stores more fat, weight and girth increase.

A number of studies have shown that genetics may be the most important determinant of how much you weigh, perhaps explaining about half the problems with obesity. Some people are more prone to weight gain than others, even when caloric intake is the same. Identical twins show similar body weight, even when they have been raised apart. Researchers conclude that genetic factors, apart from diet or lifestyle, strongly influence how much a person weighs.

Obesity tends to run in families. If both parents are obese, their children have an 80 percent chance of being obese. If neither parent is obese, the likelihood of the children being obese is no more than 14 percent. This difference could reflect genetics and/or the family's tendency to teach poor eating and exercise habits.

Three interesting theories reflect the physiological school of thought concerning obesity: the fat cell, set point, and dietary obesity theories. Obese people usually have a larger than normal number of fat cells and/or enlarged fat cells. Fat cells can be added but never subtracted, so when an obese person loses weight, the cells reduce in size, not number. The fat cell theory states that weight loss will be met with internal resistance when cells are reduced below their normal size.

Set point theory is based on the supposition that the body strives to maintain a given range of weight, fat, muscle, or related factors. Therefore, obesity results from maintaining body weight and fat at a higher than normal level. An obese individual who diets encounters strong biological resistance. Many studies show a tendency for humans to keep their weight within a fairly constant weight range.

Dietary obesity refers to a tendency to prefer calorically dense foods. Most laboratory animals fed standard foods do not overeat even when food is abundant. When these animals were offered supermarket diets of chocolate chip cookies, milk chocolate, salami, marshmallows, cheese, peanut butter, bananas, and fat, however, they gained 269 percent more weight, even when they had the option of eating their standard foods. Human beings and animals may share an inborn biological preference for calorically dense foods as a leftover survival mechanism that served a purpose when food was scarce.

Various theories speculate about why obesity occurs:
-genetics,
- fat cell theory,
- set point,
- dietary obesity theories.

MINI-SUMMARY As researchers try to figure out why some people get fat and others do not, it is becoming increasingly apparent that obesity has a variety of causes—heredity, environment, metabolism, and level of physical activity—and therefore, no single cure.

TREATMENT OF OBESITY

Before discussing the treatment of obesity, it is a good idea to discuss treatment goals. The goals of most weight-loss programs have focused on short-term weight loss. Critics of this type of goal feel that short-term weight loss is not a valid measure of success, because it is not associated with health benefits (as is long-term weight loss). Also, weight-loss goals tend to reinforce the American preoccupation with being slender, especially for women. Lastly, critics point out that weight-loss goals are often set too high when even a small weight loss can reduce the risks of developing chronic diseases. Overweight individuals who lose even relatively small amounts of weight are likely to:

- lower their blood pressure, and thereby the risks of high blood pressure
- reduce abnormally high levels of blood glucose associated with diabetes
- bring down blood levels of cholesterol and triglycerides associated with cardiovascular disease
- reduce sleep apnea or irregular breathing during sleep
- decrease the risk of osteoarthritis of the weight-bearing joints
- decrease depression
- increase self-esteem (Food and Nutrition Board, 1995).

The nondieting approach to obesity emphasizes exercise and selection of low-fat foods.

Current recommendations from the Food and Nutrition Board favor shifting from a weight-loss perspective to one of weight management in which success is judged more by the program's effect on an individual's health status than its effect on weight (Food and Nutrition Board, 1995).

Treatment of obesity generally consists of one or more of the following: diet, exercise, behavior modification, and drug therapy. Treatment programs often concentrate on two aspects of losing weight: diets and exercise. Individuals in treatment programs that just offer diets tend to regain any lost weight within 2 or 3 years (NIH Technology Assessment Conference Panel, 1993). The American Medical Association Council on Scientific Affairs has stated that a program incorporating behavior modification of both diet and exercise has the best chances of long-term weight control (Council of Scientific Affairs, 1988).

A comprehensive treatment plan for obesity needs to include:
- *diet and nutrition education,*
- *exercise,*
- *behavior modification,*
- *attitude modification,*
- *social support,*
- *and maintenance support.*

The next section will discuss each of the following components of treatment: diet and nutrition education, exercise, behavior and attitude modification, social support, and maintenance support. But first, let's take a look at a newer approach to treating obesity that doesn't use diets.

More and more health professionals are adopting a nondieting approach to treating obesity that includes eating less fat and exercising. This new approach steers clear of dieting and emphasizes helping obese people adopt a healthier lifestyle. In many cases diets simply don't work. By restricting food intake, diets often cause dieters to become obsessed with food, which may then lead to binge eating. Eating fewer fat calories and exercising can help many obese people to lose some weight and keep it off.

Diet and Nutrition Education

Basic nutrition education is crucial for dieters. They need education about fat, carbohydrate, and protein in foods and about balancing them in a lower-calorie and lower-fat diet. They need to understand variety, moderation, and nutrient density, particularly because they have to pack the same amount of nutrients into fewer calories.

Dieters need to understand seven basic concepts of nutrition education before planning their actual diets:

1. Calories should not be overly restricted during dieting because this practice decreases the likelihood of success. A dieter who normally eats 2500 calories daily and goes on a 1200-calorie diet is eating less than half of what he or she normally eats. Restricting calories by 500 each day amounts to about one pound lost in a week. In any case, calories should not be restricted below 1200 because getting adequate nutrients is impossible below this level. A progressive weight loss of 1 to 2 pounds a week is considered safe.

2. The focus should be on decreasing fat calories, since they provide more than twice the calories of carbohydrate and protein. Fat calories also tend to be stored in fat cells. In obesity research, the Flatt hypotheses states that high fat diets are related to the development and maintenance of obesity (Thomas, Peters, Reed, Abumrad, Sun, and Hill, 1992). By restricting how much fat you eat, you can cut down on how many calories you eat. This might be the only adjustment that a moderately overweight person needs to make in order to lose weight (hopefully he or she will also exercise). With the emphasis on eating less fat, keep in mind that fat-free foods still contain calories.

3. No foods should be forbidden, as that only makes them more attractive.

4. Eating three meals and one to two snacks each day is crucial to minimizing the possibility of getting hungry. People tend to overeat when hungry.

5. Portion control is vital. Measuring and weighing foods is important because "eyeballing" is not always accurate.

6. Variety, balance, and moderation are crucial to satisfying all nutrient needs.

7. Weighing is important but should not be done every day because 1- to 2-

pound weight gains and losses can occur on a daily basis due to fluid shifts. Weekly weigh-ins are more accurate and less likely to cause disappointment.

Exercise

Exercise is a vital component of any weight-control program. Research consistently shows that time spent exercising is a major predictor of long-term weight loss (Kayman, Bruvold, and Stern, 1990). Exercise not only facilitates weight loss through direct energy expenditure but burns fat both during and after exercise (Saris, 1993). Regular exercise also helps control or suppress appetite, and builds and tones muscles, which in turn raises your basal metabolic rate. But regular exercise has many benefits beyond simply losing pounds and keeping them off. Indeed, the Centers for Disease Control and Prevention and the American College of Sports Medicine recommend that every American adult should accumulate 30 minutes or more of moderate-intensity physical activity on most, preferably all, days of the week (Pate et al., 1995). Additional advantages of regular physical activity include:

1. improved functioning of the cardiovascular system
2. reduced levels of blood lipids associated with cardiovascular disease
3. increased ability to cope with stress, anxiety, and depression
4. increased stamina
5. increased resistance to fatigue
6. improved self-image

A consistent pattern of exercise is vital to achieving these beneficial results.

The key to a successful exercise program is choosing an enjoyable activity. Some questions obese people need to answer to find a good exercise include:

1. Do you like to exercise alone or with others?
2. Do you prefer to exercise outdoors or in your home?
3. Do you particularly like any activities?
4. How much money are you willing to spend for sports equipment or facilities if needed?
5. When can you best fit the activity into your schedule?

An obese person may resist starting an exercise program for several reasons. Many have had bad experiences in school physical education classes and want to avoid such activity. Some tend to be self-conscious and may not want to be seen exercising. Activity is also harder for obese people and requires more effort.

Aerobic activities such as walking, jogging, cycling, and swimming are ideal as the major component of an exercise program. Aerobic activities must be brisk enough to raise heart and breathing rates, and they must be sustained, meaning they must be done at least 15 to 30 minutes without interruption. Activities such as baseball, bowling, and golf are not vigorous or sustained. They still have certain benefits—they can be enjoyable, help improve coordination and muscle tone, and help relieve tension—but they are not aerobic.

Any exercise program for sedentary and overweight people must be started slowly, with enjoyment and commitment as the major goals. A buildup in intensity and duration should be gradual and progressive, depending to a large extent on how overweight an individual is. Aerobic capacity improves when exercise increases the heart rate to a target zone of 65 to 80 percent of the maximum heart rate, which is the fastest the heart can beat. Maximum heart rate can be calculated by subtracting your age from 220. One goal of the exercise program should be to build up to this intensity of exercise. Exercise between 65 and 80 percent of the maximum heart rate conditions the heart and lungs, besides burning calories (Table 9-4). To determine whether your heart rate is in the target zone, take your pulse as follows:

1. When you stop exercising, quickly place the tip of your third finger lightly over one of the blood vessels on your neck located to the left or right of your Adam's apple. (Another convenient pulse spot is the inside of your wrist just below the base of your thumb.)
2. Count your pulse for 30 seconds and multiply by 2.
3. If your pulse is below your target zone, exercise a little harder the next time. If you are above your target zone, exercise a little easier. If it falls within the target zone, you are doing fine.
4. Once you are exercising within your target zone, you should check your pulse at least once each week.

Exercise should take place at least three times per week and include a warm-up period, the exercise itself, and then a cooling-down period. To warm up before exercising, do stretching exercises slowly and in a steady, rhythmic way. Start at a medium pace and gradually increase. Next, begin jumping rope or jogging in place slowly before starting any vigorous activities to ease the cardiovascular system into the aerobic exercise. The exercise part of the session should burn at least 300 calories, which can be achieved with 15 to 30 minutes of aerobic activity in the target zone or 40 to 60 minutes of lower-intensity activity, such as leisurely walking. After exercising, slowing down the exercise activity or changing to a less vigorous

TABLE 9-4. Calories burned per hour by a 150-pound person (reduce the calories 1/3 for a 100-pound person and multiply by 1 1/3 for a 200-pound person).

Activity	Calories Burned Per Hour
Bicycling at 6 mph	240
Bicycling at 12 mph	410
Cross-country skiing	700
Jogging at 5.5 mph	740
Jogging at 7 mph	920
Running in place	650
Jumping rope	750
Swimming 25 yards/minute	275
Swimming 50 yards/minute	500
Tennis, singles	400
Walking at 2 mph	240
Walking at 3 mph	320
Walking at 4.5 mph	440

Source: U.S. Department of Health and Human Services. 1983. *Exercise and Your Heart.* Washington, D.C.: U.S. Government Printing Office.

activity for 5 to 10 minutes is important to allow the body to relax gradually.

Beyond the exercise program, obese people should be encouraged to schedule more activity into their daily routines. For instance, they should use stairs, both up and down, instead of elevators or escalators. They can also park or get off public transportation a distance away from their destination to allow more walking.

Behavior and Attitude Modification

Behavior modification deals with identifying and changing behaviors that affect weight gain, such as raiding the refrigerator at midnight. Elements of behavior and attitude modification can be grouped into several categories: self-monitoring, stimulus or cue control, eating behaviors, reinforcement or self-reward, self-control, and attitude modification.

Self-monitoring. Self-monitoring involves keeping a food diary or daily record of types and amounts of foods and beverages consumed as well as time and place of eating, mood at the time, and degree of hunger felt. Its purpose is, of course, to increase awareness of what is actually being eaten and whether it is in response to hunger or other stimuli.

Once harmful patterns that encourage overeating are identified, negative behaviors can be changed to more positive ones. Figure 9-2 contains a sample food diary page.

Cue or Stimulus Control. Through self-monitoring, cues or stimuli to overeating can be identified. For example, passing a bakery may be a cue for someone to stop and buy a dozen cookies. Examples of behavioral modification techniques for cue or stimulus control follow.

Food purchasing, storage, and cooking.

1. Plan meals a week or more ahead.
2. Make a shopping list.
3. Do food shopping after eating, that is, on a full stomach.
4. Do not shop for food with someone who will pressure you to buy foods you do not need.
5. If you feel you must buy high-calorie foods for someone else in the family who can afford the calories, buy something you do not like or let them buy, store, and serve the particular food.
6. Store food out of sight and limit storage to the kitchen.
7. Keep low-calorie snacks on hand and ready to eat.
8. When cooking, keep a small spoon such as a half-teaspoon on hand to use if you must taste while cooking.

Mealtime.

1. Do not serve food at the table or leave serving dishes on the table.
2. Leave the table immediately after eating.

Holidays and parties.

1. Eat and drink something before you go.
2. Drink fewer alcoholic beverages.
3. Bring a low-calorie food to the party.
4. Decide what you will eat before eating.
5. Stay away from the food as much as possible.
6. Concentrate on socializing.
7. Be polite but firm and persistent when refusing another portion or drink.

Eating Behaviors. Eating behaviors need to be modified to discourage overeating. First, one or two eating places, such as the kitchen and dining room tables, need to be set up so that eating occurs in only these predesignated locations. Eat only while sitting at the table and make the

Figure 9-2. Food diary form

Time?	What Was Eaten?	Where?	How Much?	Hungry?	With Whom?	Mood?

environment as attractive as possible. Do not read, watch television, or do anything else while you eat, because you can easily form associations between certain activities and food, such as television and snacking. Do not eat while standing at cabinets or refrigerators.

Second, plan three meals and at least two snacks daily, preferably at certain times of the day. Third, eat slowly by putting your fork down between bites, eating your favorite foods first, talking to others, eating a high-fiber food that requires time to chew, and drinking a no-calorie beverage to help you fill up. In addition, take smaller bites, savor each bite, use a smaller plate to make the food look bigger, and leave a bite or two on your plate. If you clean your plate, you are responding to the sight of food, not to real hunger. When you want a snack, postpone it for 10 minutes.

Reinforcement or Self-reward. Reward yourself for positive steps taken to lose weight, but do not use food as a reward. Other rewards could include reading a good book or magazine, doing a hobby such as sewing, taking a long bubble bath, picking some fresh flowers, or calling a friend.

Self-control. Overeating sometimes occurs in reaction to stressful situations, emotions, or cravings. The food diary is very useful in identifying these situations. Then you can handle these situations in new ways. You can express your feelings verbally if you are overeating in response to frustration or similar stressful emotions. You can exercise or use relaxation techniques to relieve stress, or you can switch to a new activity, such as taking a walk, knitting, reading, or engaging in a hobby to help you take your mind off food. If you allow yourself five minutes before getting something to eat, you often will go on to something else and forget about the food. Positive self-talk is important for good self-control. Instead of repeating a negative statement such as "I cannot resist that cookie," say, "I will resist that cookie."

Attitude Modification.   The most common attitude problem obese people have is thinking of themselves as either on or off a diet. Being "on a diet" implies that at some point the diet will be over, resulting in weight gain if old habits are resumed. Dieting should not be so restrictive or have such unrealistic goals that the person cannot wait to get "off the diet." When combined with exercise, behavior and attitude modification, social support, and a maintenance plan, dieting is really a plan of sensible eating that allows for periodic indulgences.

Another attitude that needs modification revolves around using words such as **always**, **never**, or **every**. The following are examples of unrealistic statements using these terms.

> I will always control my desire for chocolates.
> I will never eat more than 1500 calories each day.
> I will exercise every day.

Goals stated in this manner decrease the likelihood that you will ever accomplish them, and thus result in discouragement and thoughts of failure.

Setting realistic goals, followed by monitoring and self-reward when appropriate, is crucial to the success of any weight-loss program. Through goal setting, complex behavior changes can be broken down into a series of small, successive steps. Goals need to be reasonable and stated in a positive, behavioral manner. For example, if a problem behavior is buying a chocolate bar every afternoon at work, a goal may be to bring an appropriate afternoon snack from home. If this goal is not truly attainable, perhaps one chocolate bar per week should be allowed and worked into the diet.

Even with reasonable goals, occasional lapses in behavior occur. This is when having a constructive attitude is critical. After eating and drinking too much at a party one night, for example, feelings of guilt and failure are common. However, they do nothing to help people get back on their feet. Instead, the dieter must stay calm, realize that what is done is done, and that no one is perfect.

Two other attitudes that often need correcting concern hunger and foods that are "bad for you." Hunger is a physiological need for food, whereas appetite is a psychological need. Eating should be in response to hunger, not to appetite. Although obese people frequently regard certain foods as "good" or "bad," they must realize that no food is inherently good or bad. Some foods do contain more nutrients per calorie, and some are mostly empty calories with few nutrients. However, no food is so bad that it can never be eaten.

Social Support

In general, obese people are more likely to lose weight when their families and friends are supportive and involved in their weight-loss plans. As social support increases, so does a person's chances of maintaining weight loss (Parham, 1993). When possible, obese people need to enlist the help of someone who is easy to talk to, understands and empathizes with the problems of losing weight, and is genuinely interested in helping. Supporters can model good eating habits and give praise and encouragement. The obese person needs to tell others exactly how to be supportive by, for example, not offering high-calorie snacks. Requests need to be specific and positive.

Maintenance Support

Not enough is known about factors associated with weight-maintenance success or what support is needed during the first few months of weight maintenance, when a majority of dieters begin to relapse. Being at a normal, or more normal, weight can bring about stress as adjustments are made. Food is no longer a focal point, and old friends and activities may not fit into the new lifestyle. Support and encouragement from significant others will probably diminish. A formal maintenance program can help deal with those issues as well as others.

Strategies that appear to support weight maintenance include:

1. Determining how many calories are needed for weight maintenance and working out a livable diet
2. Learning skills for dealing with high-risk situations when a lapse in eating behavior may occur, and what to do when a relapse occurs
3. Continued self-monitoring
4. Continued exercise
5. Continued social support
6. Continued use of other strategies that were useful during weight loss
7. Dealing with unrealistic expectations about being thin

These strategies can be used during formal maintenance programs and after treatment is terminated.

Mini-Summary A comprehensive treatment plan for obesity needs to include diet and nutrition education, exercise, behavior and attitude modification, social support, and maintenance support. A newer, non-dieting approach de-emphasizes dieting because dieting works in so few cases. This approach emphasizes exercise and fewer fat calories.

MENU PLANNING FOR WEIGHT LOSS AND MAINTENANCE

1. Cut down on fats; they are loaded with calories. Menu planning for foods lower in fat, saturated fat, and cholesterol can be found in Chapters 12 and 13.
2. De-emphasize protein foods as the central part of a meal, especially as entrees. Instead highlight complex carbohydrates rich in starch and high in fiber. Menu planning guidelines for foods high in complex carbohydrates also appear in Chapter 12.
3. Be sure to suggest snacks that are healthy and not too high in calories. Try fresh fruit and vegetables, popcorn without added fat and sprinkled with garlic or chili powder, regular and soft pretzels, bread sticks, muffins or quick breads, whole-grain cookies (preferably homemade), graham crackers, vanilla wafers, gingersnaps, small amounts of peanut butter or cheese on whole-grain crackers, unsweetened ready-to-eat cereals, puddings such as rice or bread made with skim milk, frozen yogurt, some commercial frozen fruit and pudding bars with less than 100 calories per serving, plain low-fat yogurt, skim or low-fat milk, diet soft drinks, bottled waters, fruit spritzers (fruit juice with bottled water), coffee, tea, and herbal tea.

THE PROBLEM OF UNDERWEIGHT

A person is considered *underweight* if he or she weighs 10 percent below the listing in the height-weight tables. Although anyone who has seriously dieted may think the underweight person is problem free, this is hardly the case. Underweight persons who have trouble gaining weight have very real concerns. Just as some people cannot seem to lose weight, so some people have trouble putting on a few extra pounds. The cause could be genetics, metabolism, or environment. However, some thin people, if they were to gain weight, would feel uncomfortable. Anyone who is underweight due to wasting diseases such as cancer or eating disorders also has a problem: malnutrition.

Gaining weight can be as hard for underweight people as it is for obese people to lose weight.

The following list contains tips on gaining weight.

1. If you find you cannot eat large meals, do not get discouraged. You can increase your intake by eating smaller meals frequently.

Food Facts: A Guide to Healthy Snacking

Snacking between meals may not be as bad as many people believe. In fact, there is nothing wrong with it at all, if you use snack time to eat nutritious foods without consuming too many calories. In any case, snacking is a way of life in the United States, from young children who are often unable to consume all the food they need in three regular meals, to teenagers with busy schedules, to adults at work or at home who often welcome snacking as a needed break and an occasion to socialize.

Snack foods eaten most often include fresh fruit, ice cream, cookies, cheese, crackers, popcorn, potato chips, and peanut butter. Your snack choices can provide an important percentage of the RDAs for calories and nutrients.

To make the most out of your snacks, note which foods you are most likely to eat as a snack, then ask yourself the following questions:

1. Do you make varied choices, or do you always snack on the same foods?
2. Do you choose lots of fruits, vegetables, and grain products, or higher in fat choices such as cookies, cupcakes, and chips?
3. Do you plan snacks as part of your total calories for the day?

Following are some ideas to make snack time interesting, and nutritious as well!

1. Hard and soft pretzels are good snack choices as they are very low in fat and a good source of complex carbohydrate. Pretzels using whole-wheat flour and coated with sesame seeds (rather than salt) are even more nutritious.
2. Popcorn is a good choice served with a minimal amount of melted margarine, and is an even better choice without adding any fat! Instead use garlic, onion or chili powder, grated very hard cheese or another seasoning.

2. Avoid drinking low-calorie beverages such as coffee, tea, or water, especially with meals. Try fruit juices, milk, and milkshakes for more calories.
3. Add additional calories to your meals by using margarine, mayonnaise, oil, salad dressing, cream, sour cream, cream cheese, gravy, cream sauces, and the like. For example, spread margarine on bread, put cream on cereal with fruit, or use whipped cream on desserts and fruits.
4. Add skim milk powder to soups, sauces, gravies, mixed casseroles, scrambled eggs, and hot cereals. It adds both calories and protein. It can also be blended with milk at the rate of 2 to 4 tablespoons of powder to 1 cup of milk.

3. To make a healthy pizza snack, use lowfat cheeses, such as skim-milk mozzarella, and top with fresh vegetables like green peppers, mushrooms and zucchini. Minipizzas can be made with pita bread, a little Parmesan cheese, vegetables, garlic powder, and oregano.

4. Fresh fruits and vegetables are popular snack foods. Raw vegetables with dip and fruit with low-fat cheese, such as cottage cheese, are great combinations. Or make a dip for fruit with 8 ounces plain low-fat yogurt, 3 tablespoons no-sugar added strawberry jam, and 1/2 teaspoon cinnamon.

5. The sour cream or cream used in many dips for vegetables can be replaced with plain lowfat yogurt, reduced calorie cream cheese and/or soft tofu. Good dips to make using these alternate ingredients include onion, chives, spinach, or artichoke dip. Other good dip choices are bean dip such as hummus (made from chickpeas) or salsa (a tomato-based Mexican dip that is hot).

6. Breads and crackers are great snack choices. Try whole-grain breads and crackers, pita bread, bread sticks made with a minimum of oil, mini-rolls, quick breads and muffins. You may want to spread a thin layer of peanut butter or a thin slice of low-fat cheese on breads and crackers, or you can stuff a pita pocket with lettuce, tomato, and any other vegetable and top with diet dressing. Tortilla chips can be made by cutting tortillas and baking them, then sprinkling with garlic, onion or chili powder or small amounts of grated cheese. Serve with salsa.

7. For a beverage try skim milk, fruit juice, bottled water with a twist of lemon or lime, or carbonated water with fruit juice.

5. Add cheese to favorite sandwiches. Use grated cheese on top of casseroles, salads, soups, sauces, and baked potatoes.

6. Try breaded and fried foods.

7. Use cream in soups, sauces, egg dishes, batters, puddings, and custards. Put it on cereal and into cocoa. Add it to mashed potatoes. Substitute cream for milk in recipes.

8. Eat regular yogurt, peanut butter or cheese with crackers, nuts, milkshakes, and whole-grain cookies and muffins as snacks.

9. Add regular cottage cheese to casseroles or egg dishes such as quiche, scrambled eggs, and souffles. Add it to spaghetti or noodles.

10. Make every mouthful count!

The primary fuels for exercise are carbohydrates and fat.

NUTRITION FOR THE ATHLETE

The amount of energy required by the athlete depends on the type of activity and its duration, frequency, and intensity. In addition, the athlete's BMR, body composition, age, and environment must be taken into account. Many athletes require between 3000 and 6000 calories daily.

Carbohydrates and fat are the primary fuel sources for exercise. Protein plays a minor role. An appropriate diet for many athletes consists of 60 to 65 percent of calories as carbohydrates, 30 percent or less as fat, and enough protein to provide between 1 to 1.5 grams per kilogram body weight (The American Dietetic Association and The Canadian Dietetic Association, 1993).

The most crucial nutrient for athletes is water.

Although many athletes take vitamin and mineral supplements, they will not enhance performance unless there is a deficiency. Most athletes get plenty of vitamins and minerals in their regular diets, although young athletes and women need to pay special attention to iron and calcium.

Water is the most crucial nutrient for athletes. They need about 1 liter of water for every 1000 calories consumed. For moderate exercise without extreme temperatures or duration, cold water is the choice for replacing fluids. Cold water both cools the body and empties quicker from the stomach. Athletes need 2 cups of water about 15 to 20 minutes before endurance exercise and at regular intervals during exercise. A good way to determine how much fluid to replace after exercising is to weigh in before and after exercise and also the next morning. For every pound that is lost, the athlete needs to drink 2 cups, or 16 ounces, of water.

For endurance events, some carbohydrates in fluids taken before and during competition may be helpful in maintaining normal blood sugar levels.

Carbohydrate loading involves gradually exercising less for 3 to 6 days before the event (with one full day of rest the day before) and gradually increasing carbohydrate intake from 60 to 70 percent and fluid intake (add 4 more cups) during this time.

Carbohydrate or glycogen loading is a regimen involving 3 or more days of decreasing amounts of exercise and increased consumption of carbohydrates before an event to increase glycogen stores. The theory is that increased glycogen stores (which increase between 50 to 80 percent) will enhance performance by providing more energy during lengthy competition.

Here are some menu-planning guidelines for athletes.

1. Offer a variety of foods from all four food groups: meat, poultry, and seafood; milk and dairy products; fruits and vegetables; and grain products.
2. Good sources of complex carbohydrates to emphasize on menus include pasta, rice, other grain products such as breads and cereals, legumes, and fruits and vegetables. On the eve of the New York City Marathon each year, marathon officials typically host a pasta dinner

Hot Topic: Sports Drinks

A topic of much interest to athletes is whether sports drinks, such as Gatorade or Exceed, are needed during an event or workout. Sports drinks contain a dilute mixture of carbohydrate and electrolytes. Most contain about 50 calories per cup (or about 12 grams of carbohydrate) and small amounts of sodium and potassium. Sports drinks are purposely made to be weak solutions so they can empty faster from the stomach and the nutrients in it are therefore available quicker to the body. They are primarily designed to be used during exercise, although there are some specially formulated sports drinks with slightly more sugar that can be used just prior to exercising.

During exercise lasting 90 minutes or more, sports drinks can help replace water and electrolytes and provide some carbohydrates for energy. During an endurance event or workout, you increasingly rely on blood sugar for energy as your muscle glycogen stores diminish. Carbohydrates taken during exercise can help you maintain a normal blood sugar level and enhance (as well as lengthen) performance. Athletes often consume between 1/2 to 1 cup of sports fluids every 15 to 20 minutes during exercise.

Some sports drinks tout that they contain glucose polymers, which are chains of glucose. It was thought that sports drinks with glucose polymers emptied from the stomach faster than solutions with sucrose or glucose, but it turned out that each of these solutions empties at approximately the same rate and provides the same positive affects on performance as long as the carbohydrate concentration is between 5 to 8 percent (which it usually is).

Although sports drinks clearly can help the athlete in lengthy events or workouts, are there other products that can do much the same? Long before sports drinks were even available, athletes had their own homemade sports drinks: flat or defizzed cola, tea with honey, and dilute lemonade. Which works best?—whichever satisfies you best both physically and psychologically.

for runners featuring spaghetti with marinara sauce and cold pasta primavera. Complex carbohydrates such as pasta also provide needed B vitamins, minerals, and fiber. Whole-grain products such as whole-wheat bread contain more nutrients than refined products such as white bread. If using refined products, be sure they are enriched (the thiamin, riboflavin, niacin, and iron have been replaced). Here are some ways to include complex carbohydrates in your menu.

At breakfast, offer a variety of pancakes, waffles, cold and hot cereals, breads, and rolls.

At lunch, make sandwiches with different types of bread, such as pita pockets, raisin bread, onion rolls, and brown bread. Also, have a variety of breads and rolls available for nonsandwich items.

Serve pasta and rice as a side or main dish with, for example, chicken and vegetables. Cold pasta and rice salads are great too.

Potatoes, whether baked, mashed, or boiled, are excellent sources of carbohydrates.

Always have available as many types of fresh fruits and salads as possible.

Don't forget to use beans and peas in soups, salads, entrees, and side dishes.

Nutritious desserts emphasizing carbohydrates are frozen yogurt with fruit toppings, oatmeal cookies, and fresh fruit.

3. Don't offer too much protein and fat in the thought that athletes need the extra calories. They do, but much of those extra calories should come from complex carbohydrates. The days of steak-and-egg dinners are over for athletes. The protein and fat present in these meals does nothing to improve performance. Here are some ways to moderate the amount of fat and protein.

   Use lean, well-trimmed cuts of beef.

   Offer chicken, turkey, and fish—all lower in fat than beef. Broiling, roasting, and grilling are preferred cooking methods, with frying being acceptable occasionally.

   Offer larger serving sizes of meat, poultry, and fish, perhaps 1 to 2 ounces more, but don't overdo it!

   Offer fried food in moderation.

   Offer low-fat and skim milk.

   Offer high-fat desserts, such as ice cream and many types of sweets, in moderation. Frozen yogurt and ice milk generally contain less fat than ice cream and can be topped with fruit or crushed oatmeal cookies. Fruit ice and sorbet contain no fat.

4. Offer a variety of fluids, not just soft drinks and other sugared drinks. Good beverage choices include fruit juices, iced tea, and iced coffee (preferably freshly brewed decaffeinated), and plain and flavored mineral and seltzer water, spritzers (fruit juice and mineral water), and milkshakes made with yogurt or ice milk and fruit. Soft drinks and juice drinks—both loaded with sugar—should be offered in moderation.

5. Make sure iodized salt is on the table.

6. Be sure to include sources of iron at each meal. Good iron sources include liver, red meats, legumes, and iron-fortified breakfast cereal. Moderate iron sources include raisins, dried fruit, bananas, nuts, whole-grain and fortified grain products. Be sure to include good

vitamin C sources at each meal as vitamin C helps iron absorption. Vitamin C sources include citrus fruits and juices, cantaloupe, strawberries, broccoli, potatoes, and brussels sprouts.

7. The most important meal is the one closest to the competition, commonly called the *precompetition meal*. The functions of this meal include getting the athlete fueled up, both physically and psychologically, helping settle the stomach, and preventing hunger. The meal should consist of mostly complex carbohydrates (they digest easier and faster and help maintain blood sugar levels), and should be low in fat. High-fat foods take longer to digest and can cause sluggishness. Substantial precompetition meals are usually served 3 to 4 hours prior to competition in order to allow enough time for stomach emptying (to avoid cramping and discomfort during the competition). Menus might include: cereals with low-fat or skim milk topped with fresh fruit, low-fat yogurt with muffins and juice, or 1 to 2 eggs with toast and jelly and juice. The meal should include 2 to 3 cups of fluid for hydration and typically provide 300 to 1000 calories. Smaller precompetition meals may be served 2 to 3 hours before competition. Many athletes have specific "comfort" foods that they enjoy before competition.

8. After competition and workouts, again emphasize complex carbohydrates to ensure glycogen restoration. The sooner an athlete fuels up after exercising, the more glycogen will be stored in the muscle. Food is also important to restore the minerals lost in sweating.

KEY TERMS

Body mass index (BMI)
Carbohydrate (glycogen) loading
Height–weight tables
Mild obesity
Moderate obesity
Obesity
Overweight
Precompetition meal
Severe obesity

REVIEW QUESTIONS

1. Describe the three classifications of obesity.
2. How is degree of obesity measured?

3. List seven health concerns for which obese individuals are at increased risk.

4. Describe possible causes of obesity.

5. What are the elements of a comprehensive treatment plan for obesity? Give an example of each.

6. What are the important elements of nutrition for athletes?

7. What should be included in a precompetition meal?

ACTIVITIES AND APPLICATIONS

1. Quiz

Check your answers with these.

1. False
2. True
3. False
4. False
5. True
6. False
7. False
8. False
9. True
10. False

2. Your Desirable Weight

Using Tables 9-1 and 9-2, determine your desirable weight using both the 1959 and 1983 height–weight charts. What is the difference between the figures? Using body mass index, determine whether you are overweight, as well as your desirable weight. Determine how many pounds you would have to weigh to be 20 percent and 40 percent overweight. If you are overweight, find out from your family if you have a family history of any of the medical conditions discussed in the section on health and obesity.

3. Low-Calorie Menu Planning

A national chain of steak and seafood restaurants has asked you to design lower-calorie menu items as follows: two appetizers, two soups, three entrees, and one dessert. Their emphasis is freshly made traditional American cooking. Provide recipes that include calorie information.

4. Using a Food Diary

Using the food diary form, complete a three-day food diary. Then examine it to increase your awareness of how much and how often you are eating and whether you are eating in response to moods, people, and/or activities. Write down five insights you gained about your eating habits.

5. Box Lunches

Design three complete box lunches for calorie- and fat-conscious customers of a gourmet take-out deli with complete kitchen facilities in a major U.S. city. The meal must be balanced and provide a main dish, side dish, dessert, and beverage.

6. Precompetition Meals

Devise a menu for a precompetition meal for long-distance runners on a university track team who will compete at 4 P.M. Have alternate menu items available (one for each item you offer).

REFERENCES

Adams, Simone O., Kathleen E. Grady, Claudia H. Wolk, and Carrie Mukaida. 1986. Weight loss: A comparison of group and individual interventions. *Journal of The American Dietetic Association* 86(4): 485–489.

American Dietetic Association and Canadian Dietetic Association. 1993. Position of the The American Dietetic Association and The Canadian Dietetic Association: Nutrition for physical fitness and athletic performance for adults. *Journal of The American Dietetic Association* 93(6): 691–696.

Brownell, Kelly D. 1984. The psychology and physiology of obesity: implications for screening and treatment. *Journal of The American Dietetic Association* 84(4): 406–414.

Brownell, Kelly D. 1986. A program for managing obesity. *Dietetic Currents* 13(3): 1–5.

Brownell, Kelly D., and Christopher G. Fairburn (eds). 1995. *Eating Disorders and Obesity: A Comprehensive Handbook.* New York: Guilford Press.

Cassell, Jo Anne, 1995. Social anthropology and nutrition: A different look at obesity in America. *Journal of The American Dietetic Association* 95(4): 424–427.

Council of Scientific Affairs, American Medical Association, 1988. Treatment of obesity in adults. *Journal of The American Medical Association* 260(17): 2547–2551.

Danforth, Elliot. 1985. Diet and obesity. *American Journal of Clinical Nutrition* 41(5 Suppl.): 1132–1145.

Duncan, Karen H., Jane A. Bacon, and Roland L. Weinsier. 1983. The effects of high and low energy density diets on satiety, energy intake, and eating time of obese and nonobese subjects. *American Journal of Clinical Nutrition* 37(5): 763–767.

Fisher, Michele C., and Paul A. Lachance. 1985. Nutrition evaluation of published weight-reducing diets. *Journal of The American Dietetic Association* 85(4): 450–454.

Food and Nutrition Board Committee to Develop Criteria for Evaluating the Outcomes of Approaches to Prevent and Treat Obesity, Institute of Medicine, National Academy of Sciences. 1995. Summary: Weighing the Options–criteria for evaluating weight-management programs. *Journal of The American Dietetic Association* 95(1): 96–105.

Frankle, Reva T. 1985. Obesity a family matter: creating new behavior. *Journal of The American Dietetic Association* 85(5): 597–601.

Frankle, Reva T., and Mei-Uih Yang, eds. 1988. *Obesity and Weight Control, The Health Professional's Guide to Understanding and Treatment.* Baltimore: Aspen Publishing.

Haus, Gail, Sharon L. Hoerr, Brian Mavis, and Jon Robison, 1994. Key modifiable factors in weight maintenance: Fat intake, exercise, and weight cycling. 94(4): 409–413.

Holli, Betsy B. 1988. Using behavior modification in nutrition counseling. *Journal of The American Dietetic Association* 88(12): 1530–1536.

Kayman, S., W. Bruvold, and J. S. Stern. 1990. Maintenance and relapse after weight loss in women: behavioral aspects. *American Journal of Clinical Nutrition* 52: 800–807.

Mathus-Vliegen, Lisbeth M. H., and Annemieke M. A. Res. 1993. Dexfenfluramine influences dietary compliance and eating behavior, but dietary instruction may overrule its effect on food selection in obese subjects. *Journal of The American Dietetic Association* 93(10): 1163–1165.

NIH Technology Assessment Conference Panel. 1993. Methods for voluntary weight loss and control. *Annals of Internal Medicine* 119: 764–770.

Parham, Ellen S. 1993. Enhancing social support in weight loss management groups. *Journal of The American Dietetic Association* 93(10): 1152–1156.

Parham, Ellen S. 1993. Nutrition education research in weight management among adults. *Journal of Nutrition Education* 25(5): 258–268.

Pate, R. R., M. Pratt, S. N. Blair, W. L. Haskell, C. A. Macera, C. Bouchard, D. Buckner, W. Ettinger, G. W. Heath, A. C. King, A. Kriska, A. S. Leon, B. H. Marcus, J. Morris, R. S. Paffenbarger, K. Patrick, M. L. Pollock, J. M. Rippe, J. Sallis, and J. H. Wilmore. 1995. Physical activity and public health; A recommendation from the Centers for Disease Control and Prevention and the American College of Sports Medicine. *Journal of The American Medical Association* 273(5): 402–407.

Pavlou, Konstantin N., William P. Steffee, Robert H. Lerman, and Belton A. Burrows. 1985. Effects of dieting and exercise on lean body mass, oxygen uptake, and strength. *Medicine and Science in Sports and Exercise* 17(4): 466–471.

Petre, Kay, and Joanne Gatto. 1987. Lifesteps: weight management program. *Journal of The American Dietetic Association* 87(9 Suppl.): S26–S29.

Robison, Jonathan, I., Sharon L. Hoerr, John Strandmark, and Brian Mavis. 1993. Obesity, weight loss, and health. *Journal of The American Dietetic Association* 93(4): 445–449.

Robison, Jonathan, I., Sharon L. Hoerr, Karen A. Petersmarck, and Judith V. Anderson. 1993. Redefining success in obesity intervention: The new paradigm. *Journal of The American Dietetic Association* 95(4): 422–423.

Rock, Cheryl L., and Ann M. Coulston. 1988. Weight-control approaches: A review by the California Dietetic Association. *Journal of The American Dietetic Association* 88(1): 44–48.

Stunkard, Albert, and Eliot Stellar, eds. 1984. *Eating and Its Disorders.* New York: Raven Press.

Sullivan, Ann C., Susan Hogan, and Joseph Triscari. 1987. New developments in pharmacological treatments for obesity. *Annals of the New York Academy of Sciences* 499: 269–276.

Thomas, C. D., J. C. Peters, G. W. Reed, N. N. Abumrad, M. Sun, and J. O. Hill. 1992. Nutrient balance and energy expenditure during ad libitum feeding of high fat and high carbohydrate diets in humans. *American Journal of Clinical Nutrition* 55:934–942.

Volkmar, Fred R., Albert J. Stunkard, Joseph Wollston, and Robert A. Bailey. 1981. High attrition rates in commercial weight reduction programs. *Archives of Internal Medicine* 141(4): 426–28.

Zelasko, Chester J. 1995. Exercise for weight loss: What are the facts? *Journal of The American Dietetic Association* 95(12): 1414-1417.

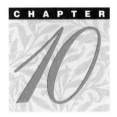

CHAPTER 10

Menu Planning for the Vegetarian

**KEY
QUESTIONS**

1. Are there different types of vegetarians?
2. Why does someone become a vegetarian?
3. Can a vegetarian diet be well balanced and adequate in all nutrients?
4. How do you plan balanced and varied menus for vegetarians that go beyond macaroni and cheese?

QUIZ

Quiz
Circle the correct answer.

1. Vegetarianism is a passing fad.	*True*	*False*
2. To get enough protein on a daily basis, you must eat some animal products, such as meat, chicken, eggs, and/or milk.	*True*	*False*
3. Protein from plant sources usually contains less fat than animal protein.	*True*	*False*
4. Vegetarians enjoy certain health benefits from their diets.	*True*	*False*
5. Pasta, bread, and beans contain protein.	*True*	*False*
6. Tofu, an excellent plant source of protein, is made from split peas.	*True*	*False*
7. A vegetarian diet that includes dairy products is likely to be deficient in some nutrients.	*True*	*False*

INTRODUCTION

The number of vegetarians in the United States has been increasing, and they now number about 12 million, or 7 percent of our population. Vegetarians do not eat food that requires the death of, or injury to, an animal. Instead of eating the meat entrees that have traditionally been the major source of protein in the American diet, they dine on main dishes emphasizing legumes (dried beans and peas), grains, and vegetables. Vegetarian entrees, such as red beans and rice, can supply adequate protein with less fat and cholesterol, and more fiber than their meat counterparts (see Table 10-1).

On any given day, about 5 percent of people eating out will order a vegetarian dish. This figure goes up to 15 percent for college students eating on campus. But vegetarian dishes aren't just for vegetarians. Nonvegetarians are also selecting meatless meals. Luckily, more and more restaurants are offering meatless options, and their dishes are quite varied and, at times, sophisticated.

How about this for a sophisticated vegetarian dish: wild mushroom strudel with shallot and sherry.

Animal Foods	Fat (grams)	Saturated Fat (grams)	Protein (grams)	Cholesterol (milligrams)
Beef, ground broiled, 3 oz.	16	6	21	74
Chicken breast, roasted, 3 oz.	3	1	27	73
Cod, baked, 3 oz.	1	0	19	47
Milk, 2%, 8 fl. oz.	5	3	8	18
Cheese, American, 1 oz.	9	6	6	27
Egg, 1	6	2	6	274

Plant Foods	Fat (grams)	Saturated Fat (grams)	Protein (grams)	Cholesterol (milligrams)
Lentils, cooked, 1/2 cup	0	0	9	0
Brown rice, cooked, 1/2 cup	1	0	2	0
Spaghetti, whole wheat, 1 cup	1	0	7	0
Whole wheat bread, 2 slices	2	0	5	0
Broccoli, chopped 1 cup	0	0	6	0
Apple, 1 medium	0	0	0	0

TABLE 10-1. Fat, saturated fat, protein, and cholesterol in animal and plant foods.

Sources: United States Department of Agriculture Handbooks. Numbers 8-1, 8-5, 8-13, 8-15, 8-20

After discussing the different types of vegetarian eating styles, this chapter goes on to explain why individuals choose to be vegetarian, the nutritional adequacy of these diets, and menu planning.

ARE THERE DIFFERENT KINDS OF VEGETARIAN EATING STYLES?

Whereas vegetarians do not eat meat, poultry, or fish, the largest group of vegetarians, referred to as **lacto-ovovegetarians**, do consume animal products in the form of eggs (ovo) and milk and milk products (lacto).

Hot Topic: Pesticides and Organic Foods

Pesticides are chemicals used to control insects, diseases, weeds, fungi, mold, and other pests on plants, vegetables, fruits, and animals. Examples include insecticides (designed to kill insects) and fungicides (designed to kill fungi). Pesticides are normally applied to crops as a spray, fog, or dust to protect the crops from damage and increase their yields. The Environmental Protection Agency (EPA) is responsible for setting safety levels and for approving pesticides and other chemicals used in growing food. The FDA then monitors for compliance with EPA tolerance levels for most foods. Each year, the FDA tests thousands of shipments of all foods , both domestic and imported (except meat and poultry), for pesticide residues.

Over the years the EPA has banned the use of a wide variety of carcinogenic pesticides, and it continues to study others to determine their safety. For pesticides deemed safe to use, it establishes minimum exposure standards, or tolerances, that have a built-in safety level.

The goal of organic farming is to preserve the natural fertility and productivity of the land. Organic foods are foods that have been grown without nearly all synthetic insecticides, fungicides, herbicides, and fertilizers. Natural methods are used to get rid of bugs. These include rotating crops, weeding manually, and using bugs, such as ladybugs, to eat harmful bugs. Organic alternatives to synthetic fertilizers include animal manure, compost, and crop rotation, which helps to replenish the soil's nutrients.

Animals raised for organic meat and poultry are not given antibiotics or hormones. Organic dairy cows are not given hormones to increase milk production either. Organic packaged foods, such as soups and salad dressings, must contain all (or almost all) organically grown ingredients. These foods are also not permitted to contain artificial additives or preservatives, and they must be organically processed. For example, if skins need to be peeled off a fruit or vegetable before canning, a natural method such as steaming must be used instead of chemicals.

There are many different vegetarian eating styles based on which foods they will eat, and which they won't. Using the categories here helps give some order to the topic.

Another group of vegetarians, **lactovegetarians**, consume milk and milk products but forego eggs.

Most vegetarians are either lacto-ovovegetarians or lactovegetarians. **Vegans**, a third group of vegetarians, do not eat eggs or dairy products and therefore rely exclusively on plant foods to meet protein and other nutrient needs. Vegans are a small group, and it is estimated that only 4 percent of vegetarians are vegans (Johnston, 1995).

In addition, some vegetarians (**pescovegetarians**) eat seafood. Also, some vegetarian diets restrict certain foods and beverages such as highly

The exact meaning of the term *organic* has varied from one part of the United States to another. By 1997, the United States hopes to implement national standards for organic foods and agriculture as required by the Organic Foods Production Act. These standards prohibit the use of certain materials, such as mostly synthetic fertilizers, and mandate certain practices, such as those that enrich the soil. By looking at labels on produce, dairy, meats, poultry, and packaged and canned goods, you'll be able to see whether the product is certified organic.

Many vegetarians prefer buying organic products to decrease their exposure to pesticides. Other steps you can take include:

Removing the outer leaves of leafy vegetables, such as lettuce.

Washing produce carefully using a brush, to remove some (but not all) residues. Although pesticides are often found on the fruit surfaces, some pesticides do concentrate in the interior of fruits and vegetables.

Peeling carrots, waxed cucumbers, apples, peaches, and pears because these foods are more likely to contain hazardous pesticide residues.

Buying less imported produce, since it often contains more pesticides.

Buying produce from a local farmer's market, since it is probably treated with less pesticide than produce traveling from state to state.

Trimming fat and skin from meat, poultry, and fish. Pesticides in animal feed can concentrate in animal fat. Skim fat from pan drippings, broths, sauces, and soups.

Eating a varied diet so that no one food dominates.

The green color found under the skin of the potato is not due to pesticides but is a natural toxin that is not destroyed during cooking. Since it is toxic, it is best to cut it out. By storing potatoes in a dark and cool area, it is less likely to develop.

processed foods containing certain additives and preservatives, foods that contain pesticides and/or have not been grown organically, or caffeinated or alcoholic beverages.

MINI-SUMMARY Most vegetarians are either lactovegetarians or lacto-ovovegetarians. Vegans, who eat only plant foods, are the smallest group.

WHY BECOME A VEGETARIAN?

So why does someone choose to eat as a vegan, lactovegetarian, or lacto-ovovegetarian? The number one reason people give for being vegetarian is health. Being a vegetarian has health benefits. Vegetarians tend to be leaner and keep their body weight and blood lipid levels closer to desirable levels than nonvegetarians. Vegetarians tend to be at lower risk for the following diseases (American Dietetic Association, 1993).

1   Hypertension
2. Coronary artery disease
3. Breast cancer
4. Colon cancer
5. Non-insulin-dependent (Type II) diabetes mellitus
6. Osteoporosis
7. Diverticular disease of the colon

A comprehensive study of rural Chinese suggested that eating much less animal protein and fat (and more complex carbohydrates) results in reductions of blood cholesterol levels and the chronic degenerative diseases (such as heart disease and cancer) associated with high blood cholesterol levels (Campbell and Junshi, 1994).

Being vegetarian does not necessarily mean that you automatically get these benefits. There are vegetarians who eat well-balanced and varied diets and then there are vegetarians who eat eggs for breakfast, peanut butter for lunch, and pizza for supper. In other words, it is possible to be a vegetarian and still eat too much fat, saturated fat, and cholesterol. It's probably the exception, rather than the rule, but it is still possible. Being vegetarian does not guarantee that your diet will meet current dietary recommendations. Some other reasons for becoming vegetarian include the following.

1. *Ecology.* For ecological reasons, vegetarians choose plant protein because livestock and poultry require much land, energy, water, and plant food (such as soybeans), which they consider wasteful. According to the North American Vegetarian Society, grains and soybeans that are fed to U.S. livestock could feed 1.3 billion people. Livestock product also wastes loads of water—it takes 2500 gallons of water to produce one pound of meat, but only 25 gallons to produce one pound of wheat (Clark, 1994).
2. *Economics.* A vegetarian diet is more economical—in other words, less expensive. This fact can be easily demonstrated by the fact that in a

typical foodservice operation, the largest component of food purchases is for meats, poultry, and fish.

3. *Ethics.* Vegetarians do not eat meat for ethical reasons; they believe that animals should not suffer or be killed unnecessarily. They feel that animals suffer real pain in crowded feed lots and cages, and that both their transportation to market and their slaughter are traumatic.

4. *Religious beliefs.* Some vegetarians, such as the Seventh Day Adventists, practice vegetarianism as a part of their religion, which also encourages exercise and forbids smoking and drinking alcohol.

MINI-SUMMARY   Reasons for becoming vegetarian may be related to health benefits, ecology, economics, ethics, or religious beliefs.

IS A VEGETARIAN DIET NUTRITIONALLY ADEQUATE?

Vegetarian diets are consistent with the Dietary Guidelines for Americans and can meet Recommended Dietary Allowances for nutrients. You can get enough protein from a vegetarian diet as long as the variety and amounts of foods consumed are adequate. Meat, fish, and poultry are major contributors of iron, zinc, and B vitamins in most American diets, and vegetarians should pay special attention to these nutrients. Vegans eat only foods of plant origin. Because animal products are the only food sources of vitamin B_{12}, vegans must supplement their diets with a source of this vitamin. (*Dietary Guidelines for Americans*, Fourth Edition, 1995.)

In 1995, the Dietary Guidelines finally addressed the topic of vegetarian diets, with assurances that they can be nutritionally adequate when varied and adequate in calories (except for vegan diets, which need supplementation with vitamin B_{12}). Most vegetarians get enough protein, and their diets are typically lower in fat, saturated fat, and cholesterol.

As discussed in Chapter 4, most plant proteins are considered incomplete proteins, but this doesn't mean they are low quality. When plant proteins are eaten with other foods, the food combinations usually result in complete protein. For example, when peanut butter and whole-wheat bread are eaten over the course of a day, the limiting amino acid in each of these foods is supplied by the other food. Such combinations are called complementary proteins. Eating complementary proteins at different meals during the day generally assures a balance of dietary amino acids. Some vegetable proteins, such as the grains amaranth and quinoa and protein from soybeans are complete proteins.

Meat analogs are imitation meat products made from a variety of ingredients such as soy protein, wheat gluten, and wheat germ. These ingredients can be used to make foods that look like hamburgers, hotdogs, and sausage.

Let's take a look at some of the nutrients that need some special attention.

1. *Vitamin B$_{12}$.* Vitamin B$_{12}$ is found only in animal foods. Lacto-ovovegetarians usually get enough of this vitamin unless they limit their intake of dairy products and eggs. Vegans definitely need either a supplement or vitamin B$_{12}$–fortified foods, such as most ready-to-eat cereals, most meat analogs, some soy beverages, and some brands of nutritional yeasts.

2. *Vitamin D.* Milk is fortified with vitamin D, and vitamin D can be made in the skin with sunlight. Generally, only vegans without enough exposure to sunlight need a supplementary source of vitamin D. Some ready-to-eat breakfast cereals and some soy beverages are fortified with vitamin D.

3. *Calcium.* Lactovegetarians and lacto-ovovegetarians generally don't have a problem here, but vegans sometimes do if they don't eat enough other calcium-rich foods. Good choices include calcium-fortified soy milk or orange juice and tofu made with calcium. Some green leafy vegetables (such as spinach, beet greens, Swiss chard, sorrel, and parsley) are rich in calcium but they also contain a binder (called oxalic acid) that prevents some of the calcium from being absorbed. Dried beans and peas are moderate sources of calcium. Without calcium-fortified drinks or calcium supplements, it can be difficult to take in enough calcium.

4. *Iron.* Interestingly enough, vegetarians do not experience any more problems with iron-deficiency anemia than their meat-eating counterparts–don't forget, meat is rich in iron (Craig, 1994). Iron is widely distributed in plant foods, and its absorption is greatly enhanced by vitamin C–containing fruits and vegetables. Vegetarians get iron from eating dried beans and peas, green leafy vegetables, dried fruits, many nuts and seeds, and enriched and whole-grain products.

5. *Zinc.* Zinc is found in many plant foods, such as whole grains, legumes, and nuts and seeds (especially peanut butter). Its absorption into the body is reduced by plant substances, such as phytate. Children may need zinc supplements.

Infants, children, and adolescents can follow vegetarian diets, even vegan diets. For growing youngsters, however, vegetarian diets need to be well planned, varied, and adequate in calories. In the case of a vegan diet, special attention should be focused on getting enough calories, vitamin B$_{12}$, vitamin D, calcium, iron, and zinc. A reliable source of vitamin B$_{12}$

TABLE 10-2. Legumes.

Bean, Pea, or Lentil	Size/Shape/Color	Flavor	Soaking Required	Cooking Time	Cups Liquid for Cooking	Yield*	Uses
Black beans (Turtle beans)	Small, pea-shaped, black	Full, mellow	Yes Yes	1½ hours	4	2 2	Mediterranean cuisine, soups (black bean soup), chilies, salads with rice
Black-eye peas (Cowpeas, black eyed beans)	Small, oval, creamy white with black spot	Earthy, absorb other flavors	No	50–60 minutes	3	2	Casseroles, with rice, with pork, Southern dishes
Chick-peas (Garbanzo beans, ceci beans)	Round, tan, large	Nutty	Yes	3 hours	4	4	Salads, soups, casseroles, hors d'oeuvres, hummus and other Middle East dishes
Fava beans, whole	Large, round, flat, off white or tan	Full	Yes	3 hours	2½	4	Soups, casseroles, salads
Great Northern beans	Large, oval, white	Mild	Yes	2 hours	3½	2	Soups, casseroles, baked beans, and mixing with other varieties
Kidney beans	Large, kidney-shaped, red or white (red is much more common)	Rich, meaty sweet	Yes	1–1½ hours	3	2	Chili, casseroles, salads, soups, a favorite in Mexican and Italian cooking
Lentils	Small, flat, disc-shaped, green, red, or brown, split or whole	Mild, earthy	No	30–45 minutes	2	2¼	Soups, stews, salads, casseroles, stuffing, sandwiches, spreads, with rice
Lima beans	Flat, oval, cream or greenish, large or baby size	Large–full; Baby–mild	Yes	1½ hours (large) 1 hour (baby)	2	1¼	Soups, casseroles, side dishes
Navy beans (Pea beans)	Small to medium, round to oval, white	Mild	Yes	1½ hours	3	2	Baked beans, soups, salads, side dishes, casseroles
Peas, split	Small, flat on one side, green or yellow	Rich, earthy	No	1½ hours	3	2¼	Soups, casseroles
Peas, whole	Small-medium, round yellow or green	Rich, earthy	Yes	1 hour 40 minutes	3	2¼	Soups, casseroles, Scandinavian dishes
Pinto beans	Medium, kidney-shaped, pinkish brown	Rich, meaty	Yes	1½ hours	3	2	A favorite for chili, refried beans, and in other Mexican cooking
Pink beans	Medium, oval, pinkish brown	Rich, meaty	Yes	1 hour	3	2	Popular in barbecue-style dishes
Soybeans	Medium, oval-round, creamy, yellow	Distinctive	Yes	3½ hours or more	3	2	Soups, stews, casseroles

*From 1 cup of uncooked beans, pea, or lentil.

is particularly essential. Soy milk that has been fortified with calcium and vitamin D will help meet the needs for those vitamins. Meat analogs, soy products, legumes, and nut butters are valuable sources of protein, and some provide iron and/or zinc. If inadequate amounts of these nutrients are taken in from food, supplements are always available.

MINI-SUMMARY Vegetarian diets can be nutritionally adequate when varied and adequate in calories, except for vegan diets, which need supplementation with vitamin B_{12}. Nutrients of special interest to vegetarians are vitamin B_{12}, vitamin D, calcium, iron, and zinc.

HOW TO PLAN MEALS FOR VEGETARIANS

Before going into menu-planning guidelines, let's first take a look at foods commonly eaten by vegetarians, some of which may be new to you.

Legumes, Grains, Nuts, and Seeds

Legumes (LEG-yooms or le-GYOOMS) include dried beans, peas, and lentils (Table 10-2). They are all seeds of leguminous plants, and have either been allowed to dry in their pods before being picked or have been dried after being shelled. Green beans and green peas are also legumes, but they are picked in their immature state and are not as rich nutritionally as legumes. Legumes are good sources of some B vitamins and iron and average 22 percent protein by weight (except for soybeans, which are 40 percent protein). They contain no cholesterol, and most are low in fat (except for soybeans, which still contain considerably less fat and saturated fat than meats).

Don't forget that chili con carne is another international dish using beans.

Many natives of the United States are not aware that legumes have been food staples in other parts of the world for centuries. Some examples of meatless international dishes using legumes include Mexican refried beans and Middle Eastern hummus (chickpea puree). In the United States, legumes are seen mostly in baked beans and split pea, navy bean, or lentil soup (usually with pork added!). Beans, peas, and lentils are quite versatile and can be used in soups, salads, casseroles, and sandwich spreads.

The soybean plant was first domesticated in China 3000 years ago. The Chinese call it the "yellow jewel" or the "great treasure" for several reasons. Soybeans are easy to farm, and the plants do not deplete the soil. They are inexpensive to buy, contain the most and best quality protein of all legumes (with no cholesterol), and are a very versatile food. When merely boiled, however, they have a strong taste with a metallic aftertaste.

TABLE 10-3.   Other soybean products.

Tempeh, a white cake made from culturing soybeans with a certain bacteria, is a pleasant-tasting, high-protein food that can be barbecued, fried, or cut into pieces to add to soups or stews. Tempeh is cultured like cheese and yogurt and therefore must be used when fresh.

Soy protein concentrate and **soy protein isolate** are used in **meat analogs** (imitation meat products) and as extenders and binders in actual meat products. They contain mostly the protein from the soybean, and both taste rather bland. Meat analogs contain little or no fat and cholesterol but are often high in sodium. They can be made from a variety of ingredients such as soy, wheat gluten, and wheat germ. Some are fortified with vitamin B_{12} and iron. They are offered in meat-like forms such as hamburgers, hot dogs, bacon, ham, and chicken chunks. They can be expensive, and their acceptability is variable.

Textured vegetable protein (TVP) is made of granules of isolated soy protein that must be rehydrated before using in recipes. It can replace up to one-quarter of the meat in a recipe without being unacceptable to most consumers. It is a highly concentrated source of protein and is almost fat-free. It's most successful use is in highly flavored dishes such as chili and curries.

Soy milk can be used for drinking and cooking. When fortified with calcium, vitamin D, and vitamin B_{12}, soy milk is an important part of the diet.

Soybean sprouts, similar to other bean sprouts, can be grown and refrigerated for up to 5 days.

Soynuts, similar to roasted peanuts, are made from soaked soybeans that are roasted with or without the skin.

Brands of **tofu ice cream** can be run through a soft-serve machine and are available to the foodservice operator.

Soy sauce combines fermented soy and wheat. The wheat is first roasted and contributes both the soy sauce's brown color and its sharp, distinctive flavor.

Miso is similar to soy sauce but pasty in consistency. It is made by fermenting soybeans with or without rice or other grains. A number of varieties are available from light-colored and sweet to dark and robust. It is used in soups and gravies, as a marinade for tofu, as a seasoning, and as a spread on sandwiches and fried tofu.

This is perhaps the reason soybeans have been used to make a wide variety of products, including soy oil and tofu.

Soybeans are grown in abundance in the United States (they are the second leading crop), but most are sold as animal feed after being processed for their oil, or are exported. Almost all the oil used in prepared dressings in the United States is soy oil, and soy oil is used extensively in margarines and cooking oils.

Another important soybean product, particularly for vegetarians, is **tofu**, or bean curd. Tofu, invented by a Chinese scholar in 164 B.C., is the most important of the soybean-based foods. Tofu is made in a process similar to making cheese. Soybeans are crushed to produce soy milk, which is then coagulated, causing solid curds (the tofu) and liquid whey to form.

Tofu is white in color and bland in taste but readily picks up other flavors; it is therefore a great choice in mixed dishes such as lasagne. Tofu is available in many supermarkets, typically in the produce department. It is shaped in cakes of varying textures (soft, medium, or firm) and packed in water, which must be changed daily to keep it fresh.

Soft tofu is good to use in blenderized recipes to make dips, cream pies, spreads, puddings, and cream soups. Medium and firm tofu hold their shape better during preparation and cooking. Hard tofu is best for slicing, deep-fat frying, or crumbling. Regular and hard tofu can be used in casseroles, in Italian recipes to replace ricotta cheese, and in a variety of other dishes. Other soybean products are listed in Table 10-3.

Cereal grains are the fruits or seeds of cultivated grasses and include wheat, corn, rice, rye, barley, oats, millet, and sorghum. Buckwheat, although not a true cereal grain (it is not a member of the grass family), is considered to be one because of its grasslike structure. Cereal grains are made into hot and cold breakfast cereals, baking flours, starches used in thickening foods such as puddings and gravies, and dried pastes used to make pastas such as macaroni, spaghetti, and egg noodles.

Cereal grains are good sources of iron and B vitamins, particularly thiamin, riboflavin, and niacin. Whole grains that have not been milled or refined are also good sources of fiber and minerals. Cereal grains are discussed in more detail in Chapter 2.

Although nuts are high in fat, most of the fat is polyunsaturated or monounsaturated, with only small amounts of saturated fat. Nuts are also a good source of fiber.

Nuts and seeds are commonly used as snacks in the vegetarian diet, but also are used as toppings on cooked vegetables and grains and in baked goods, salads, casseroles, vegetarian loaves, and stuffing. Some are toasted lightly to bring out flavors. Nut and seed butters, such as peanut butter, can be used as spreads for sandwiches and crackers. Nuts and seeds play a minor role in menu planning for vegetarians as compared to legumes, grains, and vegetables, probably in part due to their high fat content (about 50 percent) and their relatively high cost.

Vegetarian Food Pyramid

The Food Guide Pyramid (Figure 7-1), when modified as described here, works well for vegetarians (Haddad, 1994).

The Food Guide Pyramid can be altered to suit different eating styles.

1. *Breads, cereals, rice, and pasta* (6–11 servings per day). This group stays the same. Whole-grain products are recommended. Vitamin B$_{12}$-fortified breakfast cereals are important for vegans. Some vegans with large calorie needs may eat more than 11 servings.
2. *Fruits* (2 or more servings). This group also stays the same except that no limit is placed on consumption.

TABLE 10-4.	**Good sources of vitamin B$_{12}$, vitamin D, calcium, iron and zinc.**
Vitamin B$_{12}$:	Dairy products, eggs, fortified cereals, and meat analogs
Vitamin D:	Fortified milk, eggs, fortified cereals, and soy milk
Calcium:	Milk and milk products, canned salmon and sardines (with bones), oysters, calcium-fortified juice or soy milk, broccoli, collards, kale, greens
Iron:	Liver, meats, breads and cereals, green leafy vegetables, legumes, dried fruits
Zinc:	Whole grains, legumes, nuts and seeds, peanut butter

3. *Vegetables* (3 or more servings).   Like fruits, no limit is placed on the number of servings.
4. *Meat substitutes* (2–3 servings).   This group obviously omits any meats, poultry, or fish and instead concentrates on substitutes such as cooked dry beans, peas, or lentils; tofu and other soybean products; nuts and seeds and butters made from them; meat analogs; and eggs for lacto-ovovegetarians. One serving is 1/2 cup of cooked beans, peas, or lentils; 4 ounces of tofu; 1/4 cup of shelled nuts; 1/8 cup of seeds; 2 tablespoons of peanut butter; or 1 egg. One serving of legumes should be served daily.
5. *Milk, cheese, and yogurt* (2 servings for adults, 3 servings for pregnant and lactating women, teenagers, and young adults up to age 24).   This group is enlarged to include soy milk fortified with calcium and vitamin D (and vitamin B$_{12}$ for vegans), and soy cheese fortified with calcium and vitamin D. One serving is 1 cup of fortified soy milk or 1½ ounces of soy cheese. One cup of cooked broccoli or greens can be substituted for 1 cup of milk. If a vegan does not drink soy milk or eat soy cheese, a carefully planned diet with sources of the missed nutrients, or supplements, is necessary.

Menu Planning Guidelines

1. *Variety is a key word to remember when planning vegetarian menu items.* Macaroni and cheese, pizza, and grilled cheese are fine to serve—

especially if made with vegetables too—but much more variety (and less fat and saturated fat) is needed.

2. *Use a variety of plant protein sources at each meal: legumes, grain products (preferably whole-grain), nuts and seeds, and/or vegetables.* Vegetarian entrees commonly use cereal grains such as rice or bulgur wheat (precooked and dried whole wheat) in combination with legumes and/or vegetables. Use small amounts of nuts and seeds in dishes.

3. *Use a wide variety of vegetables.* Steaming, stir-frying, or microwaving vegetables retains flavor, nutrients, and color.

4. *Offer entrees that are acceptable to lactovegetarians and lacto-ovovegetarians and an entree for vegans.* Although lactovegetarians and lacto-ovovegetarians will eat vegan entrees, vegans won't eat entrees with any dairy products or eggs.

5. *Choose low-fat and nonfat varieties of milk and milk products and limit the use of eggs.* This is important to prevent a high intake of saturated fat, found in whole milk, low-fat milk, regular cheeses, eggs, and other foods.

6. *Offer dishes made with soybean-based products, such as tofu and tempeh.* Soybeans are unique: They are the only plant protein that is nutritionally equivalent to animal protein.

7. *Provide foods that contain nutrients of special importance to vegetarians.* Table 10-4 lists good sources of vitamin B_{12}, vitamin D, calcium, iron, and zinc.

Breakfast menu ideas can be found in this chapter's "Food Facts." Figure 10-1 gives menu ideas for lunch and dinner.

MINI-SUMMARY Legumes, grains, nuts, and seeds are important foods for vegetarians. Vegetarians can still follow the Food Pyramid concept by concentrating on meat substitutes in the Meat/Meat Substitute group and adding fortified soy milk and soy cheeses to the dairy group. Menu-planning guidelines are given.

KEY TERMS

Lacto-ovovegetarian
Lactovegetarian
Legumes
Pescovegetarians
Pesticides
Tofu
Vegans

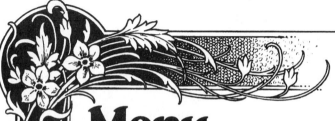

Menu

Vegetarian Menu Ideas

Sandwiches

Mexican Bean Sandwich
Garbanzo Bean Spread
Chili-Cheddar Spread
Tahini-Peanut Butter Spread
Tricolor Pepper Cream Cheese Spread
Egg Salad Supreme
Pita Veggie Pockets
Fruit and Cheese Pockets

Soups

Split Pea and Barley Soup
Classic Bean Soup
Bean and Corn Soup
Brown Rice & Black Bean Soup
Creamy Broccoli Soup
Eight-Vegetable Soup
Minestrone Soup
Potato Cheese Soup
Chilled Soups: Gazpacho and Fruit Soup

Salads

California Tossed Salad
Apple-Cabbage Slaw
Zucchini, Tomato, and Wheat Berry Slaw
Southwestern Bean Salad
Potato Vegetable Salad with Yogurt
Bulgur with Raisins and Apple Salad
Broccoli and White Bean Salad
Pineapple-Bulgur Wheat Salad
Four Bean Salad
Spinach and Mushroom Salad
Marinated Garden Vegetable Salad
Pasta Primavera Salad

Pastas

Cheesy Manicotti
Whole Wheat Pasta Primavera
Fusilli with Fresh Tomato Sauce
Four Vegetable Tortilla Lasagna
Pasta with Beans and Tomatoes
Stuffed Shells Florentine
Fettucine with Low-Fat Cheese Sauce

Entrees

Spinach and Cheese Calzones
Broiled Veggie Burger
Not-Sloppy Joes
Spicy Red Beans and Rice
Veggie Jambalaya
Four Bean Enchiladas
Tostadas
Eggplant Parmesan
Three Bean Casserole
Apple Mac-and-Cheese
Black Bean Chili
Vegetable Pot Pie
Stuffed Baked Potatoes
Vegetable Stir-Fry with Tofu
Veggie Stuffed Tomatoes
Spaghetti Squash Casserole
Curried Apple and Lentil Stew
Buttons & Bowties
Brown Rice Pilaf
Three Bean-Apple Bake
Boston Baked Beans
White Bean Casserole
Vegetable Confetti Rice
Fresh Vegetable Risotto

Side Dishes

Baked Squash
Tomato-Zucchini Casserole
Green Bean Casserole
Grilled Tomatoes
Apple-Yam Casserole
Creamed Spinach
Carrot-Apple Sauté
Sweet Potatoes with Pineapple
Honeyed Butternut Squash
Grilled Vegetable Kabobs

FIGURE 10-1. Vegetarian menu ideas

REVIEW QUESTIONS

1. Use the following chart to check the foods each type of vegetarian will eat.

	Fish	Eggs	Dairy	Fruit	Vegetable	Grains
Lacto-ovovegetarian						
Lactovegetarian						
Pescovegetarian						
Vegan						

2. List five possible health benefits of being vegetarian. Give other reasons why someone might decide to become vegetarian.
3. Is a vegetarian diet nutritionally adequate for adults? For growing children? If so, under what conditions? Give your answer for lacto-ovovegetarians and for vegans.
4. Name five legumes, five cereal grains, two nuts, and two seeds that may be a part of the vegetarian diet.
5. Draw a Food Pyramid for vegetarians that names each food group, gives three examples of foods for each group, and gives the recommended number of daily servings.
6. List the menu planning guidelines for vegetarian diets.

ACTIVITIES AND APPLICATIONS

1. Quiz

Check your answers with these.

1. False
2. False
3. True
4. True
5. True
6. False
7. False

2. Myth Busting

Explain why each of the following statements about vegetarians is a myth.

Vegetarians eat only vegetables.

Vegetarian recipes are always healthy.

Cheese is healthier to eat than meat.

No legumes have the high-quality protein that meat has.

3. Menu Planning

With the help of vegetarian cookbooks, trade publications such as *Restaurants USA* and *Restaurants & Institutions*, magazines such as *Vegetarian Times*, or the newspaper, suggest two vegetarian entrees and desserts for use at each of the following establishments: a casual-themed restaurant for younger people, a college cafeteria, and a dining room for bank personnel.

4. Cooking with Tofu

Experiment with tofu by using it in a recipe for soup, an Italian entree such as lasagna, or a dessert such as chocolate cream pie.

5. Vegetarian Interview

Interview a vegetarian and find out why he or she is a vegetarian, what type of vegetarian he or she is, and what types of foods he or she eats.

6. Vegetarian Meal

Plan a vegetarian meal for yourself and your classmates. Have each class member bring in something. Plan the meal so that there are items for both lacto-ovovegetarians and vegans. Use the menu-planning guidelines in deciding what foods to have.

REFERENCES

Akers, Keith. 1983. *A Vegetarian Source.* Arlington, VA: Vegetarian Press.

American Dietetic Association. 1993. Position of the American Dietetic Association: Vegetarian diets. *Journal of The American Dietetic Association* 93(11): 1317–1319.

Beilin, Lawrence J. 1994. Vegetarian and other complex diets, fats, fiber, and hypertension. *American Journal of Clinical Nutrition* 59 (Suppl.): 1130S–1135S.

Burke, Kenneth. 1995. The use of soy foods in a vegetarian diet. *Topics in Clinical Nutrition* 10(2): 37–43.

Clark, Amy Rosenbaum. 1994. 20 good reasons to be vegetarian. *Vegetarian Times* (Nov): 100–103.

Craig, Winston J. 1994. Iron status of vegetarians. *American Journal of Clinical Nutrition* 59 (Suppl.): 1233S–1237S.

Fisher, Marc, Peter H. Levine, Bonnie Weiner, Ira S. Ockene, Brian Johnson, Mark H. Johnson, Anita M. Natale, Christine H. Vaudreuil, and James Hoogasian. 1986. The effect of vegetarian diets on plasma lipid and platelet levels. *Archives of Internal Medicine* 146(6): 1193–1197.

Freeland-Graves, Jeanne H., Sue A. Greninger, Glenn R. Graves, and Robert K. Young. 1986. Health practices, attitudes, and beliefs of vegetarians. *Journal of The American Dietetic Association* 86(7): 913–918.

Freeland-Graves, Jeanne H., M. Lavone Ebangit, and Pamela W. Bodzy. 1980. Zinc and copper content of foods used in vegetarian diets. *Journal of The American Dietetic Association* 77(6): 648–654.

Gibson, Rosalind S. 1994. Content and bioavailability of trace elements in vegetarian diets. *American Journal of Clinical Nutrition* 59(Suppl.): 1223S–1232S.

Gussow, J. D. 1994. Ecology and vegetarian considerations: Does environmental responsibility demand the elimination of livestock? *American Journal of Clinical Nutrition* 59(Suppl.): 1110S–1116S.

Haddad, Ella H. 1994. Development of a vegetarian food guide. *American Journal of Clinical Nutrition* 59(Suppl.): 1248S–1254S.

Haddad, Ella H. 1995. Meeting the RDAs with a vegetarian diet. *Topics in Clinical Nutrition* 10(2): 7–16.

Hapgood, Fred. 1987. Soybean. *National Geographic* 72(1): 65–91.

Helman, Anthony D., and Ian Darnton-Hill. 1987. Vitamin and iron status in new vegetarians. *American Journal of Clinical Nutrition* 45(4): 785–789.

Hodgkin, Georgia. 1994. Osteoporosis and vegetarian diets. *Topics in Clinical Nutrition* 10(2): 34–36.

Janelle, K. Christina, and Susan I. Barr. 1995. Nutrient intakes and eating behavior scores of vegetarian and nonvegetarian women. *Journal of The American Dietetic Association* 95(2): 180–186, 189.

Johnston, Patricia K. 1995. Vegetarians among us: Implications for health professionals. *Topics in Clinical Nutrition* 10(2): 1–6.

Lappé, Frances Moore. 1982. *Diet for a Small Planet.* New York: Ballantine Books.

Lewis, Stephen. 1994. An opinion on the global impact of meat consumption. *American Journal of Clinical Nutrition* 59(Suppl.): 1099S–1102S.

Margetts, Barrie M., Lawrence J. Beilin, Robert Vandongen, and Bruce K. Armstrong. 1986. Vegetarian diet in mild hypertension: A randomised controlled trial. *British Medical Journal* 293(6560): 1468–1471.

McGruter, Patricia Gaddis. 1979. *The Great American Tofu Cookbook.* Brookline, MA: Autumn Press.

McNeill, Deborah A., Perveen S. Ali, and Young S. Song. 1985. Mineral analyses of vegetarian, health, and conventional foods: magnesium, zinc, copper and manganese content. *Journal of The American Dietetic Association* 85(5): 569–572.

Mills, P. K., W. L. Beeson, R. L. Phillips, and G. E. Fraser. 1994. Cancer incidence among California Seventh-Day Adventists, 1976–1982. *American Journal of Clinical Nutrition* 59(Suppl.): 1136S–1142S.

Robertson, Laurel, Carol Flinders, and Brian Ruppenthal. 1986. *The New Laurel's Kitchen*. Berkeley, CA: Ten Speed Press.

Sanders, T. A. B., and S. Reddy. 1994. Vegetarian diets and children. *American Journal of Clinical Nutrition* 59(Suppl.): 1176S–1181S.

Solomon, Jay. 1993. Robust vegetarian meals. *Restaurants USA* 13(9): 23–27.

Swarner, Julia. 1995. The vegetarian diet and cancer prevention. *Topics in Clinical Nutrition* 10(2): 17–21.

Walkup, Carolyn. 1995. Vegetarian menu items sprout at mainstream restaurants. *Nation's Restaurant News* (Dec. 11): 33.

Weaver, Connie M. and Karen L. Plawecki. 1994. Dietary calcium: Adequacy of a vegetarian diet. *American Journal of Clinical Nutrition* 59(Suppl.): 1238S–1241S.

Webster, Wendy A. 1994. Meatless menus win high marks on campus. *Restaurants USA* 14(6): 11–12.

Whitten, Crystal. 1995. Vegetarian diets and ischemic heart disease. *Topics in Clinical Nutrition* 10(2): 27–33.

Young, Vernon R. and Peter L. Pellett. 1994. Plant proteins in relation to human protein and amino acid nutrition. *American Journal of Clinical Nutrition* 59(Suppl.): 1203S–1212S.

Sources of Meat Analogs and Tofu Products

Legume (frozen tofu dinners)
P.O. Box 288
Caldwell, NJ 07006
(201)882-9190

Loma Linda Foods
11503 Pierce Street
Riverside, CA 92515
(714)687-7800

Morningstar Farms
Worthington Foods, Inc.
Worthington, OH 43085
(614)885-9511

Food Facts: Vegetarian Breakfast Possibilities

Cereals

Cereals are made from grains, the most popular being wheat, corn, oats, and rice. Ready-to-eat cereals are made by grinding the grain into a paste, forming it into desired shapes, and toasting it to make flakes, puffs, and other familiar forms.

The huge variety of cereals on the market can make choosing one confusing, so keep in mind these helpful tips.

1. Choose whole-grain cereals. Examples of whole grains to look for on cereal labels include:
   - Whole wheat
   - Whole oats or rolled oats
   - Whole corn
   - Brown rice
   - Whole barley

   Whole grains have more copper, potassium, and magnesium.

2. Choose a cereal with at least 4 grams of fiber per serving. The National Cancer Institute recommends 20 to 30 grams of fiber each day.

3. Choose a cereal with 5 grams or less of added sugar per serving. In presweetened cereals, sugar replaces other more valuable nutrients such as starch and fiber. Instead of buying presweetened cereals, make cereal naturally sweet with fresh, canned, or dried fruit.

4. If you like granola or muesli (granola's untoasted European counterpart), choose a brand that is labeled "low-fat". Granola-type cereals are made with much more fat than other ready-to-eat cereals. Low-fat versions of some granola cereals are now available. Choose one with 3 grams or less of fat per serving.

Breakfast cereals are perfect candidates for a wide variety of toppings. Toppings not only add flavor and texture but can provide important nutrients. Use one or more of these suggestions to give your morning cereal a little variety, and maybe a big crunch!

- Dried fruit such as raisins
- Cut-up fresh fruit such as sliced bananas or sliced peaches
- Canned fruit such as fruit cocktail or crushed pineapple
- Wheat germ
- Chopped nuts
- Small seeds such as sunflower seeds
- Shredded coconut

Some additional toppings work especially well on hot cereal.

- Low-fat or nonfat yogurt
- Low-fat or nonfat cottage cheese
- Buttermilk, low-fat milk or skim milk
- Fruit sauce
- Fruit spread
- A pinch of cinnamon or nutmeg or 1 tablespoon of brown sugar, honey, or maple syrup

Breakfast Breads and Spreads

When buying or making breakfast breads, keep in mind the following tips.

1. Choose whole-grain breads. For more nutrients and fiber, pick up (or make) one of these whole-grain breads.

- 100% whole-wheat bread
- Stone ground whole-wheat bread
- Cracked wheat bread
- Whole-wheat pita bread
- Corn tortillas
- Oatmeal bread
- Whole-wheat English muffins
- Whole-wheat bagels

Although you may think that breads labeled *multigrain, rye,* or *pumpernickel* are made from whole grains, most contain little whole-grain flour. If white or wheat flour is the first ingredient on these products (the first ingredient is always the major ingredient), the bread contains little whole-grain flour.

2. Choose in moderation those breads that are high in fat. Most yeast breads are low in fat (about 2 grams of fat per slice). Some breads and bread products are made with quite a bit more fat. These include croissants, brioche, cheese bread, cornbread, popovers, and many biscuits. Most of these breads can be made at home with much less fat.

3. Choose muffins with 5 grams or less of fat per medium muffin. If you are baking your own muffins or other quick breads such as banana bread, choose recipes that have 5 grams or less of fat per serving.

Let your bread become the foundation of a nutritious breakfast by topping it with one or more of the following.

- Peanut butter (Peanut butter contains much fat but is a good source of protein and other nutrients. For less fat, mix equal amounts of peanut butter and mashed bananas, or use reduced-fat peanut butter.)
- Sesame butter mixed with honey
- Apple butter or strawberry butter (Despite their names, these spreads contain no fat.)
- Fruit spread
- Yogurt or cottage cheese
- Cheese, preferably reduced in fat.
- Tomato sauce and grated cheese (Make a breakfast pizza!)

Although margarine and butter are popular spreads, they provide only fat. Butter is especially high in saturated fats. Cream cheese is also high in fat but provides a small amount of protein. Choose margarine, butter, and cream cheese in moderation or choose reduced-fat brands.

Flapjacks

Flapjacks (better known as pancakes), French toast, and waffles can be the basis of a healthy breakfast. Whether you like to make your own or microwave frozen versions for a speedy breakfast, choose one (or more) of the following toppings for a super breakfast.

- Nonfat sour cream and berries
- Fruit butters
- Fruit sauce
- Pureed fruit (Use the blender or food processor and process fruit until smooth.)
- Sliced fresh fruit and powdered sugar
- Real maple syrup
- Nut butters (peanut butter, almond butter)
- Honey and raisins
- Mashed banana and honey
- Yogurt or ricotta cheese with sliced fruit

If you like to make your own pancakes or French toast but don't have time in the morning, you can prepare the pancake batter or soak the bread the night before and cook them in the morning. You can also prepare them in advance and reheat them in the morning. If you like fruited pancakes, soak fresh apple rings in the pancake batter overnight.

Yummy Yogurt

Although yogurt is an ancient food, it has become popular in the United States only during the past 20 years. Yogurt is a good source of protein, calcium, and vitamin B$_{12}$. Whole-milk yogurt contains the same amount of fat per cup as one cup of whole milk (about 8 grams). Yogurt made from low-fat milk contains between 0.5 and 2 grams of fat, and nonfat yogurt contains only a trace of fat.

Some toppings for plain yogurt include:

- Any fresh, canned, or chopped dried fruit
- Any fruit sauce or fruit spread
- Chopped nuts or seeds
- Wheat germ
- Granola
- A pinch of nutmeg or cinnamon or a dash of vanilla extract to develop flavor

If you don't have enough time to top your own yogurt, check out the yogurt section at the supermarket to find some yogurts that come with their own topping.

Shake It Up!

If you like to drink your breakfast, try a blender breakfast. The perfect recipe for a breakfast shake includes one or more liquid ingredients, solid ingredients, and flavorings.

Liquid Ingredients	Solid Ingredients	Flavorings
Skim or low-fat milk	Fresh fruit	Honey
Fruit juice or nectar	Canned fruit	Maple syrup
Nonfat low-fat yogurt	Wheat germ	Vanilla extract

To complete your breakfast, include a serving from the bread, cereal, rice, or pasta group.

Sunny Side Up

Eggs are very nutritious and full of high-quality protein, vitamins, and minerals. The current concern with overconsumption of eggs stems from the fact that they are high in cholesterol—213 milligrams per egg (compare that to the 300-milligram suggested daily maximum). One egg also contributes 5 grams of fat, of which 1.5 grams are saturated fat. Egg consumption should be limited to 4 per week.

Eggs can be cooked in many ways: baked, hard cooked or soft cooked (in the shell), poached, fried, or scrambled. When making fried eggs, scrambled eggs, or omelets, you can reduce the amount of fat by spraying nonstick frypans with vegetable-oil cooking sprays. To further reduce fat scrambled eggs and omelets, use one whole egg and substitute two egg whites for each additional egg. Egg whites contain no fat or cholesterol (it's all in the yolk).

Leftovers Revisited

If you are one of those people who like cold pizza for breakfast, this tip's for you! Leftovers from previous lunch or dinner meals are perfect breakfast candidates. Just reheat, if desired, in the microwave and enjoy. For example, try rice pudding or custard for breakfast. Or if you have a leftover baked potato in the refrigerator, cut it into thin slices and stuff into a pita pocket along with sliced tomatoes and cheese. Then warm up to eat!

CHAPTER 11

Nutrition and Health

QUIZ

1. The following diseases are the four leading causes of death in the United States. Number them from the most prevalent to the least prevalent.
   Stroke
   Heart disease
   Diabetes
   Cancer

2. The three most important heart disease risk factors that you can do something about are smoking, elevated blood cholesterol, and high blood pressure.   *True   False*

3. Phytochemicals found in foods help high blood pressure.   *True   False*

4. Diabetes is caused by eating too much sugar.   *True   False*

5. More people are now surviving cancer.   *True   False*

6. The most effective dietary method to lower your blood cholesterol level is by eating less cholesterol.   *True   False*

7. Heart disease is the number 2 killer of women in the United States.   *True   False*

8. Physical inactivity is related to heart disease.   *True   False*

9. Blood pressure increases with age and obesity.   *True   False*

10. People with diabetes are more vulnerable to many kinds of infections and to deterioration of the kidneys, heart, blood vessels, nerves, and vision.   *True   False*

KEY QUESTIONS

1. What are the four leading causes of death in the United States? Does diet play a role in the prevention and treatment of each of them?

2. What is cardiovascular disease and what forms does it take? What are the risk factors for cardiovascular diseases?

3. What causes heart attacks and strokes?

4. What is the Step I Diet? When is it used?

5. Why is blood pressure the silent killer?

6. What lifestyle modifications are necessary to lower blood pressure?

7. What are key points in planning menus for people with cardiovascular diseases?

8. How does cancer start?

9. What are the key components of an anticancer diet?

10. What are the two forms of diabetes and the principles of diabetic diets?

INTRODUCTION

According to *The Surgeon General's Report on Nutrition and Health* (1988), approximately 2.1 million people die every year in the United States. This includes 500,000 deaths from coronary heart disease, 150,000 from stroke, and 475,000 from cancer. Overall, over 1 million Americans die each year of diet-related diseases—at tremendous expense to society in direct health-care expenditures and lost productivity. Add to this cost the yearly cost for diabetes and osteoporosis and the dollars go still higher.

This chapter discusses the four leading causes of death in the United States: coronary artery disease, cancer, stroke, and diabetes (in order from 1 to 4). All these medical problems have one element in common: diet. Prevention and treatment of all of these diseases have a dietary component. Let us first look at heart attacks and stroke, then move on to cancer and diabetes.

The four leading causes of death in the U.S., in order, are: coronary artery disease, cancer, stroke, and diabetes.

NUTRITION AND CARDIOVASCULAR DISEASE

According to current estimates, about one in four Americans have one or more forms of **cardiovascular disease (CVD)**. Cardiovascular disease is a general term for diseases of the heart and blood vessels as seen in the following.

- Coronary artery disease
- Stroke
- High blood pressure
- Rheumatic heart disease
- Congenital heart defects

About 40 percent of all deaths in 1992 were attributable to cardiovascular diseases.

Smoking, high blood pressure, and high blood cholesterol are three major **risk factors** for cardiovascular disease. A risk factor is a habit, trait, or condition associated with an increased chance of developing a disease. Preventing or controlling risk factors generally reduces the probability of illness. These three risk factors are modifiable to some extent. Other risk factors are obesity, age (CVD increases with age), a family history of premature CVD (heart attack in a father before age 55 or before 65 in a mother), and diabetes.

Major risk factors for CVD are: smoking, high blood pressure, high blood cholesterol.

The two medical conditions that lead to most cardiovascular disease are atherosclerosis and high blood pressure. Let's take a look at atherosclerosis first. **Atherosclerosis**, a condition characterized by plaque

Atherosclerosis and high blood pressure contribute to CVD.

Plaque starts to build up in the arteries during childhood.

buildup along the artery walls, is the most common form of artery disease. (*Arteriosclerosis* is a general medical term that includes all diseases of the arteries involving hardening and blocking of the blood vessels.) Atherosclerosis affects primarily the larger arteries of the body. In this condition, arterial linings become thickened and irregular with deposits called **plaque**. Plaque contains cholesterol, fat, fibrous scar tissue, calcium, and other biological debris. Why plaque deposits are formed and what role fat and cholesterol play in its formation are questions with only partial answers.

Atherosclerosis develops by a process that is totally silent. At birth the blood vessels are clear and smooth. As time goes on, plaque builds up, resulting in narrower passages and less elasticity in the vessel wall, both of which contribute to high blood pressure (Figure 11-1). What's even more dangerous is when the plaque closes off blood flow completely, or the rough plaque surface provides a place for a blood clot to form and block blood passage in a partially closed artery. If the artery takes blood to the brain, then a stroke occurs. If the closed artery is in the heart, then a heart attack occurs, the next topic.

Coronary Heart Disease

The heart is like a pump, squeezing and forcing blood throughout the body. Like all muscles in the body, the heart must have oxygen and nutrients in order to do its work. The heart cannot use oxygen and nutrients directly from the blood within the chambers of the heart. Instead, nutrients and oxygen are furnished by three main blood vessels outside the heart, referred to as coronary arteries. **Coronary heart disease (CHD)** is a broad term used to describe damage to or malfunction of the heart caused by narrowing or blockage of the coronary arteries.

More than two-thirds of a coronary artery may be filled with fatty deposits without causing symptoms. Symptoms may manifest themselves as chest pain as in **angina** or as a heart attack. Angina refers to the symptoms of pressing, intense pain in the area of the heart because the heart muscle does not get enough blood. Sometimes stress or exertion can cause angina.

Most heart attacks are caused by a clot in a coronary artery at the site of narrowing and hardening that stops the flow of blood. Clots normally form and dissolve in response to injuries in the blood vessels, but in atherosclerosis blood clots appear to form in response to plaque when they are not needed. If an area of the heart is supplied by more than one vessel, the heart muscle may live for a period of time even if one vessel becomes blocked. The extent of heart muscle damage after a heart attack depends on which vessel is blocked, whether it is big or small, and on the

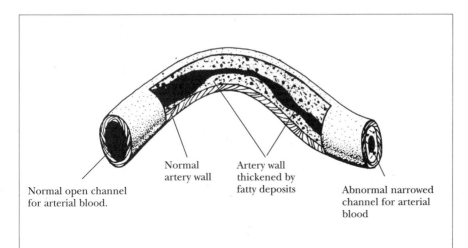

FIGURE 11-1.

Cross-sectional
representaion of
a coronary artery
partially closed
with plaque

Normal artery wall

Artery wall
thickened by
fatty deposits

Normal open channel
for arterial blood.

Abnormal narrowed
channel for arterial
blood

remaining blood supply to that area. When heart muscle does not get adequate oxygen and nutrients, it may die—this is what a heart attack actually is. A further area of heart muscle may be deprived of blood flow and oxygen to a lesser degree, causing a temporary injury called **myocardial ischemia**. This dead or injured heart muscle causes the heart to lose some of its effectiveness as a pump because reduced muscle contraction means reduced blood flow.

Coronary heart disease is the number one killer of women. Every year, just as many women as men die from coronary heart disease. Whereas heart attacks are seen in men 40 years of age and older, women do not usually experience heart attacks until after menopause.

During a heart attack, part of the heart muscle does not have enough oxygen or nutrients to do its job properly.

MINI-SUMMARY Cardiovascular disease includes diseases of the heart such as coronary artery disease. Major risk factors include smoking, high blood pressure, and high blood cholesterol. Atherosclerosis is characterized by plaque build-up on arterial walls, which can eventually close off blood circulation.

Nutrition and Coronary Heart Disease

Much research over the past 40 years has linked dietary intake of saturated fat and cholesterol to the development of CHD (American Heart Association, 1990). In response, national organizations such as the National Heart, Lung and Blood Institute and the American Dietetic Association, have recommended diets lower in fat, saturated fat, and cholesterol. In particular, reducing saturated fat intake significantly reduces CHD incidence and its associated costs (Oster and Thompson, 1996).

Cholesterol is carried in the blood in the form of substances called *lipoproteins.* CHD risk can be assessed by measuring total blood cholesterol as well as the proportions of the various types of lipoproteins. Total cholesterol refers to the overall level of cholesterol in the blood. High-density lipoprotein (HDL) is often referred to as "good" cholesterol, beause high levels of HDL are associated with lowered CHD risk. High levels of low-density lipoprotein (LDL)—often referred to as "bad" cholesterol—and very low density lipoprotein (VLDL) increase CHD risk.

The National Cholesterol Education Program (NCEP) recommends that all adults age 20 and older have their total cholesterol and HDL measured at least once every five years. For people without CHD, a total blood cholesterol level of less than 200 mg/dL is considered desirable; from 200 to 239 is borderline high; and 240 or more is high. An HDL level of less than 35 mg/dL is defined as low and is considered a CHD risk factor.

Lipoprotein analysis, which measures LDL as well as HDL, is recommended for people with CHD or for those at very high risk of developing CHD. The optimum LDL for patients with CHD is 100 mg/dL or lower. The optimum LDL for high-risk individuals is about 130 mg/dL.

The Step I Diet is suitable for anyone: 30 percent or less of calories from fat, 8 to 10 percent of calories from saturated fat, and less than 300 mg of cholesterol daily.

Dietary therapy is the mainstay of treatment of high blood cholesterol at every age. Unless a young adult (a man under age 35 or a premenopausal woman) is at very high risk of CHD with a total cholesterol of more than 300 mg/dL, the NCEP recommends that drug therapy be delayed and dietary modification and lifestyle change be attempted first.

Dietary therapy is prescribed in two steps, called the Step I and Step II Diets. These are designed to help reduce saturated fat and cholesterol intake, and to help achieve a desirable weight by eliminating excess calories. The Step I Diet is usually the starting point of dietary therapy. In the Step I Diet, no more than 8 to 10 perent of calories are in the form of saturated fat, 30 percent or less of calories come from total fat, and less than 300 mg of cholesterol are allowed each day.

If the patient is already following the Step I Diet and cholesterol continues to be above to desirable levels, then the Step II Diet should be instituted, according the NCEP report. People with high cholesterol who have CHD or other atherosclerotic disease should begin this diet immediately, with physician guidance. The Step II Diet calls for reducing daily saturated fat intake to less than 7 percent of calories and cholesterol to less than 200 mg.

Drug treatment is considered appropriate for adults who have a very high LDL level, especially if they also have other CHD risk factors (Table 11-1). The goals of drug therapy are the same as those of dietary therapy:

TABLE 11-1. Treatment decisions based on LDL cholesterol.

Dietary Therapy

	Initial Level	LDL Goal
Without CHD and with fewer than 2 risk factors	≥160 mg/dL	<160 mg/dL
Without CHD and with 2 or more risk factors	≥130 mg/dL	<130 mg/dL
With CHD	>100 mg/dL	≤100 mg/dL

Drug Treatment

	Consideration Level	LDL Goal
Without CHD and with fewer than 2 risk factors	≥190 mg/dL*	<160 mg/dL
Without CHD and with 2 or more risk factors	≥160 mg/dL	<130 mg/dL
With CHD	≥130 mg/dL**	≤100 mg/dL

*In men under 35 years of age and premenopausal women with LDL-cholesterol levels 190-219 mg/dL, drug therapy should be delayed except in high-risk patients such as those with diabetes.
**In CHD patients with LDL-cholesterol levels 100–129 mg/dL, the physician should exercise clinical judgment in deciding whether to initiate drug treatment.

Source: National Institutes of Health. 1993. *Second Report of the Expert Panel on Detection, Evaluation, and Treatment of High Blood Cholesterol in Adults.* NIH Publication No. 93-3096.

to lower LDL cholesterol to below 160 mg/dL or 130 mg/dL if two other risk factors are present.

MINI-SUMMARY The National Cholesterol Education Program recommends that all adults age 20 and older have their total cholesterol and HDL measured at least once every five years. For people without CHD, a total blood cholesterol level of less than 200 mg/dL is considered desirable; from 200 to 239 is borderline high; and 240 or more is high. An HDL level of less than 35 mg/dL is defined as low and is considered a CHD risk factor. An LDL level of 160 mg/dL is desirable. Table 11-1 shows the point at which dietary and drug treatment are suggested. On the Step I Diet, no more than 8 to 10 percent of calories from saturated fat, 30 percent or less of calories from total fat, and less than 300 mg of cholesterol are allowed. The Step II Diet calls for reducing saturated fat to less than 7 percent of calories and cholesterol to less than 200 mg.

Stroke

A **stroke** is damage to brain cells resulting from an interruption of the blood flow to the brain. The brain must have a continual supply of blood rich in oxygen and nutrients for energy. Although the brain constitutes only 2 percent of the body's weight, it uses about 25 percent of the oxygen and almost 75 percent of the glucose circulating in the blood. Unlike

Atherosclerosis contributes to many strokes.

other organs, the brain cannot store energy. If deprived of blood for more than a few minutes, brain cells die from energy loss and from certain chemical interactions that are set in motion. The functions these cells control—speech, muscle movement, comprehension—die with them. Dead brain cells cannot be revived.

The majority of strokes are caused by blockages in the arteries that supply blood to the brain. These blockages may be caused by a clot that forms on the inner lining of a brain or neck artery already partly clogged by plaque. The most serious kinds of stroke occur not from blockage but from hemorrhage, when a spot in a brain artery weakened by disease— usually atherosclerosis or high blood pressure—ruptures or begins to leak blood. If an artery inside the brain ruptures, it is called a **cerebral hemorrhage**. Hemorrhagic strokes account for less than 20 percent of all types of strokes but are far more lethal, with a death rate of over 50 percent. Strokes caused by clots or hemorrhage usually strike suddenly, with little or no warning, and do all their damage in a matter of seconds or minutes.

Because blood clots play a major role in causing strokes, drugs that inhibit blood coagulation may prevent clot formation. Physicians have several drugs at their disposal—including aspirin—to treat those at risk. Aspirin works by preventing blood platelets from sticking together. Controlling blood pressure is also important.

Most people who have had mild strokes, and about half of those who have had moderate or severe paralysis on one side, recover enough to walk out of the hospital under their own steam or with some mechanical aid and resume their lives, though with certain limitations. Others are not so lucky.

MINI-SUMMARY The majority of strokes are caused by blockages in the arteries that supply blood to the brain. Another type of stroke is called a hemorrhagic stroke, or cerebral hemorrhage.

High Blood Pressure

The medical name for high blood pressure is hypertension.

As many as 50 million Americans have high blood pressure (also called **hypertension**) or are taking antihypertensive medications. Because high blood pressure usually doesn't give early warning signs, it is known as the "silent killer." High blood pressure is one of the major risk factors for coronary heart disease and stroke. All stages of hypertension are associated with increased risk of nonfatal and fatal cerebrovascular disease and renal disease.

Arterial blood pressure is the pressure of blood within arteries as it's pumped through the body by the heart. Whether your blood pressure is

TABLE 11-2. **Classification of blood pressure for adults age 18 and older.***

Category	Systolic mm Hg	Diastolic mm Hg
Normal	<130	<85
High normal	130–139	85–89
Hypertension**		
STAGE 1 (Mild)	140–159	90–99
STAGE 2 (Moderate)	160–179	100–109
STAGE 3 (Severe)	180–209	110–119
STAGE 4 (Very Severe)	$\geq$210	$\geq$120

*Not taking antihypertensive drugs and not acutely ill. When systolic and diastolic pressure fall into different categories, the higher category should be selected to classify the individual's blood pressure status.
**Based on the average of two or more readings taken at each of two or more visits following an initial screening.

Source: National Institutes of Health and National Heart, Lung, and Blood Institute. 1994. *The Fifth Report of the Joint National Committee on Detection, Evaluation, and Treatment of High Blood Pressure.* NIH Publication No. 93-1088.

high, low, or normal depends mainly on several factors: the output from your heart, the resistance to blood flow by your blood vessels, the volume of your blood, and blood distribution to the various organs.

Everyone experiences hourly and even moment-by-moment blood-pressure changes. For example, your blood pressure will temporarily rise with strong emotions such as anger and frustration, with water retention caused by too much salty food that day, and with heavy exertion, which makes your heart beat harder and faster, increasing its output by pushing more blood into your arteries. These transient elevations in blood pressure usually don't indicate disease or abnormality.

Blood pressure is represented as a fraction, as in $\frac{120}{80}$. The top number, 120, is called the **systolic pressure**—the pressure of blood within arteries when the heart is pumping. The bottom number, 80, is called the **diastolic pressure**—the pressure in the arteries when the heart is resting between beats. Both blood pressure numbers are measured in millimeters of mercury, abbreviated mm Hg.

Normal blood pressure varies from person to person. High blood pressure occurs when the blood pressure stays too high and is defined as systolic pressure greater than 140 mm Hg and/or a diastolic pressure greater than or equal to 90 mm Hg or both. Table 11-2 classifies blood pressure readings for adults. Even though hypertension starts with a systolic reading of 140 or higher, and/or a diastolic reading of 90 or higher, optimal blood pressure is about 120/80. People with high normal pressure account for more than one-third of preventable deaths related to blood pressure.

When persistently elevated blood pressure is due to a medical problem, such as hormonal abnormality or an inherited narrowing of the aorta (the largest artery leading from the heart), it is called **secondary hypertension**. That is, the high blood pressure arises secondary to another condition. Only 5 percent of individuals with hypertension have secondary hypertension. The remaining 95 percent have what is called **primary**, or **essential**, **hypertension**. The cause of essential hypertension is unknown.

The cause of essential hypertension is not understood.

The prevalence of high blood pressure increases with age, is greater for blacks than for whites, and in both races is greater in less educated than more educated people. It is especially prevalent and devastating in lower socioeconomic groups. In young adulthood and early middle age, high blood pressure prevalence is greater for men than for women; thereafter, the reverse is true.

The following lifestyle modifications offer some hope for prevention of hypertension and are effective in lowering the blood pressure of many people who follow them (Table 11-3).

- Weight reduction
- Increased physical activity
- Moderation of dietary sodium
- Moderation of alcohol intake

These lifestyle modifications can also reduce other risk factors for premature cardiovascular disease. Their ability to reduce death and disease in those with elevated blood pressure has not been conclusively documented. However, because of their ability to improve the cardiovascular risk profile, they offer many benefits at little cost and with minimal risk.

Excess body weight is correlated closely with increased blood pressure. Weight reduction reduces blood pressure in a large proportion of hypertensive individuals who are more than 10 percent above ideal weight.

Excessive alcohol intake can raise blood pressure and cause resistance to antihypertensive therapy. Hypertensive patients who drink alcohol-containing beverages should be counseled to limit their daily intake to 1 ounce of ethanol (2 ounces of 100-proof whiskey), 8 ounces of wine, or 24 ounces of beer).

TABLE 11-3. Lifestyle modifications for hypertension control and/or overall cardiovascular risk.

- Lose weight if overweight.
- Limit alcohol intake to no more than 1 ounce of ethanol per day (24 ounces of beer, 8 ounces of wine, or 2 ounces of 100-proof whiskey).
- Exercise (aerobic) regularly.
- Reduce sodium intake to less than 2.3 grams per day.
- Maintain adequate dietary potassium, calcium, and magnesium intake.
- Stop smoking and reduce dietary saturated fat and cholesterol intake for overall cardiovascular health. Reducing fat intake also helps reduce caloric intake—important for control of weight and Type II diabetes.

Source: National Institutes of Health and National Heart, Lung, and Blood Institutes. 1994. *The Fifth Report of the Joint National Committee on Detection, Evaluation, and Treatment of High Blood Pressure.* NIH Publication No. 93–1088.

Regular aerobic physical activity, adequate to achieve at least a moderate level of physical fitness, may be beneficial both for prevention and treatment of hypertension. Sedentary and unfit individuals with normal blood pressure have a 20 to 50 percent increased risk of developing hypertension during followup when compared with their more active and fit peers.

Research documents a reduction of blood pressure in response to reduced sodium intake. Individuals vary in their blood pressure response to changes in dietary sodium chloride. Blacks, older people, and patients with hypertension are more sensitive to changes in dietary sodium chloride. Because the average American consumption of sodium is in excess of 3 grams of sodium per day, a level of less than 2.3 grams of sodium per day is recommended.

Reduced sodium intake usually reduces blood pressure.

A high dietary potassium intake may protect against developing hypertension, and potassium deficiency may increase blood pressure. Therefore, normal blood levels of potassium should be maintained, preferably from food sources.

In many but not all studies, calcium deficiency is associated with an increased prevalance of hypertension, and a low calcium intake may increase the effects of a high sodium intake on blood pressure. An increased calcium intake may lower blood pressure in some patients with hypertension. There is currently no rationale for recommending calcium intakes in excess of the recommended daily allowance to lower blood pressure (National Institutes of Health and National Heart, Lung, and Blood Institute, 1994).

When lifestyle modifications do not succeed in lowering blood pressure enough, drugs are the next step. Reducing blood pressure with drugs clearly decreases the incidence of cardiovascular death and disease. Two classes of antihypertensive drugs—diuretics and beta-blockers—are preferred for initial drug therapy.

MINI-SUMMARY High blood pressure occurs when the blood pressure stays too high and is defined as systolic pressure greater than 140 mm Hg and/or a diastolic pressure greater than or equal to 90 mm Hg or both. Table 11-2 classifies blood pressure readings for adults. Table 11-3 lists the components of lifestyle modifications that can lower blood pressure. If they do not bring blood pressure down enough, drug treatment is the next choice.

Menu Planning for Cardiovascular Diseases

Menu planning for cardiovascular diseases revolves around offering dishes rich in complex carbohydrates and fiber and using small amounts of fat, saturated fat, cholesterol, and sodium.

GENERAL RECOMMENDATIONS
- Decrease or replace salt in recipes by using vegetables, herbs, spices, and flavorings.
- Offer salt-free seasoning blends (see Table 11-3) and lemon wedges.

BREAKFAST
- Offer fresh and canned fruits and juices.
- Almost all cold and hot cereals are great choices. Granola cereals tend to be high in fat unless labeled as reduced fat.
- Most breads are low in fat except for croissants, brioche, cheese breads, and many biscuits. Bagels, low-fat muffins, and baguettes are good choices.
- Have reduced-fat margarine and light cream cheese available to spread on bagels or toast.
- Serve chicken filets, poultry sausages, low-fat ham slices, or fish as leaner sources of protein than the traditional bacon and pork sausage.
- Offer egg substitutes for scrambled eggs and other egg-based items. Egg substitutes taste better when herbs, flavorings, and/or vegetables are cooked with them. Instead of egg substitutes, you can offer to make scrambled eggs and omelets by mixing one whole egg to two egg whites.

- Serve an omelet with blanched vegetables such as chopped broccoli or spinach and low-fat cheese instead of regular cheese.
- As a spread or topping on pancakes and waffles, offer sauces combining low-fat or nonfat yogurt with a fruit puree.
- Serve a breakfast buffet with loads of fruits, low-fat dairy products, and cereals.

APPETIZERS AND SOUPS

- Offer juices and fresh sliced fruits. Fresh sliced fruits can be served with a yogurt dressing flavored with fruit juices.
- Offer raw vegetables with dips using low-fat yogurt, low-fat cottage cheese, or ricotta cheese as the base, rather than dips using sour cream, cheeses, cream, or cream cheese. Try hummus, a chickpea-based dip, or salsa made from tomatoes, onions, hot peppers, garlic, and herbs.
- Offer grilled chicken, broiled Buffalo-style chicken wings, or steamed seafood such as shrimp.
- Dish up baked (rather than fried) potato skins and baked corn tortillas for tortilla chips. Sprinkle with grated cheese, garlic, onion, or chili powder.
- Feature soups that use stock as the base and vegetables and grains as the ingredients. Dried beans, peas, and lentils make great soups when cooked and pureed, without using cream or high-fat thickeners such as roux.

SALADS

- Offer salads with lots of vegetables and fruits.
- Use only small amounts, if any, of bacon, meat, cheese, eggs, or croutons. Choose cooked beans and peas or low-fat cheeses.
- Offer reduced-calorie or non-fat salad dressings. Place on the side when desired.
- Make tuna fish salad and other similar salads with low-fat mayonnaise.
- Use cooked salad dressing that contains little fat for Waldorf and other salads. It has a tarter flavor than mayonnaise.

BREADS

- Most breads are low in fat and saturated fat. Breads with more fat include biscuits, cheese breads, croissants, popovers, brioche, corn bread, and many commercial crackers (although low-fat varieties are available or can be made with less fat).

ENTREES

- Serve combination dishes with small amounts of meat, poultry, or seafood with whole grains such as rice, legumes, vegetables, and/or fruits.
- Offer moderate portions of broiled, baked, stir-fried, or poached seafood, white-meat poultry without skin, and lean cuts of meat (see Table 12-2).
- Offer fresh meat, poultry, or seafood instead of canned, cured, smoked or salty meat, poultry, or seafood (such as ham, corned beef, smoked turkey, dried cod, and most luncheon meats). Cheeses are high in sodium, so use small amounts in sandwiches.
- Feature freshly made entrees instead of processed or prepared foods.
- Offer a hamburger, meat loaf, or other ground beef dishes made with low-fat ground beef.
- Feature one or more meatless entrees, such as vegetarian burgers. Vegetarian burgers either try to imitate beef burgers (usually through the use of soy products) or are real veggie burgers (made of vegetables, especially mushrooms).
- For sauced entrees (or side dishes), feature sauces thickened with flour, cornstarch, or vegetable purees. Salsas, chutneys, relishes, and coulis also work well.
- Offer sandwiches made with roasted turkey, chicken, water-pack tuna fish salad, lean roast beef made from the round, or a spicy bean or lentil spread.
- For sandwich spreads, use reduced-calorie mayonnaise, French or Russian-style salad dressing, mustard, ketchup, barbecue sauce, or salsa.
- Feature lots of different vegetables in sandwiches.
- Instead of high-sodium accompaniments to sandwiches such as pickles, olives, and potato chips, serve fresh vegetables, cole slaw made with reduced-calorie mayonnaise, or another healthful salad.

SIDE DISHES

- Most side dishes of vegetables, grains, and pasta are good choices as long as little fat is added during preparation.
- Serve grilled potato halves instead of French fries, as well as other grilled vegetables.

DESSERTS

- Offer fruit-based desserts such as apple cobbler.
- Spotlight sorbets, sherbets, frozen yogurt, and ice milk. All contain less fat than ice cream.

- Feature desserts made from fat-free egg whites such as angel food cake and meringues. Serve with a fruit sauce.
- Offer puddings made with skim milk.
- Serve low-fat cookies such as ladyfingers, biscotti, gingerbread, and fruit bars.

BEVERAGES
- Offer 1% or skim milk.

MINI-SUMMARY Menu planning for cardiovascular diseases revolves around offering dishes rich in complex carbohydrates and fiber and using small amounts of fat, saturated fat, cholesterol, and sodium.

NUTRITION AND CANCER

Following heart disease, **cancer** is the second leading cause of death in the United States. The good news about cancer is that people being treated for cancer are living longer. The bad news is that more of it is being diagnosed, but there is no evidence of a cancer epidemic. The most prevalent form of cancer is skin cancer, which is quite curable when treated early. More than 90 percent of skin cancers are completely cured. The most frequent malignant cancer found in women is breast cancer.

Cancer is a group of diseases characterized by unrestrained cell division and growth that can disrupt the normal functioning of an organ and spread beyond the tissue in which it started. Figure 11-2 is a diagram of this process. Cancer is basically a two-step process. First, a **carcinogen**, such as an x-ray, starts or initiates the sequence by altering the genetic material of a cell, the deoxyribonucleic acid (DNA), and causing a mutation. Such cells are generally repaired or replaced. When repair or replacement does not occur, however, **promoters** such as alcohol can advance the development of the mutated cell into a tumor. Promoters do not initiate cancer but enhance its development once initiation has occured. The tumor may disrupt normal body functions and leave the tissue for other sites, a process called **metastasis**.

Cancer is a two-step process: initiation and promotion.

Cancer develops as a result of interactions between environmental factors (such as diet, smoking, alcohol, and radiation) and genetic factors. Research suggests that diet plays a role in the cause of certain cancers. In 1989, the National Academy of Sciences report, *Diet and Health: Implications for Reducing Chronic Disease Risk,* stated that in countries with better diets, cancer rates are about half that of the United States. For example, breast cancer rates are four to seven times higher in the United

About one-third of all cancers is caused by diet: too much fat, too little fiber, and too few fruits and vegetables.

States than in Asia. This difference is not explained by genetics, because when Asian women move to the United States their risk doubles after 10 years. Estimates of how much cancer is caused by diet varies. In 1986, a National Cancer Institute report estimated that about 35 percent of all cancer deaths are associated with the typical American diet, which is high in fat and calories and low in fiber, fruits, and vegetables. The most common cancers are cancer of the lungs, breast, colon and rectum, prostate, bladder, and skin. Of these cancers, all but one (skin cancer) is associated with diet.

So what characteristics of the American diet seem to enhance certain types of cancer? Basically our diet has: too much fat, too much saturated fat, too little fiber, and too few fruits and vegetables. The National Cancer Institute estimates that significant reductions in cancer incidence could be achieved by the year 2000 if all Americans adopted and maintained a low-fat, high-fiber, and high fruit and vegetable diet. The National Cancer Institute estimates that the following reductions in cancer incidence could be achieved by dietary changes.

- 50% reduction in colon and rectal cancer
- 25% reduction in breast cancer
- 15% reduction in cancers of the prostate, endometrium, and gallbladder
- Possible reductions in cancers of the stomach, esophagus, pancreas, ovaries, liver, lung, and bladder.

Let's take a look at why some of these dietary changes are recommended.

- Although dietary fat does not initiate cancer, it promotes its development once started. It may be that certain forms of fat promote cancer more than others. Monounsaturated fatty acids (found in olive oil) and omega-3 fatty acids (found in fatty fish) may be protective, whereas linoleic acid, an omega-6 fatty acid found in many vegetable oils, may be a promoter.
- Fiber may help prevent certain cancers, such as cancers of the colon and rectum, by:
  - Reducing the length of time for feces formation and elimination and therefore decreasing the time the bowel is exposed to potential carcinogens.
  - Retaining water in the intestinal tract, increasing stool bulk, which may dilute carcinogenic concentrations in the colon.
  - Binding with bile acids in the intestinal tract, some of which can be converted by colonic organisms into cancer-causing compounds.

Hot Topic: Carotenoids and Disease Prevention

Until 1994, research on beta carotene (the most abundant of the carotenoids) consistently showed that it could reduce cancer risk and possibly heart disease risk too. Studies revealed a lower risk of cancer in people who ate a diet rich in beta-carotene foods such as broccoli. Even smokers eating beta-carotene fruits and vegetables seemed to be at less risk for lung cancer.

Then studies were done on human subjects that took beta carotene in supplement form rather than in foods. This time, the results changed. In a research study of 30,000 male smokers in Finland, those who received beta-carotene supplements actually had a higher risk of lung cancer. Then, another major research study of mostly smokers and ex-smokers (called the CARET for Beta Carotene and Retinol Efficacy Trial)

was called off before it was completed. It seems that the smokers taking both beta carotene and vitamin A supplements had a 28 percent increase in the number of lung cancers over the smokers not getting the supplements. In a third research study, the twelve-year Physicians' Health Study, 22,000 men (89 percent nonsmokers) took beta carotene supplements. The supplements didn't harm the subjects, but did not provide any cancer-prevention benefits either.

So what can be said about beta carotene and health? Eat your fruits and vegetables. There are no doubt substances in them that decrease cancer risk, or it might be that fruits and vegetables often replace fats in your diet. Also, avoid beta carotene supplements with more than the RDA. Even if they don't hurt, they don't seem to help either.

- Fruits and vegetables help reduce the risk of cancer because they are rich sources of carotenoids, vitamin C, and fiber. Beta-carotene, the most abundant carotenoid, may inhibit the initiation and promotion of cancers because it is a powerful antioxidant. Antioxidants combine with oxygen, so oxygen is not available to oxidize, or destroy, important substances. Antioxidants prevent the oxidation of unsaturated fatty acids in the cell membrane, DNA (the genetic code), and other cell parts that substances called free radicals try to destroy. In the absence of antioxidants, free radicals may destroy cells (possibly accelerating the aging process) and alter DNA (possibly increasing the risk for cancerous cells to develop). Free radicals are produced in the body through normal metabolism or as a result of exposure to cigarette smoke, radiation, ultraviolet light, air pollutants, some pesticides, or alcohol.

Beta-carotene, vitamin C, and vitamin E are antioxidants that may protect against cancer.

Vitamin C also acts as an antioxidant by preventing the oxidation of certain chemicals, such as nitrosamines, to active carcinogens. Nitrates and nitrites are used in the curing of cold cuts, frankfurters, bacon, and other cured meats. Nitrates can be converted to nitrites by bacteria in the mouth or gastrointestinal tract. Nitrites can then be converted into nitrosamines in the mouth, stomach, and colon. Vitamin C inhibits nitrosamine formation in the gastrointestinal tract.

- Some vegetables, as well as other plant foods (such as fruits, grains, herbs, and spices), contain **phytochemicals**, minute plant compounds that fight cancer formation. For instance, broccoli contains the chemical sulforaphane, which seems to initiate increased production of cancer-fighting enzymes in the cells. Isoflavonoids, found mostly in soy foods, are known as plant estrogens or phytoestrogens because they are similar to estrogen and interfere with its actions (estrogen seems to promote breast tumors). Members of the cabbage family (cabbage, broccoli, cauliflower, mustard greens, kale) also called **cruciferous vegetables**, contain phytochemicals such as indoles and dithiolthiones. They activate enzymes that destroy carcinogens.

- Fruits and vegetables are also low in fat (with the exceptions of coconut, avocados, and olives).

Some consumers are concerned about eating more fruits and vegetables that may contain carcinogenic pesticides. The National Academy of Sciences, along with other organizations, feel that the health benefits of eating fresh fruits and vegetables far outweigh any risk associated with pesticide residues. The federal government strictly regulates the kinds and amounts of pesticides used on field crops. The tiny amounts of pesticide residues found on produce are set hundreds of times lower than the amounts that would actually pose any health threat.

MINI-SUMMARY   Cancer begins as depicted in Figure 11-2. The components of the American diet that raise our cancer risk include too much fat, too much saturated fat, too little fiber, and too few fruits and vegetables. Dietary fat is probably a promoter of cancer. Fiber, fruits, and vegetables lower cancer risk. Beta-carotene and vitamin C in fruits and vegetables act as antioxidants. Some fruits and vegetables also contain phytochemicals thought to fight the formation of cancer.

Menu Planning to Lower Cancer Risk

In the long run, prevention of cancer, and therefore eating a healthy diet, will play the major role in its control. Use the following guidelines to plan menus to lower cancer risk.

1. Offer lower-fat menu items. See Chapters 3 and 12 for tips on lowering fat and saturated fat. Also offer more plant-based menu items.

2. Avoid salt-cured, smoked, and nitrite-cured foods. These foods, which are also high in fat, include anchovies, bacon, corned beef, dried chipped beef, herring, pastrami, processed lunch meats such as bologna and hot dogs, sausage such as salami and pepperoni, and smoked meats and cheeses. Conventionally smoked meats and fish contain tars that are thought to be carcinogenic due to the smoking process. Nitrites are known carcinogens.

3. Offer high-fiber foods. For example:
   - Use beans and peas as the basis for entrees, and add them to soups, stews, casseroles, and salads. Nuts and seeds are high in fiber but also contain a significant amount of fat and calories, so use them sparingly.
   - Serve whole-grain breads, rolls, crackers, cereals, and muffins. Bran or wheat germ can be added to some baked goods to increase the fiber content.
     High-fiber grains such as brown rice and bulgur (cracked wheat) can be used as side dishes instead of white rice.
   - Leave skins on potatoes, fruits, and vegetables as much as possible.
   - Offer salads using lots of fresh fruits and vegetables. Omit shredded cheese, chopped eggs, and bacon bits, all of which contribute fat.

4. Include lots of vegetables, especially cruciferous vegetables. Cruciferous vegetables contain substances that are natural anti-carcinogens. These vegetables include broccoli, brussels sprouts, cabbage, cauliflower, bok choy, kale, collards, kohlrabi, mustard, rutabagas, spinach, and watercress.

5. Offer foods that are good sources of beta-carotene and vitamins C and E. Excellent sources of beta-carotene include dark green, yellow, and orange vegetables and fruits such as broccoli, cantaloupe, carrots, spinach, squash, and sweet potatoes. Good sources include apricots, beet greens, brussels sprouts, cabbage, nectarines, peaches, tomatoes, and watermelon. Excellent sources of vitamin C include citrus fruits and juices, any other juices with vitamin C added, strawberries, tomatoes, and broccoli. Good vitamin C sources include berries, brussels sprouts, cabbage, melons, cauliflower, and potatoes. Vitamin E is found in vegetable oils and margarines, whole-grain cereals, wheat germ, soybeans, leafy greens, and spinach.

Eat Five A Day is a national campaign to get Americans to eat five fruits and vegetables each day (see page 224 for more information).

6. Offer alternatives to alcoholic drinks. Heavy drinkers are more likely to develop cancer in the gastrointestinal tract, such as cancer of the esophagus and stomach. Chapter 15 presents nonalcoholic alternatives.

MINI-SUMMARY The keys to menu planning are lower-fat foods; foods that have not been salt-cured, nitrite-cured, or smoked; high-fiber foods, lots of fruits and vegetables including cruciferous vegetables, and nonalcoholic drinks for heavy drinkers.

NUTRITION AND DIABETES MELLITUS

Diabetes mellitus gets its name from the ancient Greek word for siphon (tube), because early physicians noted that diabetics tend to be unusually thirsty and to urinate a lot, as if a tube quickly drained out everything they drank. *Mellitus* is from the Latin version of the ancient Greek word for honey, used because doctors in centuries past diagnosed the disease by the sweet taste of the patient's urine.

Diabetes is a disease in which there is insufficient or ineffective **insulin**, a hormone that helps regulate blood sugar level. When the blood sugar is above normal, such as after eating a meal, the pancreas releases insulin. The insulin facilitates the entry of glucose into body cells to be used for energy. If there is no insulin or the insulin is not working, sugar cannot enter the cells. Thus high blood sugar levels (called **hyperglycemia**) result and sugar spills into the urine.

About 13 million Americans are diabetic—about 6 percent of the entire population. The life expectancy for a diabetic is only two-thirds that of the non-diabetic, and diabetes is the fourth leading cause of death. Risk factors for the most common type of diabetes include advanced age, family history, obesity, high waist-to-hip ratio, and a high fat/low carbohydrate diet.

Diabetics are more vulnerable to many kinds of infections and to deterioration of the kidneys, heart, blood vessels, nerves, and vision. The National Institutes of Health estimates that more than 250,000 Americans a year die from the complications of this illness, largely because it doubles their chances of having heart attacks and strokes. In addition, diabetes is the nation's leading cause of kidney failure and adult blindness. Because of the damage diabetes can do to the blood vessels and nerves of the lower limbs, only accidents necessitate more amputations of the toes, feet, and legs.

There are two types of diabetes.

1. **Type I (Insulin-dependent diabetes mellitus).**   This form of diabetes is seen mostly in children and adolescents. These patients produce no insulin at all and therefore require frequent insulin injections to maintain a normal level of blood glucose. Fewer than 10 percent of Americans who have diabetes have Type I.

2. **Type II (Noninsulin-dependent diabetes mellitus).**   This form of diabetes is a separate disease from Type I. Patients are usually older and obesity is common; in fact, 80 percent of patients weigh 20 percent or more than they should. In Type II, the person's beta cells do, in fact, produce insulin and may make too much. The problem here is that the patient's tissues aren't sensitive enough to the hormone and so use it inefficiently. Some of these patients require insulin but many do not. Treatment is with diet, weight reduction when appropriate, exercise, and if necessary, oral hypoglycemic agents (medications taken by mouth that can stimulate the release of insulin and improve the body's sensitivity to insulin). Most diabetics fall into this category.

Although both types of diabetes are popularly called "sugar diabetes," they are not caused by eating too many sweets. High sugar levels in the blood and urine are a result of these illnesses; their exact causes are unknown. What is clear is that Type II runs in families far more often than Type I does, and—unlike Type I, which cannot be prevented—can frequently be avoided by staying in shape.

Diabetes is not caused by eating too much sugar.

Symptoms of Type I diabetes typically appear abruptly and include excessive, frequent urination, insatiable hunger, and unquenchable thirst. Unexplained weight loss is also common, as are blurred vision (or other vision changes), nausea and vomiting, weakness, drowsiness, and extreme fatigue.

Type I diabetes can't be prevented.

The most immediate and life-threatening aspect of Type I diabetes is the formation of poisonous acids called *ketone bodies*. They occur as an end-product of burning fat for energy because glucose does not get into the cells to be burned for energy. Like glucose, ketone bodies accumulate in the blood and spill into the urine.

Symptoms of Type II diabetes may include any or all of those of Type I, but they are often overlooked because they tend to come on gradually and be less pronounced. Other symptoms are tingling or numbness in the lower legs, feet or hands, skin or genital itching, and gum, skin or bladder infections that recur and are slow to clear up. Again, many people fail to connect them with possible diabetes.

Measuring glucose levels in samples of the patient's blood is key to diagnosing both types of diabetes. This is first done early in the morning on an empty stomach. For more information, the blood test is repeated, usually on another day, before the patient has drunk a liquid containing a known amount of glucose and at intervals thereafter.

Treatment for either type seeks to do what the human body normally does naturally: maintain a proper balance between glucose and insulin. The guiding principle is that food makes the blood glucose level rise, whereas insulin and exercise make it fall. The trick is to juggle the three factors to avoid both hyperglycemia (a blood glucose level that is too high) and hypoglycemia (one that is too low). Either condition causes problems for the patient.

Having diabetes means having to juggle your diet, exercise, and medication to keep your blood glucose within normal limits.

The cornerstone of treatment is diet, exercise, and medication. The exact nature of the diabetic diet has changed over the years from starvation diets to more liberal diets. The current diabetic diet is based on the following principles.

- There is no one diet suitable for every diabetic. The diet needs to be individualized based on each person's type of diabetes, food preferences, culture, age, lifestyle, medication, other health concerns, education, nutrition status, medical treatment goals, and other factors.

- The goals for meal planning are to maintain the best glucose control possible, keep blood levels of fat and cholesterol in normal ranges, maintain or get body weight within a desirable range, and meet all nutrient needs.

- Sugar need not be avoided, because sucrose and other sugars do not impair blood sugar control any more than starchy foods do. Sugars can be incorporated into the diabetic diet as part of the total carbohydrate allowance. The total amount of carbohydrate consumed, rather than the source of carbohydrate, should be the priority. Because sugars appear in foods that usually contain a lot of calories and fat, sweets can be eaten occasionally.

- Instead of setting rigid percentages of protein, fat, and carbohydrates, the new guidelines recommend that protein make up 10 to 20 percent of calories consumed. Saturated fat and polyunsaturated fat should be maintained at less than 10 percent each. The remaining 60 to 70 percent of calories should come from carbohydrates and monounsaturated fats. Caloric distribution depends on the individual's nutritional assessment and treatment goals.

Mini-Summary   There are two classifications of diabetes: Type I (insulin-dependent) seen mostly in children, and Type II (non-insulin-dependent) seen mostly in overweight older adults. The life expectancy for a diabetic is only two-thirds that of the non-diabetic, and diabetes is the fourth leading cause of death. Diabetics are more vulnerable to many kinds of infections and to deterioration of the kidneys, heart, blood vessels, nerves, and vision. The cornerstone of treatment is diet, exercise, and medication. Diets are individualized for each person. Sugar need not be avoided but can be incorporated into the diabetic diet as part of the total carbohdyrate allowance.

Using the Diabetic Exchanges

The **Exchange Lists for Meal Planning** have been developed by the American Diabetes and American Dietetic Associations for use primarily by diabetics who need to regulate what and how much they eat (see Appendix D). There are seven exchange lists of like foods. Each food on a list has approximately the same amount of calories, carbohydrate, fat, and protein as another in the portions listed, so any food on a list can be exchanged, or traded, for any other food on the same list. The seven exchange lists are starch, fruit, milk, other carbohydrates, vegetables, meat and meat substitutes, and fat. Diabetics can exchange starch, fruit, or milk choices within their meal plans because they all have about the same amount of carbohydrate per serving. A patient works with the dietitian to determine an appropriate meal plan that sets up how many exchanges of each food group can be eaten at each meal and snack.

The exchange lists are also helpful for people wanting to lose weight.

Each exchange list has a typical, easy-to-remember item of a specific portion size:

Starch: 1 slice of bread, 80 calories
Meat: 1 ounce of lean meat, 55 calories
Vegetable: 1/2 cup of cooked vegetable, 25 calories
Fruit: 1 small apple, 60 calories
Milk: 1 cup of skim milk, 90 calories
Fat: 1 teaspoon of margarine, 45 calories

The meat exchange is broken down into very lean, lean, medium-fat, and high-fat meat and meat alternates. Very lean and lean meats are encouraged. The milk exchange contains skim, low-fat, and whole milk exchanges. Fats are divided into three groups, based on the main type of fat they contain: monounsaturated, polyunsaturated, and saturated. There is also a listing of free foods that contain negligible calories.

MINI-SUMMARY By using the exchange lists and a meal plan worked out with a dietitian, a diabetic can plan enjoyable, healthy meals.

<table>
<tr><td colspan="2">**KEY TERMS**</td></tr>
</table>

KEY TERMS

Angina	Hypertension
Arterial blood pressure	Insulin
Atherosclerosis	Myocardial ischemia
Cancer	Plaque
Carcinogen	Phytochemical
Cardiovascular disease (CVD)	Promoter
Cerebral hemorrhage	Risk factors
Coronary heart disease (CHD)	Secondary hypertension
Cruciferous vegetables	Stroke
Diabetes mellitus	Systolic pressure
Diastolic pressure	Type I (insulin-dependent)
Essential (primary) hypertension	diabetes mellitus
Exchange Lists for Meal Planning	Type II (noninsulin-dependent)
Hyperglycemia	diabetes mellitus

REVIEW QUESTIONS

In your own words, answer the following questions.

1. What are the four leading causes of death in the United States?
2. What do the four leading causes of death have in common?
3. List five forms of cardiovascular disease.
4. Name major and minor risk factors for cardiovascular disease.
5. What is atherosclerosis, and what forms of heart disease does it contribute to?
6. What is plaque made of?
7. Discuss briefly two forms of coronary heart disease.
8. What are desirable numbers of total blood cholesterol, LDL, and HDL?
9. What is the difference between a Step I and a Step II Diet? When is each used?
10. Define stroke and compare the two types of strokes discussed.
11. Why is hypertension a silent killer?
12. What does 120/80 mean? Is it optimal?
13. Explain the difference between primary and secondary hypertension.
14. List six lifestyle modifications for controlling high blood pressure.
15. Describe the relationship between sodium and blood pressure.
16. If lifestyle modifications do not lower blood pressure as much as needed, what is the next step?

17. What are the principles of menu planning for cardiovascular diseases?
18. Describe how cancer starts, including possible carcinogens and possible promoters.
19. What dietary changes can be made to reduce cancer risk?
20. Why is the life expenctancy for a diabetic only two-thirds that of a non-diabetic?
21. Compare the two types of diabetes.
22. Why isn't there one diet for all diabetics?
23. Why can diabetics eat sugar?
24. Explain how a diabetic uses the exchange lists.

ACTIVITIES AND APPLICATIONS

1. *Quiz*

Check your answers with the following.

1. Stroke   3
   Heart disease 1
   Diabetes   4
   Cancer   2
2. True
3. False
4. False
5. True
6. False
7. False
8. True
9. True
10. True

2. *A Diet for Disease Prevention*

You have read about several diseases and the dietary means for preventing and treating each one. Using this information, write what you would consider to be an ideal diet for disease prevention. Focus on different groups of foods and what role each would play (and why) in disease prevention.

REFERENCES

American Diabetes Association. 1994. Nutrition recommendations and principles for people with diabetes mellitus. *Diabetes Care* 17(5): 519–522.

American Heart Association. 1990. The cholesterol facts. A summary of the evidence relating dietary fats, serum cholesterol, and coronary heart disease. A joint statement by the American Heart Association and the National Heart, Lung, and Blood Institute. *Circulation.* 81: 1721–1733.

Augustin, Joi, and Johanna Dwyer. 1994. Coronary heart disease: Dietary approaches to reducing risks. *Topics in Clinical Nutrition* 10(1): 1–13.

Bal, Dileep G., and Susan B. Foerster. 1993. Dietary strategies for cancer prevention. *Cancer* 72(Suppl. 3): 1005–1010.

Clifford, Carolyn, and Barnett Kramer. 1993. Diet as risk and therapy for cancer. *Medical Clinics of North America* 77(4): 725–744.

Carroll, K. K. 1991. Dietary fats and cancer. *American Journal of Clinical Nutrition* 53: 10645–10675.

Diabetes Care and Education, A Practice Group of the American Dietetic Association; Tinker, L. F., Heins, J. M., and Holler, H. J. Commentary and translation: 1994 nutrition recommendations for diabetes.

Franz, M. J., E. S. Horton, J. P. Bantle, C. A. Beebe, J. D. Brunzell, A. M. Coulston, R. R. Henry, B. J. Hoogwerf, and P. W. Stacpoole. 1994. Nutrition principles for the management of diabetes and related complications. *Diabetes Care* 17(5): 490–518.

Hankin, Jean H. 1993. Role of nutrition in women's health: Diet and breast cancer. *Journal of The American Dietetic Association* 93(9): 994–999.

Hennekens, C. H. 1994. Antioxidant vitamins and cancer. *American Journal of Medicine* 97(3A): 25–45.

Levey, Wendy A., Melinda M. Manore, Linda A. Vaughan, Steven S. Carroll, Laurel Van Halderen, and James Felicetta. 1995. Blood pressure responses of white men with hypertension to two low-sodium metabolic diets with different levels of dietary calcium. *Journal of The American Dietetic Association* 95(11): 1280–1287.

Lipid Research Clinics Program. 1984. The Lipid Research Clinics Coronary Primary Prevention Trial results, I. Reduction in incidence of coronary heart disease. *Journal of the American Medical Association* 251(3): 351–364.

Lipid Research Clinics Program. 1984. The Lipid Research Clinics Coronary Primary Prevention Trial results, II. The relationship of reduction in incidence of coronary heart disease to cholesterol lowering. *Journal of the American Medical Association* 251(3): 365–374.

Lyon, Rachel B., and Debra M. Vinci. 1993. Nutrition management of insulin-dependent diabetes mellitus in adults: Review by the Diabetes Care and Education dietetic practice group. *Journal of The American Dietetic Association* 93: 309–314, 317.

National Institutes of Health. 1993. *Second Report of the Expert Panel on Detection, Evaluation, and Treatment of High Blood Cholesterol in Adults.* NIH Publication No. 93–3096.

National Institutes of Health. 1994. *So You Have High Blood Cholesterol.* NIH Publication No. 93–2922.

National Institutes of Health and National Heart, Lung, and Blood Institute. 1994. *The Fifth Report of the Joint National Committee on Detection, Evaluation, and Treatment of High Blood Pressure.* NIH Publication No. 93–1088.

Oster, Gerry, and David Thompson. 1996. Estimated effects of reducing dietary saturated fat intake on the incidence and costs of coronary heart disease in the United States. *Journal of The American Dietetic Association* 96(2): 127–131.

Tinker, Lesley Fels. 1994. Diabetes mellitus—A priority health care issue for women. *Journal of The American Dietetic Association* 94(9): 976–985.

U.S. Department of Health and Human Services. 1988. *The Surgeon General's Report on Nutrition and Health.* Washington DC: U.S. Government Printing Office.

Food Facts: Choosing Oils and Margarines

When choosing vegetable oils, choose those high in monounsaturated fats, such as olive oil, canola oil, peanut oil, and other nut oils. Olive oil is the best choice because it is 73 to 77 percent monounsatuated fat.

The color of olive oil varies from pale yellow to green and its flavor varies from sweet to a full, fruity taste. The color and flavor of olive oil depend on the olive variety, level of ripeness, and processing method. When buying olive oil, look for these terms on the label.

1. *Extra virgin* and *virgin olive oil* have a strong olive taste that is good for flavoring finished dishes and in salad dressings, but they tend to burn when cooked.
2. *Pure olive oil* can be used for sautéing and in salad oils. It is not as strong in taste as extra virgin or virgin olive oil.
3. *Light* or *extra-light olive oil* refers only to color or taste. These olive oils lack the color and much of the flavor found in the other products. Light olive oil is good for sautéing, deep frying, or baking because the oil is used mainly to transfer heat rather than enhance flavor.

Polyunsaturated fats, such as corn oil, safflower oil, sunflower oil, and soybean oil, are also good choices, but not as good as monounsaturated fats. Polyunsaturated fats and monounsaturated fats both lower LDL levels (the bad cholesterol) in the body, but polyunsaturated fat also lowers HDL (the good cholesterol that you want plenty of). Monounsaturated fats, such as olive oil, do not seem to affect the HDL levels.

Vegetable oil is also available in a convenient spray form that can be used as a nonstick spray coating for cooking and baking with a minimal amount of fat. Vegetable oil cooking sprays come in a variety of flavors (butter, olive, Oriental, Italian, mesquite), and a quick two-second spray adds about 1 gram of fat to the product. To use, spray the pan first away from any open flames (the spray is flammable), heat up the pan, then add the food.

Tables 11-4 and 11-5 give information on various oils. Be prepared to spend more money for the more exotic oils, such as almond, hazelnut, sesame, and walnut oils. Because these oils tend to be cold pressed (meaning they are processed without heat), they are not as stable as the all-purpose oils and should be purchased in small quantities (they are strong, so you don't need to use much of them). Don't purchase these oils to cook with—they burn easily.

Margarine was first made in France in the late 1800s to provide an economical fat for Napoleon's army. It didn't become popular in the United States until World War II, when it was introduced as a low-cost replacement for butter. Margarine must contain vegetable oil and water and/or milk or milk solids. Flavorings, coloring, salt, emulsifiers, preservatives, and vitamins are usually added. The mixture is heated and blended, then firmed by exposure to hydrogen gas at very high temperatures, a process known as hydrogenation (see page 106). The firmer the margarine, the greater the degree of hydrogenation and the longer its shelf life.

TABLE 11-4. **Vegetable oils.**

Oil	Characteristics/Uses	Oil	Characteristics/Uses
Canola oil	Light yellow color Bland flavor Good for frying, sautéing, and in baked goods Good oil for salad dressings	Peanut oil	Pale yellow color Mild nutty flavor Good for frying and sautéing Good oil for salad dressings
Corn oil	Golden color Mild flavor Good for frying, sautéing, and in baked goods Too heavy for salad dressings	Safflower oil	Golden color Bland flavor Has a higher concentration of polyunsaturated fatty acids than any other oil Good for frying, sautéing, and in baked goods Good oil for salad dressings
Cottonseed oil	Pale yellow color Bland flavor Good for frying, sautéing, and in baked goods Good oil for salad dressings	Sesame oil	Light gold flavor Distinctive, strong flavor Good for sautéing Good for flavoring dishes and in salad dressings Use in small amounts Expensive
Hazelnut oil	Dark amber color Nutty and smoky flavor Not for frying or sautéing as it burns easily Good for flavoring finished dishes and salad dressings Use in small amounts Expensive	Soybean oil	More soybean oil is produced than any other type, used in most blended vegetable oils and margarines Light color Bland flavor Good for frying, sautéing, and in baked goods Good oil for salad dressings
Olive oil	Varies from pale yellow with sweet flavor to greenish color and fuller flavor to full, fruity taste (color and flavor depend on olive variety, level of ripeness, and how they were processed) Extra virgin or virgin olive oil—do not cook with it because it burns, good for flavoring finished dishes and in salad dressings, strong olive taste Pure olive oil—can be used for sautéing and in salad oils, not as strong an olive taste as extra virgin or virgin	Sunflower oil	Pale golden color Bland flavor Good for frying, sautéing, and in baked goods Good oil for salad dressings
		Walnut oil	Medium yellow to brown color Rich, nutty flavor For flavoring finished dishes and in salad dressings Use in small amounts Expensive

				Grams	Grams
Fat or Oil	Calories/ Tablespoon	Grams Fat/ Tablespoon	Grams Saturated Fat/Tablespoon	Monounsaturated Fat/Tablespoon	Polyunsaturated Fat/Tablespoon
Coconut oil	120	14	12	1	0
Palm kernel oil	120	14	11	2	0
Palm oil	120	14	7	5	1
Butter, stick	108	12	8	4	0
Lard	115	13	5	6	1
Cottonseed oil	120	14	4	2	7
Olive oil	119	14	2	10	1
Canola oil	120	14	1	8	4
Peanut oil	119	14	2	6	4
Safflower oil	120	14	1	2	10
Corn oil	120	14	2	3	8
Soybean oil	120	14	2	3	8
Sunflower oil	120	14	1	6	6
Shortening	106	12	3	6	3
Margarine, stick	102	11	2	5	4
Margarine, soft tub	102	11	2	4	5
Margarine, liquid	102	11	2	3	6
Margarine, whipped	70	7	2	2	3
Margarine spread	78	9	1	5	3
Margarine diet	51	6	1	2	2
Margarine fat-free	0	0	0	0	0

TABLE 11-5. Total calories and fat in selected fats and oils.

Source: U.S. Department of Agriculture and manufacturers.

Like butter, margarine is at least 80 percent fat and is fortified with vitamin A. Butter is made from cream and milk. They both supply the same amount of fat, but margarine's fat is much higher in polyunsaturates than butter, which is high in saturates. Butter also contains much cholesterol.

There are a variety of margarines available.

- Stick margarine. These are made by hydrogenating plant oils and adding water, milk solids, flavoring, and coloring to make a product similar to butter.

- Soft tub margarine. These contain more polyunsaturated fatty acids than stick margarines, so they melt at lower temperatures and are easier to spread.

- Whipped margarine. These are stick margarines that have been whipped. They contain more air and therefore fewer calories per tablespoon (don't substitute for regular butter or margarine in recipes— they contain a lot of air and water).

- Liquid margarine. These are packaged in squeeze bottles in which the margarine is truly liquid, even in the refrigerator.
- Margarine spread. These are soft margarines with water, gums, gelatins, and various starches added. They contain less than 80 percent fat by weight so they are classified as spreads.
- Light margarine. More water is added to this product, which contains about 40 to 60 percent fat.
- Diet margarine. This product has about 45 percent fat and therefore more air and water than margarine spreads and light margarine. It contains half to one-third the fat of regular margarine. Also called reduced–calorie margarine.
- Fat-free margarine. If you are wondering how they make a margarine fat free, here's the answer: gelatin. Gelatin is what is used in Promise Ultra Fat Free and Promise Extra Light margarines. Rice starch is also used in the fat-free version.

In addition to margarines and spreads, you will also find blends and butter-flavored buds at the supermarket. Blends are part margarine and part butter (about 15 to 40 percent). They are made of vegetable oil, milk fat, and other dairy ingredients added to make the product taste like butter. Blends may have as much fat as regular margarine or butter (in other words, at least 80 percent fat) or they may be reduced in fat, like spreads. Butter-flavored buds are made from carbohydrates and a small amount of dehydrated butter. They are virtually fat-free and cholesterol-free. They are designed to melt on hot, moist foods such as a baked potato. They can also be mixed with water to make butter-flavored sauces.

Here are some tips for buying margarine.

- Read the margarine label for calories, calories from fat, and fat grams, and compare labels of different products.
- If the margarine you choose has water as the first ingredient, don't use it for cooking or baking; it won't produce the same results as regular margarine.
- Avoid margarines in which the first ingredient is a hydrogenated or partially hydrogenated fat.
- Pick a margarine that meets your needs in terms of fat and taste.
- For the least amount of trans fats, choose diet tub margarine. Trans fats are unsaturated fats created during the process in which liquid oils are made solid into margarines. Because they raise blood cholesterol levels, intake should be limited.

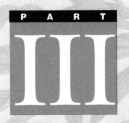

PART
III

Nutrition in
Restaurants
and
Foodservices

CHAPTER 12

Nutrition and Menu Planning

1. What percentage of diners are looking for healthy menu selections when eating out?
2. How are healthy menus developed, and what considerations should be kept in mind?
3. What menu items would you consider for each area of your menu to meet any one or more of the following nutrition objectives: lower in fat, saturated fat and cholesterol; lower in refined sugar; lower in sodium; or higher in complex carbohydrates?

QUIZ

Quiz

1. What percentage of diners choose health and nutrition when they eat out?
   a. 10 percent
   b. 25 percent
   c. 33 percent
   d. 50 percent
2. To develop a healthy menu, you could
   a. use existing menu items that are healthy
   b. modify existing menu items
   c. develop new recipes
   d. all of the above
3. Taste is the key to customer acceptance and the successful marketing of healthy menu items.   *True   False*
4. Most appetizers and soups are low in refined sugar.   *True   False*
5. Which would be a good low-fat dip for vegetables?
   a. sour cream with chives
   b. cheddar cheese dip
   c. salsa
   d. none of the above
6. A low-fat cookie could include
   a. gingerbread
   b. ladyfingers
   c. fruit bars
   d. all of the above
7. The following breads are healthy choices for sandwiches *except*
   a. whole-wheat bread
   b. croissant
   c. pita bread
   d. Italian bread

8. An entree high in complex carbohydrates is
   a. lentil burritos
   b. low-fat meat loaf stuffed with spinach and cheese
   c. tuna salad with tomato in a pita pocket
   d. cheese omelet
9. Which menu category contains the most sugar?
   a. entrees
   b. side dishes
   c. desserts
   d. appetizers
10. Which of the following sandwich condiments is high in sodium?
    a. pickles
    b. olives
    c. chips
    d. all of the above

INTRODUCTION

Every year, more and more Americans see the importance of good nutrition, especially as it relates to health (Morreale and Schwartz, 1995). Nutrition is no longer considered a trend—a fad that is here today and gone tomorrow. However, whereas more Americans recognize the importance of nutrition, they tend to make food choices based on taste, which means they often choose less-than-healthy foods.

For example, in the 1993 Survey of American Dietary Habits, 82 percent of Americans reported that nutrition was at least moderately important, yet only about half that number said they were doing all they could to eat healthfully. In other words, Americans are ambivalent about their beliefs or attitudes (that nutrition is important) and their behaviors (such as eating too few fruits and vegetables, eating too many calories, and so on).

American's nutrition ambivalence is evident to many chefs and food-service managers who have prepared tasty, nutritious meals in response to customers' requests only to see these wonderful dishes not sell up to expectations. Despite the lukewarm response, most quick-service restaurants and about half of table-service restaurants do offer nutritious choices. A 1988 survey by the National Restaurant Association showed that almost all table-service restaurants surveyed will alter preparation methods on request, serve sauces or salad dressings on the side, cook without salt, and cook with vegetable oil or margarine instead of butter or shortening. As the editorial board of *Nation's Restaurant News* stated in 1995:

Restaurants at virtually every price level and of almost every type have made at least token nods to the low-fat trend.

In a survey of non-commercial foodservices, 76 percent of operators reported building healthier menus and 49 percent reported expanding their low-fat dessert choices (Murray, 1996).

National Restaurant Association research shows that about a third of diners are choosing health and nutrition when they eat out. Americans eat out about three to four times each week, for breakfast, lunch, or dinner (National Restaurant Association, 1994). If you consider that half of all adults are foodservice customers each day, that's plenty of grilled chicken sandwiches and salads!

THE HEALTHY MENU

The healthy menu provides nutritious options.

The healthy menu provides choice: nutritious dishes are available for guests who want them. The guest is responsible for taking charge of his or her own eating habits. The foodservice can help by offering some healthy choices and meals emphasizing balance, variety, and moderation. So what is a healthy dish? Can it be defined? The answer to that question is yes and no. Some foodservice operators simply look to the U.S. Dietary Guidelines (see page 194) for guidance, whereas others develop more specific guidelines such as:

A nutritious entree will have no more than
- 30 percent of its total calories from fat
- 10 percent of its total calories from saturated fat
- 150 milligrams of cholesterol
- 1000 milligrams or less of sodium

That's pretty well defined!

A healthy menu may simply highlight two or more entrees and one or two appetizers and desserts. To develop some nutritious menu items, the first step is to look seriously at your existing menu while engaging in some old-fashioned menu planning. You may go in one of three directions.

1. **Use existing items on your menu.** Certain menu selections, such as fresh vegetable salads or grilled skinless chicken, may already meet your needs.

2. **Modify existing items to make them more nutritious.** For example, broil fish instead of baking it with a butter sauce. In general, modification centers on ingredients, preparation, and cooking techniques.

Modifying an existing item may simply mean offering a half-portion. The next chapter gives specifics on modifying recipes.

3. **Create new selections.** Many light and nutritious cookbooks, as well as magazines such as *Cooking Light* and *Eating Well,* are on the market. Quantity healthy cookbooks are also available, some of which are listed at the end of this chapter.

Start simply by offering only a few quality items; then evaluate their sales and profitability.

Whenever you are involved in menu planning, keep in mind the following considerations.

1. Is the menu item tasty? Taste is the key to customer acceptance and the successful marketing of these items. If the food does not taste delicious and look out of this world, then no matter how nutritious it may be, it is not going to sell.

   Taste is a primary consideration in choosing which foods to eat.

2. Does the menu item blend with and complement the rest of the menu?
3. Does the menu item meet the food habits and preferences of the guests?
4. Is the food cost appropriate for the price that can be charged?
5. Does each menu item require a reasonable amount of preparation time?
6. Is there a balance of color in the foods themselves and in the garnishes?
7. Is there a balance of texture—soft and crisp versus firm-textured foods?
8. Is there a balance of shape, with different-sized pieces and shapes of foods?
9. Are flavors varied?
10. Are the food combinations acceptable?
11. Are cooking methods varied?
12. Can each menu item be prepared properly by the cooking staff?

Table 12-1 describes the roles of foodservice managers and chefs in developing a healthy menu.

Up to this point, guidelines for developing healthy menu options have been discussed. The remainder of this chapter gives menu-planning guidelines for each section of the menu so you can plan menu items in the following categories.

- Low in fat, saturated fat, and cholesterol
- High in complex carbohydrates

> **TABLE 12-1.** **Role of foodservice managers and chefs in developing healthy menus.**
>
> - Develop insight into customers' food habits and preferences.
> - Choose appropriate recipes to test.
> - Use culinary knowledge to modify recipes so they are both healthy and tasty.
> - Evaluate final products.
> - Work with registered dietitians to ensure that the final product is tasty and healthy.
> - Keep up to date on trends and techniques of healthy cooking.

- Low in refined sugar
- Low in sodium

Keep in mind that when *Restaurants & Institutions* asked consumers which healthful dishes they wanted at restaurants, 47 percent of respondents asked for more salads, vegetables, seafood, poultry, fresh fruit, and vegetarian dishes.

MINI-SUMMARY A healthy menu offers nutritious options for customers to choose. To guide you in selecting or creating nutritious dishes, you can follow the Dietary Guidelines for Americans (1995) or set nutrient limits on calories, fat, saturated fat, cholesterol, and/or sodium. When working on developing healthy menu items, you may find existing menu items that meet your nutrition goals, modify menu items to meet your goals, or develop new dishes. When menu planning, don't ever forget that taste is still more important than nutrition. Healthy foods must taste, and look, great.

PLANNING MENU ITEMS LOW IN FAT, SATURATED FAT, AND CHOLESTEROL

Breakfast
- Offer fresh and canned fruits and juices.
- Almost all cold and hot cereals are great choices. Granola cereals tend to be high in fat unless labeled "reduced fat."
- Most breads are low in fat except for croissants, brioche, cheese breads, and many biscuits. Bagels, low-fat muffins, and baguettes are good choices.

- Have reduced-fat margarine and light cream cheese available to spread on bagels or toast.
- Serve chicken filets, poultry sausages, low-fat ham slices, or fish as leaner sources of protein than the traditional bacon and pork sausage.
- Offer egg substitutes for scrambled eggs and other egg-based items. Egg substitutes taste better when herbs, flavorings, and/or vegetables are cooked with them. Instead of egg substitutes, you can offer to make scrambled eggs and omelets by mixing one whole egg to two egg whites.
- Serve an omelet with blanched vegetables such as chopped broccoli or spinach and low-fat cheese instead of regular cheese.
- As a spread or topping on pancakes and waffles, offer sauces combining low-fat or nonfat yogurt with a fruit puree.
- Serve a breakfast buffet with loads of fruits, low-fat dairy products, and cereals.

Appetizers and Soups
- Offer juices and fresh sliced fruits. Fresh sliced fruits can be served with a yogurt dressing flavored with fruit juices.
- Offer raw vegetables with dips using low-fat yogurt, low-fat cottage cheese, or ricotta cheese as the base, rather than dips using sour cream, cheeses, cream, or cream cheese. Try **hummus**, a chickpea-based dip, or **salsa** made from tomatoes, onions, hot peppers, garlic, and herbs.
- Offer grilled chicken, broiled Buffalo-style chicken wings, or steamed seafood such as shrimp.
- Dish up baked (rather than fried) potato skins and baked corn tortillas for tortilla chips. Sprinkle with grated cheese, garlic, onion, or chili powder.
- Feature stock-based soups with vegetables and grains as the ingredients. Dried beans, peas, and lentils make great soups when cooked and pureed, without using cream or high-fat thickeners such as roux.

Salads
- Offer salads with lots of vegetables and fruits.
- Use only small amounts, if any, of bacon, meat, cheese, eggs, or croutons. Choose cooked beans and peas or low-fat cheeses.
- Offer reduced-calorie or nonfat salad dressings (placed on the side when desired).
- Make tuna fish salad and other similar salads with low-fat mayonnaise.
- Use cooked salad dressing that contains little fat for Waldorf and other salads. It has a tarter flavor than mayonnaise.

TABLE 12-2.   Lean cuts of meat.

Beef

Top round (roasted for roast beef, cut into cubes for kebabs, marinated to make London broil)
Eye of round (roasted for roast beef or braised for pot roast)
Tip round (cut into cubes for kebabs)
Strip loin steak (broiled to make New York strip steak, club steak, and so on)
Top sirloin butt steak (broiled to make sirloin steak, cut into cubes for kebabs, or marinated to make London broil)
Flank steak (marinated and broiled to make London broil)
Tenderloin steak (broiled to make filet mignon)

Pork (each cut has less than 9 grams of fat per 3 ounces cooked)

Boneless loin roast
Boneless rib roast
Center rib chop
Center loin chop
Top loin chop
Sirloin roast
Boneless sirloin chop
Tenderloin

Veal

Almost all cuts are low in fat.

Lamb

Sirloin roast
Shank half of leg roast
Loin chops
Blade chops
Foreshank

Breads

- Most breads are low in fat and saturated fat. Breads with more fat include biscuits, cheese breads, croissants, popovers, brioche, corn bread, and many commercial crackers (although some are low in fat or can be made with less fat).

Entrees

- Serve combination dishes with small amounts of meat, poultry, or seafood and lots of whole grains such as rice, legumes, vegetables, and/or fruits.

Food Facts: Low-Fat Hamburgers

Low-fat ground beef, currently being used in some fast-food hamburgers, contain on average about 7 grams of fat in a 3-ounce cooked hamburger. This is about half the fat of a normal hamburger. To be more accurate, low-fat ground beef should really be called lower-fat ground beef. A low-fat hamburger still gets about 40 percent of its calories from fat—hardly the definition of low-fat but certainly a better profile than a regular hamburger, which gets over 60 percent of its calories from fat.

Low-fat ground beef uses fat replacers to cut back on the amount of fat. A popular fat replacer is carrageenan, a carbohydrate from red seaweed. Oat bran, oat fiber, and soy protein (from soybeans) are also used. In addition to taking the place of fat, fat replacers help maintain the normal texture and moisture of regular beef. If some of the fat were simply removed from hamburgers and not replaced, the meat would be very dry and fall apart during cooking.

Low-fat ground beef can be prepared using the same cooking methods as regular beef; however, it is different from regular ground beef in several ways.

1. Because low-fat beef has less fat, it cooks quicker than regular beef, dries out faster, and doesn't hold together as well. Low-fat beef looks and tastes best when cooked to order and not overcooked.
2. Overmixing low-fat ground beef creates a firm, compact texture that is undesirable. Because this product can easily be overworked, many foodservice operators buy pre-made hamburger patties.
3. Low-fat ground beef shrinks less during cooking because there is less fat. This fact may help make up for its generally higher price.
4. When cooking low-fat hamburgers, avoid squishing them—it will take out the moisture and make them dry.

When handled, cooked, and held properly, low-fat beef can be used quite successfully, as it has been at foodservices as big as Walt Disney World in Orlando, Florida.

- Offer moderate portions of broiled, baked, stir-fried, or poached seafood, white-meat poultry without skin, and lean cuts of meat (see Table 12-2).
- Offer a hamburger, meat loaf, or other ground beef dishes made with low-fat ground beef.
- Feature one or more meatless entrees, such as vegetarian burgers. Vegetarian burgers either imitate beef burgers (usually through the use of soy products) or are veggie burgers (made of vegetables, especially mushrooms).

Popular brands of vegetarian burgers include Gardenburger (made by Wholesome and Hearty Foods Inc.) and Garden Patties T.M. (made by Morningstar Farms).

Chutney, such as tomato-coconut chutney, is made from fruits, vegetables, and herbs, and comes from India originally. Relish is a spicy condiment, often made from pickles but also made with other ingredients; corn relish for example.

- For sauced entrees (or side dishes), feature sauces thickened with flour, cornstarch, or vegetable purees. Salsas, **chutneys**, **relishes**, and coulis also work well.
- Offer sandwiches made with roasted turkey, chicken, water-pack tuna fish salad, lean roast beef made from the round, or a spicy bean or lentil spread.
- For sandwich spreads, use reduced-calorie mayonnaise, French or Russian-style salad dressing, mustard, ketchup, barbecue sauce, or salsa.
- Feature lots of different vegetables in sandwiches.

Side Dishes

- Most side dishes of vegetables, grains, and pasta are good choices as long as little fat is added during preparation.
- Serve grilled potato halves instead of French fries, as well as other grilled vegetables.

Desserts

- Offer fruit-based desserts such as apple cobbler.
- Spotlight sorbets, sherbets, frozen yogurt, and ice milk. All contain less fat than ice cream.
- Feature desserts such as angel food cake and meringues made from fat-free egg whites. Serve with a fruit sauce.
- Offer puddings made with skim milk.

Biscotti means "twice baked." They are a hard-textured cookie from Italy.

- Serve low-fat cookies such as ladyfingers, biscotti, gingerbread, and fruit bars.

Beverages

- Offer 1 percent or skim milk.

MINI-SUMMARY By using lean meats, poultry without the skin, seafood, low-fat or nonfat dairy products, egg whites, fruits, vegetables, grains, and legumes with little or no fat, you can create many menu items that are low in fat, saturated fat, and cholesterol.

PLANNING MENU ITEMS HIGH IN COMPLEX CARBOHYDRATES

Breakfast

- Offer fruit in many different ways. Fruit is the most requested breakfast food for guests concerned about eating a nutritious breakfast.

- Serve freshly made fruit and vegetable juices, such as carrot and apple juice.
- Feature whole-grain and multigrain toast, muffins (bran muffins are high in fiber), bagels, breads and rolls, and even pancakes, French toast, waffles, and crepes.
- Offer different varieties of cooked and cold cereals, especially whole-grain cereals containing whole wheat, oats, or other whole grains. Cereals with bran contain much fiber. Be sure to use fresh fruit for a topping as well as raisins and other dried fruits.

Appetizers and Soups
- Select soups rich in split peas, beans, lentils, vegetables, grains, or pasta. In the summer, feature a cold fruit soup.
- Serve soups with high-fiber crackers such as rye krisps, whole-wheat melba toast, or others made with whole grains and/or bran.

Salads
- Most salads are good sources of complex carbohydrates.
- Feature pasta salads with lots of fresh vegetables and/or fruits.
- Dish up salads with grains such as bulgur or wild rice, dried fruits, and small amounts of nuts or seeds.

Whole-wheat grains that have been steamed, dried, and cracked into small pieces are called bulgur.

Breads
- Breads are great for complex carbohdyrates. Feature whole-grain breads such as oat bread and whole-wheat parkerhouse rolls.
- In bread baskets, be sure to include fiber-rich muffins or biscuits containing whole grains, bran, nuts, fruits, or vegetables such as pumpkin.

Entrees
- Dish up pasta dishes, preferably using whole-wheat pasta for more fiber.
- Feature main dishes using grains, such as quinoa Mexican style, or legumes, such as lentil tacos.
- Spotlight a veggie whole-wheat pizza.
- Top sandwiches with lettuce, tomatoes, sprouts, cucumbers, onions, hot peppers, green pepper rings, and mushrooms. Use whole-grain breads, rolls, or tortillas.

Side Dishes
- Feature a variety of vegetables and fruits (keep skins on)—they are all good sources of complex carbohydrates.

- Dish up side dishes using grains such as brown rice, and cooked or canned dry beans and peas. (See the Food Facts on page 63 for information on grains.)
- Spotlight potatoes in all their cooked forms.

Desserts

For desserts, offer

- fruits in any form.
- cakes or cookies using whole-grain flours, nuts, fruits, or vegetables, such as oatmeal raisin bars or carrot pineapple cake.
- rice pudding (use brown rice and add cherries), tapioca pudding, or bread pudding.
- fruit-filled cobblers and tarts with whole grains such as oats used in the cobbler topping or tart shell.
- fruit toppings on cakes.

MINI-SUMMARY Menu items high in complex carbohydrates include lots of fruits, vegetables, legumes, grains, and products made with grains, such as breads and cereals.

PLANNING MENU ITEMS LOW IN REFINED SUGAR

Breakfast

- Offer 100 percent fruit juices. Products labeled "fruit drink" or "fruit beverage" contain added sugars and often contain little juice.
- In addition to pure fruit juices, have on hand fresh fruits and canned fruits packed in their own juice.
- Offer unsweetened breakfast cereals. For each four grams listed under "Sugars" on a label there is one teaspoon of sugar. For less sugar, choose cereals with less than 4 grams of sugar per serving, unless the sugar comes from a dried fruit such as raisins.
- Jams, jellies, and pancake syrup contain much refined sugar. Have on hand low-sugar jams and jellies or fruit spreads made from 100 percent fruit. Other toppings for toast or pancakes include sliced or chopped fresh fruit, unsweetened applesauce, or other unsweetened fruit sauce.

Appetizers and Soups

- Most appetizers and soups are low in refined sugar.

Salads

- Most salads are not high in sugar, except for those made with regular commercial gelatin mixes. Use gelatin mixes that contain aspartame or another sugar substitute.

Breads

- Most breads are low in refined sugar.

Entrees

- Most entrees are low in refined sugar.

Side Dishes

- Most side dishes are low in refined sugar.

Desserts

- Spotlight fruits in desserts. Fresh fruit can be baked (as in baked apples), poached (as in poached pears), broiled, or made into compote. Select fruits packed in their own juice rather than fruits packed in light or heavy syrup. One-half cup of fruit canned in heavy syrup contains about 4 teaspoons of sugar.
- Have sugarless puddings available.
- Offer baked goods sweetened mostly with fruits, such as fruit bars.

Beverages

- Offer bottled waters, sugar-free soft drinks, fruit and vegetable juices, and unsweetened iced tea.
- Have sugar substitutes available for beverages.

MINI-SUMMARY Many menu items are already low in refined sugar. Lower-in-sugar choices are important in the dessert and beverage menu sections. Fresh fruits and sugarless puddings are good dessert choices. Unsweetened and diet beverages work well for beverages.

PLANNING MENU ITEMS LOW IN SODIUM

General Recommendations

- Decrease or replace salt in recipes by using vegetables, herbs, spices, and flavorings.
- Offer salt-free seasoning blends (see Table 12-3) and lemon wedges.

Most whole, unprocessed foods are not high in sodium.

TABLE 12-3.   Salt-free seasoning blends.

Herb Blend

1½ teaspoons celery seed
2½ tablespoons dried crushed thyme
5 tablespoons garlic powder
1 tablespoon ground white pepper
5 tablespoons mustard powder
10 tablespoons onion powder
5 tablespoons paprika
Combine and mix well (makes 6 shakers).

Saltless Surprise

2 teaspoons garlic powder
1 teaspoon basil
1 teaspoon oregano
1 teaspoon powdered lemon rind
Blend ingredients well and place in a shaker.

Tangy Salt Substitute

3 teaspoons basil
2 teaspoons savory
2 teaspoons celery seed
2 teaspoons ground cumin seed
2 teaspoons sage
2 teaspoons marjoram
1 teaspoon lemon thyme
Mix well, powder with a mortar and pestle, and place in a shaker.

Spicy Saltless Seasoning

1 teaspoon cloves
1 teaspoon pepper
1 teaspoon crushed coriander seed
2 teaspoons paprika
1 tablespoon rosemary
Mix ingredients in a blender. Store in an airtight container.

Breakfast

- All fruits and juices are naturally low in sodium. Canned tomato or vegetable juice is high in sodium unless labeled "low sodium."
- Serve hot cereals, pancakes, French toast, and waffles without adding salt during preparation. Garnish with fruit toppings.
- Toast, bagels, and muffins contain moderate amounts of sodium.

Appetizers and Soups

- Offer unsalted crackers, chips, and pretzels.
- Feature a low-sodium soup made without commercial bases or salt. Use made-from-scratch stocks and use herbs and spices for seasoning.

Salads

- Most salad ingredients are low in sodium, except for bacon, bacon bits, and croutons (unless homemade with little or no salt).
- Offer low-sodium homemade salad dressings.

Breads

- Salt is a necessary ingredient in breads. Breads contain a moderate amount of sodium.

Entrees

- Offer fresh meat, poultry, or seafood instead of canned, cured, smoked or salty meat, poultry, or seafood (such as ham, corned beef, smoked turkey, dried cod, and most luncheon meats). Cheeses are high in sodium, so use small amounts in sandwiches.
- Feature freshly made entrees instead of processed or prepared foods.
- Offer freshly prepared salsas and other low-sodium sauces.
- Feature a home-made low-sodium pasta sauce.
- Instead of high-sodium accompaniments to sandwiches such as pickles, olives, and potato chips, serve fresh vegetables, cole slaw made with reduced-calorie mayonnaise, or another healthful salad.

Side Dishes

- Offer fresh or frozen vegetables seasoned with lemon juice, flavored vinegars, herbs, or spices instead of canned or pickled products.

Desserts

- Offer fruits, sorbets, sherbets, frozen yogurt, and homemade baked goods made with moderate amounts of sodium (avoid self-rising flour— it's high in sodium).

MINI-SUMMARY Using fresh foods combined with herbs, spices, and low-sodium flavorings provides many low-sodium menu choices.

RESETTING THE AMERICAN TABLE: AN INNOVATIVE PROJECT

The Resetting the American Table: Creating a New Alliance of Taste & Health project is an effort by chefs, dietitians, food and health writers, educators, physicians, product developers, and researchers to bridge the gap between taste and nutrition, as well as between culinary professionals and health professionals. The project started in 1989 with a national conference sponsored by the American Institute of Wine and Food and Julia Child. The American Institute of Wine and Food continues to manage the project and perform outreach activities. Members of the 1989 conference developed the following four core values.

1. Taste is a primary determinant of food choices.
2. Don't regard foods as good or bad but look at the overall diet.
3. Healthful diets begin at home.
4. Dietary recommendations should respect various cultural and ethnic culinary traditions.

The project's axiom is a good way to end this chapter.

In matters of taste, consider nutrition and in matters of nutrition, consider taste. And in all cases, consider individual needs and preferences.

MINI-SUMMARY   The Resetting the American Table: Creating a New Alliance of Taste & Health project focuses on bridging the gap between taste and nutrition as well as between culinary professionals and health professionals.

KEY TERMS   Chutney
Hummus
Relish
Resetting the American Table: Creating a New Alliance
  of Taste & Health project
Salsa

In your own words, answer the following questions.

1. Do most Americans feel that nutrition is important? Explain why or why not?
2. Explain what is meant by "nutrition ambivalence."
3. How often does the average American eat out each week? How many of these individuals choose health and nutrition when eating out?
4. Describe two ways to decide whether a menu item is healthy.
5. If you were in charge of developing a healthy menu, what three steps would you take? What considerations would you keep in mind?
6. Who is involved in the Resetting the American Table: Creating a New Alliance of Taste & Health project, and what do they do?

1. *Quiz*

1.	c	6.	d
2.	d	7.	b
3.	True	8.	a
4.	True	9.	c
5.	c	10.	d

2. *Eating Out Style*

To better understand the nutrition ambivalence of Americans and the foods you select when you eat out, answer the following questions.

1. How often do you go out to eat each week?
2. For what reasons do you go out to eat: convenience, celebration, socializing, business, and so on?
3. When you go out to eat, what influences what you decide to order?
4. During which eating out occasions do you order healthy menu items?
5. Do you eat a light meal and then order something rich and sinful for dessert?

3. *Menu Planning Exercise: Business and Industry Cafeteria*

The menu featured in Figure 12-1 is for an employee cafeteria in a large bank. The manager has asked you to add two healthy items in each of these categories: appetizers, entrees, and desserts. The manager's main concern is responding to customers' request for low-fat food. Using your nutrition knowledge and the information in this chapter, write up a list of recommendations.

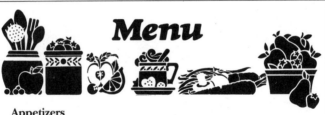

Appetizers

Mozzarella Sticks   Pizza Rolls
French Onion Soup   Buffalo Wings

The Main Event (Half Portions Available)
6 oz. Charbroiled Cheeseburger on Kaiser Roll
   Toppings: Onions, Lettuce, Tomato, Peppers, Bacon
Barbecued Chicken Breast
Veal Parmesan with Spaghetti
Fresh Crab Cakes
Stuffed Shells Florentine
Spaghetti & Meatballs
Chicken Parmesan Sandwich
Big Sweet Italian Sausage Hoagie
Baked or French fried potatoes and salad with Main Events

The Sweeter Side
Ice Cream – Today's Cake or Pie — Brownie Sundae

FIGURE 12-1.
Menu from
a cafeteria
(Courtesy: The
Wood Company)

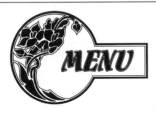

Appetizers
New England Clam Chowder   Soup of the Day
Fresh Fruit Cup   Tomato Juice

Entrees
Rotisserie Chicken – Quarter Chicken Breast with Wing
Double Sauced Meat Loaf
Open-Faced Hot Turkey Sandwich with Gravy
Carved Honey Ham
Chef's Specials

Salads
Tossed Green Salad   Chef's Salad   Salad of the Day

Desserts
Freshly Baked Chocolate Chip Cookie
Ice Cream   Sherbet   Baker's Special

FIGURE 12-2.   Menu from a lifecare community (Courtesy: The Wood Company)

4. Menu Planning Exercise: Lifecare Community

Figure 12-2 features a menu for a restaurant open primarily for dinner in a lifecare community of elderly residents. Each day three Chef's Specials (choice of three entrees, one soup of the day, one salad of the day, two desserts) are offered in addition to the regular menu. For this coming weekend, write up these items for Saturday and Sunday. The nutrition goals in the lifecare community include having low-fat, low-sugar, and low- sodium dishes available, because many of the residents have heart conditions, diabetes, and high blood pressure.

REFERENCES

DiDomenico, Pat. 1994. Portion size: How much is too much? *Restaurants USA* 14(6): 18–21.

Morreale, Sandra J., and Nancy E. Schwartz. 1995. Helping Americans eat right: Developing practical and actionable public nutrition education messages based on the ADA Survey of American Dietary Habits. *Journal of The American Dietetic Association* 95(3): 305–308.

Murray, J. 1996. Lowfat: More items move onto the serving line. *Foodservice Director* February 15: 15–65.

National Restaurant Association. 1990. *Nutrition Awareness and the Foodservice Industry.* Washington, DC: National Restaurant Association.

National Restaurant Association. 1994. *Foodservice Industry Pocket Factbook, 1995–96.* Washington, DC: National Restaurant Association.

Nation's Restaurant News' Editorial Board. 1995. Face the fats: Lean menus may help operators broaden markets. *Nation's Restaurant News,* May 1, 1995.

Palmer, Jeannette, and Carolyn Leontos. 1995. Nutrition training for chefs: Taste as an essential determinant of choice. *Journal of The American Dietetic Association* 95(12): 1418–1421.

Parks, Sara C., Karen A. Lechowich, and James F. Halling. 1994. President's Page: Challenging the future—Changing consumer eating habits create new opportunities in commercial foodservice. *Journal of The American Dietetic Association* 94(8): 908–909.

Restaurant Industry Operation Report. 1992. Chicago, IL: National Restaurant Association and Deloitte & Touche.

Somerville, Sylvia. 1995. Getting diners off to a healthy start. *Restaurants USA* 15(1): 32–36.

Somerville, Sylvia. 1996. How the public's healthy eating trends are influencing restaurants internationally. *Perspectives* 11(1) 1–8.

Survey of American Dietary Habits, 1993 Executive Summary. 1993. Chicago: The American Dietetic Association with Kraft General Foods.

Welland, Diane. 1992. A new age for beef. *Restaurants USA* 12(4): 17–18.

Hot Topic: How Are Americans Making Food Choices?: The Results of One Study[1]

It is recognized widely that American consumers, and consequently American media, are fascinated with food. Open any newspaper or magazine, or turn on the television or radio and inevitably a story about food and the relationship between diet and health will appear.

Although these are hot topics, what consumers know and how that information influences their food choices is somewhat unclear. To better understand consumers' perceptions, the Gallup Organization conducted a survey for the Information Council (IFIC) and the American Dietetic Association (ADA) to assess Americans' attitudes, concerns, and behavior regarding diet and health; their sources for and confidence in nutrition and health information; their confidence in their own ability to select a healthy diet; their perceived barriers to eating a healthy diet; and their attitudes toward physical activity as well as other topics related to health and nutrition.

The survey results are based on telephone interviews conducted in 1993 with a national sample of 754 adults. For results based on samples of this size, there is a 95 percent confidence level that the error attributable to sampling and other random effects could be plus or minus 4 percentage points.

Nutrition and Health

Americans are genuinely interested and concerned about the role foods play in their overall health. Participants were asked, "How concerned are you that what you eat may affect your future health." Eighty-four percent of those responding said they were either concerned or very concerned that what they ate could have an effect on their future health.

The majority of respondents believe in their ability to select a healthful diet, with 48 percent saying they are very confident and 40 percent somewhat confident in their ability to select a healthful diet.

Most consumers recognized that taste does not have to be compromised for health benefits. Seventy-two percent of respondents disagreed with the statement "To improve my diet, I have to eliminate my favorite foods," and 70 percent disagreed that "Foods that are good for me usually don't taste good."

Nutrition Confusion

When asked if they feel confused about knowing how to eat a healthy diet, 45 percent said they are not at all confused and 27 percent responded that they are not very confused. However, 27 percent reported feeling very or somewhat confused.

Balance, Variety, and Moderation

Despite these feelings, 94 percent of those surveyed agreed that balance, variety, and moderation are the keys to healthy eating. This figure was the same in the 1990 survey.

Consumers also understand the concepts associated with these terms. Sixty percent of those surveyed agreed that higher-fat foods can be part of a healthy diet if balanced with low-fat choices, a slight increase from 56 percent who agreed with this idea in 1990.

Almost all participants agreed that controlling the portions or serving sizes of food is important to maintaining a healthy diet. A little more than half of those surveyed also agreed that any food can be part of a total, healthy diet.

Consumers also are becoming better informed about food and nutrition, with 30 percent reporting that they are familiar with the Food Guide Pyramid. Those who are college educated were more likely to report knowing of the Pyramid.

Misconceptions

Although 56 percent agreed that any food can be part of the diet, 67 percent believe that there are "good foods" and "bad" foods, even though health authorities advise that there are only good and bad diets. This was similar to the 1990 responses.

Many consumers are also confused about the amount of fat in individual foods. Sixty-nine percent say that foods should contain 30 percent or less calories from fats. It seems that consumers are applying the 30-percent principle to individual foods rather than to total diet.

Information Sources

Americans continue to rely on the media for their food and nutrition information. When asked an unaided question about their sources for nutrition and food information, respondents mentioned magazines (34 percent), newspapers (16 percent), and television reports (16 percent) as the top sources.

This reliance on the media is also reflected in how consumers react to what they hear. Sixty-eight percent of those surveyed said they are very or somewhat likely to change their food selections based on media information.

Although they rely on the media for information, 75 percent of respondents agreed that there are too many conflicting nutrition reports, and 75 percent also agreed that the information about how to eat a healthy diet is too confusing.

When presented with conflicting reports

about the same nutrition issue, 42 percent of those surveyed said they would seek additional information, 27 percent said they would feel confused, 15 percent said they would ignore all the reports, and 5 percent reported that they would not believe any of the reports.

Physicians and registered dietitians are less common sources of food and nutrition information than the media, with approximately half of those surveyed getting information from a doctor and fewer than one-quarter from a dietitian. Of those who have received nutrition information from health professionals:

- They are more likely to rate the advice from registered dietitians (70 percent) and physicians (68 percent) as very useful.
- They are likely to say they will change their eating habits if advised to do so by a doctor (68 percent) or registered dietitian (65 percent).

Physical Activity

In addition to applying balance, variety, and moderation to their food chocies, 85 percent of respondents said that physical activity is very important to maintaining their health. When asked to list the types of physical activity they do at least a few times each week, more than half (55 percent) reported walking, the most popular response for both men and women.

Summary

Overall, Americans have a healthy attitude toward food and nutrition. They are concerned about what they eat and recognize that food choices may impact their future health. They do seek nutrition information but tend to get confused by information overload. Unfortunately, a number of nutrition misconceptions linger on, and more Americans need to learn nutrition basics such as the Food Guide Pyramid.

[1]Adapted from International Food Information Council, "How Are Americans Making Food Choices?," 1994.

CHAPTER

13

Developing Healthy Recipes

**KEY
QUESTIONS**

1. In what ways can you modify a recipe to make it healthier? What are the steps involved?
2. What prepreparation techniques can be used to reduce fat?
3. Which cooking methods can be used to produce healthy foods?
4. What are the three ways to modify ingredients?
5. What lower-fat ingredients can be substituted for fatty meats, regular dairy products, fatty sauces, fats, and oils?
6. What ingredients can be used to increase complex carbohydrates, including fiber, in recipes?
7. What ingredients can be used to decrease the amount of refined sugar in recipes?
8. What ingredients can be used to decrease the amount of sodium in recipes?
9. What are common ingredient substitutions used in baking?
10. What are seasonings, flavorings, herbs, and spices, and how and why are they used in developing healthy recipes?

QUIZ

Quiz

Modify the following recipe to make it lower in calories, fat, cholesterol, and sodium and higher in fiber.

Monte Cristo Sandwich   Yield: 100 portions

Ingredients	Amount
Ham, cooked, boneless	100 1-oz. slices
Turkey, cooked, boneless	100 1-oz. slices
Swiss cheese	100 1-oz. slices
White bread	200 slices
Whole milk	6 cups
Salt	2 teaspoons
Eggs, whole, slightly beaten	2 quarts (48 eggs)
Shortening, melted	1 quart

DIRECTIONS: Place one slice each of ham, turkey, and cheese on one slice of bread and top with a second slice. Blend milk, eggs, and salt. Dip each side of the sandwich into the egg and milk mixture; drain. Grill each sandwich on well-greased griddle about 2 minutes on each side or until golden brown and cheese is melted.

INTRODUCTION

You can modify a recipe for many reasons, such as to reduce the amount of calories, fat, saturated fat, cholesterol, sodium, or sugar. You may also modify a recipe to get more of a nutrient, such as fiber or vitamin A. Whether modifying a recipe to get more or less, there are four basic ways to go about it.

1. Use healthy prepreparation techniques.
2. Use healthy cooking techniques.
3. Change an ingredient by reducing it, eliminating it, or replacing it.
4. Add a new ingredient.

The first four sections of this chapter look at each one of these topics, followed by examples of modified recipes.

Of course, if you don't want to go through the trouble (which is sometimes a little and sometimes a lot) of modifying recipes, you can select and test recipes from healthy cookbooks. A listing of excellent healthy cookbooks, along with tips on selecting them, is given at the end of this chapter.

If you do decide to modify a recipe, follow these steps.

1. Examine the nutritional analysis of the product and decide how and how much you want to change the product's nutrient profile. For example, for a meat loaf recipe, you may decide to decrease its fat content to less than 40 percent and increase its complex carbohydrate content to 10 grams per serving.
2. Once you have set your nutrition goals, think about your taste goals. You may want the new product to mimic the taste of its original version, or you may want to introduce a new flavor.
3. Next, actually modify the recipe using any or all of the four methods listed above, making sure you reach your nutrition goals.
4. Now it is time to test the recipe to see whether you met your taste goals. This step generally leads to another slight recipe modification and another testing of the recipe. Be prepared to test the recipe a number of times before it is acceptable, and remember that some modified recipes will never be quite acceptable.

Each of the following sections of this chapter will help you make good recipe-modification decisions.

MINI-SUMMARY You can modify a recipe in any of four different ways: use healthy prepreparation techniques; use healthy cooking techniques; change an ingredient by reducing it, eliminating it, or replacing it; or add a new ingredient. By setting nutrition and taste goals for a recipe, you can test and retest the recipe until the final product is acceptable.

HEALTHY PREPREPARATION TECHNIQUES

Trimming meats of visible fat and using rubs and marinades are simple preprepenation techniques that decrease calories, fat, and cholesterol. Of course, even after trimming fat off meats, the meat still contains invisible fat. Studies performed on cooked poultry have shown that poultry cooked with the skin on (where most of the fat lurks) does not significantly add fat to the poultry meat itself and does help prevent the meat from drying out. So it's a good idea to cook poultry with the skin on, then remove it before serving.

Flavorful **rubs** and **marinades** for meats and poultry allow new and creative flavor options. Rubs combine dry spices, such as cinnamon, and finely cut herbs such as cilantro. Rubs may be dry or wet. Wet rubs, also called *pastes*, make use of liquid ingredients such as mustard or vinegar. Pastes produce a crust on the food. Wet or dry seasoning rubs work particularly well with beef and can range from a mesquite barbecue seasoning rub to Jamaican jerk rub. To make a rub, mix together various seasonings and spread or pat evenly on the meat just before cooking or up to 5 hours in advance. The larger the piece of meat or poultry, the longer the rub can stay on. Before cooking, the rubs may be scraped off.

Marinades are useful for flavoring as well as tenderizing meat and poultry. Fish can also be marinated. Although fish is already tender, a short marinating time (about 30 minutes) can develop a unique flavor. A marinade always contains an acidic ingredient, such as wine, beer, vinegar, citrus juice, or plain yogurt, to break down the tough meat or poultry. The other ingredients add flavor. Oil is often used in marinades for flavor but isn't essential. Fat-free salad dressings such as Italian work well in marinades. To add flavor to marinated foods, try minced fruits and vegetables, low-sodium soy sauce, mustard, herbs, and spices instead of oil. For example, fruit juice marinades can be flavored with Asian seasonings such as ginger and lemon grass.

MINI-SUMMARY Healthy preprepenation techniques include trimming of visible fat from meat and using rubs and marinades, preferably made with little or no oil. Poultry skin should be removed after cooking.

HEALTHY COOKING TECHNIQUES

Healthy cooking techniques do not add fat and/or they allow fat to drip away. First, we will look at dry-heat and then moist-heat cooking methods.

Dry Heat Cooking Methods

Dry-heat cooking methods, except traditional frying, are acceptable cooking methods when heat is transferred with little or no fat and excess fat is allowed to drip away from the food being cooked. Frying, both pan- and deep-frying, adds varying amounts of fat, calories, and perhaps cholesterol, depending on the source of the fat, and is therefore not an acceptable cooking method. Successful frying methods will be discussed later.

Dry heat cooking methods:
bake/roast
broil
pan broil
grill
pan fry
deep-fry
saute

When roasting or baking, always place meat, poultry, or seafood on a rack so that the drippings fall to the bottom of the pan. For meat loaf, use a perforated pan over another pan that collects the fat. When broiling, grilling, or barbecuing, be sure to allow fat to drip down away from the piece of meat, poultry, or fish. In addition to meat, poultry, and seafood, vegetables can be roasted, broiled, or grilled rather than fried. The browning that occurs during these cooking processes adds rich flavors. For example, potato wedges or slices can be seasoned and roasted.

Broiling is wonderful for cooking beef steaks, chicken breast, and fish with a little more fat such as salmon, tuna, or swordfish. The more well done you want the product, or the thicker it is, the longer the cooking time and the farther from the heat source it should be. Otherwise, the outside of the food will be cooked but the inside will not be done.

Grilling is an excellent no-fat-added way to cook meat, poultry, seafood, and vegetables. Once thought to be a tasty way to prepare hamburgers, steaks, and fish, grilling is now used to prepare a wide variety of dishes from around the world. For example, chicken is grilled to make fajitas (Tex-Mex style of cooking) or to make jerk barbecue (Jamaican style of cooking). Grilling is also an excellent method to bring out the flavors of many vegetables. Grill them with a little margarine, lemon juice, and selected seasonings.

Grilling foods properly requires much cooking experience to get the grilling temperature and timing just right. Some general rules to follow include:

1. Cook meat and poultry at higher temperatures than seafood and vegetables.
2. For speedy cooking, use boneless chicken that has been pounded out and meats that are no more than 1/2-inch thick. Fat should be trimmed off meats.

Hot Topic: Fusion Cooking

The term **"fusion cooking"** was first used in 1989 by Norman Van Aken in a speech to the Society for Cuisine in America. He borrowed the term "fusion" from the musical world where it means to blend two different styles. In the cooking world, fusion cooking means to blend ingredients, flavors, and techniques from various cuisines. For example, roast chicken breast Mediter-Asian blends Mediterranean and Asian cuisines. The chicken is marinated in Asian ingredients such as Asian chile sauce and oyster sauce and is then served with a Mediterranean sauce of onions, tomatoes, mushrooms, and Parmesan cheese.

As with most other innovations, fusion cooking has both supporters and critics. Chefs who support fusion cooking point to the fact that just as the Pilgrims blended their cooking style with the foods found in the New World, new ingredients and techniques from other cultures are now being discovered and used. Fusion cooking does not abandon old cuisines, but simply changes some recipes, adds new recipes, and lets poor recipes fade away.

Critics of fusion cooking chide chefs who combine foods from various cultures without understanding their ingredients or history. They mock chefs who experiment with cross-cultural cooking, as fusion cooking is sometimes called, to surprise, rather than please, their guests. Perhaps what critics are more upset about is that chefs frequently and deliberately use fusion cooking (without adequate knowledge in some cases) to purposely create something different when the evolution of cuisines is not always so deliberate and is certainly slower.

For fusion cooking to work, chefs need to

1. have an excellent foundation in foods, including food history and cooking techniques.
2. be knowledgeable about the cuisine(s) they are working with.
3. use all their senses to understand how the food is changing during cooking and its flavor, texture, and color.
4. be subtle with flavor.

3. Don't try to grill thin fish fillets, such as haddock, because they will fall apart. Firm-fleshed, thicker pieces of fish, such as swordfish and tuna, do much better on the grill.
4. Keep the grill clean.

Reports link outdoor grilling to a possible increased risk of cancer. Whenever foods are cooked at high temperatures, hazardous or cancer-causing chemicals can be produced. In addition, the smoke produced when fat drips to the coals or other heating element is a source of cancer-causing chemicals (called **carcinogens**). The risks involved in eating grilled foods are small and neither the American Cancer Society or the National Cancer Institute recommend that we avoid grilled foods. To limit your risk, the National Cancer Institute has made these suggestions:

1. Choose leaner cuts of meat and trim meat of outside fat to reduce the fat that drips on the coals. Also remove skin from poultry before grilling.
2. Meats containing more fat, such as spareribs or ground beef, should be precooked to remove some of the fat before grilling. You can also partially cook any food so that the grilling time is reduced.
3. Raise the level of the grill so that the meat is as far away from the heat as possible.
4. Cook meats medium—avoid well-done—so that the grilling time is decreased.
5. Cut meats into small pieces, as in kebobs, so they cook quicker.
6. Clean the grill frequently.

Deep-fried foods have a unique flavor that is never quite the same when you use healthy frying techniques. But certain tips and techniques can make great-tasting dishes. When foods are deep-fat fried, they are cooked at very high temperatures that really bring out the foods' flavors. Other high-temperature cooking methods, such as sautéing and stir-frying, yield similar results when a small amount of a strong oil or simply vegetable-oil cooking spray and a nonstick cooking pan are used.

Nonstick finishes such as Silverstone or Teflon require less fat for cooking and also clean up quicker and more easily. Pans made with anodized aluminum, such as Calphalon (the best-selling brand of anodized aluminum cookware), also require little or no fat for sautéing.

Vegetable-oil cooking sprays come in a variety of flavors (butter, olive, Oriental, Italian, mesquite), and a quick two-second spray adds about 1 gram of fat to the product. To use these sprays, spray the pan first away from any open flames (the spray is flammable), heat up the pan, then add the food.

If browning is not important, you can simmer the ingredient in a small amount of fat-free liquid, such as wine, vermouth, flavored vinegar, or defatted stock, to bring out the flavor. Vegetables naturally high in water content, such as tomatoes or mushrooms, can be cooked with little or no added fluid.

Stir-frying—cooking small-size foods over high heat in a small amount of oil—preserves the crisp texture and bright color of vegetables and cooks strips of poultry, meat, or fish quickly. Typically, stir-frying cooking is done in a **wok**—a round-bottom metal pan that fits over a gas or electric burner. Steam-jacketed kettles and tilt frying pans can also be used to make quantity stir-fry menu items. To stir-fry successfully, be sure to follow these tips.

- Cut ingredients into thin strips or diced portions.
- Coat the cooking surface with a thin layer of oil. Peanut oil works well because it has a strong flavor (so you can use just a little) and a high smoking point.
- Preheat the equipment to a high temperature.
- Stir the food rapidly during cooking and don't overfill the pan.

Oven-frying is another way to get a little bit of the fried flavor without all the fat. For oven-fried chicken and fish, dip the meat or fish in egg whites, coat with seasoned bread crumbs or crushed whole-grain cereal, and bake in a pan coated with vegetable-oil cooking spray.

Moist-Heat Cooking Methods

Moist heat cooking methods:
boil
simmer
poach
steam
braise

Moist-heat cooking methods involve water or a water-based liquid as the vehicle of heat transfer and are often used when meat or poultry is lean and not very tender. When moist-heat cooking meat or poultry, the danger is that the fat in the meat or poultry, although leaner, stays in the cooking liquid. This problem can be resolved to a large extent by chilling the cooking liquid so the fat separates and can be removed before the liquid is used. If the liquid needs to be chilled quickly, put ice cubes in it. The fat will stick to the ice cubes, which can then be removed.

When boiling, simmering, or poaching, you don't need to add fat to the water. Although directions may say to add fat, such as a tablespoon of vegetable oil when boiling grains or pasta, it is not necessary. This instruction is often included to help keep these foods from sticking together during cooking. Simply using 2 cups of water for each cup of long-grained rice, and 1 gallon of water for each pound of pasta will resolve that problem.

Steaming has been the traditional method of cooking vegetables in many quantity kitchens because it is quick and results in an excellent product. It's healthy too, because it requires no fat. Fish can also be steamed and looks great when steamed *en papillote* (in parchment) or in grape or cabbage leaves.

Braising involves two steps: browning the food (usually meat) in a small amount of oil or its own fat and then adding liquid and simmering until done. When browning meat for braising, brown in as little fat as possible without scorching, and then simmer in a small amount of liquid. Fat can be skimmed or removed from the liquid by using a **fat-separator pitcher** or **fat-off ladle**. Another way to remove the fat is to refrigerate the liquid. The fat will naturally congeal (become solid and white), and then can easily be removed.

Microwaving is another wonderful method for cooking vegetables because no fat is necessary and the vegetables' color, flavor, texture, and nutrients are retained. Boiling or simmering vegetables is not nearly as desirable as steaming or microwaving because nutrients are lost in the cooking water. Boiling and simmering also require more time.

MINI-SUMMARY Healthy cooking methods include baking, roasting, broiling, grilling, stir-frying, sautéing with little or no oil, boiling, simmering, poaching, microwaving, and braising when the fat is removed from the cooking liquid.

HEALTHY INGREDIENTS

You can modify ingredients in one of three ways: reduce the amount of an ingredient, eliminate an ingredient, or find an acceptable substitute. You can also add new ingredients, the topic of the next section. In the recipe at the beginning of the chapter, for example, you can reduce the amount of shortening needed by using a nonstick pan, eliminate the salt (there's enough salt in the ham and cheese to give it flavor), substitute 1 percent milk for whole milk, and add a seasoning.

When thinking about modifying ingredients, think: reduce, eliminate, substitute, or add.

To make intelligent decisions about modifying ingredients, ask yourself these key questions:

1. What functions does this ingredient perform? Is it there for appearance, flavor, texture, and so on?
2. What would happen if less or none of the ingredient were used? At which point would the quality of the finished product suffer?
3. What would happen if a healthy substitute, such as skim milk, were used in place of a less healthy ingredient, such as whole milk?
4. What can I add to this recipe to make it truly flavorful?

Once you have decided how you want to modify the ingredients, don't think the work is done. On the contrary, it is just beginning. The following tips and hints on modifying ingredients are culled from my own cooking background as well as from many chefs, cooks, dietitians, and healthy cookbooks. The tips are listed by menu category to make it easy to use.

Breakfast
• Substitute light cream cheese for regular cream cheese as a spread. Nonfat cream cheese is available, but it is not an acceptable spread unless mixed with fruit. Substitute whipped margarine in place of butter as a spread. (These substitutes can all be mixed with fruit purees,

jellies, jams, syrups, or honey for a delicious taste with even less fat.) Other-lower-in fat spreads include jam, jelly, preserves, marmalade, fruit butters (they don't include butter—only fruit), and honey.

- Use egg substitutes to make scrambled eggs and omelets. Most egg substitutes are made from egg whites, gums, and coloring to make them look and taste like real eggs. They still contain varying amounts of fat. You can also substitute 2 egg whites and 1 whole egg for 2 whole eggs.
- Fill omelets with vegetables and low-fat cheese instead of full-fat cheese.
- Substitute lean smoked ham, Canadian bacon, grilled chicken, poultry sausages, or fish for bacon and pork sausage.
- Use fruit as a topping for cereals, pancakes, waffles, and the like.
- Cut the fat in hash browns by using a vegetable-oil cooking spray instead of fat.

Appetizers

- Instead of sour cream for dips, substitute nonfat plain yogurt or sour cream made with less or no fat. Or use a noncreamy dip such as salsa, which can be made from a variety of fruits and vegetables, or dips based on pureed beans, peas, or lentil, such as spicy black bean dip. Reduced-calorie or fat-free salad dressings, such as peppercorn ranch, also work well as dips.
- Substitute grilled meats, poultry, and seafood for fried versions.

Soups

Great whole grains in soups include barley, kash or roasted buckwheat, rice, and bulgur.

- To thicken soups, see the discussion about thickeners under "Sauces."
- Substitute defatted stocks for regular stocks.
- Use vegetables, pasta, whole grains, and legumes instead of fatty meats.
- Instead of using cream or whole milk to make cream soups, substitute evaporated skim milk, nonfat buttermilk, low-fat milk, or skim milk. Cooked vegetable purees, such as mashed potatoes, can be used for thickening. When topped with a dollop of cream or a dash of wine, a low-fat cream soup can be quite delicious.
- Add rich ingredients through garnishes such as small amounts of shredded cheeses, croutons, sour cream, or filled pasta shapes to add splashes of color, texture, and flavor.

Salads

- Use small amounts of bacon bits, croutons, regular cheeses, and hard-boiled eggs. Substitute homemade croutons made with little fat, low-fat cheeses, and cooked beans, peas, and lentils.

- Substitute low-fat or nonfat commercial salad dressings or salsa for regular salad dressings.
- When making your own dressings, select small amounts of flavorful oils such as extra virgin olive oil, peanut oil, sesame oil, or walnut oil.
- Use flavorful vinegars, such as raspberry or rice vinegar, that require less oil to make a great salad dressing. Try using only 2 tablespoons of oil per cup of dressing.
- Substitute nonfat yogurts, blenderized low-fat cottage cheese, or low-fat sour cream for cream or sour cream in creamy salad dressings.
- Substitute equal amounts of nonfat plain yogurt and low-fat mayonnaise, or try using cooked salad dressing in place of regular mayonnaise in cold salads such as chicken or potato salad.

Breads
- Substitute yeast breads and rolls (preferably whole grain) in place of biscuits, cheese breads, **croissants**, **popovers**, **brioche**, and corn bread. Low-fat recipes are available for cheese breads, popovers, and corn bread.
- Instead of butter or margarine as spreads on bread, see the lower-fat spreads mentioned under "Breakfast."

Entrees and Sandwiches
- Substitute lean cuts of beef, pork, and lamb (see Table 13-1) for higher-fat cuts. When appropriate, use smaller portions.
- Substitute whole grains, legumes, vegetables, and/or fruits for some of the meat or poultry in entrees.
- For mixed dishes that include ground beef or pork, substitute 2 cups of cooked beans for each pound of ground meat. Substitute low-fat ground beef (read Food Facts on page 395) or ground chicken or turkey. You can also replace some of the ground meat with fillers such as grains (rolled oats), vegetables (onion, bell peppers), or dried fruits (such as currants).
- Substitute vegetable oils for butter and tropical oils (that is, palm, palm kernel, and coconut oil) in cooking. If some butter flavor is needed, mix whipped butter with an equal amount of vegetable oil. Or use small amounts of flavorful oils (such as walnut oil or extra-virgin olive oil) or infused oils (see the next section for a discussion on infused oils).
- Use yeast bread dough instead of pie crust for pot pies.
- For regular cheeses, substitute ones lower in fat (see Table 13-2) or use small amounts of a strong-flavored cheese as a garnish to give a great appearance and add flavor.

Great legumes in entress include kidney beans, Great Northern beans, navy beans, pinto beans, and black beans.

TABLE 13-1.   Guide to lean cuts of meat.

Beef

Top round (roasted for roast beef, cubed for kebabs, marinated to make London broil)

Eye of round (roasted for roast beef or braised for pot roast)

Tip round (cubed for kebabs)

Strip loin steak (broiled to make New York strip steak, club steak, and others)

Top sirloin butt steak (broiled to make sirloin steak, cubed for kebabs, or marinated to make London broil)

Flank steak (marinated and broiled to make London broil)

Tenderloin steak (broiled to make filet mignon)

Pork (Each cut has less than 9 grams of fat per 3-ounce cooked serving)

Boneless loin roast

Boneless rib roast

Center rib chop

Center loin chop

Top loin chop

Sirloin roast

Boneless sirloin chop

Tenderloin

Veal

Almost all cuts are low in fat.

Lamb

Sirloin roast

Shank half of leg roast

Loin chops

Blade chops

Foreshank

TABLE 13-2. Guide to cheeses.*	
Low in Fat (0–3 grams of fat/ounce	*Medium Fat (4–5 grams of fat/ounce)*
Cottage cheese, dry curd, 1/4 cup	Light cream cheese (1 ounce
Cottage cheese, 1/4 cup, 1%	equals 2 tablespoons)
Cottage cheese, 1/4 cup, 2%	Grated Parmesan cheese (1 ounce
Sap sago (a hard aged cheese	equals 3 tablespoons)
made from skim milk)	Mozzarella, part skim
Pot cheese (also known as	Ricotta, 1/4 cup, part skim
bakers' cheese or farmers' cheese)	String cheese, part skim
Some special low-fat brands	Some reduced-fat brands
High Fat (6–7 grams of fat/ounce)	*Very High Fat (8–10 grams of fat/ounce)*
American cheese food	American cheese
Brie	Blue cheese
Camembert	Brick
Edam	Cheddar
Feta	Colby
Gouda	Cream cheese (1 ounce
Jarlsberg	equals 2 tablespoons)
Limburger	Fontina
Mozzarella, whole milk	Gruyère
Provolone	Longhorn
Romano (1 ounce equals 3	Monterey Jack
tablespoons)	Muenster
Swiss	Port Salut
Swiss cheese food	Ricotta, 1/4 cup, whole milk
	Roquefort

* Fat grams are based on a 1-ounce serving size unless otherwise stated.

Food Facts: Good Looking Healthy Dishes

Once upon a time, you could rely on slathering an entree with cream sauce to hide any problems in its appearance or taste. Today, however, special attention needs to be paid to plating healthy dishes so that they look wonderful (after all, the guest eats first with his eyes), plentiful, and retain their appropriate temperature. Some general rules to enhance attractiveness include the following (Welland, 1993).

1. Use high-quality, fresh ingredients.
2. Prepare the dish according to the recipe and portion it accurately.
3. Keep all garnishes simple. Some dishes, such as angel food cake with a fruit sauce, are already garnished, although you may top with a slice or two of fruit.
4. Use some of the following tricks to make less look like more.

When you are serving smaller portions of meat, poultry, or seafood, various techniques can be used to make the portion size look larger. By slicing meat or poultry thin, you can fan out the slices on the plate to make less look like more. You can also arrange a piece of meat, poultry, or seafood on a bed of grains, vegetables, and/or fruits, or cover it with sautéed vegetables. In addition, you can stuff hamburgers with vegetables such as sliced mushrooms and onions, and use vegetables as fillers in other dishes such as meat loaf or flounder florentine. Serving larger portions of side dishes with the entree also makes the plate look more full.

A common problem that crops up when plating healthy foods is that many dishes lose heat quickly and dry out fast. High-fat sauces help keep a dish hot. By slicing meat for presentation, the meat loses more juice and heat, so it dries out quicker. To overcome this problem, chefs often place foods close together on the plate, putting the densest food in the center to keep the other foods warm. When slicing meats for plating, you can slice just part of the meat for appearance and then leave the remaining piece whole for the guest to cut.

- A naturally fat-free cheese, called **fromage blanc**, is a wonderful substitute for whole-milk fresh cheeses such as ricotta and cottage cheese. Fromage blanc is made by heating buttermilk until the curd begins to separate, then draining the curd.
- Instead of using bread crumbs for breading, crush some whole-grain cereal or crackers and mix with appropriate seasonings.
- Sweeten dishes with unsweetened fruit juice concentrates or fruit purees.
- Substitute roasted, broiled, or grilled lean meats and poultry for cold cuts and hot dogs at lunch time. Mashed cooked beans, peas, or

TABLE 13-3.	Guide to condiments.		
Condiment*	Calories	Fat (grams)	Saturated Fat (grams)	Cholesterol (milligrams)
Spreads				
Butter	102	11	7	31
Stick margarine	101	11	2	0
Soft tub	101	11	2	0
Imitation, about 40% fat	50	6	1	0
Cream cheese	50	5	3	16
Light cream cheese	35	2.5	2	8
Mayonnaise	99	11	1	51
Low-fat	25	1	0	0
Low-fat plain yogurt	9	0	0	1
Nonfat plain yogurt	8	0	0	0
Sweeteners				
Jam/jelly/preseves	52	0	0	0
Honey	65	0	0	0
Apple butter	33	0	0	0
Sauces				
Barbecue	16	0	0	0
Soy	11	0	0	0
Salsa	8	0	0	0
Tartar	70	8	NA	5
Teriyaki	15	0	0	0
Worcestershire	11	0	0	0
Salad Dressings				
Blue cheese	77	8	1.5	0
French	67	6	1.5	0
Reduced-calorie	22	1	0	0
Italian	69	7	1	0
Reduced-calorie	16	1.5	0	0
Russian	76	8	1	0
Reduced-calorie	23	1	0	0
Thousand Island	59	6	1	0
Reduced-calorie	24	1.5	0	2
Other				
Ketchup	15	0	0	0
Mustard, yellow	15	0	0	0
Pickle relish	20	0	0	0

*Serving size is 1 tablespoon unless otherwise noted.
Source: United States Department of Agriculture.

lentils, when mixed with spices and low-calorie salad dressing, make a tasty sandwich spread for pita bread or tortillas.

- Substitute mustard, ketchup, barbecue sauce, relish, salsa, low-fat or fat-free mayonnaise or salad dressing for butter or margarine on sandwich bread. Table 13-3 is a guide to condiments. Also add colorful, crunchy vegetables, such as red-tipped leaf lettuce, tomatoes, cucumbers, and bean sprouts.
- Instead of pepperoni and sausage on pizzas, heap on such vegetables as broccoli, mushrooms, and green peppers.
- To tenderize tough meats without using commercial tenderizers (they are high in sodium), marinate instead.

Side Dishes

- Use herbs, spices, garlic, small amounts of toasted nuts or seeds, low-sodium soy sauce, and the like, instead of butter or margarine, to flavor vegetables and other side dishes.
- On baked potatoes, substitute nonfat or reduced-fat sour cream or plain nonfat yogurt for regular sour cream. Mix with herbs, spices, or vegetables for flavor.
- Mash potatoes with light sour cream, evaporated skim milk, or nonfat buttermilk instead of butter and whole milk.
- Use flavorful rices, such as Basmati rice, instead of long-grain white rice.
- Add grains to vegetable dishes, such as brown rice with stir-fried vegetables.

Sauces

Instead of roux, use flour, cornstarch, arrowroot, and cooked vegetable purees to thicken. Use new low or no-fat sauces such as salsa, chutney, relishes, and coulis.

- Instead of thickening with roux (fat and flour) or liaison (egg yolks and cream), healthy thickening agents include:
- Flour. When flour is mixed with a cold liquid such as water, it is called a **slurry**. When flour is used as a thickener, it must be completely cooked to remove its starchy flavor.
- Cornstarch. Like flour, cornstarch must first be mixed with a cold liquid before it can be used to thicken. Cornstarch produces a translucent product that doesn't hold up well during long cooking or holding periods.
- Arrowroot. Although expensive, arrowroot has many advantages. It thickens at lower temperature than other thickeners, it has no starchy taste, and it makes a shiny sauce.
- **Purees of cooked vegetables**. Cooked vegetable purees are good thickeners for soups and stews, but can be chosen carefully to thicken sauces too. Use a little olive oil to finish these sauces and give them flavor.

- Instead of using thickening agents, reduce the juices from cooked meat, poultry, or seafood (boil or simmer until the volume is decreased). At this point, the flavors will be quite concentrated. Fat is removed from the juices by chilling the liquid in the refrigerator and then removing the congealed (solid) fat, chilling the liquid with ice cubes (if time is short) and then removing the ice cubes on which the fat is sticking, or using special fat-off ladles or fat-separator pitchers. In a fat-separator pitcher, the spout is at the bottom because the fat will float to the top, allowing you to pour out fat-free juices.
- So who says a sauce has to be a traditional white sauce, brown sauce, or the like? The hottest new sauce in the United States is salsa. Traditional Mexican salsa is made from tomatoes, onion, chili peppers, garlic, and herbs such as cilantro. Salsas can be made from a limitless combination of fruits, vegetables, and/or beans and peas, such as roasted corn and black bean salsa.
- Other vegetable and fruit sauces include chutneys, relishes, and **coulis**. They have the following in common: They are made from fruits and/or vegetables, they have primarily a sweet, tart, and/or spicy flavor, and they are used as condiments to complement the main dish.
- If a sauce calls for sour cream, use low-fat or no-fat sour cream or substitute skim-milk ricotta cheese, low-fat cottage cheese, or plain nonfat yogurt. When cooking with yogurt, use only low heat. High temperatures may cause it to separate and curdle. To prevent this, blend one tablespoon of cornstarch (or two tablespoons of flour) with a cup of yogurt before cooking. If overmixed, yogurt becomes too thin, so avoid overstirring it.
- Instead of cream, use skim milk or evaporated skim milk.

Coulis is a sauce consisting primarily of a thick puree, usually of vegetables but it can also be of fruit. Flavorings, such as fresh herbs, and a liquid, such as broth, give it taste and body.

Desserts
- Substitute frozen yogurt or ice milk for regular ice cream.
- Substitute whipped evaporated skim milk for whipped cream. To do so, whip cold evaporated skim milk with chilled beaters in a chilled bowl. Fold in vanilla and/or cinnamon for flavor.
- Substitute 1 percent or skim milk for whole milk in puddings or custards. Add a spice, such as cinnamon or nutmeg, to increase the flavor.
- Baked, stewed, or poached fruits are good substitutes for sweet desserts.
- Use fresh sliced fruits and fruit sauces instead of frosting on cakes or other desserts.

Ice milk is like a reduced-fat ice cream. Much soft-serve ice cream is really ice milk.

TABLE 13-4. Functions of baking ingredients.					
Function	Flour	Sugar	Fat	Eggs	Water
Structure	X			X	
Flavor		X	X	X	
Tenderness		X	X	X	
Moist product		X	X		
Color		X			
Freshness		X	X		
Moistens ingredients		X	X	X	X

Beverages

- Substitute skim and 1 percent milk for regular milk.
- In milkshakes, substitute **ice milk** or frozen yogurt for ice cream and skim or 1 percent milk for regular milk.
- Add fruit, such as bananas, to milkshakes to make a fruit smoothie.

Baking

The best low-fat baked goods are those in which the originals do not rely on vast amounts of fat and the low-fat versions use some fat as well as flavoring ingredients to make up for lost flavor. Modifying baking recipes is trickier than other types of recipes because slight differences in proportions of ingredients (or procedures) can make big differences in the end product. That's why bakers prefer to call their recipes by another name: formulas.

Most baking requires several of these ingredients: flour, sugar, fat, eggs, water or milk, and leavenings. When modifying baking recipes, keep in mind what function each of these performs in baking (Table 13-4).

- Substitute vegetable-oil cooking spray or vegetable oil for shortening when preparing pans. Then flour the pans as you normally would.
- Substitute whole-wheat pastry flour for one-third of the all-purpose flour called for in a baking recipe. Avoid using whole-wheat flours in sponge or fine-grained layer cakes because the whole-wheat product is too heavy. Experiment with other whole-grain flours such as barley, rye, and oat by substituting them for part of the wheat flour in a recipe.
- Try using a new whole-wheat flour called **white whole-wheat flour**. It is made from a variety of wheat that has the same nutritional value as regular whole wheat but with a much lighter taste. Milled from hard white winter wheat, it lacks the strong, almost bitter, flavor associated with the types of wheat used for classic whole-wheat flour. White

wheat, nicknamed "sweet wheat" by the farmers who grow it, is a lighter-colored, sweeter-tasting wheat that can be substituted for all-purpose flour in baking recipes.

To purchase white whole-wheat flour, call King Arthur Flour Company at 1-800-827-6836.

- Substitute a low-fat crumb topping or a few decorative dough pieces for the top crust on pies.
- Substitute phyllo dough for traditional pie crust. Instead of used melted fat to separate the phyllo dough sheets, use a butter-flavored cooking spray. Phyllo dough can also be substituted for puffed pastry dough to make desserts such as strudels.
- Meringue shells, made with egg whites and sugar, make excellent crusts for a variety of fruit and other fillings.
- Instead of the traditional high-fat pie crust, make a graham cracker crust. Use less melted margarine or butter to make crumb crusts and add water and honey to help the shell keep its shape and taste good.
- Substitute jams, jellies, fruit spreads, fruit sauces, or powdered sugars for cake frostings.
- When making baked Alaska, substitute angel food cake for sponge cake and substitute ice milk, frozen yogurt, sherbet, or sorbet for the regular ice cream.

Sherbet is a mixture of fruit, fruit juice, and low-fat milk. It contains 2 to 4 grams of fat per cup. Sorbet is a mixture of pureed fruit, fruit juice, and sugar with little or no fat or cholesterol.

- Substitute coconut extract for grated coconut and top the baked goods with some toasted coconut.
- Reduce the amount of toasted nuts and seeds.
- Substitute 3 tablespoons of cocoa powder plus 1 tablespoon (or less) of vegetable oil for each ounce of baking chocolate. Cocoa powder has excellent flavor and much less fat and saturated fat than baking chocolate.
- Substitute skim or 1 percent milk for regular milk.
- Substitute equal portions of 1 percent milk and evaporated skim milk for light cream.
- Substitute low-fat or nonfat yogurt for sour cream or heavy cream.
- Substitute 1 whole egg and 2 egg whites for every 2 whole eggs. Using just egg whites gives the baked good a rubbery texture.
- Substitute stick margarine for butter. Avoid using margarines, such as reduced-fat varieties, that list water as the first ingredient. Because of their high water content, they do not perform the same, or as well as, regular fats in baking.
- When a recipe calls for melted butter or melted shortening, substitute oil. Oil can also be used in soft, moist, bar cookies. When creaming fat and sugar, such as in making cakes, substitute an oil (such as canola oil) for half the solid fat. The texture will be a little more dense but acceptable.

- Substitute half the volume or weight of fat called for with prune puree. Amazingly enough, pureed prunes have been shown to be a good fat substitute. Their flavor is quite subtle—just a fruity nuance—when pureed and baked into a cake. Prunes work best in baked goods with strong flavors, such as brownies and peanut butter cookies. Once worked into a batter, the prunes have only a light tan color so they work well in any baked good that doesn't have to be white. Fruit sugar attracts and holds moisture well, so baked goods stay fresh longer. The natural sugar in pureed prunes also reduces the amount of refined sugar needed to sweeten the baked good.
- Light cream can be used in place of regular cream cheese in many baked goods, but don't substitute nonfat cream cheese in baking or frostings because it falls apart.
- Reduce refined sugar in recipes by one-fourth to as much as one-third (use about 1/4 cup sugar per cup of flour,) and use sweet spices and extracts to make up for lost flavor.
- To add flavor, texture, color, and nutritional value, try adding fruits to baked goods.
- Reduce the salt in recipes, except breads, by one-half.

MINI-SUMMARY You can modify ingredients in one of three ways: reduce the amount of an ingredient, eliminate an ingredient, or find an acceptable substitute. You can also add new ingredients. There are many ways to modify ingredients in recipes to achieve certain nutritional goals.

GETTING THE TASTE BACK: SEASONINGS AND FLAVORINGS

Seasonings and **flavorings** (Figure 13-1) are very important in modified recipes because they help replace missing ingredients such as fat and salt in satisfying the taste buds. Seasonings are used to bring out flavor already present in a dish, whereas flavorings add a new flavor or modify the original one. The difference between them is one of degree. Examples of seasonings and flavorings include herbs, spices, lemon juice, onions, garlic, chives, scallions, shallots, carrots, celery, prepared mustard, plain and flavored vinegars, and grated lemon and orange rind. Seasonings such as garlic salt, onion salt, monosodium glutamate (MSG), and soy sauce are all high in sodium. Salt substitutes should not be used in cooking because they become bitter. Also, sodium in many salt substitutes is replaced by potassium—a hazard for people on certain types of blood pressure medications. Due to this potential problem, staying away from salt substitutes is advisable.

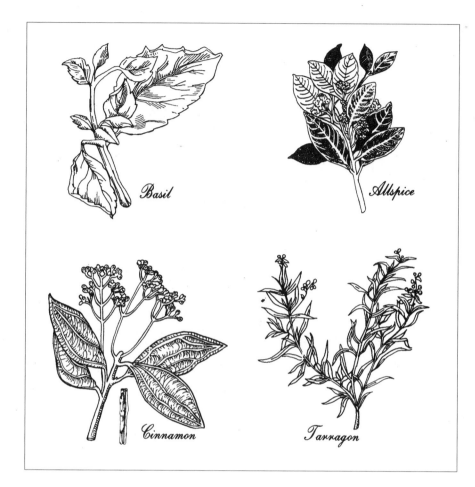

Herbs are the leaves of certain plants grown in temperate climates. **Spices** are dried bits of bark, leaves, and berries from tropical climates (Table 13–5). Although herbs and spices are available dried, more food-service operators are buying or growing their own fresh herbs for better quality and flavor. Here are some tips for seasoning and flavoring with herbs and spices.

1. Use only good-quality seasonings and flavorings.
2. Store all herbs and spices in cool, dry areas away from light and moisture, which deteriorate them at a faster rate.
3. Whole herbs and spices need heat to release their flavors. Ground herbs and spices release their flavors quickly and should be added toward the end of the cooking process. Whole spices are excellent in long-cooking dishes such as stews because they take longer to release

TABLE 13-5. Herb and spice reference chart.

Product	Description	Product Notes
Allspice (spice)	Dried, dark brown berries of an evergreen tree.	Clove-like flavor, but smoother, mellower; undertones of cinnamon, nutmeg, hence name; also called "pimento."
Anise Seed (herb seed)	Small, gray-brown seeds of plant of the parsley family.	Licorice-like flavor. Its oil is heavily used for licorice flavoring, though true licorice is from the roots of another plant.
Star Anise (spice)	Large, brown, star-shaped fruit of an evergreen tree. Each point contains a seed; whole fruit is used.	Anise-like flavor. Old-time pickling favorite, now available again since China trade embargo was lifted.
Basil (herb)	Bright green leaves of an herb of the mint family.	Special affinity for tomato flavored dishes; currently enjoying fastest popularity growth of an herb.
Bay Leaves (herb)	Large, olive-green leaves of the sweet-bay or laurel tree.	An important product; only dried herb to come in original, whole-leaf form, Also "laurel."
Caraway Seed (herb seed)	Hard, brown, scimiter-shaped seeds of an herb of the parsley . family.	The seed of "seeded rye bread"; essential in the liqueur kummel; German sauerkraut favorite.
Cardamom Seed (spice)	Pod and dark brown seeds of a plant of the ginger family.	Scandinavian bakery goods; Indian foods; worldwide biggest use is in Middle East coffee.
Celery Seed (herb seed)	Tiny brown seeds of the smallage, or wild celery plant.	Strong celery flavor; heavy use in salad dressings, sauces, vegetable cocktails.
Chervil (herb)	Lacy, fern-like leaves of a plant of the parsley family.	Much like parsley, but sweeter and more aromatic; anise-like fragrance with slight pepper flavor.
Chives (herb)	Tubular green leaves of a member of the onion family.	Normally freeze-dried to protect fragile quality and vibrant green color; product is tiny lengths of tubular shoots.
Cinnamon/ Cassia (spice)	Bark of various evergreen trees of the cinnamomum family.	Two main types: Zeylanicum (Ceylon) is tan colored, thin bark, mild, sweet flavor. Cassia is reddish brown, thicker bark, strong cinnamon flavor, most popular in U.S.

Product	Description	Product Notes
Cloves (spice)	Dried, unopened flower buds of an evergreen tree.	Intriguing, nail-like shape makes exotic garnish. Ground cloves very strong flavored.
Coriander Leaves (herb)	Green leaves of a plant of the parsley family.	Most frequently called "cilantro." Strong, exotic flavor, associated with Mexican food.
Coriander Seed (herb seed)	Small, round, buff-colored seeds of the coriander plant.	Mild, delicately fragrant aroma with lemony/sage undertone.
Cumin Seed (herb seed)	Small, elongated, yellowish-brown seeds of a plant of the parsley family	Also "comino." The aromatic flavor note in chili powder and essential in curries.
Dill Seed (herb seed)	Small, oval-shaped, tan seed of a member of the parsley family.	Principal flavor of dill pickles, also used in dips, sauces, sausages.
Dill Weed (herb)	Green, feathery leaves of the dill plant.	Dill weed is much used in sauces for fish, cheese dips, salads, dressings.
Fennel Seed (herb seed)	Small, yellowish-brown, watermelon-shaped seeds of a member of the parsley family.	Anise-like flavor. The distinctive note in Italian sausages (both sweet and hot).
Fenugreek Seed (herb seed)	Very small, reddish-brown seeds of a member of the pea family.	Pleasantly bitter flavor with curry-like aroma. Essential in curry powder; basis of imitation maple.
Ginger (spice)	Dried roots (rhizomes) of a member of the zingiber family.	Root pieces are called "hands." Smooth, straw-colored ones have been peeled, bleached.
Mace (spice)	Lacy, scarlet-colored aril (orange when dried) that surrounds the seed of the nutmeg fruit.	Flavor is stronger than nutmeg. Ground mace is often chosen for light-colored products, such as pound cake.
Marjoram (herb)	Grayish-green leaves of a member of the mint family	A cousin of oregano but with milder, sweeter flavor.
Mint Flakes (herb)	Dark green leaves of either the peppermint or spearmint plant.	Spearmint is the mint usually packed as mint flakes for retail and food service; peppermint is also available to industrial customers.
Mustard Seed (spice)	Tiny yellow or brownish seeds of a member of the cabbage family.	Yellow (or white) seeds have sharp bite, but no aromatic pungency. Brown (and oriental) seeds are aromatically pungent as well as biting (i.e., Chinese restaurant mustard).

Product	Description	Product Notes
Nutmeg (spice)	The brown seed of the fruit of an evergreen tree.	Of the two sources, Indonesian and West Indian compare favorably in aroma, but higher fixed oil in the W.I. restricts its use in some applications.
Oregano (herb)	Light green leaves of members of the mint family.	Two distinct types: Mediterranean (Italian/Greek foods); Mexican (chili, Mexican, TexMex foods).
Paprika (spice)	Powder milled from the flesh of pods of certain capsicum plants.	Extractable color is principal evaluation of paprika. Flavor can range from sweet-mild to mildly pungent.
Parsley (herb)	Bright green leaves of parsley plant.	About 12 pounds of de-stemmed parsley leaves are required to make one pound of parsley flakes.
Black Peppercorns (spice)	Dried, mature berries of a tropical vine.	The whole dried berry (peppercorn) is used for black pepper.
Chili Pepper (spice)	Large, mildly pungent pods of Anaheim (or "California-type") peppers and the newer "6–4" variety (New Mexican-type).	Spice industry reserves "chili peppers" for these mild pods; "chillies" for the hot little pods (see Red Pepper).
Green Peppercorns	Immature berries (dried or freeze-dried) of the pepper vine.	Pepper berries are picked while still green, resulting in somewhat milder flavor.
Pink Peppercorns	Dried, red berries of a shrub-like evergreen of the Anareardiacease.	No relation to black pepper. Proper label is Rose Baises (Red Berries).
Red Pepper (spice)	Dried fruit (pods) of various small, hot peppers. Whole pods are called "chillies."	"Red pepper" is today's industry designation for any ground hot pepper product. "Cayenne" is being phased out.
White Peppercorns	Light tan-colored seed of the pepper berry from which the dark outer husk has been removed.	White pepper has the heat but not the total bouquet of black. Often chosen for light colored soups, soups, sauces.
Poppy Seed (herb seed)	Tiny, gray-blue seeds of the poppy plant.	The same plant produces opium and morphine. but the seeds have no drug significance.
Rosemary (herb)	Green, needle-like leaves of a shrub of the mint family.	Rosemary and lamb are closely associated, but it's also important in Italian herb blends, sauces and salad dressings. Has natural antioxidant properties.

Product	Description	Product Notes
Saffron (herb)	Dried flower stigmas of a member of the crocus family.	By the pound, our most expensive spice, but a pinch does so much flavoring and coloring that it is not prohibitive.
Sage (herb)	Long, slender leaves (silver-gray when dried) of a member of the mint family.	Three types: "Cut" is used for end products where sage should show. "Rubbed" is minimally ground and coarsely sieved to a fluffy consistency. "Ground" is sieved to a fine degree.
Savory (herb)	Small, brownish-green (when dried) leaves of a summer savory—a member of the mint family.	So good with green beans, its German name translates to "bean herb." Also in poultry seasoning and other herb blends.
Sesame Seed (herb seed)	Small, oval, pearly white seeds of a member of the.Pedaliacae family.	Also "benne." Needs toasting or high heat of baking to develop its nutty flavor.
Tarragon (herb)	Slender, dark green leaves of a member of the aster family.	Distinctive for its hint of anise flavor. Hallmark of sauce bearnaise, salad dressings, vinegars.
Thyme (herb)	Grayish green leaves of a member of the mint family.	One of the strongest herbs. Manhattan-style clam chowder and innumerable herb blends.
Tumeric (spice)	Orange colored roots (rhizomes) of a member of the ginger family.	Provides color for prepared mustards, curry powder, mayonnaise, sauces, pickles, relishes.

Source: American Spice Trade Association.

their flavor. Wrap whole spices in a cheesecloth or muslin bag for easy removal and add at the beginning of the cooking process. Too much cooking results in flavor loss because spices evaporate during cooking. The kitchen may smell wonderful, but the food is losing its taste.

4. When adding herbs and spices to cold foods such as salads and dressings, allow several hours or overnight for the flavors to develop.

5. Dried herbs and spices are much stronger than fresh ones. A useful formula is: 2 to 3 teaspoons fresh herbs = 1 teaspoon dried.

6. When adding herbs or spices to a dish, add 1/4 teaspoon at a time per pound of meat or pint of sauce or soup until the desired taste is achieved. Add only 1/8 teaspoon at a time of red pepper.

7. Periodically test the foods being seasoned and adjust as needed.

8. Pair intense herbs, such as tarragon and rosemary, with richly flavored foods.

9. Citrus fruits, flavored vinegars, and chilies also make excellent seasonings and flavorings.

Figure 13-2 is a seasoning and flavoring guide.

Various types of vinegars can add flavor to a wide variety of dishes from salads to sauces. They have a light, tangy taste, and add flavor without fat. Popular vinegars include **wine vinegars** (made from white wine, red wine, rose wine, rice wine, champagne, or sherry), **cider vinegar** (made from apples) and **balsamic vinegar**. Balsamic vinegar, a dark brown vinegar with a rich sweet-sour flavor, is made from the juice of a very sweet white grape and is aged for at least ten years. Vinegars can also be infused, or flavored, with all sorts of ingredients, such as chili peppers, roasted garlic, or any herbs, vegetables, and fruits. These types of vinegars are called **flavored**, or **infused vinegars**. For example, lemon vinegar works well in salad dressings and cold sauces.

Like vinegar, oils can be infused with ingredients such as fresh herbs, ground spices, and fresh roots. Small amounts of **flavored oils** can add much flavor to sauces or even be used alone as a sauce for both hot and cold foods. To make a flavored oil, place the ingredient into a bland oil such as canola, corn, or safflower oil until the oil has taken on the desired flavor.

Alcoholic beverages can also add flavor. For example, **sherry** and **brandies** add flavor to low-fat sauces. **Liqueurs**, wines, and brandies are frequently used in baked goods. For example, a liqueur such as kahlua or amaretto is used in cheesecakes, and brandy may be used in custards and creams.

Other ingredients can also be used to get flavor back into products

To make an infused vinegar, boil the vinegar and ingredients, then simmer for 2 to 20 minutes - depending on how strong you want it to be. Heat releases the flavor. Cool and use.

Sherry is a fortified wine. Brandy is a distilled spirit made from wine or other fermented fruit juice. A liqueur, also called cordial, is a brandy or other spirit sweetened and flavored with natural flavorers.

LOW SODIUM SEASONING CHART

Try These Spice Combinations

Poultry

► Rosemary and thyme
► Tarragon, marjoram and onion and garlic powders
► Cumin, bay leaf and saffron (or turmeric)
► Ginger, cinnamon and allspice
► Curry powder, thyme and onion powder

Fish and Seafood

► Cumin and oregano
► Tarragon, thyme, parsley flakes and garlic powder
► Thyme, fennel, saffron and red pepper
► Ginger, sesame and white pepper
► Cilantro, parsley flakes, cumin and garlic powder

Beef

► Thyme, bay leaf and instant minced onion
► Ginger, dry mustard and garlic powder
► Dill, nutmeg and allspice
► Black pepper, bay leaf and cloves
► Chili powder,* cinnamon and oregano

Pork

► Caraway, red pepper and paprika
► Thyme, dry mustard and sage
► Oregano and bay leaf
► Anise, ginger and sesame
► Tarragon, bay leaf and instant minced garlic

Vegetables

Beans (green) – Marjoram and rosemary; caraway and dry mustard
Broccoli – Ginger and garlic powder; sesame and nutmeg
Cabbage – Celery seeds and dill; curry powder and nutmeg
Carrots – Cinnamon and nutmeg; ginger and onion powder
Corn – Chili powder* and cumin; dill and onion powder
Peas – Anise and onion powder; rosemary and marjoram
Spinach – Curry powder and ginger; nutmeg and garlic powder
Squash (summer) – Mint and parsley flakes; tarragon and garlic powder
Squash (winter) – Cinnamon and nutmeg; allspice and red pepper
Tomatoes – Basil and rosemary; cinnamon and ginger

Potatoes, Rice and Pasta

Potatoes – Dill, onion powder and parsley flakes; caraway and onion powder; nutmeg and freeze-dried chives
Rice – Chili powder* and cumin; curry powder, ginger and coriander; cinnamon, cardamom and cloves
Pasta – Basil, rosemary and parsley flakes; cumin, turmeric and red pepper; oregano and thyme

Fruits

Apples – Cinnamon, allspice and nutmeg; ginger and curry powder
Bananas – Allspice and cinnamon; nutmeg and ginger
Peaches – Coriander and mint flakes; cinnamon and ginger
Oranges – Cinnamon and cloves; poppy and onion powder
Pears – Ginger and cardamom; black (or red) pepper and cinnamon
Cranberries – Allspice and coriander; cinnamon and dry mustard
Strawberries or Kiwi fruit – Cinnamon and ginger; black pepper and nutmeg

Note: Black pepper may be routinely used in all dishes including some fruits as a basic seasoning. When listed in this chart, it's intended to be a major flavoring.

*No salt variety available.

Tips For Seasoning Low Sodium Dishes

WHEN ELIMINATING SALT:
► Double the marinating time for poultry and meat for more complete flavor penetration.
► Increase the amount of spices and herbs in recipes by about 25 percent.
► With long cooking dishes, reserve about 25 percent of the seasonings to add during the last ten minutes of cooking; herbs should be finely crushed.

For best flavor results, keep spices in tightly covered containers away from heat and light. Check them regularly. As soon as they lose their aroma and color they should be replaced.

Prepared by the American Spice Trade Association

FIGURE 13-2. Seasoning and flavoring guide (courtesy American Spice Trade Association)

with less fat, such as baked goods or sauces. They include dried fruits, **zests** of citrus fruits (the grated skin), fruit jams and jellies, sweet herbs and spices, extracts such as vanilla and almond, instant coffee, cocoa powder, and highly flavored sugars such as brown sugar and molasses.

MINI-SUMMARY Seasonings and flavoring are important in modified recipes because they help replace missing ingredients such as fat and salt in satisfying the taste buds. Seasonings are used to bring out flavors already present in a dish, whereas flavorings add a new flavor or modify the original flavor. The difference between them is one of degree. Flavored vinegars, flavored oils, and certain alcoholic beverages can be used successfully as flavorings in certain dishes.

MODIFYING ACTUAL RECIPES

Monte Cristo Sandwich

Let's start with the Monte Cristo sandwich given at the beginning of the chapter.

Original Monte Cristo Sandwich	*Yield: 100 portions*
Ingredients	*Amount*
Ham, cooked, boneless	100 1-oz. slices
Turkey, cooked, boneless	100 1-oz. slices
Swiss cheese	100 1-oz. slices
White bread	200 slices
Whole milk	6 cups
Salt	2 teaspoons
Eggs, whole, slightly beaten	2 quarts (48 eggs)
Shortening, melted	1 quart

DIRECTIONS: Place one slice each of ham, turkey, and cheese on one slice of bread and top with a second slice. Blend milk, eggs, and salt. Dip each side of the sandwich into the egg and milk mixture; drain. Grill each sandwich on a well-greased griddle about 2 minutes on each side or until golden brown and the cheese is melted.

Here are some modifications you can make.

1. For less fat and saturated fat, select low fat turkey ham instead of regular ham and use less of it. Also, either roast your own turkey breast or make sure the brand you purchase is low in fat.
2. Like the ham, the Swiss cheese adds much of the distinctive flavor to this sandwich. To reduce the fat and saturated fat, you can use less than

      1 ounce of Swiss—about 1/2 to 3/4 ounce should be enough.

3.   If you wish to add fiber (and more nutrients), use a whole-grain bread instead of white bread. It will also add flavor, especially if it is an interesting vegetable or seed bread.

4.   Instead of dipping the sandwich in eggs and whole milk, use egg substitutes or egg whites and skim milk.

5.   A quicker, and healthier, way to cook the sandwiches would be to place them on a sheet pan coated with butter-flavored cooking spray and bake them in a moderate-high oven.

6.   Salt is not really needed in the recipe because the turkey ham, cheese, and bread already contain moderate to higher amounts of sodium.

7.   One way to add back some flavor to this sandwich is to add some grilled vegetables, such as onions and peppers, or use them as an accompaniment on the plate.

Chicken Pot Pie

Original Pot Pie

Yield: 4 individual pot pies

Ingredients for the crust:	*Amount*
Flour	1 cup
Salt	¼ teaspoon
Lard	⅓ cup
Cold water	2 tablespoons

For the pie:	
Potatoes, diced	⅓ cup
Carrots, sliced	⅓ cup
Frozen green peas	⅓ cup
Celery, chopped	¼ cup
Onion, chopped	1 tablespoon
Butter	¼ cup
Flour	¼ cup
Salt	½ teaspoon
Pepper	⅛ teaspoon
Poultry seasoning	⅛ teaspoon
Turkey broth, unsalted	1⅓ cups
Light cream	⅔ cup
Chicken, cooked, diced	1½ cups

DIRECTIONS: For pie crust, mix flour and salt thoroughly. Cut the lard in until the mixture is crumbly. Add cold water and form the dough into a ball. Divide the dough into 4 pieces and roll each piece between 2 sheets of waxed paper until it is at least 1/2 inch wider than the baking dishes.

For filling, add the vegetables to boiling water and boil gently until the vegetables are just tender, about 6 minutes, then drain. Melt the butter, then stir in the flour and seasonings. Add the broth and milk slowly, stirring constantly. Cook until thickened. Stir in the turkey and vegetables. Pour into four 1-cup baking dishes. Put one piece of rolled pastry on each dish and fold the edges under. Flute the edges of the dough with fingers or press lightly with the tines of a fork. Cut several small slits in the dough for steam to escape during baking. Bake at 400 degrees F. until crusts are browned and filling is bubbly, about 40 minutes.

Some modifications you can make include the following:

1. Make only half the pie crust recipe (it needs some changes too) and lay an attractive lattice top on each pot pie.
2. For each cup of flour for the pie crust, you need only 3 tablespoons of fat—not 1/3 cup. To give the crust its characteristic flakiness, split the 3 tablespoons equally between vegetable shortening and margarine. Lard is a highly saturated fat and can easily be replaced with other fats. When using this formulation, you will need a little more water—between 3 to 4 tablespoons.
3. A healthier way to cook the vegetables is to steam them.
4. For the roux use 2 tablespoons of margarine instead of 1/4 cup of butter. Other thickeners, such as flour with water or vegetable purees, could be used.
5. Instead of light cream, use evaporated skim milk, which has 50 percent of its water content removed.
6. For more flavor, more onions would help, perhaps along with some sherry.

Beef Stroganoff
Original Beef Stroganoff

Original Beef Stroganoff	*Yield: 4 servings*
Ingredients	*Amount*
Beef round steak, cut in strips	1 pound
Flour	2 ounces
Salt	1 teaspoon
Pepper	¼ teaspoon
Butter	4 tablespoons
Onion, chopped	¼ cup
Mushrooms, sliced	½ cup
Beef stock	1 cup
Sour cream	6 ounces

DIRECTIONS: Dredge the meat in the flour, salt, and pepper, and brown it in butter. Add the onions and mushrooms and sauté. Pour the beef stock in and simmer 1½ hours until the meat is tender. Turn off the heat and stir in the sour cream until thickened. Serve over noodles.

Some modifications you can make include the following:

1. Use less meat—12 ounces would be fine for 4 servings.
2. Cut the beef into bite-size strips and stir-fry in oil instead of butter.
3. Use more fresh mushrooms and tomatoes for flavor and body.
4. Use defatted beef stock and tomato paste for a sauce.
5. Use plain nonfat yogurt stabilized with cornstarch and flavored with wine instead of sour cream.

MINI-SUMMARY The techniques described in this section can reduce the fat in a recipe and add flavor.

EVALUATING HEALTHY COOKBOOKS

Many more cookbooks with nutrition and health as their theme are new on the market. Because the quality of these cookbooks can vary immensely, here are some guidelines for choosing the best ones.

1. Dismiss those that promise miracles such as adding years to your life.
2. Evaluate the recipes from a nutrition standpoint. Just because a cookbook is advertised as containing healthy or diet recipes does not mean this is the case. Check to see if the recipes include a nutrient analysis. Such analyses are helpful in answering these questions:
     Are carbohydrates emphasized over fat and protein?
     Are high-fiber foods emphasized?
     Are lean meats, poultry, and fish emphasized?
     Are desserts still high in fat?
     Are the recipes in low-sodium cookbooks also low in fat?
     Are the recipes in low-sugar cookbooks also low in fat?
3. Do the recipes seem appealing? Would they meet customers' needs? Do they require too much preparation time? Are the ingredients readily available? Is special cooking equipment required?
4. If you like the answers to these questions, buy the book!

MINI-SUMMARY Choose healthy cookbooks with appealing and truly nutritious recipes that fit your needs.

KEY TERMS

Balsamic vinegar
Brandy
Brioche
Carcinogens
Cider vinegar
Coulis
Croissants
Fat-off ladle
Fat-separator pitcher
Flavored oils
Flavored (infused) vinegars
Flavorings
Fromage blanc
Fusion cooking
Herbs

Ice milk
Liqueurs
Marinades
Nonstick pans
Popovers
Purees of cooked vegetables
Rubs
Seasonings
Sherry
Slurry
Spices
White whole-wheat flour
Wine vinegars
Wok
Zests

REVIEW QUESTIONS

1   List four ways to modify a recipe.
2. List three prepreparation techniques that either reduce fat or add flavor.
3. Is it necessary to remove poultry skin before cooking to reduce fat content? Explain why or why not.
4. What is a rub and how is it used?
5. What is a marinade and how is it used?
6. Which dry-heat and moist-heat cooking methods do not add fat and/or allow fat to drip away?
7. How can you make frying more acceptable?
8. Describe the four ways you can modify ingredients.
9. What questions do you need to consider when you modify ingredients?
10. Complete the following substitution table.

Instead of	*Use*
Butter	
Whole milk	
Cream	
Sour cream	
Cream cheese	
Cheddar cheese	
Whole egg	
Ice cream	
Roux	
Fatty meats	

11. How much sugar and salt can be reduced in a baking recipe without affecting quality?
12. What can you add to increase the amount of fiber in baked goods?
13. Can you use reduced-fat margarines and nonfat cream cheese successfully in baking? Describe why or why not?
14. What is white whole-wheat flour?
15. Define seasoning, flavoring, herb, and spice.
16. What are infused vinegars and oils? How can they be used?

1. Modifying Home Recipes

Collect three recipes from cookbooks, newspapers, or home recipe collections as follows: 1 main dish, 1 side dish, and 1 dessert. Detail how each recipe could be modified using tips and guidelines given in this chapter. If possible, test a modified recipe.

2. Design a Salad Bar

You are to design a new salad bar for a quick-service operation in California that emphasizes fresh, nutritious foods. Come up with 2 selections of salad greens, 16 selections of toppings, and 4 salad dressings that would be appropriate.

3. Seasonings and Flavorings in Recipes

Pick out ten recipes and write down the names of seasonings and flavorings used in each.

4. Supermarket Sleuth

Visit your local supermarket and check out the lower-in-fat options available in the milk, sour cream, yogurt, cream cheese, cheese, margarine, salad dressing, and baked goods sections. Write down two examples from each section.

5. Low-Fat Brownies

List the function of each of the ingredient in the following recipe. Next, modify the recipe so it has less fat. Try out your recipe and evaluate the results.

Regular Brownies	**Makes 16**
Ingredients	*Amount*
Butter	½ cup
Unsweetened chocolate	2 squares (2 ounces)
Sugar	1 cup

Eggs	2
Vanilla	1 teaspoon
All-purpose flour	¾ cup
Chopped nuts	½ cup

DIRECTIONS: Melt the margarine and chocolate over a low heat. Remove from the heat and stir in the sugar, eggs, and vanilla. Beat lightly by hand just until combined. Next, stir in the flour and nuts. Spread the batter in a greased 8-inch square baking pan and bake at 350 degrees F. for 30 minutes. Cool.

6. Computerized Nutrient Analysis

Do a nutrient analysis of a recipe from a cookbook that has all the recipes analyzed. Compare your results to the book's nutrient analysis. Are they close? Why or why not?

REFERENCES

Carpenter, Hugh, and Teri Sandison. 1994. *Fusion Cooking.* New York: Artisan.

Culinary Institute of America. 1996. *The New Professional Chef.* New York: Van Nostrand Reinhold.

Egan, Maureen, and Susan Davis Allen. 1992. *Healthful Quantity Baking.* New York: John Wiley & Sons.

Kapoor, Sandy. 1995. *Professional Healthy Cooking.* New York: John Wiley & Sons.

Regan, Claire. 1986. Revising recipes to improve nutritional quality. *Restaurants USA* 6(7): 18.

Ruggiero, Tina. 1995. The war on fat: An update from the frying front. *Restaurants USA* 15(2): 18–22.

Solomon, Jay. 1992. The art of global grilling. *Restaurants USA* 12(5):14-17.

Somerville, Sylvia. 1994. Fusion cuisine: A decade of melding cultures has sparked creativity and controversy. *Restaurants USA* 14(8): 22–26.

Welland, Diane. 1993. Making a healthy plate look great. *Restaurants USA* 13(7): 20–23.

Welland, Diane. 1993. Splash on some flavored vinegars. *Restaurants USA* 13(2): 12–14.

Woodier, Olwen. 1987. A taste of herbs and spices. *Food Management* 22(6): 140–146.

Healthy Cookbooks

Culinary Institute of America. 1993. *Techniques of Healthy Cooking.* New York: Van Nostrand Reinhold.

Egan, Maureen, and Susan Davis Allen. 1992. *Healthful Quantity Baking.* New York: John Wiley & Sons.

Kapoor, Sandy. 1995. *Professional Healthy Cooking.* New York: John Wiley & Sons.

Moosewood Collective. 1996. *Moosewood Restaurant Cooks for a Crowd: Recipes with a Vegetarian Emphasis for 24 or More.* New York: John Wiley & Sons.

1995 Cooking Light Cookbook. 1995. Birmingham: Oxmoor House.

Purdy, Susan. 1993. *Have Your Cake and Eat It Too.* New York: William Morrow and Company.

Turner, Stephanie, and Vivienne Aronowitz. 1990. *Healthwise Quantity Cookbook.* Washington DC: Center for Science in the Public Interest.

Winston, Mary, ed. 1991. *American Heart Association Cookbook,* 5th ed. New York: Random House.

CHAPTER

14

Marketing Healthy Menu Options

**KEY
QUESTIONS**

1. What methods can foodservice operators use to determine the needs and wants of the clientele for healthy foods?
2. How can you make your customers aware of the healthy dishes that are available?
3. What can be done to promote nutritious menu items?
4. Which staff members need to be trained before offering menu options, and what topics need to be included in the training?
5. How do you evaluate the success or failure of healthy menu items?

QUIZ

Quiz
1. Marketing includes
   a. finding out what consumers want and need.
   b. developing a product consumers want and need.
   c. promoting the product.
   d. all of the above
2. When hearing descriptions of healthy menu entrees, most customers
   a. want complete nutrient information.
   b. want fat, saturated fat, and cholesterol information.
   c. want good descriptions of the ingredients, portion size, and method of preparation.
   d. none of the above
3. When you tout foods as "heart healthy," you are approaching customers in a negative manner.
   True   False
4. An example of publicity is
   a. radio advertising.
   b. a press release.
   c. recipes from a food association.
   d. a point-of-purchase display.
5. When you evaluate the success or failure of a healthy menu, you need to get feedback from
   a. customers.
   b. staff.
   c. managers.
   d. all of the above

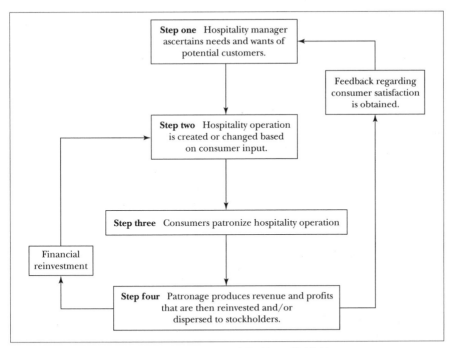

From Robert Reid. 1989. *Hospitality Marketing Management.* New York: Van Nostrand Reinhold.

INTRODUCTION

Before discussing how to market healthy menu options, let's first define **marketing**.

Hospitality marketing is defined as encompassing the following activities.
- Ascertaining consumer needs and wants
- Creating the product-service mix that satisfies these needs and wants
- Promoting and selling the product-service mix in order to generate a level of income satisfactory to the management and stockholders of the organization (Reid, 1989)

These steps are illustrated in Figure 14-1, the **marketing cycle**, and will be discussed in this chapter as they relate to marketing healthy menu options. Resources for developing healthy menu options are listed in Appendix E.

MINI-SUMMARY Marketing means finding out what your customers need and want, developing what they need and want, and then promoting what will hopefully be a successful program.

GAUGING CUSTOMERS' NEEDS AND WANTS

Most foodservice operators who have successfully implemented healthy menu options have done so through reviewing eating trends, examining what other operators are doing, and keeping abreast of their customers' requests for healthy foods. To determine customer wants, foodservice operators could interview the waitstaff about customer requests, for example, for light foods such as broiled meat, poultry, or fish; dishes prepared without salt; sauces and gravies removed or served on the side; butter substitutes; reduced-calorie salad dressing; or skim or low-fat milk.

Another way to gauge customer needs is to do a survey as shown in Figure 14-2. At the same time, answers to the following questions need to be considered.

When doing customer surveys, more customers will respond if they receive something, like a free beverage, for filling out the survey form.

1. What are the majority of requests made during a certain meal?
2. Which items are most frequently requested?
3. How much time does your cooking staff and waitstaff have to meet these special requests?
4. Which requests are easy to meet? Which are very time-consuming?

Answers to these questions can help you decide which types of healthy menu items to offer.

If market research demonstrates a sizable need for healthy entrees and the like, and there is enough time and staff to commit to this project, then now may be the time to do more than meet customers' special requests.

MINI-SUMMARY   Customer interest in nutritious menu items can be gauged through waitstaff feedback and customer surveys.

DEVELOPING AND IMPLEMENTING HEALTHY MENU OPTIONS

Various personnel are normally involved in the development and implementation phase: foodservice operators, directors, and managers; chefs and cooking staff; and nutrition experts such as registered dietitians. Chefs and cooking staff are valuable resources in modifying recipes or creating new ones, and may be given much of this responsibility. Nutrition experts are needed to provide accurate nutrient analysis data as well as suggestions for modifying dishes. In larger companies, personnel responsible for training, advertising and publicity, marketing, menu planning, and recipe development may also be involved.

Chapters 12 and 13 covered the basics of developing healthy menu items and modifying recipes. Once you know what you want to offer, you

Figure 14-2.

Customer survey

1. How often do you visit this restaurant?
   First visit
   Once or twice a year
   Once every three months
   Once every two months
   Once a month
   Two or three times a month
   Once a week
   More than once a week
2. Today I came for:
   Breakfast
   Lunch
   Dinner
   Snack
3. Are you here during your work day?
   Yes No
4. Are you here for social reasons?
   Yes No
5. Have you ever been to a restaurant that offers light and nutritious menu choices?
   Yes No
6. Would you order light and nutritious foods if they were offered here?
   Yes, frequently
   Yes, sometimes
   No
   Not sure
7. How likely would you be to try the following nutritious menu choices?

Menu Choice	Very Likely	Likely	Unlikely
A. Broiled fish without butter			
B. Reduced calorie salad dressing			
C. Vegetables with no added salt			

need to think about how to inform your clientele of these options. Here are some suggestions.

1. Highlight nutritious menu selections with symbols or words such as "light." For example, put a picture of wheat next to nutrition selections that meet specific nutrition goals, usually described at the bottom of the menu (Figure 14-3).

2. Include a special, separate section on the regular menu. With this format, customers are certain to see the nutritious options, and see them as being integrated into the foodservice concept. A heading for this section might be "Fit Fare."

Hot Topic: Alcohol and Nutrition

Alcohol is a depressant drug that slows the nervous system. Its effects may include, depending on the level of alcohol consumed:

Loss of inhibition
Slurred speech
Loss of some muscle coordination
Aggressiveness
Unconsciousness, if too much alcohol is consumed

When you drink alcoholic beverages, the alcohol passes from the stomach and intestine into the blood, where it travels all around your body. If you drink on an empty stomach, the alcohol will pass into your blood in about 20 minutes. Many factors affect the absorption of alcohol into the blood, including

Amount of alcohol consumed
Rate of consumption
Weight (a given amount of alcohol affects small people more intensely than heavier people)
Sex (alcohol is absorbed quicker in women than men)
Whether you eat before or while drinking (food slows the stomach's emptying rate, dilutes the alcohol, and slows its absorption)

An accurate way to determine how much alcohol has been consumed is through a Blood Alcohol Concentration (BAC) test. At 0.10 level, a customer is legally intoxicated in many states and driving ability is impaired. At 0.20, a customer is 100 times more of a traffic risk.

About two-thirds of all American adults drink alcohol at least occasionally. Current evidence suggests that moderate drinking is associated with a lower risk for coronary heart disease in some individuals. However, higher levels of alcohol intake raise the risk for high blood pressure, stroke, heart disease, certain cancers, accidents, violence, suicides, birth defects, and overall mortality. About 7 percent of individuals who drink alcohol will develop moderate to serious symptoms of alcohol dependence. Too much alcohol may cause inflammation of the pancreas, damage to the brain and heart, **fatty liver**, and **cirrhosis** of the liver.

Fatty liver is the first stage of liver deterioration seen in heavy drinkers. The liver tissue starts to break down and becomes filled with fat. Eventually the fat chokes off the blood supply to the liver and liver cells die. All functions of the liver, such as making glucose and processing alcohol and drugs, decrease. In the next stage of liver disease, scar tissue develops. Up to this point, if the alcoholic stays away from alcohol and gets proper nutrition, the damage is mostly reversible. The final stage of liver disease is cirrhosis. At this point liver cells harden and die, and the damage is irreversible. Symptoms of cirrhosis include nausea, poor appetite, weight loss, weakness, and stomach pain.

Heavy drinkers are also at risk of developing non-insulin-dependent diabetes and malnutrition. Alcohol contains calories that often substitute for those in more nutritious foods. Almost 100 percent of alcoholic patients with serious liver problems also suffer from malnutrition. Deficiencies of many nutrients are common, including thiamin, niacin, folate, and vitamins A, B_6, C, and D. Some of these deficiencies result from a poor diet, whereas others are due to liver malfunction and problems with digesting foods and absorbing nutrients.

A popular screening device for alcohol abuse uses the following questions.

1. Have you ever felt you ought to cut down on drinking?
2. Have people annoyed you by criticizing your drinking?
3. Have you ever felt bad or guilty about your drinking?
4. Have you ever had a drink first thing in the morning to steady your nerves or get rid of a hangover?

If just one question is answered with a "yes," it could mean an alcohol problem.

Some people should not drink alcoholic beverages at all. These include

- Children and adolescents

- Individuals of any age who cannot restrict their drinking to moderate levels. This is a special concern for recovering alcoholics and people with a family history of alcohol problems.
- Women who are trying to conceive or who are pregnant. Major birth defects, including fetal alcohol syndrome, have been attributed to heavy drinking by the mother while pregnant. Although there is no conclusive evidence that an occasional drink is harmful to the fetus or to the pregnant woman, a safe level of alcohol intake during pregnancy has not been established.
- Individuals who plan to drive or take part in activities that require attention or skill. Most people retain some alcohol in the blood for as long as 2 to 3 hours after a single drink.
- Individuals using prescription and over-the-counter medications. Alcohol may alter the effectiveness or toxicity of medicines. Also, some medications may increase blood alcohol levels or increase the adverse effect of alcohol on the brain.

If you drink alcoholic beverages, do so in moderation, with meals, and when consumption does not put you or others at risk.

3. Add a clip-on to the regular menu and/or a blackboard or lightboard. This method requires no alterations to the menu and is particularly useful in that it is flexible and inexpensive. Healthy selections can be changed without involving much time or money. In some operations, treating the nutrition selections like daily specials has increased their selling power.
4. Use the waitstaff to offer and describe nutritious menu options. In some instances, healthier preparation methods can be suggested for regular menu items.

No matter which method you use to include healthy selections on the menu, you must consider how thorough a description is appropriate. In general, customers do not want calorie counts, fat, cholesterol, or sodium content on the menu, but prefer simply a good description of the ingredients, portion size, and preparation method. Menu items are more effectively promoted by emphasizing quality and variety rather than nutrition.

Market healthy foods in a positive, not negative, way.

Marketing healthy menu items can be done either positively or negatively. When you tout foods as "heart healthy," you are approaching customers in a negative manner. For example, when you market freshly squeezed fruit juices, you are approaching customers in a positive manner.

Promotion

Three methods of promoting a nutrition program are advertising, sales promotion, and publicity. Advertising can be done through magazines and newspapers, radio and television, outdoor displays (posters and signs), indoor table tents and posters, direct mail, and novelties (such as matchboxes). Direct mail works well when targeted to current customers.

Advertising messages should say something desirable, beneficial, distinctive, and believable about the nutritious dining program. For example, the new menu selections could be advertised as healthy and using only the freshest, most exotic ingredients. Because foodservice operators need to get the best advertising for the money, hiring a reputable advertising company may be the best option.

Sales promotions can include coupons, point-of-purchase displays (such as a blackboard at the dining room entrance listing the nutrition selections), or contests (such as having customers guess the number of calories in a nutritious dining entree to win a free meal).

Publicity involves obtaining free editorial space or time in various media. Many foodservice operators do their own publicity. However, if you wish to obtain the advice of outside publicity consultants, O'Dwyers Directory includes most public relations firms. Here are some ideas for publicizing your nutrition program.

St. Andrew's Cafe

Starters
(Small / Large)

Mussels Steamed in White Wine, Shallots and Saffron 5.25 / 9.50

Wood-grilled Shrimp with Spicy Carrot and Tarragon Juice 5.95 / 10.90

Lobster and Shrimp Ravioli with Shellfish-Chervil Broth 6.95 / 12.90

☙ Wild Mushroom Risotto with White Truffle Oil 5.95/10.90

Cold Smoked Moulard Duck Breast with Root Vegetable Salad and Black Currant Sauce 5.25

Soups and Salads

☙ Chestnut Soup with Ginger Cream 3.50

Woodlands Duck and Wild Rice Soup 3.50

☙ "Salad Lorette" with Bibb Lettuce, Celeriac, Beet Root, Apples, and Walnut Dressing 3.75

☙ Pickled Beet and Baby Lettuce Salad with Blue Cheese and Red Onion 3.75

☙ Dressed Local Organic Lettuces 3.00
Choice of Lemon-Thyme Vinaigrette, Creamy Blue Cheese or Creamy Herb Dressing

Wood-fired Pizzas
(Small 4.25 or Large 5.75)

☙ Mediterranean-style with Sun-dried Tomatoes, Artichokes, Fennel,
Calamata Olives and Romano Cheese

☙ White-style Pizza with Coach Farm Goat Cheese and Wild Mushrooms

Pizza Selection of the Day

At St. Andrew's Cafe, we believe that eating wisely should be enjoyable. Menus are planned to follow guidelines of balance, nutrition, and taste. Our aim is that each dish be moderate in terms of the amount of calories, fat, cholesterol, and sodium it contains but also be prepared according to the good culinary principles of taste and presentation. ☙ The Culinary Institute of America has served as a leader for many advances in the foodservice and hospitality industry, including the incorporation of nutrition into fine cuisine. The General Foods Nutrition Center and St. Andrew's Cafe are examples of our commitment to the constant refinement of our educational mission. ☙ St. Andrew's Cafe is one of four award-winning, student-staffed restaurants open to the public at The Culinary Institute of America. All are staffed by students in the final semester of the school's associate degree programs. We hope you enjoy your meal and encourage you to dine with us often.
For restaurant reservations and information, call (914) 471-6608.

Main Courses

Caramelized Baby Red Snapper Fillet Provençal 13.75

☙ Garbanzo Bean Stew with Portabella Mushroom and Grilled Flat Bread 8.95

Pan-seared Venison Loin Noisettes with Apples, Pears and Port Wine Jus 17.00

Wood-Grilled Main Courses

Breast of Chicken with Black Bean Sauce, Curried Onions
and Roasted Eggplant and Mango Relishes 10.50

Prosciutto-wrapped Quail with Sun-dried Figs and Soft Polenta 15.75

Peppered Tenderloin of Double J Ranch Limousin Beef with Oven-roasted Potatoes
and Stone Ground Mustard Sauce 15.25

Atlantic Salmon Fillet with Lentil Ragout, Braised Greens, Fennel and Horseradish Cream 14.50

Side-Dish Selections

☙ Marinated Mushrooms 1.50

Cous Cous with Black Bean Sauce 1.50

☙ Chilled Grilled Bell Peppers 1.50

☙ Parsnip and Potato Puree with Vegetable Gravy 1.50

☙ **Indicates Vegetarian Selections**

NOT-FOR-PROFIT STATEMENT

The Culinary Institute of America is an independent, not-for-profit educational organization pursuing its mission of providing the highest quality culinary education. This not-for-profit status enables us to focus on the quality of education rather than on satisfying the investment expectations of any shareholders.
St. Andrew's Cafe is a non-smoking restaurant. Thank you for your cooperation.

AMERICA'S CENTER FOR CULINARY EDUCATION SINCE 1946

433 Albany Post Road, Hyde Park, NY 12538-1499

FIGURE 14-3.
St. Andrew's
Cafe menu.
Courtesy: The
Culinary Institute
of America,
Hyde Park, NY

A press or news release is sent to various news media in hopes that they may pick up your story and use it. The first paragraph often tells the who, what, when, where, and why of your story.

1. Send a **press release** about your healthy dining options to the appropriate contact person by name, not title, as indicated in the following list.

    Television and radio news: Assignment editor or specialty reporters appropriate to your story, such as health and food editors

    Television and radio talk shows: Producer

    Newspapers: Section editors (food, health and science, lifestyle), or city desk editor for special events

    Magazines and trade publications: Managing editor, articles editor, or specialty editors appropriate to your story

    Local publications and newsletters: Corporate employee or customer newsletters, or supermarket, utility company, bank, school, and church publications

    Follow up each press release with a phone call. Editors are always looking for article ideas and just may pick up on your story.

2. Offer to write a column on nutritious meal preparation for a local newspaper.
3. Offer cooking demonstrations or on-site classes, or volunteer to conduct classes for health associations, retail stores, and supermarkets.
4. Invite local media and community leaders for the opening day of your new program and let them taste some nutritious menu selections.
5. Contact the foodservice director of a medical center or the public relations director of a health maintenance organization and offer to cosponsor a health or nutrition event such as a bike race or health fair. Check for local health and sporting events in which you can participate.
6. Contact your local American Heart Association and ask if it has a "Dining Out Guide" in which to feature your restaurant.
7. Develop a newsletter for your operation and use it to publicize the new program (include some of your nutritious recipes). Newsletters help to build loyal customers.

There are many sources for promotional materials such as table tents, posters, buttons, menu clip-ons, point-of-sale materials, and artwork (Appendix E). Food manufacturers, foodservice distributors, and food marketing boards and associations are excellent sources of promotional materials. Each year, Restaurants and Institutions publishes a listing of food boards and associations that provide recipes and other promotional materials, many of which feature healthful dining.

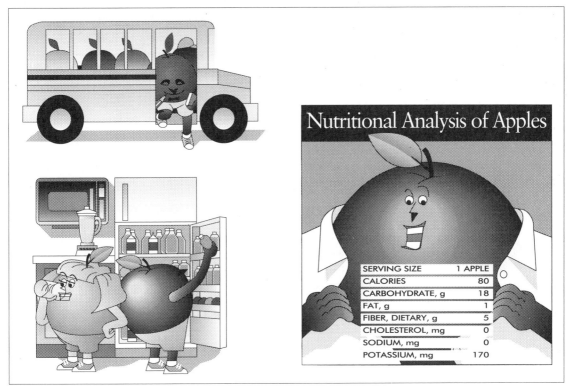

FIGURE 14-4. Artwork from International Apple Institute

Staff Training

Staff training centers on the waitstaff and the cooking staff. Before training begins, involve the waitstaff as much as possible in developing your nutrition program so that they feel a part of it and take some ownership. They can be a valued resource in designing the program because they make daily contact with the customers both in selling and serving as well as in listening to requests, compliments, and complaints. During training, the waitstaff needs to understand:

- the scope and rationale for the nutrition program.
- grand opening details.
- the ingredients, preparation, and service for each menu item.
- some basic food and nutrition concepts so they can help guests with special dietary concerns such as food allergies (see page 128 for a full discussion on food allergies).

Figure 14-4 shows artwork available from the International Apple Institute that can be used, particularly by schools, to promote apples.

TABLE 14-1. Learning objectives for service staff.

1. Servers must be able to respond to consumer health concerns by providing menu suggestions that meet their dietary needs. They should be able to make menu suggestions for the following dietary restrictions:

   Low calorie

   Low sodium

   Low cholesterol and low fat

   Low sodium, low cholesterol, and low fat

   High fiber

2. The wait staff should be able to describe healthful dining options in straightforward, appropriate language to patrons. Servers must be able to provide information on ingredients, methods of preparation, portion sizes, and how the menu items are served.

   Ingredients: The wait staff should be knowledgeable about details regarding ingredient usage: addition of fat or the type of fat used in cooking, the use of salt or high-sodium seasonings, cuts of meats used, the type of liquids used to prepare menu items, fats and thickening agents used in sauces, and the use of sugar or sugar substitutes.

   Cooking methods: Patrons commonly need to know not only what the composition of a menu item is but how it was prepared. Was the food fried in vegetable oil or animal shortening? Was the food prepared by pan frying, broiling, baking, poaching or sautéing? Can the item be broiled without added butter? Is fat removed form meat juices or stocks before using them for sauces or soups?

   Presentation and portions: Patrons frequently want to know how the item will be served when making their menu selections. The waitstaff should be prepared to answer the following questions: What is the portion size of the item? What accompaniments are served with the item? Are special food items available to accompany the item? For example, is light syrup available for the light pancakes? Is a fruit spread available instead of jam for the whole-wheat brads? Can toast be served dry instead of buttered? Can salad dressing be served on the side?

3. The waitstaff should be able to explain the nutritional basis for menu items designated as light or healthful in terms of caloric, fat, cholesterol, and/or sodium content. They may need to answer questions about the program rationale. They should know the nutritional guidelines (US dietary guidelines, American Heart Association guidelines, and/or National Cancer Institute recommendations) that provide the basis for the program.

4. Servers should be able to respond to patron inquiries about the availability of special foods or beverages. Does the restaurant serve brewed decaffeinated coffee? Are diet salad dressings available for the light salad entrees? Is margarine available instead of butter? Are herb seasonings available instead of salt for adjusting seasonings at the table? Does the restaurant serve skim milk?

5. The waitstaff should be able to respond to questions concerning substitutions of meal accompaniments. Can an entree be served with two vegetables instead of a vegetable and a starch? Can a salad be substituted for the starch or vegetable served with the entree? Can a fruit appetizer be served for dessert?

6. The wait staff need to know what special requests the foodservice operation can accommodate. For example, can margarine or vegetable oil be used instead of butter in preparing foods? Can entrees be broiled instead of fried? Are smaller portion sizes available? Can sauces and salad dressing be served on the side?

7. The wait staff should be able to recommend other foods and beverages that complement menu choices, including appetizers, soups, salads, desserts, and beverages that are light or meet the dietary restrictions of the patron.

8. The waitstaff should be knowledgeable about what is served with light menu items and what the correct portion sizes are for these items. Servers will act as the final quality control agents prior to the service of the foods. If light menu items are similar to traditional offerings, the waitstaff should be able to distinguish between the two items.

9. Staff members should respond politely and accurately to guest questions about healthful dining options. It should be emphasized that the proper response to a patron's inquiry is "I can find out for you," not "I don't know." When uncertain of the answer, the staff member should ask the kitchen manager, manager, or chef.

Source: Ganem, Beth Carlson. 1990. *Nutrition Menu Concepts for the Hospitality Industry.* New York: Van Nostrand Reinhold.

TABLE 14-2. How employees learn best.

1. When employees participate in their own training, they tend to identify with and retain the concepts being taught. To get employees involved, choose appropriate training methods.

2. Employees learn best when training material is practical, relevant, useful, and geared to an appropriate level. Learning is facilitated, too, when the material is well organized and presented in small, easy-to-grasp steps. Adult learners are selective about what they will spend time learning, and learning must be especially pertinent and rewarding for them. Adults also need to be able to master new skills at their own pace.

3. Employees learn best in an informal, quiet, and comfortable setting. Your effort in selecting and maintaining an appropriate training environment shows employees that you think their training is important. When employees are stuffed into a crowded office or a noisy part of the kitchen, or when the trainer is interrupted by phone calls, they may rightly feel that their training isn't really important. Employees like to feel special; so, when possible, find a quiet setting. Of course, much training, such as on-the-job training, necessarily takes place in the work environment.

4. Employees learn best when they are being paid for time spend in training.

5. Employees learn best with a good trainer. Although you may not ever find a person with all these qualities, you can use this list to evaluate potential trainers:

Characteristics of a Successful Trainer
- Is knowledgeable
- Display enthusiasm
- Has a sense of humor
- Communicates clearly, concisely, straightforwardly
- Is sincere, caring, respectful, responsive to employees
- Encourages employee performance; is patient
- Sets an appropriate role model
- Is well organized
- Maintains control, frequent eye contact with employees
- Listens well
- Is friendly and outgoing
- Keeps calm; is easygoing
- Tries to involve all employees
- Facilitates learning process
- Positively reinforces employees

6. Employees learn best when they receive awards or incentives. For example, on successful completion of training for the position of cook, you can send a letter of recognition to the employee, which can also be put into the personnel file. The largest franchisee of Arby's awards employees a progression of bronze, silver, and gold name tags, as well as pay increases, as they learn each area of the restaurant. When the employee has learned all areas, he or she is promoted to the position of crew leader.

7. Employees learn best when they are coached on their performance on the job.

Source: Drummond, Karen. 1992. *Retraining Your Foodservice Employees.* New York: Van Nostrand Reinhold.

- how to handle special customer requests such as orders for half-portions.
- merchandising and promotional details.

Table 14-1 gives specific learning objectives for the service staff.

A poorly trained waitstaff will confuse the customer and, quite frankly, doom the program instead of knowledgeably promoting it. Conversely, a properly trained waitstaff can function as excellent sales agents and solicit feedback, including customer recommendations.

The cooking staff also needs training. Their training needs center on

- the scope and rationale for the nutrition program.
- grand opening details.
- the ingredients, preparation, portion size, and plating of each new menu item.
- some basic food and nutrition concepts so they can help guests with special dietary concerns such as food allergies.
- how to respond to special dietary requests.

Table 14-2 explains seven ways that employees learn best.

The cooking staff need to understand the prime importance of using only the freshest ingredients, using standardized recipes, measuring and weighing accurately, and attractive presentation.

Training the cooking staff to prepare healthy dishes correctly can be challenging. As managers have found during nutrient-content analysis, cooks do not always prepare recipes exactly as called for. Perhaps a key ingredient was unavailable, time was tight, or the cook forgot a step. Healthy menu items often are more labor-intensive, and more training and coaxing are needed. In any case, cooking staff need training not only in making new menu items but also in the importance of following recipes and serving the correct portion size.

In 1995, the Center for Science in the Public Interest analyzed seventeen healthy entrees from seven of the largest restaurant chains (including T.G.I. Friday's, Denny's, Chili's, Chi Chi's, and the Olive Garden) (Hurley and Liebman, 1995). Although the healthy items had less fat, fewer calories, and more vegetables and fruit than other menu items, several promised less fat than was actually found in the entrees. For example, a fajita from a the menu of a Mexican restaurant was supposed to have only 17 grams of fat but actually had 30 grams of fat. Problems such as this point to the importance of training and retraining cooking staff.

Food Facts: Computerized Nutrient Analysis

Computers are becoming popular tools for analyzing a recipe's nutrient content. Small wonder since a task that used to take a half an hour or more can be completed in less than 5 minutes in front of the computer. Before computers, it was necessary to look up the nutritional content of each recipe ingredient and record it by hand. If ingredient amounts differed, you would have to perform tedious calculations on all the nutrient values to come up with the right numbers. Then, you would have to add up all your columns to get totals. In the final step, you would divide the totals by the yield of the recipe to get the amount of nutrients per serving. Sounds complicated! It sure is, and time-consuming too.

The computer has done a lot to speed up this process and increase its accuracy. Computerized nutrient-analysis programs contain nutrient information on hundreds of items. Just type in the name of an ingredient and the computer will list similar ingredients so that you can choose exactly which one is appropriate. Then simply type in the amount of the ingredient you want analyzed, such as 1 cup. After inputing all the ingredients, you can ask the computer to divide the results by the yield, such as twelve portions. The computer will tell you exactly how much of each nutrient (and the percent of the RDA) is contained in one portion. Most computer-analysis programs also provide a percentage breakdown of calories from protein, fat, carbohydrate, and alcohol. Of course, these figures can be printed out and/or stored in memory. A sample recipe analysis is given in Figure 14-5.

Appendix G lists computer-analysis programs that are currently on the market. When considering such a program, some key questions to answer are:

- What functions does the program perform, and how many of these functions do I need?
- Is my computer system able to run this software?
- How large is the nutrient database? (Databases may contain from several hundred to 30,000 or more foods. The average is about 3000.)
- Can foods be added to the database? If so, how many?
- How is output presented (graphs, tables, pie charts, and so on), and how easily can it be printed?
- How easy is it to use this program?
- How much does this software cost?
- What service and support are available once I purchase the program? Is on-line help available?

Many companies offer demonstration software at no cost. This is a real benefit because you can try out the program before buying it.

Breakfast: 4 Foods

Item	Food Name	Serving	Portion	Amount
441	Pancakes, Home Recipe	3.00	Items	81.00 Gms
3354	Syrup — Pancake w/Maple	1.00	Tbsp	20.07 Gms
648	Sausage — Turk Brkfast	2.00	Ounces	56.80 Gms
362	Orange Juice — From Conc	1.00	Cup	250.00 Gms

Nutrient Values

Kilocalories	454 KC	21% of RDA
Protein	19.50 Gm	39%
Carbohydtate	67.73 Gm	25%
Fat	14.66 Gm	19%
Saturated Fat	1.42 Gm	6%
Cholesterol	109.00 Gm	37%
Fiber — Dietary	1.78 Gm	8%
Vitamin A	37.98 RE	5%
Vitamin C	96.69 Mg	161%
Vitamin D	0.00 Ug	0%
Sodium	934.34 Mg	39%
Potassium	572.22 Mg	29%
Iron	1.35 Mg	10%

Percent of Kcals from Protein: 16%   Carb: 57%   Fat: 26%
Diabetic Exchanges: Milk: 0.0   Veg: 0.0   Fruit: 2.0   Bread: 2.0   Meat:1.8   Fat:1.8

FIGURE 14-5.   Sample computerized nutrient analysis output. (Courtesy First Data Bank, San Bruno, California)

Opening Night

By the time opening night rolls around, everyone is ready and excited. But until everyone gets used to making and serving the new menu items flawlessly, managers and supervisors need to spend much time observing how things are going in order to jump in and give guidance when needed. Close supervision in the dining room and kitchen will help ensure the program's success.

MINI-SUMMARY   Once the menu planning is completed, you need to decide how to inform customers about the new menu items. You can highlight them on the menu with symbols or words such as "light," include them in a separate section of the menu, feature them on a menu clip-on and/or a blackboard or lightboard, or have waitstaff announce them. The program can be communicated to the public via promotional activities that may include advertising, sales promotion, and publicity. Training is a crucial component, and waitstaff and cooking staff need hands-on, comprehensive training.

PROGRAM EVALUATION

The healthy menu program should be evaluated much like any other program. Key questions for evaluation include:

1. How did the program do operationally? Did the cooks prepare and plate foods correctly? Did the waitstaff promote the program and answer questions well?
2. Did the food look good and taste good?
3. How well did each of the healthy menu options sell? How much did each item contribute to profits? How did the overall program affect profitability?
4. Did the program increase customer satisfaction? What was the overall feedback from customers? Did the program create repeat customers?

A popular method used to evaluate the sales and profits of menu items is menu engineering.

Proper program evaluation requires much time observing and talking with staff and customers, as well as going over written records, such as sales records.

Once a program has been evaluated, certain changes to fine tune the program might be necessary. Here are some suggestions.

- Develop ongoing promotions to maintain customer interest.
- Add, modify, or delete certain menu items.
- Change pricing.
- Improve the appearance of healthy items.
- Listen to customers more to get future menu and merchandising ideas.

MINI-SUMMARY Evaluation is needed to determine program effectiveness from customer, the employee, and management viewpoints.

KEY TERMS

Marketing
Marketing cycle
Press release
Publicity

REVIEW QUESTIONS AND EXERCISES

1. List the steps in the marketing cycle.
2. How can you gauge customer wants and needs for healthy menu options?
3. List the ways a restaurant can make customers aware of the availability of healthy menu options.
4. What is the best way to describe healthy foods on a menu?

5. What constitutes advertising, sales promotion, and publicity? Give an example of each.
6. Describe three ways to publicize a healthy menu.
7. How should you train cooking staff in the correct preparation of healthy menu items?
8. List five training topics for waitstaff.
9. What is needed on opening night to ensure a successful launch?
10. How do you evaluate the healthy menu after it has been implemented for at least several months?

1. Quiz
Check your answers.
1. d
2. c
3. True
4. b
5. d

2. Restaurant Menu Check
Study the menus from five different foodservices, including quick-service, and identify any menu items that are healthy. How do menu items appear on the menu? Would customers know they are healthy? What information is included?

3. Restaurant Promotion
Check restaurant advertisements in the newspaper and check to see if they have healthy and nutritious foods. What do the advertisements say? Have you heard any radio advertisements for healthy menu options? If so, describe.

4. Restaurant Visit
Visit a local restaurant that offers healthy menu options. Find out how it uses the marketing cycle to develop, implement, and evaluate their nutrition program.

REFERENCES

A balance of tastes. 1995. *Food Management* 30(10): 74–88.

American Dietetic Association. 1986. *The Competitive Edge: Marketing Strategies for the Registered Dietitian.* Chicago: American Dietetic Association.

Carlson, Beth L. 1987. Promoting nutrition on your menu: Three myths, eight tarnished rules, and five hot tips. *The Cornell H.R.A. Quarterly* 27(4): 18–21.

Carlson, Beth L., and Mary H. Tabacchi. 1986. Meeting consumer nutrition information needs in restaurants. *Journal of Nutrition Education* 18(5): 211–214.

Chernoff, R., ed. 1986. *Communicating as Professionals.* Chicago: American Dietetic Association.

DiDomenico, Pat. 1994. Portion size: How much is too much? *Restaurants USA* 14(6): 18–21.

Food and Drug Administration. 1986. *F.D.A. Health and Diet Survey.* Washington, DC: Food and Drug Administration.

Forster-Coull, Lisa, and Doris Gillis. 1988. A nutrition education program for restaurant patrons. *Journal of Nutrition Education* 20(1): 22B–22C.

Gallup survey: Nutrition plays strong role in dining decisions. 1986. *Nation's Restaurant News* 21 (July 14): 13.

Ganem, Beth Carlson. 1990. *Nutrition Menu Concepts for the Hospitality Industry.* New York: Van Nostrand Reinhold.

Hurley, Jayne, and Bonnie Liebman. 1995. Healthier restaurant food. *Nutrition Action Healthletter* 22(10): 11–13.

Mautner, J., and N. Ryan. 1985. Public relations: Do you need it? *Restaurants and Institutions* 95 (October 16): 189.

National Restaurant Association. 1986. *Consumer Nutrition Concerns and Restaurant Choices* (Summary), Volume 1. Washington, DC: National Restaurant Association.

National Restaurant Association. 1986. *A Nutrition Guide for the Restaurateur.* Washington, DC: National Restaurant Association.

National Restaurant Association. 1987. *Ingredient and Nutrition Information, Guidelines for Providing Facts to Foodservice Patrons.* Washington, DC: National Restaurant Association.

Regan, Claire. 1986. New developments in beef production. *NRA News* 6(6): 29.

Regan, Claire. 1987. Promoting nutrition in commercial foodservice establishments: A realistic approach. *Journal of The American Dietetic Association* 87(4): 486–488.

Reid, Robert. 1989. *Hospitality Marketing Management,* 2nd ed. New York: Van Nostrand Reinhold.

Somerville, Janice. 1988. Faster, lighter lunches build bigger hotel profits. *Hotel and Restaurants International* 22(1): 50–52.

Somerville, Sylvia. 1995. The skinny on restaurant nutrition claims. *Restaurants USA* 15(5): 36–38.

Straus, Karen. 1994. The healthy menu, part III: What do customers really want? *Restaurants & Institutions* 104(15): 36–46.

Weiss, Steve. 1994. The healthy menu, part II: The restaurateur's dilemma. *Restaurants & Institutions* 104(13): 122–134.

Hot Topics: Nutrition Labeling in Restaurants

Consumer groups have been making increased demands for ingredient and nutrition information from foodservices. They contend that, since nearly half of consumer food dollars are spent in restaurants, consumers have a right not to be misled by health and nutritional claims on restaurant menus.

The National Restaurant Association believes that consumers have a right to know what is in their food, but is opposed to mandatory ingredient and nutrition labeling because it is not practical and can be financially burdensome. In the past the Food and Drug Administration and other federal agencies have also rejected labeling for restaurants for these reasons. Mandatory labeling could very well be costly for the operator who, for example, serves six different kinds of soft drinks in three sizes. This would require 18 different cups to be purchased, stocked, and used appropriately by staff. The problem gets worse if you consider an item such as pizza, which comes in many different sizes and has many types of crusts and toppings. The possible combinations are endless.

The National Restaurant Association asserts that restaurants are not like supermarkets, so labeling can't be done in the same manner. Many restaurants vary their menu from day to day, depending on available ingredients, and in some settings the menu varies from meal to meal.

Although the restaurant industry opposes mandatory labeling, a growing number of foodservice operators are making nutrition information available to consumers, and the National Restaurant Association has been working with its members to do so. Nutrition information is available to many customers through a variety of means: printed material in the restaurant, toll-free telephone numbers, wall posters, and so on.

Under the Nutrition Education and Labeling Act of 1990, any nutrient or health claim made on a poster, sign, or table tent must abide by the same rules as claims made on food labels (see Chapter 1 for a discussion on food labels). Therefore, if an entree is advertised on a table tent as "low fat," it must have no more than 3 grams of fat per serving. Menus were exempt from this requirement until a federal judge ordered the Food and Drug Administration to include menus and establish regulations in mid-1996. Proof of a dish's nutrient content can be documented through a computerized nutrient analysis or food testing, also called *proximate analysis*, in which a laboratory analyzes the food for its nutrient content. To avoid incorrect nutrition claims, which the media has repeatedly jumped on, the terms and definitions set by the Food and Drug Administration (See Table 7-15) must be used.

CHAPTER
15

Light Beverages and Foods for the Beverage Operation

**KEY
QUESTIONS**

1. What trends have occurred in the area of beverage management and what forces were behind them?
2. What drinks can be offered that are lower in calories and alcohol than most others?
3. What healthy foods can be offered in a beverage operation?
4. How can a beverage operator market healthy foods and lower-calorie drinks?
5. What are dramshop acts and how do they affect beverage service?

QUIZ

Quiz

1. Which is lower in calories?
   (a) 12 fluid ounces of light beer
   (b) 7 fluid ounces of gin and tonic
   (c) 6 fluid ounces of white wine
   (d) 12 fluid ounces of tonic water
2. Drinks that taste like mixed drinks but contain no alcohol are called
   (a) coolers.
   (b) dealcoholized spirits.
   (c) mocktails.
   (d) smoothies.
3 The emphasis in beverage operations has changed to
   (a) food.
   (b) theme events.
   (c) entertainment.
   (d) participative events.
   (e) all of the above
4. Which of the following foods could not be served as a nutritious appetizer?
   (a) vegetables with yogurt dip
   (b) soft pretzels
   (c) vegetarian pizza on pita bread
   (d) deep-fried zucchini
5. In many states, if a bartender serves alcoholic beverages to a minor, he or she could be subject to criminal prosecution as well as lawsuits by any individuals injured by the drunk minor.
   True   False

INTRODUCTION

Heavy foods and strong alcoholic beverages were a way of life in most beverage operations until about 1970. At that time, the sale of spirits began to decline, whereas sales of "lighter" drinks, such as beer and wine, began to increase. Next, beer went light—a well received change—and wine by the glass was promoted. Mocktails—nonalcoholic beverages—began to appear as well, as part of the movement against alcohol abuse. In addition, the drinking age was raised to 21 in many states, warning labels appeared on liquor bottles, and successful lawsuits were waged against beverage operations by victims of drunk drivers—all part of a movement aimed not at the use but the abuse of alcohol. There is a big difference between alcohol abuse and moderate use. In fact, the 1995 edition of the Dietary Guidelines for Americans, for the first time, indicated that moderate drinking is associated with a lower risk for coronary heart disease in some individuals.

Alcoholic beverages are any liquids containing a type of alcohol called ethanol.

In an effort to curb drunk-driving accidents, beverage operations have changed their emphasis from all-you-can-drink specials (and the like) to foods, entertainment, music, contests, games, and theme parties, in order to overcome an association with heavy drinking. Themes might be international, such as Mexican, with tacos and burritos and staff dressed in Mexican outfits. A Workout Night theme might involve asking customers to come dressed in their workout clothes.

This chapter first looks at lower-calorie and lower-alcohol beverages and nutritious food choices, then goes on to discuss marketing these selections. A discussion on alcohol and the law completes the chapter.

Mini-Summary Due to increased efforts to fight alcohol abuse, beverage operations emphasize foods, entertainment, music, contests, games, and theme parties.

LOWER-CALORIE AND LOWER-ALCOHOL DRINK OPTIONS

Bar customers who want a lower-calorie beverage or a drink with little or no alcohol have a number of choices: fruit juices and fruit-juice-based beverages, creamy drinks, **dealcoholized wines**, **light** and **nonalcoholic beers**, **mocktails**, **bottled waters**, and other beverages. As Table 15-1 indicates, when the alcohol content of a drink increases, so do calories. Alcohol contains 7 calories per gram, compared to 4 calories per gram of carbohydrate or protein.

Alcoholic beverages represent empty calories as they do not contain any significant amounts of any nutrients.

Fruit Juices and Fruit Juice-Based Beverages

Fruit juices serve as a base for make many different nonalcoholic drinks, such as fruit juice served with seltzer (water with bubbles or carbonation). Fruit may serve as the basis for blended drinks such as strawberry coolers made with fresh strawberries, sugar, sparkling water, and ice cubes.

Alcohol-free grape juices, made to resemble wines, are available, either sparkling or still, in red, pink, and white varieties. Nonalcoholic sparkling cider, a soft, fruity, and light drink, is made in France and in the United States.

Creamy Drinks

Ice milk is like a reduced-fat ice cream. Much soft-serve ice cream is really ice milk.

Creamy drinks are made with milk, yogurt, cream, ice cream, or other dairy products. A good example is a category of creamy drinks called **fruit smoothies**, frozen blends of fruit, milk, and/or fresh or frozen yogurt. When regular dairy products such as cream and ice cream are used, these drinks are not low in calories; however, low-fat or nonfat yogurt, ice milk, and skim or 1 percent milk can be used to make drinks with fewer calories and less fat.

Dealcoholized Wines

Dealcoholized wine contains up to 0.5 percent alcohol and is available in red, pink, and white varieties, either still or sparkling. Varietal wines with one predominant grape variety, such as gamay or Riesling, are available as well. One of these products even won a wine contest!

Wine coolers are a mix of wine, fruit flavor, and carbonated or plain water. They usually contain fructose or high-fructose corn syrup for sweetening, and a few also have preservatives added. They generally have half the alcohol content of wine. Many flavors are on the market, and some brands are available in kegs. Wine coolers can also be made on site and served on the rocks or over shaved ice. **Wine spritzers** are made with wine and club soda and are mixed at the bar.

Light and Nonalcoholic Beers

Several varieties of beer with varying alcohol and calorie contents are available, as seen in Table 15-1. Different brands of light beer can vary tremendously in calorie content, but most have one-third to one-half the alcohol and calories of regular beers. Nonalcoholic beers, produced by removing the alcohol after brewing or by stopping the fermentation process before alcohol forms, contain one-half of 1 percent or less of alcohol. In either case, these beers have about half the calories of regular beer and two-third the calories of light beer.

People buy **bottled water** for what it does not have—calories, caffeine, additives, preservatives, and, in most cases, not too much sodium. The bottled water market just continues to grow and grow. Per-person consumption was about 10 gallons in 1995, up approximately 15 percent from 1994. Over three-quarters of fine-dining and midrange restaurants and hotels now offer bottled water.

The Food and Drug Administration (FDA) has published standard definitions for different types of bottled water to promote honesty and fair dealing in the marketplace. Bottled water, like all other foods regulated by the FDA, must be processed, packaged, shipped, and stored in a safe and sanitary manner and be truthfully and accurately labeled. Bottled water products must also meet specific FDA quality standards for contaminants, set in response to requirements that the Environmental Protection Agency (EPA) has set for tap water.

To help resolve possible confusion, the FDA has set the following definitions.

- **Spring water** is water collected as it flows naturally to the surface, or when pumped through a hole from the spring source. The FDA regulation allows labeling to describe how the water came to the surface, for example, "naturally flowed to the surface, not extracted."
- **Mineral water** must come from a protected underground source and contain at least 250 parts per million in total dissolved solids. Mineral water was previously exempt from bottled water quality standards but must now meet them.
- Water bottled from municipal water supplies must be clearly labeled as such, unless it is processed sufficiently to be labeled as "distilled" or "purified" water.

Different mineral and carbonation levels of bottled waters make them appeal to different customers and eating situations. For instance, a heavily carbonated (also called sparkling) water such as Perrier is excellent as an aperitif, yet some customers may prefer the lighter sparkle of San Pellegrino. Still waters such as Evian are generally more popular and appropriate to have on the table during the meal.

FDA regulations for bottled waters do not cover any soft drinks or similar beverages that do not highlight a water ingredient. Like all other foods, such beverages must be safe and truthfully labeled, but if the water ingredient is highlighted in any way, that water must meet bottled water standards. Some popular beverages that are not regulated by the FDA include:

- **Seltzer** is filtered, artificially carbonated tap water that generally has no added mineral salts. It is available with assorted flavor essences, including vanilla cream, black cherry, orange, raspberry, lemon lime, root beer, and cola. If seltzer contains sweeteners (and therefore calories), it must be called a "flavored soda."
- **Club soda**, sometimes called "soda water" or "plain soda," is filtered, carbonated tap water to which mineral salts are added to give it a unique taste. Most average 30 to 70 milligrams of sodium per 8 ounces.
- **Tonic water** is not really water or low in calories. It contains 84 calories per 8 ounces. Diet tonic water that uses sugar substitutes is available.

TABLE 15-1. Calories in alcoholic and nonalcoholic beverages.

Beverage	Amount (fluid ounces)	Calories	Alcohol
Mixed Drinks			
Bloody Mary	5 fl. oz.	116	11.7%
Bourbon and soda	4 fl. oz.	105	16.1%
Daiquiri	2 fl. oz.	111	28.3%
Gin and tonic	7.5 fl. oz.	171	8.8%
Manhattan	2 fl. oz.	128	36.9%
Martini	2.5 fl. oz.	156	38.4%
Piña colada	4.5 fl. oz	262	12.3%
Screwdriver	7 fl. oz.	174	8.2%
Tequila sunrise	5.5 fl. oz.	189	13.5%
Tom collins	7.5 fl. oz.	121	9.0%
Whiskey sour	3 fl. oz.	123	20.6%
Distilled Liquors			
Gin, 90 proof	1.5 fl. oz.	110	45%
Rum, 80 proof	1.5 fl. oz.	97	40%
Vodka, 80 proof	1.5 fl. oz.	97	40%
Whiskey, 86 proof	1.5 fl. oz.	105	43%
Wine			
Table wine, red	3.5 fl. oz.	74	11.5%
Table wine, rose	3.5 fl. oz.	73	11.5%
Table wine, white	3.5 fl. oz.	70	11.5%
Beer			
Beer	12 fl. oz.	146	4.5%
Light beer	12 fl. oz.	100	2.2–4.4%
Dealcoholized beer	12 fl. oz.	50	Less than 0.5%
Nonalcoholic Beverages			
Cola	12 fl. oz.	151	
Ginger ale	12 fl. oz.	124	
Lemon-lime soda	12 fl. oz.	149	
Orange soda	12 fl. oz.	177	
Root beer	12 fl. oz.	152	
Tonic water	12 fl. oz.	125	
Club soda, seltzer, mineral or sparkling waters	12 fl. oz.	0–10	
Cranberry-apple juice drink	6 fl. oz.	123	
Cranberry juice cocktail	6 fl. oz.	108	
Grape juice drink	6 fl. oz.	94	
Lemonade	8 fl. oz.	100	
Tomato vegetable juice cocktail	8 fl. oz.	44	

Source: United States Department of Agriculture Handbook #8–14.

Mocktails

Mocktails are much more than just a Virgin Mary, a bloody Mary without the vodka, or simply tomato juice! Mocktails attempt to imitate the real thing. For instance, a mockarita, an imitation margarita, is blenderized with lemonade, lime juice, and ice cubes and served in a margarita glass with a salted rim. Hot mocktails, such as mock Irish coffee, can be made as well. Some bartenders substitute lower-proof products in cocktails, such as Chablis for tequila to make a white wine margarita, although such drinks are not true mocktails. This substitution lowers both alcohol and calories.

Other Choices

Other lower-calorie and/or no-alcohol alternatives include bottled waters (see the Food Facts in this chapter), vegetable juices, diet soft drinks, iced tea flavored with lemon or other fruit juice, and some specialty coffees such as **espresso** or **cafe latte** (see Table 8-18). Other flavorings for lower-alcohol drinks include vanilla and rum extracts or nonalcoholic fruit syrups such as cassis.

Cassis is black currant liqueur. It is sweet and is popular to flavor desserts.

MINI-SUMMARY Drinks with fewer calories and less alcohol include fruit juices and fruit-juice-based beverages, creamy drinks, dealcoholized wines, light and nonalcoholic beers, mocktails, bottled waters, vegetable juices, diet soft drinks, iced tea, and specialty coffees.

HEALTHY FOOD CHOICES

Nutritious food choices for beverage operations need not be dull, monotonous, or unappetizing. Some food choices already being offered are lower in calories, such as fresh vegetables with yogurt dip. Other foods may require altering a cooking method, such as broiling chicken wings rather than frying them or modifying an ingredient.

Following are some more nutritious food ideas.

1. Soft pretzels can be made from scratch or from frozen dough and topped with sesame or poppy seeds instead of salt. Pretzel sticks can be mixed with crunchy, ready-to-eat cereals and a few peanuts and then tossed with a small amount of oil, Worcestershire sauce, and garlic powder to make a tasty snack food.

2. Popcorn is a good choice served with a minimal amount of melted margarine, and is an even better choice without adding any fat! Instead, use garlic, onion, or chili powder, grated hard cheese, or other seasoning.

See chapters 12
and 13 for more
menu ideas.

3. To make a healthy pizza, use low-fat cheeses such as skim-milk mozzarella, and top with fresh vegetables such as green peppers, mushrooms, and zucchini. Mini-pizzas can be made with pita bread, a little Parmesan cheese, vegetables, garlic powder, and oregano. Mini-calzones can be stuffed with part-skim ricotta or mozzarella cheese and vegetables.

4. Fresh vegetables and fruits are popular and can be attractively presented. Raw vegetables with dip, fruit with low-fat cheese cubes, and grilled vegetables are also possibilities. Instead of deep-frying potato skins, season and bake them. Wrap vegetables in thin puff pastry or phyllo dough and bake them as an alternate to deep-fried vegetables.

5. The sour cream or cream used in many dips can be replaced with plain low-fat yogurt, low-fat cream cheese, and/or soft tofu. Good dips using these alternate ingredients include blue cheese, chives, onion, spinach, or artichoke dip. Other good dip choices are bean dips such as hummus (made from chickpeas) and salsa (a tomato-based, hot Mexican dip).

6. Tortilla chips can be made by cutting tortillas, baking them, and then sprinkling with garlic, onion, or chili powder or small amounts of grated cheese. Serve with salsa.

7. Healthier protein choices include steamed or broiled shellfish, chicken wings broiled instead of fried, and mini-burritos stuffed with beans in sauce and topped with fresh vegetables.

MINI-SUMMARY Some healthy food options can be prepared without too much fuss and satisfy the needs of some customers.

MARKETING LIGHT BEVERAGES AND FOODS

The first step in marketing light beverages and foods involves analyzing the surrounding market and clientele needs and wants; projecting sales volume, pricing, and profit structures; and seeing how such options would fit into the operation in terms of ordering, inventory, and menus. A beverage operator might start by choosing five items, perhaps a wine cooler, a de-alcoholized wine and beer, a mineral water, and a juice-based drink. In a more developed market, the choices might be enlarged. Using cookbooks or other resources such as those listed at the end of Chapter 13, you can select, implement, and evaluate lower-calorie foods that fit well into your operation. The production staff must be involved in these decisions. For both drinks and food, variety and quality are of the utmost importance.

Presentation of lower-calorie and/or lower-alcohol drinks is just as important as it is for regular drinks. For instance, serve sparkling cider in stemmed glasses or champagne flutes, and garnish with an apple ring and a sprig of mint.

Bartenders and servers need to be trained about the new offerings as well as taste them. A well-trained staff can suggest options appropriately, but they must learn to present lower-calorie and/or lower-alcohol drinks as positively as regular drinks. If servers lose tips by selling these new items, a bonus or incentive may be needed in order for the program to be successful.

The proposed program must be merchandised with flair during good selling times to enhance its success. During these times, menu clip-ons, blackboards, lightboards, table tents, posters, or other techniques let customers know what is available. A special dinner menu may be used, and promotions such as water tastings and "nonalcoholic beer of the month" offerings can be effective.

Once the program is launched, getting customer feedback is very important, as well as analyzing sales and profits. After enough time, the success of the program needs to be evaluated, just like any other program.

MINI-SUMMARY As with other programs, light beverages and foods must first be selected and developed to meet clientele needs and wants and, hopefully, to make money. Staff must be trained, and merchandising and promotion techniques selected before the program is launched. When the program has been in place long enough, sales and profits can be evaluated.

ALCOHOL AND THE LAW

Read the following story. Did The Tavern break any laws? Can they be sued by the injured parties (commonly called third parties)?

At The Tavern, Jane serves drinks and Jim bartends. They both work part-time while going to college. One evening, Jane sees a young couple sit down at a table in her section and takes their beverage order. While waiting for Jim to fill the drink order, Jane wonders aloud whether the petite young lady was asked for proof of age at the front door. She just looks so young. Jim says not to worry, that's the responsibility of the manager, who monitors the traffic at the front door. Jane serves the couple several rounds of drinks and, as they leave, notices that the young lady needs some assistance walking. Since the young man seemed fine, Jane hoped he was going to be the one driving home. Indeed, the young man did drive the car as they left, but he drove his girlfriend back to the parking lot at work, where they had left from earlier, so she could then drive herself home. On her way home, she had an accident that sent a 43-year-old man and his 8-year-old daughter to the hospital. Her blood alcohol content was above the legal limit and her driver's license showed that she was 19 in a state where the minimum drinking age is 21.

Yes, The Tavern broke a law: serving a minor, and because of this, both managers and employees are liable and can be sued in most states.

Alcohol-related liability is generally covered through court interpretation of state liquor laws or state **dramshop acts**. In most states, serving minors, intoxicated persons, known alcoholics, or habitual drunkards is against state laws. There are virtually no defenses to knowingly serving alcohol to minors. When foodservice operators violate state laws, they (meaning both involved managers and employees) leave themselves open to criminal prosecution and penalties as well as liability lawsuits. The establishment can also lose its liquor license. When innocent third parties, such as the man and his daughter in the foregoing story, are hurt by intoxicated customers and sue, resulting lawsuits can be quite expensive.

Dramshop acts are state acts that define liability for liquor sales to customers who injure or kill third parties. Most states do allow third parties injured by intoxicated customers the right to sue licensed alcohol vendors. However, dramshop acts usually require the injured third party to prove that the alcohol was illegally sold (such as to a minor), the seller caused or contributed to the intoxication, and the sale resulted in injury to the victim. In a few states, it does not matter whether or not the alcohol was sold illegally.

Learn how to serve alcohol responsibly. You could save someone's life.

The best defense against these third-party liability suits is a policy of responsible alcohol service, including practices such as the following.

All guests' identification should be properly checked, using identification with photos, before serving.

All servers need to be trained to spot a guest who is becoming intoxicated and (1) inform the guest that alcohol service is no longer legal and (2) offer a nonalcoholic drink.

Sponsor a designated driver program.

Provide transportation home to intoxicated guests.

Serve food.

Serve only one drink at a time.

Refrain from promotional activities that promote excessive drinking.

MINI-SUMMARY Alcohol-related liability is generally covered through court interpretation of state liquor laws or state dramshop acts. In most states, serving minors, intoxicated persons, known alcoholics, or habitual drunkards is against state laws. When foodservice operators violate state laws, they (meaning both involved managers and employees) leave themselves open to criminal prosecution and penalties, loss of liquor licenses, as well as liability lawsuits. The best defense is a policy of responsible alcohol service.

Bottled waters	Espresso	Nonalcoholic beers	**KEY TERMS**
Cafe latte	Fatty liver	Seltzer	
Cirrhosis	Fruit smoothies	Spring water	
Club soda	Light beers	Tonic water	
Dealcoholized wines	Mineral water	Wine coolers	
Dramshop acts	Mocktails	Wine spritzers	

In your own words, answer the following questions.

REVIEW QUESTIONS

1. Why have beverage operations put more emphasis on activities that do not involve drinking?
2. List six categories of beverages that have fewer calories and less alcohol than regular alcoholic beverages. Give two examples of each category.
3. List five nutritious choices for a beverage operation.
4. Describe the steps involved in marketing light beverages and foods.
5. Where is alcohol-related liability covered in most states?
6. Who is it against the law to serve?
7. What are dramshop acts?
8. Describe some practices that help prevent third-party liability suits.
9. How does excessive drinking affect an individual's nutrition status and health?
10. Who should avoid drinking alcoholic beverages?

1. Quiz

ACTIVITIES AND APPLICATIONS

Check your answers with the following.
1. a
2. c
3. e
4. d
5. True

2. Dramshop Laws

Find out more about your state's dramshop laws by calling the Small Business Administration.

3. Supermarket Sleuth

Go to a large supermarket and examine the selection of bottled waters, fruit juices made to resemble wine, and dealcoholized beers and wines.

4. Taste Testing: Dealcoholized Beer and Wine

Have a taste-testing of dealcoholized beers and wines. Examine the dealcoholized beers in terms of how close they taste to real beer, calories per bottle, appearance, foam, and flavor. Examine the dealcoholized wines in terms of how close they taste to real wine, calories per serving, sweetness or dryness, and appearance.

4. Taste Testing: Bottled Waters

Have a taste-testing of bottled waters, including at least two from each of these categories: mineral water, spring water, seltzer, and club soda.

5. Develop Light Beverage and Food Options

You are in charge of developing ten food and ten beverage selections to be featured in a special Friday night promotion using a workout night theme. Customers will be asked to come in their workout clothes and more healthful food and beverage selections will be featured.

REFERENCES

Backas, Nancy. 1987. Slake the "mocktail" thirst. *Restaurants and Institutions* 97(12): 270–271.

Bottled (flavored) waters get the "bottoms up" sign. 1987. *Nation's Restaurant News*, Secion 2, 21(24): 30–32.

Cianci, Maria. 1986. High potential for low-alcohol. *Restaurant Business* 85(2): 143–144.

Crouch, Dorothy. 1985. *Entertaining Without Alcohol.* Washington, DC: Acropolis Books.

Hochstein, Mort. 1987. Non-alcoholic beverage market spurred by customer demand. *Nation's Restaurant News* 21(42): 5.

Making a comeback? Some still call it "happy hour." 1987. *Nation's Restaurant News*, Secion 2, 21(35): 18.

Scarpa, Jim. 1987. No- and low-alcohol alternatives. *Restaurant Business* 86(12): 219–220.

Sherry, John E. H. 1994. *Legal Aspects of Hospitality Management*, 2nd ed. Chicago: Educational Foundation of the National Restaurant Association.

Slater, David. 1988. Bottled water: The beverage of the future? *Restaurants USA* 8(1): 11–15.

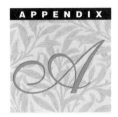

Nutritive Value of Foods

This table shows the nutritive value of 908 common foods. The foods are grouped under the following main headings:

Beverages	Meat and meat products
Dairy products	Mixed dishes and fast foods
Eggs	Poultry and poultry products
Fats and oils	Soups, sauces, and gravies
Fish and shellfish	Sugars and sweets
Fruits and fruit juices	Vegetables and vegetable products
Grain products	Miscellaneous items
Legumes, nuts, and seeds	

Most of the foods are listed in ready-to-eat form. Some are basic products widely used in food preparation, such as flour, fat, and cornmeal.

Source: The Nutritive Value of Foods. USDA Home and Garden Bulletin no. 72, 1989.

(Tr indicates nutrient present in trace amount.)

Item No.	Foods, approximate measures, units, and weight (weight of edible portion only)			Water	Food energy	Pro-tein	Fat	Fatty acids		
								Satu-rated	Mono-unsatu-rated	Poly-unsatu-rated
			Grams	Per-cent	Cal-ories	Grams	Grams	Grams	Grams	Grams
	Beverages									
	Alcoholic:									
	Beer:									
1	Regular	12 fl oz	360	92	150	1	0	0.0	0.0	0.0
2	Light	12 fl oz	355	95	95	1	0	0.0	0.0	0.0
	Gin, rum, vodka, whiskey:									
3	80-proof	1-1/2 fl oz	42	67	95	0	0	0.0	0.0	0.0
4	86-proof	1-1/2 fl oz	42	64	105	0	0	0.0	0.0	0.0
5	90-proof	1-1/2 fl oz	42	62	110	0	0	0.0	0.0	0.0
	Wines:									
6	Dessert	3-1/2 fl oz	103	77	140	Tr	0	0.0	0.0	0.0
	Table:									
7	Red	3-1/2 fl oz	102	88	75	Tr	0	0.0	0.0	0.0
8	White	3-1/2 fl oz	102	87	80	Tr	0	0.0	0.0	0.0
	Carbonated:[2]									
9	Club soda	12 fl oz	355	100	0	0	0	0.0	0.0	0.0
	Cola type:									
10	Regular	12 fl oz	369	89	160	0	0	0.0	0.0	0.0
11	Diet, artificially sweetened	12 fl oz	355	100	Tr	0	0	0.0	0.0	0.0
12	Ginger ale	12 fl oz	366	91	125	0	0	0.0	0.0	0.0
13	Grape	12 fl oz	372	88	180	0	0	0.0	0.0	0.0
14	Lemon-lime	12 fl oz	372	89	155	0	0	0.0	0.0	0.0
15	Orange	12 fl oz	372	88	180	0	0	0.0	0.0	0.0
16	Pepper type	12 fl oz	369	89	160	0	0	0.0	0.0	0.0
17	Root beer	12 fl oz	370	89	165	0	0	0.0	0.0	0.0
	Cocoa and chocolate-flavored beverages. See Dairy Products (items 95-98).									
	Coffee:									
18	Brewed	6 fl oz	180	100	Tr	Tr	Tr	Tr	Tr	Tr
19	Instant, prepared (2 tsp powder plus 6 fl oz water)	6 fl oz	182	99	Tr	Tr	Tr	Tr	Tr	Tr
	Fruit drinks, noncarbonated:									
	Canned:									
20	Fruit punch drink	6 fl oz	190	88	85	Tr	0	0.0	0.0	0.0
21	Grape drink	6 fl oz	187	86	100	Tr	0	0.0	0.0	0.0
22	Pineapple-grapefruit juice drink	6 fl oz	187	87	90	Tr	Tr	Tr	Tr	Tr
	Frozen:									
	Lemonade concentrate:									
23	Undiluted	6-fl-oz can	219	49	425	Tr	Tr	Tr	Tr	Tr
24	Diluted with 4-1/3 parts water by volume	6 fl oz	185	89	80	Tr	Tr	Tr	Tr	Tr
	Limeade concentrate:									
25	Undiluted	6-fl-oz can	218	50	410	Tr	Tr	Tr	Tr	Tr
26	Diluted with 4-1/3 parts water by volume	6 fl oz	185	89	75	Tr	Tr	Tr	Tr	Tr
	Fruit juices. See type under Fruits and Fruit Juices.									
	Milk beverages. See Dairy Products (items 92-105).									
	Tea:									
27	Brewed	8 fl oz	240	100	Tr	Tr	Tr	Tr	Tr	Tr
	Instant, powder, prepared:									
28	Unsweetened (1 tsp powder plus 8 fl oz water)	8 fl oz	241	100	Tr	Tr	Tr	Tr	Tr	Tr
29	Sweetened (3 tsp powder plus 8 fl oz water)	8 fl oz	262	91	85	Tr	Tr	Tr	Tr	Tr

[1]Value not determined.
[2]Mineral content varies depending on water source.

							Vitamin A value						
Cho-les-terol	Carbo-hydrate	Calcium	Phos-phorus	Iron	Potas-sium	Sodium	(IU)	(RE)	Thiamin	Ribo-flavin	Niacin	Ascorbic acid	Item No.
Milli-grams	Grams	Milli-grams	Milli-grams	Milli-grams	Milli-grams	Milli-grams	Inter-national units	Retinol equiva-lents	Milli-grams	Milli-grams	Milli-grams	Milli-grams	
0	13	14	50	0.1	115	18	0	0	0.02	0.09	1.8	0	1
0	5	14	43	0.1	64	11	0	0	0.03	0.11	1.4	0	2
0	Tr	Tr	Tr	Tr	1	Tr	0	0	Tr	Tr	Tr	0	3
0	Tr	Tr	Tr	Tr	1	Tr	0	0	Tr	Tr	Tr	0	4
0	Tr	Tr	Tr	Tr	1	Tr	0	0	Tr	Tr	Tr	0	5
0	8	8	9	0.2	95	9	(1)	(1)	0.01	0.02	0.2	0	6
0	3	8	18	0.4	113	5	(1)	(1)	0.00	0.03	0.1	0	7
0	3	9	14	0.3	83	5	(1)	(1)	0.00	0.01	0.1	0	8
0	0	18	0	Tr	0	78	0	0	0.00	0.00	0.0	0	9
0	41	11	52	0.2	7	18	0	0	0.00	0.00	0.0	0	10
0	Tr	14	39	0.2	7	[3]32	0	0	0.00	0.00	0.0	0	11
0	32	11	0	0.1	4	29	0	0	0.00	0.00	0.0	0	12
0	46	15	0	0.4	4	48	0	0	0.00	0.00	0.0	0	13
0	39	7	0	0.4	4	33	0	0	0.00	0.00	0.0	0	14
0	46	15	4	0.3	7	52	0	0	0.00	0.00	0.0	0	15
0	41	11	41	0.1	4	37	0	0	0.00	0.00	0.0	0	16
0	42	15	0	0.2	4	48	0	0	0.00	0.00	0.0	0	17
0	Tr	4	2	Tr	124	2	0	0	0.00	0.02	0.4	0	18
0	1	2	6	0.1	71	Tr	0	0	0.00	0.03	0.6	0	19
0	22	15	2	0.4	48	15	20	2	0.03	0.04	Tr	[4]61	20
0	26	2	2	0.3	9	11	Tr	Tr	0.01	0.01	Tr	[4]64	21
0	23	13	7	0.9	97	24	60	6	0.06	0.04	0.5	[4]110	22
0	112	9	13	0.4	153	4	40	4	0.04	0.07	0.7	66	23
0	21	2	2	0.1	30	1	10	1	0.01	0.02	0.2	13	24
0	108	11	13	0.2	129	Tr	Tr	Tr	0.02	0.02	0.2	26	25
0	20	2	2	Tr	24	Tr	Tr	Tr	Tr	Tr	Tr	4	26
0	Tr	0	2	Tr	36	1	0	0	0.00	0.03	Tr	0	27
0	1	1	4	Tr	61	1	0	0	0.00	0.02	0.1	0	28
0	22	1	3	Tr	49	Tr	0	0	0.00	0.04	0.1	0	29

[3]Blend of aspartame and saccharin; if only sodium saccharin is used, sodium is 75 mg; if only aspartame is used, sodium is 23 mg.
[4]With added ascorbic acid.

(Tr indicates nutrient present in trace amount.)

Item No.	Foods, approximate measures, units, and weight (weight of edible portion only)		Grams	Water Per-cent	Food energy Cal-ories	Pro-tein Grams	Fat Grams	Fatty acids		
								Saturated Grams	Mono-unsaturated Grams	Poly-unsaturated Grams
	Dairy Products		Grams	Per-cent	Cal-ories	Grams	Grams	Grams	Grams	Grams
	Butter. See Fats and Oils (items 128-130).									
	Cheese:									
	Natural:									
30	Blue-----------------------	1 oz-----------	28	42	100	6	8	5.3	2.2	0.2
31	Camembert (3 wedges per 4-oz container)-----------------	1 wedge--------	38	52	115	8	9	5.8	2.7	0.3
	Cheddar:									
32	Cut pieces----------------	1 oz-----------	28	37	115	7	9	6.0	2.7	0.3
33		1 in³----------	17	37	70	4	6	3.6	1.6	0.2
34	Shredded------------------	1 cup----------	113	37	455	28	37	23.8	10.6	1.1
	Cottage (curd not pressed down):									
	Creamed (cottage cheese, 4% fat):									
35	Large curd---------------	1 cup----------	225	79	235	28	10	6.4	2.9	0.3
36	Small curd---------------	1 cup----------	210	79	215	26	9	6.0	2.7	0.3
37	With fruit--------------	1 cup----------	226	72	280	22	8	4.9	2.2	0.2
38	Lowfat (2%)--------------	1 cup----------	226	79	205	31	4	2.8	1.2	0.1
39	Uncreamed (cottage cheese dry curd, less than 1/2% fat)--------------------	1 cup----------	145	80	125	25	1	0.4	0.2	Tr
40	Cream-----------------------	1 oz-----------	28	54	100	2	10	6.2	2.8	0.4
41	Feta------------------------	1 oz-----------	28	55	75	4	6	4.2	1.3	0.2
	Mozzarella, made with:									
42	Whole milk----------------	1 oz-----------	28	54	80	6	6	3.7	1.9	0.2
43	Part skim milk (low moisture)----------------	1 oz-----------	28	49	80	8	5	3.1	1.4	0.1
44	Muenster--------------------	1 oz-----------	28	42	105	7	9	5.4	2.5	0.2
	Parmesan, grated:									
45	Cup, not pressed down-----	1 cup----------	100	18	455	42	30	19.1	8.7	0.7
46	Tablespoon----------------	1 tbsp---------	5	18	25	2	2	1.0	0.4	Tr
47	Ounce--------------------	1 oz-----------	28	18	130	12	9	5.4	2.5	0.2
48	Provolone-------------------	1 oz-----------	28	41	100	7	8	4.8	2.1	0.2
	Ricotta, made with:									
49	Whole milk----------------	1 cup----------	246	72	430	28	32	20.4	8.9	0.9
50	Part skim milk-----------	1 cup----------	246	74	340	28	19	12.1	5.7	0.6
51	Swiss-----------------------	1 oz-----------	28	37	105	8	8	5.0	2.1	0.3
	Pasteurized process cheese:									
52	American-------------------	1 oz-----------	28	39	105	6	9	5.6	2.5	0.3
53	Swiss----------------------	1 oz-----------	28	42	95	7	7	4.5	2.0	0.2
54	Pasteurized process cheese food, American --------------	1 oz-----------	28	43	95	6	7	4.4	2.0	0.2
55	Pasteurized process cheese spread, American-------------	1 oz-----------	28	48	80	5	6	3.8	1.8	0.2
	Cream, sweet:									
56	Half-and-half (cream and milk)	1 cup----------	242	81	315	7	28	17.3	8.0	1.0
57		1 tbsp---------	15	81	20	Tr	2	1.1	0.5	0.1
58	Light, coffee, or table-------	1 cup----------	240	74	470	6	46	28.8	13.4	1.7
59		1 tbsp---------	15	74	30	Tr	3	1.8	0.8	0.1
	Whipping, unwhipped (volume about double when whipped):									
60	Light-----------------------	1 cup----------	239	64	700	5	74	46.2	21.7	2.1
61		1 tbsp---------	15	64	45	Tr	5	2.9	1.4	0.1
62	Heavy-----------------------	1 cup----------	238	58	820	5	88	54.8	25.4	3.3
63		1 tbsp---------	15	58	50	Tr	6	3.5	1.6	0.2
64	Whipped topping, (pressurized)	1 cup----------	60	61	155	2	13	8.3	3.9	0.5
65		1 tbsp---------	3	61	10	Tr	1	0.4	0.2	Tr
66	Cream, sour----------------------	1 cup----------	230	71	495	7	48	30.0	13.9	1.8
67		1 tbsp---------	12	71	25	Tr	3	1.6	0.7	0.1

							Vitamin A value						
Cho-les-terol	Carbo-hydrate	Calcium	Phos-phorus	Iron	Potas-sium	Sodium	(IU)	(RE)	Thiamin	Ribo-flavin	Niacin	Ascorbic acid	Item No.
Milli-grams	Grams	Milli-grams	Milli-grams	Milli-grams	Milli-grams	Milli-grams	Inter-nationa, units	Retinol equiva-lents	Milli-grams	Milli-grams	Milli-grams	Milli-grams	
21	1	150	110	0.1	73	396	200	65	0.01	0.11	0.3	0	30
27	Tr	147	132	0.1	71	320	350	96	0.01	0.19	0.2	0	31
30	Tr	204	145	0.2	28	176	300	86	0.01	0.11	Tr	0	32
18	Tr	123	87	0.1	17	105	180	52	Tr	0.06	Tr	0	33
119	1	815	579	0.8	111	701	1,200	342	0.03	0.42	0.1	0	34
34	6	135	297	0.3	190	911	370	108	0.05	0.37	0.3	Tr	35
31	6	126	277	0.3	177	850	340	101	0.04	0.34	0.3	Tr	36
25	30	108	236	0.2	151	915	280	81	0.04	0.29	0.2	Tr	37
19	8	155	340	0.4	217	918	160	45	0.05	0.42	0.3	Tr	38
10	3	46	151	0.3	47	19	40	12	0.04	0.21	0.2	0	39
31	1	23	30	0.3	34	84	400	124	Tr	0.06	Tr	0	40
25	1	140	96	0.2	18	316	130	36	0.04	0.24	0.3	0	41
22	1	147	105	0.1	19	106	220	68	Tr	0.07	Tr	0	42
15	1	207	149	0.1	27	150	180	54	0.01	0.10	Tr	0	43
27	Tr	203	133	0.1	38	178	320	90	Tr	0.09	Tr	0	44
79	4	1,376	807	1.0	107	1,861	700	173	0.05	0.39	0.3	0	45
4	Tr	69	40	Tr	5	93	40	9	Tr	0.02	Tr	0	46
22	1	390	229	0.3	30	528	200	49	0.01	0.11	0.1	0	47
20	1	214	141	0.1	39	248	230	75	0.01	0.09	Tr	0	48
124	7	509	389	0.9	257	207	1,210	330	0.03	0.48	0.3	0	49
76	13	669	449	1.1	307	307	1,060	278	0.05	0.46	0.2	0	50
26	1	272	171	Tr	31	74	240	72	0.01	0.10	Tr	0	51
27	Tr	174	211	0.1	46	406	340	82	0.01	0.10	Tr	0	52
24	1	219	216	0.2	61	388	230	65	Tr	0.08	Tr	0	53
18	2	163	130	0.2	79	337	260	62	0.01	0.13	Tr	0	54
16	2	159	202	0.1	69	381	220	54	0.01	0.12	Tr	0	55
89	10	254	230	0.2	314	98	1,050	259	0.08	0.36	0.2	2	56
6	1	16	14	Tr	19	6	70	16	0.01	0.02	Tr	Tr	57
159	9	231	192	0.1	292	95	1,730	437	0.08	0.36	0.1	2	58
10	1	14	12	Tr	18	6	110	27	Tr	0.02	Tr	Tr	59
265	7	166	146	0.1	231	82	2,690	705	0.06	0.30	0.1	1	60
17	Tr	10	9	Tr	15	5	170	44	Tr	0.02	Tr	Tr	61
326	7	154	149	0.1	179	89	3,500	1,002	0.05	0.26	0.1	1	62
21	Tr	10	9	Tr	11	6	220	63	Tr	0.02	Tr	Tr	63
46	7	61	54	Tr	88	78	550	124	0.02	0.04	Tr	0	64
2	Tr	3	3	Tr	4	4	30	6	Tr	Tr	Tr	0	65
102	10	268	195	0.1	331	123	1,820	448	0.08	0.34	0.2	2	66
5	1	14	10	Tr	17	6	90	23	Tr	0.02	Tr	Tr	67

(Tr indicates nutrient present in trace amount.)

Item No.	Foods, approximate measures, units, and weight (weight of edible portion only)		Grams	Water Per-cent	Food energy Cal-ories	Pro-tein Grams	Fat Grams	Fatty acids Satu-rated Grams	Mono-unsatu-rated Grams	Poly-unsatu-rated Grams
	Dairy Products—Con.									
	Cream products, imitation (made with vegetable fat):									
	Sweet:									
	Creamers:									
68	Liquid (frozen)------------	1 tbsp----------	15	77	20	Tr	1	1.4	Tr	Tr
69	Powdered-------------------	1 tsp-----------	2	2	10	Tr	1	0.7	Tr	Tr
	Whipped topping:									
70	Frozen--------------------	1 cup----------	75	50	240	1	19	16.3	1.2	0.4
71		1 tbsp----------	4	50	15	Tr	1	0.9	0.1	Tr
	Powdered, made with whole									
72	milk---------------------	1 cup----------	80	67	150	3	10	8.5	0.7	0.2
73		1 tbsp----------	4	67	10	Tr	Tr	0.4	Tr	Tr
74	Pressurized---------------	1 cup----------	70	60	185	1	16	13.2	1.3	0.2
75		1 tbsp----------	4	60	10	Tr	1	0.8	0.1	Tr
76	Sour dressing (filled cream type product, nonbutterfat)--	1 cup----------	235	75	415	8	39	31.2	4.6	1.1
77		1 tbsp----------	12	75	20	Tr	2	1.6	0.2	0.1
	Ice cream. See Milk desserts, frozen (items 106-111).									
	Ice milk. See Milk desserts, frozen (items 112-114).									
	Milk:									
	Fluid:									
78	Whole (3.3% fat)-------------	1 cup----------	244	88	150	8	8	5.1	2.4	0.3
	Lowfat (2%):									
79	No milk solids added-------	1 cup----------	244	89	120	8	5	2.9	1.4	0.2
80	Milk solids added, label claim less than 10 g of protein per cup----------	1 cup----------	245	89	125	9	5	2.9	1.4	0.2
	Lowfat (1%):									
81	No milk solids added-------	1 cup----------	244	90	100	8	3	1.6	0.7	0.1
82	Milk solids added, label claim less than 10 g of protein per cup----------	1 cup----------	245	90	105	9	2	1.5	0.7	0.1
	Nonfat (skim):									
83	No milk solids added-------	1 cup----------	245	91	85	8	Tr	0.3	0.1	Tr
84	Milk solids added, label claim less than 10 g of protein per cup----------	1 cup----------	245	90	90	9	1	0.4	0.2	Tr
85	Buttermilk-----------------	1 cup----------	245	90	100	8	2	1.3	0.6	0.1
	Canned:									
86	Condensed, sweetened---------	1 cup----------	306	27	980	24	27	16.8	7.4	1.0
	Evaporated:									
87	Whole milk-----------------	1 cup----------	252	74	340	17	19	11.6	5.9	0.6
88	Skim milk------------------	1 cup----------	255	79	200	19	1	0.3	0.2	Tr
	Dried:									
89	Buttermilk-----------------	1 cup----------	120	3	465	41	7	4.3	2.0	0.3
	Nonfat, instantized:									
90	Envelope, 3.2 oz, net wt.[6]	1 envelope------	91	4	325	32	1	0.4	0.2	Tr
91	Cup-----------------------	1 cup----------	68	4	245	24	Tr	0.3	0.1	Tr
	Milk beverages:									
	Chocolate milk (commercial):									
92	Regular--------------------	1 cup----------	250	82	210	8	8	5.3	2.5	0.3
93	Lowfat (2%)----------------	1 cup----------	250	84	180	8	5	3.1	1.5	0.2
94	Lowfat (1%)----------------	1 cup----------	250	85	160	8	3	1.5	0.8	0.1

[5]Vitamin A value is largely from beta-carotene used for coloring.
[6]Yields 1 qt of fluid milk when reconstituted according to package directions.

Cholesterol	Carbohydrate	Calcium	Phosphorus	Iron	Potassium	Sodium	Vitamin A value		Thiamin	Riboflavin	Niacin	Ascorbic acid	Item No.
							(IU)	(RE)					
Milligrams	Grams	Milligrams	Milligrams	Milligrams	Milligrams	Milligrams	International units	Retinol equivalents	Milligrams	Milligrams	Milligrams	Milligrams	
0	2	1	10	Tr	29	12	[5]10	[5]1	0.00	0.00	0.0	0	68
0	1	Tr	8	Tr	16	4	Tr	Tr	0.00	Tr	0.0	0	69
0	17	5	6	0.1	14	19	[5]650	[5]65	0.00	0.00	0.0	0	70
0	1	Tr	Tr	Tr	1	1	[5]30	[5]3	0.00	0.00	0.0	0	71
8	13	72	69	Tr	121	53	[5]290	[5]39	0.02	0.09	Tr	1	72
Tr	1	4	3	Tr	6	3	[5]10	[5]2	Tr	Tr	Tr	Tr	73
0	11	4	13	Tr	13	43	[5]330	[5]33	0.00	0.00	0.0	0	74
0	1	Tr	1	Tr	1	2	[5]20	[5]2	0.00	0.00	0.0	0	75
13	11	266	205	0.1	380	113	20	5	0.09	0.38	0.2	2	76
1	1	14	10	Tr	19	6	Tr	Tr	Tr	0.02	Tr	Tr	77
33	11	291	228	0.1	370	120	310	76	0.09	0.40	0.2	2	78
18	12	297	232	0.1	377	122	500	139	0.10	0.40	0.2	2	79
18	12	313	245	0.1	397	128	500	140	0.10	0.42	0.2	2	80
10	12	300	235	0.1	381	123	500	144	0.10	0.41	0.2	2	81
10	12	313	245	0.1	397	128	500	145	0.10	0.42	0.2	2	82
4	12	302	247	0.1	406	126	500	149	0.09	0.34	0.2	2	83
5	12	316	255	0.1	418	130	500	149	0.10	0.43	0.2	2	84
9	12	285	219	0.1	371	257	80	20	0.08	0.38	0.1	2	85
104	166	868	775	0.6	1,136	389	1,000	248	0.28	1.27	0.6	8	86
74	25	657	510	0.5	764	267	610	136	0.12	0.80	0.5	5	87
9	29	738	497	0.7	845	293	1,000	298	0.11	0.79	0.4	3	88
83	59	1,421	1,119	0.4	1,910	621	260	65	0.47	1.89	1.1	7	89
17	47	1,120	896	0.3	1,552	499	[7]2,160	[7]646	0.38	1.59	0.8	5	90
12	35	837	670	0.2	1,160	373	[7]1,610	[7]483	0.28	1.19	0.6	4	91
31	26	280	251	0.6	417	149	300	73	0.09	0.41	0.3	2	92
17	26	284	254	0.6	422	151	500	143	0.09	0.41	0.3	2	93
7	26	287	256	0.6	425	152	500	148	0.10	0.42	0.3	2	94

[7]With added vitamin A.

(Tr indicates nutrient present in trace amount.)

Item No.	Foods, approximate measures, units, and weight (weight of edible portion only)		Water	Food energy	Pro-tein	Fat	Fatty acids		
							Satu-rated	Mono-unsatu-rated	Poly-unsatu-rated
	Dairy Products—Con.	Grams	Per-cent	Cal-ories	Grams	Grams	Grams	Grams	Grams
	Milk beverages:								
	Cocoa and chocolate-flavored beverages:								
95	Powder containing nonfat dry milk----------------------	1 oz------------	28	1	100	3	1	0.6	0.3	Tr
96	Prepared (6 oz water plus 1 oz powder)-------------	1 serving-------	206	86	100	3	1	0.6	0.3	Tr
97	Powder without nonfat dry milk----------------------	3/4 oz----------	21	1	75	1	1	0.3	0.2	Tr
98	Prepared (8 oz whole milk plus 3/4 oz powder)------	1 serving-------	265	81	225	9	9	5.4	2.5	0.3
99	Eggnog (commercial)------------	1 cup------------	254	74	340	10	19	11.3	5.7	0.9
	Malted milk:								
	Chocolate:								
100	Powder---------------------	3/4 oz ---------	21	2	85	1	1	0.5	0.3	0.1
101	Prepared (8 oz whole milk plus 3/4 oz powder)----	1 serving-------	265	81	235	9	9	5.5	2.7	0.4
	Natural:								
102	Powder---------------------	3/4 oz----------	21	3	85	3	2	0.9	0.5	0.3
103	Prepared (8 oz whole milk plus 3/4 oz powder)----	1 serving-------	265	81	235	11	10	6.0	2.9	0.6
	Shakes, thick:								
104	Chocolate-------------------	10-oz container	283	72	335	9	8	4.8	2.2	0.3
105	Vanilla---------------------	10-oz container	283	74	315	11	9	5.3	2.5	0.3
	Milk desserts, frozen:								
	Ice cream, vanilla:								
	Regular (about 11% fat):								
106	Hardened-------------------	1/2 gal---------	1,064	61	2,155	38	115	71.3	33.1	4.3
107		1 cup-----------	133	61	270	5	14	8.9	4.1	0.5
108		3 fl oz---------	50	61	100	2	5	3.4	1.6	0.2
109	Soft serve (frozen custard)	1 cup-----------	173	60	375	7	23	13.5	6.7	1.0
110	Rich (about 16% fat), hardened-------------------	1/2 gal---------	1,188	59	2,805	33	190	118.3	54.9	7.1
111		1 cup-----------	148	59	350	4	24	14.7	6.8	0.9
	Ice milk, vanilla:								
112	Hardened (about 4% fat)------	1/2 gal---------	1,048	69	1,470	41	45	28.1	13.0	1.7
113		1 cup-----------	131	69	185	5	6	3.5	1.6	0.2
114	Soft serve (about 3% fat)----	1 cup-----------	175	70	225	8	5	2.9	1.3	0.2
115	Sherbet (about 2% fat)---------	1/2 gal---------	1,542	66	2,160	17	31	19.0	8.8	1.1
116		1 cup-----------	193	66	270	2	4	2.4	1.1	0.1
	Yogurt:								
	With added milk solids:								
	Made with lowfat milk:								
117	Fruit-flavored[8]------------	8-oz container--	227	74	230	10	2	1.6	0.7	0.1
118	Plain---------------------	8-oz container--	227	85	145	12	4	2.3	1.0	0.1
119	Made with nonfat milk-------	8-oz container--	227	85	125	13	Tr	0.3	0.1	Tr
	Without added milk solids:								
120	Made with whole milk---------	8-oz container--	227	88	140	8	7	4.8	2.0	0.2
	Eggs								
	Eggs, large (24 oz per dozen):								
	Raw:								
121	Whole, without shell---------	1 egg-----------	50	75	80	6	6	1.7	2.2	0.7
122	White-----------------------	1 white---------	33	88	15	3	Tr	0.0	0.0	0.0
123	Yolk------------------------	1 yolk----------	17	49	65	3	6	1.7	2.2	0.7
	Cooked:								
124	Fried in butter-------------	1 egg-----------	46	68	95	6	7	2.7	2.7	0.8
125	Hard-cooked, shell removed---	1 egg-----------	50	75	80	6	6	1.7	2.2	0.7
126	Poached---------------------	1 egg----------	50	74	80	6	6	1.7	2.2	0.7
127	Scrambled (milk added) in butter. Also omelet--------	1 egg-----------	64	73	110	7	8	3.2	2.9	0.8

[8]Carbohydrate content varies widely because of amount of sugar added and amount and solids content of added flavoring.

Nutrients in Indicated Quantity

Cholesterol	Carbohydrate	Calcium	Phosphorus	Iron	Potassium	Sodium	Vitamin A value (IU)	Vitamin A value (RE)	Thiamin	Riboflavin	Niacin	Ascorbic acid	Item No.
Milligrams	Grams	Milligrams	Milligrams	Milligrams	Milligrams	Milligrams	International units	Retinol equivalents	Milligrams	Milligrams	Milligrams	Milligrams	
1	22	90	88	0.3	223	139	Tr	Tr	0.03	0.17	0.2	Tr	95
1	22	90	88	0.3	223	139	Tr	Tr	0.03	0.17	0.2	Tr	96
0	19	7	26	0.7	136	56	Tr	Tr	Tr	0.03	0.1	Tr	97
33	30	298	254	0.9	508	176	310	76	0.10	0.43	0.3	3	98
149	34	330	278	0.5	420	138	890	203	0.09	0.48	0.3	4	99
1	18	13	37	0.4	130	49	20	5	0.04	0.04	0.4	0	100
34	29	304	265	0.5	500	168	330	80	0.14	0.43	0.7	2	101
4	15	56	79	0.2	159	96	70	17	0.11	0.14	1.1	0	102
37	27	347	307	0.3	529	215	380	93	0.20	0.54	1.3	2	103
30	60	374	357	0.9	634	314	240	59	0.13	0.63	0.4	0	104
33	50	413	326	0.3	517	270	320	79	0.08	0.55	0.4	0	105
476	254	1,406	1,075	1.0	2,052	929	4,340	1,064	0.42	2.63	1.1	6	106
59	32	176	134	0.1	257	116	540	133	0.05	0.33	0.1	1	107
22	12	66	51	Tr	96	44	200	50	0.02	0.12	0.1	Tr	108
153	38	236	199	0.4	338	153	790	199	0.08	0.45	0.2	1	109
703	256	1,213	927	0.8	1,771	868	7,200	1,758	0.36	2.27	0.9	5	110
88	32	151	115	0.1	221	108	900	219	0.04	0.28	0.1	1	111
146	232	1,409	1,035	1.5	2,117	836	1,710	419	0.61	2.78	0.9	6	112
18	29	176	129	0.2	265	105	210	52	0.08	0.35	0.1	1	113
13	38	274	202	0.3	412	163	175	44	0.12	0.54	0.2	1	114
113	469	827	594	2.5	1,585	706	1,480	308	0.26	0.71	1.0	31	115
14	59	103	74	0.3	198	88	190	39	0.03	0.09	0.1	4	116
10	43	345	271	0.2	442	133	100	25	0.08	0.40	0.2	1	117
14	16	415	326	0.2	531	159	150	36	0.10	0.49	0.3	2	118
4	17	452	355	0.2	579	174	20	5	0.11	0.53	0.3	2	119
29	11	274	215	0.1	351	105	280	68	0.07	0.32	0.2	1	120
274	1	28	90	1.0	65	69	260	78	0.04	0.15	Tr	0	121
0	Tr	4	4	Tr	45	50	0	0	Tr	0.09	Tr	0	122
272	Tr	26	86	0.9	15	8	310	94	0.04	0.07	Tr	0	123
278	1	29	91	1.1	66	162	320	94	0.04	0.14	Tr	0	124
274	1	28	90	1.0	65	69	260	78	0.04	0.14	Tr	0	125
273	1	28	90	1.0	65	146	260	78	0.03	0.13	Tr	0	126
282	2	54	109	1.0	97	176	350	102	0.04	0.18	Tr	Tr	127

(Tr indicates nutrient present in trace amount.)

Item No.	Foods, approximate measures, units, and weight (weight of edible portion only)			Water	Food energy	Pro-tein	Fat	Fatty acids		
								Satu-rated	Mono-unsatu-rated	Poly-unsatu-rated
	Fats and Oils		Grams	Per-cent	Cal-ories	Grams	Grams	Grams	Grams	Grams
	Butter (4 sticks per lb):									
128	Stick-------------------------	1/2 cup---------	113	16	810	1	92	57.1	26.4	3.4
129	Tablespoon (1/8 stick)---------	1 tbsp----------	14	16	100	Tr	11	7.1	3.3	0.4
130	Pat (1 in square, 1/3 in high; 90 per lb)-------------	1 pat-----------	5	16	35	Tr	4	2.5	1.2	0.2
131	Fats, cooking (vegetable shortenings)--------------------	1 cup-----------	205	0	1,810	0	205	51.3	91.2	53.5
132		1 tbsp----------	13	0	115	0	13	3.3	5.8	3.4
133	Lard---------------------------	1 cup-----------	205	0	1,850	0	205	80.4	92.5	23.0
134		1 tbsp----------	13	0	115	0	13	5.1	5.9	1.5
	Margarine:									
135	Imitation (about 40% fat), soft	8-oz container--	227	58	785	1	88	17.5	35.6	31.3
136		1 tbsp----------	14	58	50	Tr	5	1.1	2.2	1.9
	Regular (about 80% fat): Hard (4 sticks per lb):									
137	Stick----------------------	1/2 cup---------	113	16	810	1	91	17.9	40.5	28.7
138	Tablespoon (1/8 stick)-----	1 tbsp----------	14	16	100	Tr	11	2.2	5.0	3.6
139	Pat (1 in square, 1/3 in high; 90 per lb)---------	1 pat-----------	5	16	35	Tr	4	0.8	1.8	1.3
140	Soft-----------------------	8-oz container--	227	16	1,625	2	183	31.3	64.7	78.5
141		1 tbsp----------	14	16	100	Tr	11	1.9	4.0	4.8
	Spread (about 60% fat): Hard (4 sticks per lb):									
142	Stick----------------------	1/2 cup---------	113	37	610	1	69	15.9	29.4	20.5
143	Tablespoon (1/8 stick)-----	1 tbsp----------	14	37	75	Tr	9	2.0	3.6	2.5
144	Pat (1 in square, 1/3 in high; 90 per lb)---------	1 pat-----------	5	37	25	Tr	3	0.7	1.3	0.9
145	Soft-----------------------	8-oz container--	227	37	1,225	1	138	29.1	71.5	31.3
146		1 tbsp----------	14	37	75	Tr	9	1.8	4.4	1.9
	Oils, salad or cooking:									
147	Corn-------------------------	1 cup-----------	218	0	1,925	0	218	27.7	52.8	128.0
148		1 tbsp----------	14	0	125	0	14	1.8	3.4	8.2
149	Olive------------------------	1 cup-----------	216	0	1,910	0	216	29.2	159.2	18.1
150		1 tbsp----------	14	0	125	0	14	1.9	10.3	1.2
151	Peanut-----------------------	1 cup-----------	216	0	1,910	0	216	36.5	99.8	69.1
152		1 tbsp----------	14	0	125	0	14	2.4	6.5	4.5
153	Safflower--------------------	1 cup-----------	218	0	1,925	0	218	19.8	26.4	162.4
154		1 tbsp----------	14	0	125	0	14	1.3	1.7	10.4
155	Soybean oil, hydrogenated (partially hardened)---------	1 cup-----------	218	0	1,925	0	218	32.5	93.7	82.0
156		1 tbsp----------	14	0	125	0	14	2.1	6.0	5.3
157	Soybean-cottonseed oil blend, hydrogenated----------------	1 cup-----------	218	0	1,925	0	218	39.2	64.3	104.9
158		1 tbsp----------	14	0	125	0	14	2.5	4.1	6.7
159	Sunflower--------------------	1 cup-----------	218	0	1,925	0	218	22.5	42.5	143.2
160		1 tbsp----------	14	0	125	0	14	1.4	2.7	9.2
	Salad dressings: Commercial:									
161	Blue cheese------------------	1 tbsp----------	15	32	75	1	8	1.5	1.8	4.2
	French:									
162	Regular-------------------	1 tbsp----------	16	35	85	Tr	9	1.4	4.0	3.5
163	Low calorie---------------	1 tbsp----------	16	75	25	Tr	2	0.2	0.3	1.0
	Italian:									
164	Regular-------------------	1 tbsp----------	15	34	80	Tr	9	1.3	3.7	3.2
165	Low calorie---------------	1 tbsp----------	15	86	5	Tr	Tr	Tr	Tr	Tr
	Mayonnaise:									
166	Regular-------------------	1 tbsp----------	14	15	100	Tr	11	1.7	3.2	5.8
167	Imitation-----------------	1 tbsp----------	15	63	35	Tr	3	0.5	0.7	1.6
168	Mayonnaise type-------------	1 tbsp----------	15	40	60	Tr	5	0.7	1.4	2.7
169	Tartar sauce---------------	1 tbsp----------	14	34	75	Tr	8	1.2	2.6	3.9
	Thousand island:									
170	Regular-------------------	1 tbsp----------	16	46	60	Tr	6	1.0	1.3	3.2
171	Low calorie---------------	1 tbsp----------	15	69	25	Tr	2	0.2	0.4	0.9

[9]For salted butter; unsalted butter contains 12 mg sodium per stick, 2 mg per tbsp, or 1 mg per pat.
[10]Values for vitamin A are year-round average.

| | | | | | | | Nutrients in Indicated Quantity | | | | | | |

Cholesterol	Carbohydrate	Calcium	Phosphorus	Iron	Potassium	Sodium	Vitamin A value		Thiamin	Riboflavin	Niacin	Ascorbic acid	Item No.
							(IU)	(RE)					
Milligrams	Grams	Milligrams	Milligrams	Milligrams	Milligrams	Milligrams	International units	Retinol equivalents	Milligrams	Milligrams	Milligrams	Milligrams	
247	Tr	27	26	0.2	29	[9]933	[10]3,460	[10]852	0.01	0.04	Tr	0	128
31	Tr	3	3	Tr	4	[9]116	[10]430	[10]106	Tr	Tr	Tr	0	129
11	Tr	1	1	Tr	1	[9]41	[10]150	[10]38	Tr	Tr	Tr	0	130
0	0	0	0	0.0	0	0	0	0	0.00	0.00	0.0	0	131
0	0	0	0	0.0	0	0	0	0	0.00	0.00	0.0	0	132
195	0	0	0	0.0	0	0	0	0	0.00	0.00	0.0	0	133
12	0	0	0	0.0	0	0	0	0	0.00	0.00	0.0	0	134
0	1	40	31	0.0	57	[11]2,178	[12]7,510	[12]2,254	0.01	0.05	Tr	Tr	135
0	Tr	2	2	0.0	4	[11]134	[12]460	[12]139	Tr	Tr	Tr	Tr	136
0	1	34	26	0.1	48	[11]1,066	[12]3,740	[12]1,122	0.01	0.04	Tr	Tr	137
0	Tr	4	3	Tr	6	[11]132	[12]460	[12]139	Tr	0.01	Tr	Tr	138
0	Tr	1	1	Tr	2	[11]47	[12]170	[12]50	Tr	Tr	Tr	Tr	139
0	1	60	46	0.0	86	[11]2,449	[12]7,510	[12]2,254	0.02	0.07	Tr	Tr	140
0	Tr	4	3	0.0	5	[11]151	[12]460	[12]139	Tr	Tr	Tr	Tr	141
0	0	24	18	0.0	34	[11]1,123	[12]3,740	[12]1,122	0.01	0.03	Tr	Tr	142
0	0	3	2	0.0	4	[11]139	[12]460	[12]139	Tr	Tr	Tr	Tr	143
0	0	1	1	0.0	1	[11]50	[12]170	[12]50	Tr	Tr	Tr	Tr	144
0	0	47	37	0.0	68	[11]2,256	[12]7,510	[12]2,254	0.02	0.06	Tr	Tr	145
0	0	3	2	0.0	4	[11]139	[12]460	[12]139	Tr	Tr	Tr	Tr	146
0	0	0	0	0.0	0	0	0	0	0.00	0.00	0.0	0	147
0	0	0	0	0.0	0	0	0	0	0.00	0.00	0.0	0	148
0	0	0	0	0.0	0	0	0	0	0.00	0.00	0.0	0	149
0	0	0	0	0.0	0	0	0	0	0.00	0.00	0.0	0	150
0	0	0	0	0.0	0	0	0	0	0.00	0.00	0.0	0	151
0	0	0	0	0.0	0	0	0	0	0.00	0.00	0.0	0	152
0	0	0	0	0.0	0	0	0	0	0.00	0.00	0.0	0	153
0	0	0	0	0.0	0	0	0	0	0.00	0.00	0.0	0	154
0	0	0	0	0.0	0	0	0	0	0.00	0.00	0.0	0	155
0	0	0	0	0.0	0	0	0	0	0.00	0.00	0.0	0	156
0	0	0	0	0.0	0	0	0	0	0.00	0.00	0.0	0	157
0	0	0	0	0.0	0	0	0	0	0.00	0.00	0.0	0	158
0	0	0	0	0.0	0	0	0	0	0.00	0.00	0.0	0	159
0	0	0	0	0.0	0	0	0	0	0.00	0.00	0.0	0	160
3	1	12	11	Tr	6	164	30	10	Tr	0.02	Tr	Tr	161
0	1	2	1	Tr	2	188	Tr	Tr	Tr	Tr	Tr	Tr	162
0	2	6	5	Tr	3	306	Tr	Tr	Tr	Tr	Tr	Tr	163
0	1	1	1	Tr	5	162	30	3	Tr	Tr	Tr	Tr	164
0	2	1	1	Tr	4	136	Tr	Tr	Tr	Tr	Tr	Tr	165
8	Tr	3	4	0.1	5	80	40	12	0.00	0.00	Tr	0	166
4	2	Tr	Tr	0.0	2	75	0	0	0.00	0.00	0.0	0	167
4	4	2	4	Tr	1	107	30	13	Tr	Tr	Tr	0	168
4	1	3	4	0.1	11	182	30	9	Tr	Tr	0.0	Tr	169
4	2	2	3	0.1	18	112	50	15	Tr	Tr	Tr	0	170
2	2	2	3	0.1	17	150	50	14	Tr	Tr	Tr	0	171

[11]For salted margarine.
[12]Based on average vitamin A content of fortified margarine. Federal specifications for fortified margarine require a minimum of 15,000 IU per pound.

(Tr indicates nutrient present in trace amount.)

Item No.	Foods, approximate measures, units, and weight (weight of edible portion only)			Water	Food energy	Pro-tein	Fat	Fatty acids		
								Satu-rated	Mono-unsatu-rated	Poly-unsatu-rated
	Fats and Oils—Con.		Grams	Per-cent	Cal-ories	Grams	Grams	Grams	Grams	Grams
	Salad dressings:									
	Prepared from home recipe:									
172	Cooked type[13] ----------------	1 tbsp----------	16	69	25	1	2	0.5	0.6	0.3
173	Vinegar and oil--------------	1 tbsp----------	16	47	70	0	8	1.5	2.4	3.9
	Fish and Shellfish									
	Clams:									
174	Raw, meat only-----------------	3 oz------------	85	82	65	11	1	0.3	0.3	0.3
175	Canned, drained solids---------	3 oz------------	85	77	85	13	2	0.5	0.5	0.4
176	Crabmeat, canned----------------	1 cup-----------	135	77	135	23	3	0.5	0.8	1.4
177	Fish sticks, frozen, reheated, (stick, 4 by 1 by 1/2 in)------	1 fish stick----	28	52	70	6	3	0.8	1.4	0.8
	Flounder or Sole, baked, with lemon juice:									
178	With butter--------------------	3 oz------------	85	73	120	16	6	3.2	1.5	0.5
179	With margarine-----------------	3 oz------------	85	73	120	16	6	1.2	2.3	1.9
180	Without added fat--------------	3 oz------------	85	78	80	17	1	0.3	0.2	0.4
181	Haddock, breaded, fried[14]--------	3 oz------------	85	61	175	17	9	2.4	3.9	2.4
182	Halibut, broiled, with butter and lemon juice---------------	3 oz------------	85	67	140	20	6	3.3	1.6	0.7
183	Herring, pickled[14]---------	3 oz------------	85	59	190	17	13	4.3	4.6	3.1
184	Ocean perch, breaded, fried[14]----	1 fillet--------	85	59	185	16	11	2.6	4.6	2.8
	Oysters:									
185	Raw, meat only (13-19 medium Selects)----------------------	1 cup-----------	240	85	160	20	4	1.4	0.5	1.4
186	Breaded, fried[14]---------------	1 oyster--------	45	65	90	5	5	1.4	2.1	1.4
	Salmon:									
187	Canned (pink), solids and liquid----------------------	3 oz-----------	85	71	120	17	5	0.9	1.5	2.1
188	Baked (red)--------------------	3 oz-----------	85	67	140	21	5	1.2	2.4	1.4
189	Smoked-------------------------	3 oz-----------	85	59	150	18	8	2.6	·3.9	0.7
190	Sardines, Atlantic, canned in oil, drained solids-----------	3 oz-----------	85	62	175	20	9	2.1	3.7	2.9
191	Scallops, breaded, frozen, reheated----------------------	6 scallops------	90	59	195	15	10	2.5	4.1	2.5
	Shrimp:									
192	Canned, drained solids---------	3 oz------------	85	70	100	21	1	0.2	0.2	0.4
193	French fried (7 medium)[16]------	3 oz-----------	85	55	200	16	10	2.5	4.1	2.6
194	Trout, broiled, with butter and lemon juice------------------	3 oz-----------	85	63	175	21	9	4.1	2.9	1.6
	Tuna, canned, drained solids:									
195	Oil pack, chunk light---------	3 oz-----------	85	61	165	24	7	1.4	1.9	3.1
196	Water pack, solid white--------	3 oz-----------	85	63	135	30	1	0.3	0.2	0.3
197	Tuna salad[17]---------------------	1 cup-----------	205	63	375	33	19	3.3	4.9	9.2
	Fruits and Fruit Juices									
	Apples:									
	Raw:									
	Unpeeled, without cores:									
198	2-3/4-in diam. (about 3 per lb with cores)-----------	1 apple---------	138	84	80	Tr	Tr	0.1	Tr	0.1
199	3-1/4-in diam. (about 2 per lb with cores)-----------	1 apple---------	212	84	125	Tr	1	0.1	Tr	0.2
200	Peeled, sliced---------------	1 cup-----------	110	84	65	Tr	Tr	0.1	Tr	0.1
201	Dried, sulfured--------------	10 rings--------	64	32	155	1	Tr	Tr	Tr	0.1
202	Apple juice, bottled or canned[19]	1 cup-----------	248	88	115	Tr	Tr	Tr	Tr	0.1
	Applesauce, canned:									
203	Sweetened---------------------	1 cup-----------	255	80	195	Tr	Tr	0.1	Tr	0.1
204	Unsweetened-------------------	1 cup-----------	244	88	105	Tr	Tr	Tr	Tr	Tr

[13] Fatty acid values apply to product made with regular margarine.
[14] Dipped in egg, milk, and breadcrumbs; fried in vegetable shortening.
[15] If bones are discarded, value for calcium will be greatly reduced.
[16] Dipped in egg, breadcrumbs, and flour; fried in vegetable shortening.

							Vitamin A value						
Cho-les-terol	Carbo-hydrate	Calcium	Phos-phorus	Iron	Potas-sium	Sodium	(IU)	(RE)	Thiamin	Ribo-flavin	Niacin	Ascorbic acid	Item No.
Milli-grams	Grams	Milli-grams	Milli-grams	Milli-grams	Milli-grams	Milli-grams	Inter-national units	Retinol equiva-lents	Milli-grams	Milli-grams	Milli-grams	Milli-grams	
9	2	13	14	0.1	19	117	70	20	0.01	0.02	Tr	Tr	172
0	Tr	0	0	0.0	1	Tr	0	0	0.00	0.00	0.0	0	173
43	2	59	138	2.6	154	102	90	26	0.09	0.15	1.1	9	174
54	2	47	116	3.5	119	102	90	26	0.01	0.09	0.9	3	175
135	1	61	246	1.1	149	1,350	50	14	0.11	0.11	2.6	0	176
26	4	11	58	0.3	94	53	20	5	0.03	0.05	0.6	0	177
68	Tr	13	187	0.3	272	145	210	54	0.05	0.08	1.6	1	178
55	Tr	14	187	0.3	273	151	230	69	0.05	0.08	1.6	1	179
59	Tr	13	197	0.3	286	101	30	10	0.05	0.08	1.7	1	180
75	7	34	183	1.0	270	123	70	20	0.06	0.10	2.9	0	181
62	Tr	14	206	0.7	441	103	610	174	0.06	0.07	7.7	1	182
85	0	29	128	0.9	85	850	110	33	0.04	0.18	2.8	0	183
66	7	31	191	1.2	241	138	70	20	0.10	0.11	2.0	0	184
120	8	226	343	15.6	290	175	740	223	0.34	0.43	6.0	24	185
35	5	49	73	3.0	64	70	150	44	0.07	0.10	1.3	4	186
34	0	[15]167	243	0.7	307	443	60	18	0.03	0.15	6.8	0	187
60	0	26	269	0.5	305	55	290	87	0.18	0.14	5.5	0	188
51	0	12	208	0.8	327	1,700	260	77	0.17	0.17	6.8	0	189
85	0	[15]371	424	2.6	349	425	190	56	0.03	0.17	4.6	0	190
70	10	39	203	2.0	369	298	70	21	0.11	0.11	1.6	0	191
128	1	98	224	1.4	1	1,955	50	15	0.01	0.03	1.5	0	192
168	11	61	154	2.0	189	384	90	26	0.06	0.09	2.8	0	193
71	Tr	26	259	1.0	297	122	230	60	0.07	0.07	2.3	1	194
55	0	7	199	1.6	298	303	70	20	0.04	0.09	10.1	0	195
48	0	17	202	0.6	255	468	110	32	0.03	0.10	13.4	0	196
80	19	31	281	2.5	531	877	230	53	0.06	0.14	13.3	6	197
0	21	10	10	0.2	159	Tr	70	7	0.02	0.02	0.1	8	198
0	32	15	15	0.4	244	Tr	110	11	0.04	0.03	0.2	12	199
0	16	4	8	0.1	124	Tr	50	5	0.02	0.01	0.1	4	200
0	42	9	24	0.9	288	[18]56	0	0	0.00	0.10	0.6	2	201
0	29	17	17	0.9	295	7	Tr	Tr	0.05	0.04	0.2	[20]2	202
0	51	10	18	0.9	156	8	30	3	0.03	0.07	0.5	[20]4	203
0	28	7	17	0.3	183	5	70	7	0.03	0.06	0.5	[20]3	204

[17] Made with drained chunk light tuna, celery, onion, pickle relish, and mayonnaise-type salad dressing.
[18] Sodium bisulfite used to preserve color; unsulfited product would contain less sodium.
[19] Also applies to pasteurized apple cider.
[20] Without added ascorbic acid. For value with added ascorbic acid, refer to label.

(Tr indicates nutrient present in trace amount.)

Item No.	Foods, approximate measures, units, and weight (weight of edible portion only)		Grams	Water	Food energy	Pro-tein	Fat	Fatty acids		
								Satu-rated	Mono-unsatu-rated	Poly-unsatu-rated
			Grams	Per-cent	Cal-ories	Grams	Grams	Grams	Grams	Grams
	Fruits and Fruit Juices—Con.									
	Apricots:									
205	Raw, without pits (about 12 per lb with pits)----------------	3 apricots------	106	86	50	1	Tr	Tr	0.2	0.1
	Canned (fruit and liquid):									
206	Heavy syrup pack------------	1 cup----------	258	78	215	1	Tr	Tr	0.1	Tr
207		3 halves--------	85	78	70	Tr	Tr	Tr	Tr	Tr
208	Juice pack-------------------	1 cup----------	248	87	120	2	Tr	Tr	Tr	Tr
209		3 halves--------	84	87	40	1	Tr	Tr	Tr	Tr
	Dried:									
210	Uncooked (28 large or 37 medium halves per cup)-----	1 cup----------	130	31	310	5	1	Tr	0.3	0.1
211	Cooked, unsweetened, fruit and liquid----------------	1 cup----------	250	76	210	3	Tr	Tr	0.2	0.1
212	Apricot nectar, canned-----------	1 cup----------	251	85	140	1	Tr	Tr	0.1	Tr
	Avocados, raw, whole, without skin and seed:									
213	California (about 2 per lb with skin and seed)-----------	1 avocado-------	173	73	305	4	30	4.5	19.4	3.5
214	Florida (about 1 per lb with skin and seed)---------------	1 avocado-------	304	80	340	5	27	5.3	14.8	4.5
	Bananas, raw, without peel:									
215	Whole (about 2-1/2 per lb with peel)-----------------------	1 banana--------	114	74	105	1	1	0.2	Tr	0.1
216	Sliced----------------------------	1 cup----------	150	74	140	2	1	0.3	0.1	0.1
217	Blackberries, raw---------------	1 cup----------	144	86	75	1	1	0.2	0.1	0.1
	Blueberries:									
218	Raw----------------------------	1 cup----------	145	85	80	1	1	Tr	0.1	0.3
219	Frozen, sweetened-------------	10-oz container	284	77	230	1	Tr	Tr	0.1	0.2
220		1 cup----------	230	77	185	1	Tr	Tr	Tr	0.1
	Cantaloup. See Melons (item 251).									
	Cherries:									
221	Sour, red, pitted, canned, water pack-------------------	1 cup----------	244	90	90	2	Tr	0.1	0.1	0.1
222	Sweet, raw, without pits and stems-----------------------	10 cherries-----	68	81	50	1	1	0.1	0.2	0.2
223	Cranberry juice cocktail, bottled, sweetened-------------	1 cup----------	253	85	145	Tr	Tr	Tr	Tr	0.1
224	Cranberry sauce, sweetened, canned, strained---------------	1 cup----------	277	61	420	1	Tr	Tr	0.1	0.2
	Dates:									
225	Whole, without pits------------	10 dates--------	83	23	230	2	Tr	0.1	0.1	Tr
226	Chopped-----------------------	1 cup----------	178	23	490	4	1	0.3	0.2	Tr
227	Figs, dried----------------------	10 figs---------	187	28	475	6	2	0.4	0.5	1.0
	Fruit cocktail, canned, fruit and liquid:									
228	Heavy syrup pack---------------	1 cup----------	255	80	185	1	Tr	Tr	Tr	0.1
229	Juice pack--------------------	1 cup----------	248	87	115	1	Tr	Tr	Tr	Tr
	Grapefruit:									
230	Raw, without peel, membrane and seeds (3-3/4-in diam., 1 lb 1 oz, whole, with refuse)----	1/2 grapefruit--	120	91	40	1	Tr	Tr	Tr	Tr
231	Canned, sections with syrup----	1 cup----------	254	84	150	1	Tr	Tr	Tr	0.1
	Grapefruit juice:									
232	Raw---------------------------	1 cup----------	247	90	95	1	Tr	Tr	Tr	0.1
	Canned:									
233	Unsweetened------------------	1 cup----------	247	90	95	1	Tr	Tr	Tr	0.1
234	Sweetened--------------------	1 cup----------	250	87	115	1	Tr	Tr	Tr	0.1
	Frozen concentrate, unsweetened									
235	Undiluted---------------------	6-fl-oz can-----	207	62	300	4	1	0.1	0.1	0.2
236	Diluted with 3 parts water by volume---------------------	1 cup----------	247	89	100	1	Tr	Tr	Tr	0.1

[20] Without added ascorbic acid. For value with added ascorbic acid, refer to label.
[21] With added ascorbic acid.

							Nutrients in Indicated Quantity						
Cho-les-terol	Carbo-hydrate	Calcium	Phos-phorus	Iron	Potas-sium	Sodium	Vitamin A value		Thiamin	Ribo-flavin	Niacin	Ascorbic acid	Item No.
							(IU)	(RE)					
Milli-grams	Grams	Milli-grams	Milli-grams	Milli-grams	Milli-grams	Milli-grams	Inter-national units	Retinol equiva-lents	Milli-grams	Milli-grams	Milli-grams	Milli-grams	
0	12	15	20	0.6	314	1	2,770	277	0.03	0.04	0.6	11	205
0	55	23	31	0.8	361	10	3,170	317	0.05	0.06	1.0	8	206
0	18	8	10	0.3	119	3	1,050	105	0.02	0.02	0.3	3	207
0	31	30	50	0.7	409	10	4,190	419	0.04	0.05	0.9	12	208
0	10	10	17	0.3	139	3	1,420	142	0.02	0.02	0.3	4	209
0	80	59	152	6.1	1,791	13	9,410	941	0.01	0.20	3.9	3	210
0	55	40	103	4.2	1,222	8	5,910	591	0.02	0.08	2.4	4	211
0	36	18	23	1.0	286	8	3,300	330	0.02	0.04	0.7	[20]2	212
0	12	19	73	2.0	1,097	21	1,060	106	0.19	0.21	3.3	14	213
0	27	33	119	1.6	1,484	15	1,860	186	0.33	0.37	5.8	24	214
0	27	7	23	0.4	451	1	90	9	0.05	0.11	0.6	10	215
0	35	9	30	0.5	594	2	120	12	0.07	0.15	0.8	14	216
0	18	46	30	0.8	282	Tr	240	24	0.04	0.06	0.6	30	217
0	20	9	15	0.2	129	9	150	15	0.07	0.07	0.5	19	218
0	62	17	20	1.1	170	3	120	12	0.06	0.15	0.7	3	219
0	50	14	16	0.9	138	2	100	10	0.05	0.12	0.6	2	220
0	22	27	24	3.3	239	17	1,840	184	0.04	0.10	0.4	5	221
0	11	10	13	0.3	152	Tr	150	15	0.03	0.04	0.3	5	222
0	38	8	3	0.4	61	10	10	1	0.01	0.04	0.1	[21]108	223
0	108	11	17	0.6	72	80	60	6	0.04	0.06	0.3	6	224
0	61	27	33	1.0	541	2	40	4	0.07	0.08	1.8	0	225
0	131	57	71	2.0	1,161	5	90	9	0.16	0.18	3.9	0	226
0	122	269	127	4.2	1,331	21	250	25	0.13	0.16	1.3	1	227
0	48	15	28	0.7	224	15	520	52	0.05	0.05	1.0	5	228
0	29	20	35	0.5	236	10	760	76	0.03	0.04	1.0	7	229
0	10	14	10	0.1	167	Tr	[22]10	[22]1	0.04	0.02	0.3	41	230
0	39	36	25	1.0	328	5	Tr	Tr	0.10	0.05	0.6	54	231
0	23	22	37	0.5	400	2	20	2	0.10	0.05	0.5	94	232
0	22	17	27	0.5	378	2	20	2	0.10	0.05	0.6	72	233
0	28	20	28	0.9	405	5	20	2	0.10	0.06	0.8	67	234
0	72	56	101	1.0	1,002	6	60	6	0.30	0.16	1.6	248	235
0	24	20	35	0.3	336	2	20	2	0.10	0.05	0.5	83	236

[22] For white grapefruit; pink grapefruit have about 310 IU or 31 RE.

(Tr indicates nutrient present in trace amount.)

Item No.	Foods, approximate measures, units, and weight (weight of edible portion only)		Water	Food energy	Pro-tein	Fat	Fatty acids		
							Satu-rated	Mono-unsatu-rated	Poly-unsatu-rated
		Grams	Per-cent	Cal-ories	Grams	Grams	Grams	Grams	Grams
	Fruits and Fruit Juices—Con.								
	Grapes, European type (adherent skin), raw:								
237	Thompson Seedless	10 grapes	50	81	35	Tr	Tr	0.1	Tr	0.1
238	Tokay and Emperor, seeded types	10 grapes	57	81	40	Tr	Tr	0.1	Tr	0.1
	Grape juice:								
239	Canned or bottled	1 cup	253	84	155	1	Tr	0.1	Tr	0.1
	Frozen concentrate, sweetened:								
240	Undiluted	6-fl-oz can	216	54	385	1	1	0.2	Tr	0.2
241	Diluted with 3 parts water by volume	1 cup	250	87	125	Tr	Tr	0.1	Tr	0.1
242	Kiwifruit, raw, without skin (about 5 per lb with skin)	1 kiwifruit	76	83	45	1	Tr	Tr	0.1	0.1
243	Lemons, raw, without peel and seeds (about 4 per lb with peel and seeds)	1 lemon	58	89	15	1	Tr	Tr	Tr	0.1
	Lemon juice:								
244	Raw	1 cup	244	91	60	1	Tr	Tr	Tr	Tr
245	Canned or bottled, unsweetened	1 cup	244	92	50	1	1	0.1	Tr	0.2
246		1 tbsp	15	92	5	Tr	Tr	Tr	Tr	Tr
247	Frozen, single-strength, unsweetened	6-fl-oz can	244	92	55	1	1	0.1	Tr	0.2
	Lime juice:								
248	Raw	1 cup	246	90	65	1	Tr	Tr	Tr	0.1
249	Canned, unsweetened	1 cup	246	93	50	1	1	0.1	0.1	0.2
250	Mangos, raw, without skin and seed (about 1-1/2 per lb with skin and seed)	1 mango	207	82	135	1	1	0.1	0.2	0.1
	Melons, raw, without rind and cavity contents:								
251	Cantaloup, orange-fleshed (5-in diam., 2-1/3 lb, whole, with rind and cavity contents)	1/2 melon	267	90	95	2	1	0.1	0:1	0.3
252	Honeydew (6-1/2-in diam., 5-1/4 lb, whole, with rind and cav-ity contents)	1/10 melon	129	90	45	1	Tr	Tr	Tr	0.1
253	Nectarines, raw, without pits (about 3 per lb with pits)	1 nectarine	136	86	65	1	1	0.1	0.2	0.3
	Oranges, raw:								
254	Whole, without peel and seeds (2-5/8-in diam., about 2-1/2 per lb, with peel and seeds)	1 orange	131	87	60	1	Tr	Tr	Tr	Tr
255	Sections without membranes	1 cup	180	87	85	2	Tr	Tr	Tr	Tr
	Orange juice:								
256	Raw, all varieties	1 cup	248	88	110	2	Tr	0.1	0.1	0.1
257	Canned, unsweetened	1 cup	249	89	105	1	Tr	Tr	0.1	0.1
258	Chilled	1 cup	249	88	110	2	1	0.1	0.1	0.2
	Frozen concentrate:								
259	Undiluted	6-fl-oz can	213	58	340	5	Tr	0.1	0.1	0.1
260	Diluted with 3 parts water by volume	1 cup	249	88	110	2	Tr	Tr	Tr	Tr
261	Orange and grapefruit juice, canned	1 cup	247	89	105	1	Tr	Tr	Tr	Tr
262	Papayas, raw, 1/2-in cubes	1 cup	140	86	65	1	Tr	0.1	0.1	Tr
	Peaches:								
	Raw:								
263	Whole, 2-1/2-in diam., peeled, pitted (about 4 per lb with peels and pits)	1 peach	87	88	35	1	Tr	Tr	Tr	Tr
264	Sliced	1 cup	170	88	75	1	Tr	Tr	0.1	0.1
	Canned, fruit and liquid:								
265	Heavy syrup pack	1 cup	256	79	190	1	Tr	Tr	0.1	0.1
266		1 half	81	79	60	Tr	Tr	Tr	Tr	Tr
267	Juice pack	1 cup	248	87	110	2	Tr	Tr	Tr	Tr
268		1 half	77	87	35	Tr	Tr	Tr	Tr	Tr

[20]Without added ascorbic acid. For value with added ascorbic acid, refer to label.
[21]With added ascorbic acid.

							Vitamin A value						
Cholesterol	Carbohydrate	Calcium	Phosphorus	Iron	Potassium	Sodium	(IU)	(RE)	Thiamin	Riboflavin	Niacin	Ascorbic acid	Item No.
Milligrams	Grams	Milligrams	Milligrams	Milligrams	Milligrams	Milligrams	International units	Retinol equivalents	Milligrams	Milligrams	Milligrams	Milligrams	
0	9	6	7	0.1	93	1	40	4	0.05	0.03	0.2	5	237
0	10	6	7	0.1	105	1	40	4	0.05	0.03	0.2	6	238
0	38	23	28	0.6	334	8	20	2	0.07	0.09	0.7	[20]Tr	239
0	96	28	32	0.8	160	15	60	6	0.11	0.20	0.9	[21]179	240
0	32	10	10	0.3	53	5	20	2	0.04	0.07	0.3	[21]60	241
0	11	20	30	0.3	252	4	130	13	0.02	0.04	0.4	74	242
0	5	15	9	0.3	80	1	20	2	0.02	0.01	0.1	31	243
0	21	17	15	0.1	303	2	50	5	0.07	0.02	0.2	112	244
0	16	27	22	0.3	249	[23]51	40	4	0.10	0.02	0.5	61	245
0	1	2	1	Tr	15	[23]3	Tr	Tr	0.01	Tr	Tr	4	246
0	16	20	20	0.3	217	2	30	3	0.14	0.03	0.3	77	247
0	22	22	17	0.1	268	2	20	2	0.05	0.02	0.2	72	248
0	16	30	25	0.6	185	[23]39	40	4	0.08	0.01	0.4	16	249
0	35	21	23	0.3	323	4	8,060	806	0.12	0.12	1.2	57	250
0	22	29	45	0.6	825	24	8,610	861	0.10	0.06	1.5	113	251
0	12	8	13	0.1	350	13	50	5	0.10	0.02	0.8	32	252
0	16	7	22	0.2	288	Tr	1,000	100	0.02	0.06	1.3	7	253
0	15	52	18	0.1	237	Tr	270	27	0.11	0.05	0.4	70	254
0	21	72	25	0.2	326	Tr	370	37	0.16	0.07	0.5	96	255
0	26	27	42	0.5	496	2	500	50	0.22	0.07	1.0	124	256
0	25	20	35	1.1	436	5	440	44	0.15	0.07	0.8	86	257
0	25	25	27	0.4	473	2	190	19	0.28	0.05	0.7	82	258
0	81	68	121	0.7	1,436	6	590	59	0.60	0.14	1.5	294	259
0	27	22	40	0.2	473	2	190	19	0.20	0.04	0.5	97	260
0	25	20	35	1.1	390	7	290	29	0.14	0.07	0.8	72	261
0	17	35	12	0.3	247	9	400	40	0.04	0.04	0.5	92	262
0	10	4	10	0.1	171	Tr	470	47	0.01	0.04	0.9	6	263
0	19	9	20	0.2	335	Tr	910	91	0.03	0.07	1.7	11	264
0	51	8	28	0.7	236	15	850	85	0.03	0.06	1.6	7	265
0	16	2	9	0.2	75	5	270	27	0.01	0.02	0.5	2	266
0	29	15	42	0.7	317	10	940	94	0.02	0.04	1.4	9	267
0	9	5	13	0.2	99	3	290	29	0.01	0.01	0.4	3	268

[23]Sodium benzoate and sodium bisulfite added as preservatives.

(Tr indicates nutrient present in trace amount.)

Item No.	Foods, approximate measures, units, and weight (weight of edible portion only)		Water	Food energy	Pro-tein	Fat	Fatty acids		
							Satu-rated	Mono-unsatu-rated	Poly-unsatu-rated
		Grams	Per-cent	Cal-ories	Grams	Grams	Grams	Grams	Grams
	Fruits and Fruit Juices—Con.								
	Peaches:								
	Dried:								
269	Uncooked--------------------- 1 cup-----------	160	32	380	6	1	0.1	0.4	0.6
270	Cooked, unsweetened, fruit								
	and liquid----------------- 1 cup-----------	258	78	200	3	1	0.1	0.2	0.3
271	Frozen, sliced, sweetened------ 10-oz container	284	75	265	2	Tr	Tr	0.1	0.2
272	1 cup-----------	250	75	235	2	Tr	Tr	0.1	0.2
	Pears:								
	Raw, with skin, cored:								
273	Bartlett, 2-1/2-in diam. (about 2-1/2 per lb with cores and stems)----------- 1 pear----------	166	84	100	1	1	Tr	0.1	0.2
274	Bosc, 2-1/2-in diam. (about 3 per lb with cores and stems)--------------------- 1 pear----------	141	84	85	1	1	Tr	0.1	0.1
275	D'Anjou, 3-in diam. (about 2 per lb with cores and stems)--------------------- 1 pear----------	200	84	120	1	1	Tr	0.2	0.2
	Canned, fruit and liquid:								
276	Heavy syrup pack------------- 1 cup-----------	255	80	190	1	Tr	Tr	0.1	0.1
277	1 half----------	79	80	60	Tr	Tr	Tr	Tr	Tr
278	Juice pack------------------- 1 cup-----------	248	86	125	1	Tr	Tr	Tr	Tr
279	1 half----------	77	86	40	Tr	Tr	Tr	Tr	Tr
	Pineapple:								
280	Raw, diced--------------------- 1 cup-----------	155	87	75	1	1	Tr	0.1	0.2
	Canned, fruit and liquid:								
	Heavy syrup pack:								
281	Crushed, chunks, tidbits--- 1 cup-----------	255	79	200	1	Tr	Tr	Tr	0.1
282	Slices--------------------- 1 slice---------	58	79	45	Tr	Tr	Tr	Tr	Tr
	Juice pack:								
283	Chunks or tidbits---------- 1 cup-----------	250	84	150	1	Tr	Tr	·Tr	0.1
284	Slices--------------------- 1 slice---------	58	84	35	Tr	Tr	Tr	Tr	Tr
285	Pineapple juice, unsweetened, canned------------------------ 1 cup-----------	250	86	140	1	Tr	Tr	Tr	0.1
	Plantains, without peel:								
286	Raw--------------------------- 1 plantain------	179	65	220	2	1	0.3	0.1	0.1
287	Cooked, boiled, sliced--------- 1 cup-----------	154	67	180	1	Tr	0.1	Tr	0.1
	Plums, without pits:								
	Raw:								
288	2-1/8-in diam. (about 6-1/2 per lb with pits)---------- 1 plum----------	66	85	35	1	Tr	Tr	0.3	0.1
289	1-1/2-in diam. (about 15 per lb with pits)-------------- 1 plum----------	28	85	15	Tr	Tr	Tr	0.1	Tr
	Canned, purple, fruit and liquid:								
290	Heavy syrup pack------------- 1 cup-----------	258	76	230	1	Tr	Tr	0.2	0.1
291	3 plums---------	133	76	120	Tr	Tr	Tr	0.1	Tr
292	Juice pack------------------- 1 cup-----------	252	84	145	1	Tr	Tr	Tr	Tr
293	3 plums---------	95	84	55	Tr	Tr	Tr	Tr	Tr
	Prunes, dried:								
294	Uncooked--------------------- 4 extra large or 5 large prunes	49	32	115	1	Tr	Tr	0.2	0.1
295	Cooked, unsweetened, fruit and liquid---------------------- 1 cup-----------	212	70	225	2	Tr	Tr	0.3	0.1
296	Prune juice, canned or bottled--- 1 cup-----------	256	81	180	2	Tr	Tr	0.1	Tr
	Raisins, seedless:								
297	Cup, not pressed down---------- 1 cup-----------	145	15	435	5	1	0.2	Tr	0.2
298	Packet, 1/2 oz (1-1/2 tbsp)---- 1 packet--------	14	15	40	Tr	Tr	Tr	Tr	Tr
	Raspberries:								
299	Raw--------------------------- 1 cup-----------	123	87	60	1	1	Tr	0.1	0.4
300	Frozen, sweetened-------------- 10-oz container	284	73	295	2	Tr	Tr	Tr	0.3
301	1 cup-----------	250	73	255	2	Tr	Tr	Tr	0.2

[21] With added ascorbic acid.

Nutrients in Indicated Quantity

Cholesterol	Carbohydrate	Calcium	Phosphorus	Iron	Potassium	Sodium	Vitamin A value		Thiamin	Riboflavin	Niacin	Ascorbic acid	Item No.
							(IU)	(RE)					
Milligrams	Grams	Milligrams	Milligrams	Milligrams	Milligrams	Milligrams	International units	Retinol equivalents	Milligrams	Milligrams	Milligrams	Milligrams	
0	98	45	190	6.5	1,594	11	3,460	346	Tr	0.34	7.0	8	269
0	51	23	98	3.4	826	5	510	51	0.01	0.05	3.9	10	270
0	68	9	31	1.1	369	17	810	81	0.04	0.10	1.9	[21]268	271
0	60	8	28	0.9	325	15	710	71	0.03	0.09	1.6	[21]236	272
0	25	18	18	0.4	208	Tr	30	3	0.03	0.07	0.2	7	273
0	21	16	16	0.4	176	Tr	30	3	0.03	0.06	0.1	6	274
0	30	22	22	0.5	250	Tr	40	4	0.04	0.08	0.2	8	275
0	49	13	18	0.6	166	13	10	1	0.03	0.06	0.6	3	276
0	15	4	6	0.2	51	4	Tr	Tr	0.01	0.02	0.2	1	277
0	32	22	30	0.7	238	10	10	1	0.03	0.03	0.5	4	278
0	10	7	9	0.2	74	3	Tr	Tr	0.01	0.01	0.2	1	279
0	19	11	11	0.6	175	2	40	4	0.14	0.06	0.7	24	280
0	52	36	18	1.0	265	3	40	4	0.23	0.06	0.7	19	281
0	12	8	4	0.2	60	1	10	1	0.05	0.01	0.2	4	282
0	39	35	15	0.7	305	3	100	10	0.24	0.05	0.7	24	283
0	9	8	3	0.2	71	1	20	2	0.06	0.01	0.2	6	284
0	34	43	20	0.7	335	3	10	1	0.14	0.06	0.6	27	285
0	57	5	61	1.1	893	7	2,020	202	0.09	0.10	1.2	33	286
0	48	3	43	0.9	716	8	1,400	140	0.07	0.08	1.2	17	287
0	9	3	7	0.1	114	Tr	210	21	0.03	0.06	0.3	6	288
0	4	1	3	Tr	48	Tr	90	9	0.01	0.03	0.1	3	289
0	60	23	34	2.2	235	49	670	67	0.04	0.10	0.8	1	290
0	31	12	17	1.1	121	25	340	34	0.02	0.05	0.4	1	291
0	38	25	38	0.9	388	3	2,540	254	0.06	0.15	1.2	7	292
0	14	10	14	0.3	146	1	960	96	0.02	0.06	0.4	3	293
0	31	25	39	1.2	365	2	970	97	0.04	0.08	1.0	2	294
0	60	49	74	2.4	708	4	650	65	0.05	0.21	1.5	6	295
0	45	31	64	3.0	707	10	10	1	0.04	0.18	2.0	10	296
0	115	71	141	3.0	1,089	17	10	1	0.23	0.13	1.2	5	297
0	11	7	14	0.3	105	2	Tr	Tr	0.02	0.01	0.1	Tr	298
0	14	27	15	0.7	187	Tr	160	16	0.04	0.11	1.1	31	299
0	74	43	48	1.8	324	3	170	17	0.05	0.13	0.7	47	300
0	65	38	43	1.6	285	3	150	15	0.05	0.11	0.6	41	301

(Tr indicates nutrient present in trace amount.)

Item No.	Foods, approximate measures, units, and weight (weight of edible portion only)			Water	Food energy	Pro-tein	Fat	Fatty acids		
								Satu-rated	Mono-unsatu-rated	Poly-unsatu-rated
	Fruits and Fruit Juices—Con.		Grams	Per-cent	Cal-ories	Grams	Grams	Grams	Grams	Grams
302	Rhubarb, cooked, added sugar-----	1 cup-----------	240	68	280	1	Tr	Tr	Tr	0.1
	Strawberries:									
303	Raw, capped, whole-------------	1 cup-----------	149	92	45	1	1	Tr	0.1	0.3
304	Frozen, sweetened, sliced------	10-oz container	284	73	275	2	Tr	Tr	0.1	0.2
305		1 cup-----------	255	73	245	1	Tr	Tr	Tr	0.2
	Tangerines:									
306	Raw, without peel and seeds (2-3/8-in diam., about 4 per lb, with peel and seeds)-----	1 tangerine-----	84	88	35	1	Tr	Tr	Tr	Tr
307	Canned, light syrup, fruit and liquid----------------------	1 cup-----------	252	83	155	1	Tr	Tr	Tr	0.1
308	Tangerine juice, canned, sweet-ened----------------------	1 cup-----------	249	87	125	1	Tr	Tr	Tr	0.1
	Watermelon, raw, without rind and seeds:									
309	Piece (4 by 8 in wedge with rind and seeds; 1/16 of 32-2/3-lb melon, 10 by 16 in)	1 piece---------	482	92	155	3	2	0.3	0.2	1.0
310	Diced------------------------	1 cup-----------	160	92	50	1	1	0.1	0.1	0.3
	Grain Products									
311	Bagels, plain or water, enriched, 3-1/2-in diam.[24] ---------------	1 bagel---------	68	29	200	7	2	0.3	0.5	0.7
312	Barley, pearled, light, uncooked	1 cup-----------	200	11	700	16	2	0.3	0.2	0.9
	Biscuits, baking powder, 2-in diam. (enriched flour, vege-table shortening):									
313	From home recipe---------------	1 biscuit-------	28	28	100	2	5	1.2	2.0	1.3
314	From mix-----------------------	1 biscuit-------	28	29	95	2	3	0.8	1.4	0.9
315	From refrigerated dough--------	1 biscuit-------	20	30	65	1	2	0.6	0.9	0.6
	Breadcrumbs, enriched:									
316	Dry, grated--------------------	1 cup-----------	100	7	390	13	5	1.5	1.6	1.0
	Soft. See White bread (item 351).									
	Breads:									
317	Boston brown bread, canned, slice, 3-1/4 in by 1/2 in[25] --	1 slice---------	45	45	95	2	1	0.3	0.1	0.1
	Cracked-wheat bread (3/4 en-riched wheat flour, 1/4 cracked wheat flour):[25]									
318	Loaf, 1 lb-------------------	1 loaf----------	454	35	1,190	42	16	3.1	4.3	5.7
319	Slice (18 per loaf)----------	1 slice---------	25	35	65	2	1	0.2	0.2	0.3
320	Toasted---------------------	1 slice---------	21	26	65	2	1	0.2	0.2	0.3
	French or vienna bread, en-riched:[25]									
321	Loaf, 1 lb-------------------	1 loaf----------	454	34	1,270	43	18	3.8	5.7	5.9
	Slice:									
322	French, 5 by 2-1/2 by 1 in	1 slice---------	35	34	100	3	1	0.3	0.4	0.5
323	Vienna, 4-3/4 by 4 by 1/2 in--------------------	1 slice---------	25	34	70	2	1	0.2	0.3	0.3
	Italian bread, enriched:									
324	Loaf, 1 lb-------------------	1 loaf----------	454	32	1,255	41	4	0.6	0.3	1.6
325	Slice, 4-1/2 by 3-1/4 by 3/4 in-------------------------	1 slice---------	30	32	85	3	Tr	Tr	Tr	0.1
	Mixed grain bread, enriched:[25]									
326	Loaf, 1 lb-------------------	1 loaf----------	454	37	1,165	45	17	3.2	4.1	6.5
327	Slice (18 per loaf)----------	1 slice---------	25	37	65	2	1	0.2	0.2	0.4
328	Toasted---------------------	1 slice---------	23	27	65	2	1	0.2	0.2	0.4

[24] Egg bagels have 44 mg cholesterol and 22 IU or 7 RE vitamin A per bagel.
[25] Made with vegetable shortening.

Nutrients in Indicated Quantity

Cho-les-terol	Carbo-hydrate	Calcium	Phos-phorus	Iron	Potas-sium	Sodium	Vitamin A value		Thiamin	Ribo-flavin	Niacin	Ascorbic acid	Item No.
							(IU)	(RE)					
Milli-grams	Grams	Milli-grams	Milli-grams	Milli-grams	Milli-grams	Milli-grams	Inter-national units	Retinol equiva-lents	Milli-grams	Milli-grams	Milli-grams	Milli-grams	
0	75	348	19	0.5	230	2	170	17	0.04	0.06	0.5	8	302
0	10	21	28	0.6	247	~1	40	4	0.03	0.10	0.3	84	303
0	74	31	37	1.7	278	9	70	7	0.05	0.14	1.1	118	304
0	66	28	33	1.5	250	8	60	6	0.04	0.13	1.0	106	305
0	9	12	8	0.1	132	1	770	77	0.09	0.02	0.1	26	306
0	41	18	25	0.9	197	15	2,120	212	0.13	0.11	1.1	50	307
0	30	45	35	0.5	443	2	1,050	105	0.15	0.05	0.2	55	308
0	35	39	43	0.8	559	10	1,760	176	0.39	0.10	1.0	46	309
0	11	13	14	0.3	186	3	590	59	0.13	0.03	0.3	15	310
0	38	29	46	1.8	50	245	0	0	0.26	0.20	2.4	0	311
0	158	32	378	4.2	320	6	0	0	0.24	0.10	6.2	0	312
Tr	13	47	36	0.7	32	195	10	3	0.08	0.08	0.8	Tr	313
Tr	14	58	128	0.7	56	262	20	4	0.12	0.11	0.8	Tr	314
1	10	4	79	0.5	18	249	0	0	0.08	0.05	0.7	0	315
5	73	122	141	4.1	152	736	0	0	0.35	0.35	4.8	0	316
3	21	41	72	0.9	131	113	[26]0	[26]0	0.06	0.04	0.7	0	317
0	227	295	581	12.1	608	1,966	Tr	Tr	1.73	1.73	15.3	Tr	318
0	12	16	32	0.7	34	106	Tr	Tr	0.10	0.09	0.8	Tr	319
0	12	16	32	0.7	34	106	Tr	Tr	0.07	0.09	0.8	Tr	320
0	230	499	386	14.0	409	2,633	Tr	Tr	2.09	1.59	18.2	Tr	321
0	18	39	30	1.1	32	203	Tr	Tr	0.16	0.12	1.4	Tr	322
0	13	28	21	0.8	23	145	Tr	Tr	0.12	0.09	1.0	Tr	323
0	256	77	350	12.7	336	2,656	0	0	1.80	1.10	15.0	0	324
0	17	5	23	0.8	22	176	0	0	0.12	0.07	1.0	0	325
0	212	472	962	14.8	990	1,870	Tr	Tr	1.77	1.73	18.9	Tr	326
0	12	27	55	0.8	56	106	Tr	Tr	0.10	0.10	1.1	Tr	327
0	12	27	55	0.8	56	106	Tr	Tr	0.08	0.10	1.1	Tr	328

[26] Made with white cornmeal. If made with yellow cornmeal, value is 32 IU or 3 RE.

(Tr indicates nutrient present in trace amount.)

Item No.	Foods, approximate measures, units, and weight (weight of edible portion only)		Grams	Water Per-cent	Food energy Cal-ories	Pro-tein Grams	Fat Grams	Fatty acids		
								Satu-rated Grams	Mono-unsatu-rated Grams	Poly-unsatu-rated Grams
	Grain Products—Con.									
	Breads:									
	Oatmeal bread, enriched:[25]									
329	Loaf, 1 lb-------------------	1 loaf----------	454	37	1,145	38	20	3.7	7.1	8.2
330	Slice (18 per loaf)----------	1 slice---------	25	37	65	2	1	0.2	0.4	0.5
331	Toasted---------------------	1 slice---------	23	30	65	2	1	0.2	0.4	0.5
332	Pita bread, enriched, white, 6-1/2-in diam.--------------	1 pita----------	60	31	165	6	1	0.1	0.1	0.4
	Pumpernickel (2/3 rye flour, 1/3 enriched wheat flour):[25]									
333	Loaf, 1 lb-------------------	1 loaf----------	454	37	1,160	42	16	2.6	3.6	6.4
334	Slice, 5 by 4 by 3/8 in------	1 slice---------	32	37	80	3	1	0.2	0.3	0.5
335	Toasted---------------------	1 slice---------	29	28	80	3	1	0.2	0.3	0.5
	Raisin bread, enriched:[25]									
336	Loaf, 1 lb-------------------	1 loaf----------	454	33	1,260	37	18	4.1	6.5	6.7
337	Slice (18 per loaf)----------	1 slice---------	25	33	65	2	1	0.2	0.3	0.4
338	Toasted---------------------	1 slice---------	21	24	65	2	1	0.2	0.3	0.4
	Rye bread, light (2/3 enriched wheat flour, 1/3 rye flour):[25]									
339	Loaf, 1 lb-------------------	1 loaf----------	454	37	1,190	38	17	3.3	5.2	5.5
340	Slice, 4-3/4 by 3-3/4 by 7/16 in------------------	1 slice---------	25	37	65	2	1	0.2	0.3	0.3
341	Toasted---------------------	1 slice---------	22	28	65	2	1	0.2	0.3	0.3
	Wheat bread, enriched:[25]									
342	Loaf, 1 lb-------------------	1 loaf----------	454	37	1,160	43	19	3.9	7.3	4.5
343	Slice (18 per loaf)----------	1 slice---------	25	37	65	2	1	0.2	0.4	0.3
344	Toasted---------------------	1 slice---------	23	28	65	3	1	0.2	0.4	0.3
	White bread, enriched:[25]									
345	Loaf, 1 lb-------------------	1 loaf----------	454	37	1,210	38	18	5.6	6.5	4.2
346	Slice (18 per loaf)--------	1 slice---------	25	37	65	2	1	0.3	0.4	0.2
347	Toasted-----------------	1 slice---------	22	28	65	2	1	0.3	0.4	0.2
348	Slice (22 per loaf)--------	1 slice---------	20	37	55	2	1	0.2	0.3	0.2
349	Toasted-----------------	1 slice---------	17	28	55	2	1	0.2	0.3	0.2
350	Cubes-----------------------	1 cup----------	30	37	80	2	1	0.4	0.4	0.3
351	Crumbs, soft----------------	1 cup----------	45	37	120	4	2	0.6	0.6	0.4
	Whole-wheat bread:[25]									
352	Loaf, 1 lb-------------------	1 loaf----------	454	38	1,110	44	20	5.8	6.8	5.2
353	Slice (16 per loaf)----------	1 slice---------	28	38	70	3	1	0.4	0.4	0.3
354	Toasted---------------------	1 slice---------	25	29	70	3	1	0.4	0.4	0.3
	Bread stuffing (from enriched bread), prepared from mix:									
355	Dry type---------------------	1 cup----------	140	33	500	9	31	6.1	13.3	9.6
356	Moist type-------------------	1 cup----------	203	61	420	9	26	5.3	11.3	8.0
	Breakfast cereals:									
	Hot type, cooked:									
	Corn (hominy) grits:									
357	Regular and quick, enriched	1 cup----------	242	85	145	3	Tr	Tr	0.1	0.2
358	Instant, plain-------------	1 pkt----------	137	85	80	2	Tr	Tr	Tr	0.1
	Cream of Wheat®:									
359	Regular, quick, instant----	1 cup----------	244	86	140	4	Tr	0.1	Tr	0.2
360	Mix'n Eat, plain-----------	1 pkt----------	142	82	100	3	Tr	Tr	Tr	0.1
361	Malt-O-Meal® ----------------	1 cup----------	240	88	120	4	Tr	Tr	Tr	0.1
	Oatmeal or rolled oats:									
362	Regular, quick, instant, nonfortified-------------	1 cup----------	234	85	145	6	2	0.4	0.8	1.0
	Instant, fortified:									
363	Plain--------------------	1 pkt----------	177	86	105	4	2	0.3	0.6	0.7
364	Flavored-----------------	1 pkt----------	164	76	160	5	2	0.3	0.7	0.8

[25] Made with vegetable shortening.
[27] Nutrient added.
[28] Cooked without salt. If salt is added according to label recommendations, sodium content is 540 mg.
[29] For white corn grits. Cooked yellow grits contain 145 IU or 14 RE.
[30] Value based on label declaration for added nutrients.

Nutrients in Indicated Quantity

Cho-les-terol (Milligrams)	Carbo-hydrate (Grams)	Calcium (Milligrams)	Phos-phorus (Milligrams)	Iron (Milligrams)	Potas-sium (Milligrams)	Sodium (Milligrams)	Vitamin A value (IU) (International units)	Vitamin A value (RE) (Retinol equivalents)	Thiamin (Milligrams)	Ribo-flavin (Milligrams)	Niacin (Milligrams)	Ascorbic acid (Milligrams)	Item No.
0	212	267	563	12.0	707	2,231	0	0	2.09	1.20	15.4	0	329
0	12	15	31	0.7	39	124	0	0	0.12	0.07	0.9	0	330
0	12	15	31	0.7	39	124	0	0	0.09	0.07	0.9	0	331
0	33	49	60	1.4	71	339	0	0	0.27	0.12	2.2	0	332
0	218	322	990	12.4	1,966	2,461	0	0	1.54	2.36	15.0	0	333
0	16	23	71	0.9	141	177	0	0	0.11	0.17	1.1	0	334
0	16	23	71	0.9	141	177	0	0	0.09	0.17	1.1	0	335
0	239	463	395	14.1	1,058	1,657	Tr	Tr	1.50	2.81	18.6	Tr	336
0	13	25	22	0.8	59	92	Tr	Tr	0.08	0.15	1.0	Tr	337
0	13	25	22	0.8	59	92	Tr	Tr	0.06	0.15	1.0	Tr	338
0	218	363	658	12.3	926	3,164	0	0	1.86	1.45	15.0	0	339
0	12	20	36	0.7	51	175	0	0	0.10	0.08	0.8	0	340
0	12	20	36	0.7	51	175	0	0	0.08	0.08	0.8	0	341
0	213	572	835	15.8	627	2,447	Tr	Tr	2.09	1.45	20.5	Tr	342
0	12	32	47	0.9	35	138	Tr	Tr	0.12	0.08	1.2	Tr	343
0	12	32	47	0.9	35	138	Tr	Tr	0.10	0.08	1.2	Tr	344
0	222	572	490	12.9	508	2,334	Tr	Tr	2.13	1.41	17.0	Tr	345
0	12	32	27	0.7	28	129	Tr	Tr	0.12	0.08	0.9	Tr	346
0	12	32	27	0.7	28	129	Tr	Tr	0.09	0.08	0.9	Tr	347
0	10	25	21	0.6	22	101	Tr	Tr	0.09	0.06	0.7	Tr	348
0	10	25	21	0.6	22	101	Tr	Tr	0.07	0.06	0.7	Tr	349
0	15	38	32	0.9	34	154	Tr	Tr	0.14	0.09	1.1	Tr	350
0	22	57	49	1.3	50	231	Tr	Tr	0.21	0.14	1.7	Tr	351
0	206	327	1,180	15.5	799	2,887	Tr	Tr	1.59	0.95	17.4	Tr	352
0	13	20	74	1.0	50	180	Tr	Tr	0.10	0.06	1.1	Tr	353
0	13	20	74	1.0	50	180	Tr	Tr	0.08	0.06	1.1	Tr	354
0	50	92	136	2.2	126	1,254	910	273	0.17	0.20	2.5	0	355
67	40	81	134	2.0	118	1,023	850	256	0.10	0.18	1.6	0	356
0	31	0	29	[27]1.5	53	[28]0	[29]0	[29]0	[27]0.24	[27]0.15	[27]2.0	0	357
0	18	7	16	[27]1.0	29	343	0	0	[27]0.18	[27]0.08	[27]1.3	0	358
0	29	[30]54	[31]43	[30]10.9	46	[31,32]5	0	0	[30]0.24	[30]0.07	[30]1.5	0	359
0	21	[30]20	[30]20	[30]8.1	38	241	[30]1,250	[30]376	[30]0.43	[30]0.28	[30]5.0	0	360
0	26	5	[30]24	[30]9.6	31	[33]2	0	0	[30]0.48	[30]0.24	[30]5.8	0	361
0	25	19	178	1.6	131	[34]2	40	4	0.26	0.05	0.3	0	362
0	18	[27]163	133	[27]6.3	99	[27]285	[27]1,510	[27]453	[27]0.53	[27]0.28	[27]5.5	0	363
0	31	[27]168	148	[27]6.7	137	[27]254	[27]1,530	[27]460	[27]0.53	[27]0.38	[27]5.9	Tr	364

[31] For regular and instant cereal. `For quick cereal, phosphorus is 102 mg and sodium is 142 mg.
[32] Cooked without salt. If salt is added according to label recommendations, sodium content is 390 mg.
[33] Cooked without salt. If salt is added according to label recommendations, sodium content is 324 mg.
[34] Cooked without salt. If salt is added according to label recommendations, sodium content is 374 mg.

(Tr indicates nutrient present in trace amount.)

Item No.	Foods, approximate measures, units, and weight (weight of edible portion only)			Water	Food energy	Pro-tein	Fat	Fatty acids		
								Satu-rated	Mono-unsatu-rated	Poly-unsatu-rated
	Grain Products—Con.		Grams	Per-cent	Cal-ories	Grams	Grams	Grams	Grams	Grams
	Breakfast cereals:									
	Ready to eat:									
365	All-Bran® (about 1/3 cup)----	1 oz-----------	28	3	70	4	1	0.1	0.1	0.3
366	Cap'n Crunch® (about 3/4 cup)	1 oz-----------	28	3	120	1	3	1.7	0.3	0.4
367	Cheerios® (about 1-1/4 cup)--	1 oz-----------	28	5	110	4	2	0.3	0.6	0.7
	Corn Flakes (about 1-1/4 cup):									
368	Kellogg's®----------------	1 oz-----------	28	3	110	2	Tr	Tr	Tr	Tr
369	Toasties®-----------------	1 oz-----------	28	3	110	2	Tr	Tr	Tr	Tr
	40% Bran Flakes:									
370	Kellogg's® (about 3/4 cup)	1 oz-----------	28	3	90	4	1	0.1	0.1	0.3
371	Post® (about 2/3 cup)------	1 oz-----------	28	3	90	3	Tr	0.1	0.1	0.2
372	Froot Loops® (about 1 cup)---	1 oz-----------	28	3	110	2	1	0.2	0.1	0.1
373	Golden Grahams® (about 3/4 cup)----------------------	1 oz-----------	28	2	110	2	1	0.7	0.1	0.2
374	Grape-Nuts® (about 1/4 cup)--	1 oz-----------	28	3	100	3	Tr	Tr	Tr	0.1
375	Honey Nut Cheerios® (about 3/4 cup)-------------------	1 oz-----------	28	3	105	3	1	0.1	0.3	0.3
376	Lucky Charms® (about 1 cup)---	1 oz-----------	28	3	110	3	1	0.2	0.4	0.4
377	Nature Valley® Granola (about 1/3 cup)-------------------	1 oz-----------	28	4	125	3	5	3.3	0.7	0.7
378	100% Natural Cereal (about 1/4 cup)-------------------	1 oz-----------	28	2	135	3	6	4.1	1.2	0.5
379	Product 19® (about 3/4 cup)--	1 oz-----------	28	3	110	3	Tr	Tr	Tr	0.1
	Raisin Bran:									
380	Kellogg's® (about 3/4 cup)	1 oz-----------	28	8	90	3	1	0.1	0.1	0.3
381	Post® (about 1/2 cup)------	1 oz-----------	28	9	85	3	1	0.1	0.1	0.3
382	Rice Krispies® (about 1 cup)--	1 oz-----------	28	2	110	2	Tr	Tr	Tr	0.1
383	Shredded Wheat (about 2/3 cup)----------------------	1 oz-----------	28	5	100	3	1	0.1	0.1	0.3
384	Special K® (about 1-1/3 cup)	1 oz-----------	28	2	110	6	Tr	Tr	Tr	Tr
385	Super Sugar Crisp® (about 7/8 cup)----------------------	1 oz-----------	28	2	105	2	Tr	Tr	Tr	0.1
386	Sugar Frosted Flakes, Kellogg's® (about 3/4 cup)	1 oz-----------	28	3	110	1	Tr	Tr	Tr	Tr
387	Sugar Smacks® (about 3/4 cup)	1 oz-----------	28	3	105	2	1	0.1	0.1	0.2
388	Total® (about 1 cup)---------	1 oz-----------	28	4	100	3	1	0.1	0.1	0.3
389	Trix® (about 1 cup)----------	1 oz-----------	28	3	110	2	Tr	0.2	0.1	0.1
390	Wheaties® (about 1 cup)------	1 oz-----------	28	5	100	3	Tr	0.1	Tr	0.2
391	Buckwheat flour, light, sifted---	1 cup-----------	98	12	340	6	1	0.2	0.4	0.4
392	Bulgur, uncooked-----------------	1 cup-----------	170	10	600	19	3	1.2	0.3	1.2
	Cakes prepared from cake mixes with enriched flour:[35]									
	Angelfood:									
393	Whole cake, 9-3/4-in diam. tube cake------------------	1 cake----------	635	38	1,510	38	2	0.4	0.2	1.0
394	Piece, 1/12 of cake----------	1 piece---------	53	38	125	3	Tr	Tr	Tr	0.1
	Coffeecake, crumb:									
395	Whole cake, 7-3/4 by 5-5/8 by 1-1/4 in----------------	1 cake----------	430	30	1,385	27	41	11.8	16.7	9.6
396	Piece, 1/6 of cake----------	1 piece---------	72	30	230	5	7	2.0	2.8	1.6
	Devil's food with chocolate frosting:									
397	Whole, 2-layer cake, 8- or 9-in diam.---------------	1 cake----------	1,107	24	3,755	49	136	55.6	51.4	19.7
398	Piece, 1/16 of cake----------	1 piece---------	69	24	235	3	8	3.5	3.2	1.2
399	Cupcake, 2-1/2-in diam.------	1 cupcake-------	35	24	120	2	4	1.8	1.6	0.6
	Gingerbread:									
400	Whole cake, 8 in square------	1 cake----------	570	37	1,575	18	39	9.6	16.4	10.5
401	Piece, 1/9 of cake-----------	1 piece---------	63	37	175	2	4	1.1	1.8	1.2

[27] Nutrient added.
[30] Value based on label declaration for added nutrients.

Nutrients in Indicated Quantity

Cholesterol	Carbohydrate	Calcium	Phosphorus	Iron	Potassium	Sodium	Vitamin A value (IU)	(RE)	Thiamin	Riboflavin	Niacin	Ascorbic acid	Item No.
Milligrams	Grams	Milligrams	Milligrams	Milligrams	Milligrams	Milligrams	International units	Retinol equivalents	Milligrams	Milligrams	Milligrams	Milligrams	
0	21	23	264	[30]4.5	350	320	[30]1,250	[30]375	[30]0.37	[30]0.43	[30]5.0	[30]15	365
0	23	5	36	[27]7.5	37	213	[30]40	[30]4	[27]0.50	[27]0.55	[27]6.6	[30]0	366
0	20	48	134	[30]4.5	101	307	[30]1,250	[30]375	[30]0.37	[30]0.43	[30]5.0	[30]15	367
0	24	1	18	[30]1.8	26	351	[30]1,250	[30]375	[30]0.37	[30]0.43	[30]5.0	[30]15	368
0	24	1	12	[27]0.7	33	297	[30]1,250	[30]375	[30]0.37	[30]0.43	[30]5.0	0	369
0	22	14	139	[30]8.1	180	264	[30]1,250	[30]375	[30]0.37	[30]0.43	[30]5.0	0	370
0	22	12	179	[30]4.5	151	260	[30]1,250	[30]375	[30]0.37	[30]0.43	[30]5.0	0	371
0	25	3	24	[30]4.5	26	145	[30]1,250	[30]375	[30]0.37	[30]0.43	[30]5.0	[30]15	372
Tr	24	17	41	[30]4.5	63	346	[30]1,250	[30]375	[30]0.37	[30]0.43	[30]5.0	[30]15	373
0	23	11	71	1.2	95	197	[30]1,250	[30]375	[30]0.37	[30]0.43	[30]5.0	0	374
0	23	20	105	[30]4.5	99	257	[30]1,250	[30]375	[30]0.37	[30]0.43	[30]5.0	[30]15	375
0	23	32	79	[30]4.5	59	201	[30]1,250	[30]375	[30]0.37	[30]0.43	[30]5.0	[30]15	376
0	19	18	89	0.9	98	58	20	2	0.10	0.05	0.2	0	377
Tr	18	49	104	0.8	140	12	20	2	0.09	0.15	0.6	0	378
0	24	3	40	[30]18.0	44	325	[30]5,000	[30]1,501	[30]1.50	[30]1.70	[30]20.0	[30]60	379
0	21	10	105	[30]3.5	147	207	[30]960	[30]288	[30]0.28	[30]0.34	[30]3.9	0	380
0	21	13	119	[30]4.5	175	185	[30]1,250	[30]375	[30]0.37	[30]0.43	[30]5.0	0	381
0	25	4	34	[30]1.8	29	340	[30]1,250	[30]375	[30]0.37	[30]0.43	[30]5.0	[30]15	382
0	23	11	100	1.2	102	3	0	0	0.07	0.08	1.5	0	383
Tr	21	8	55	[30]4.5	49	265	[30]1,250	[30]375	[30]0.37	[30]0.43	[30]5.0	[30]15	384
0	26	6	52	[30]1.8	105	25	[30]1,250	[30]375	[30]0.37	[30]0.43	[30]5.0	0	385
0	26	1	21	[30]1.8	18	230	[30]1,250	[30]375	[30]0.37	[30]0.43	[30]5.0	[30]15	386
0	25	3	31	[30]1.8	42	75	[30]1,250	[30]375	[30]0.37	[30]0.43	[30]5.0	[30]15	387
0	22	48	118	[30]18.0	106	352	[30]5,000	[30]1,501	[30]1.50	[30]1.70	[30]20.0	[30]60	388
0	25	6	19	[30]4.5	27	181	[30]1,250	[30]375	[30]0.37	[30]0.43	[30]5.0	[30]15	389
0	23	43	98	[30]4.5	106	354	[30]1,250	[30]375	[30]0.37	[30]0.43	[30]5.0	[30]15	390
0	78	11	86	1.0	314	2	0	0	0.08	0.04	0.4	0	391
0	129	49	575	9.5	389	7	0	0	0.48	0.24	7.7	0	392
0	342	527	1,086	2.7	845	3,226	0	0	0.32	1.27	1.6	0	393
0	29	44	91	0.2	71	269	0	0	0.03	0.11	0.1	0	394
279	225	262	748	7.3	469	1,853	690	194	0.82	0.90	7.7	1	395
47	38	44	125	1.2	78	310	120	32	0.14	0.15	1.3	Tr	396
598	645	653	1,162	22.1	1,439	2,900	1,660	498	1.11	1.66	10.0	1	397
37	40	41	72	1.4	90	181	100	31	0.07	0.10	0.6	Tr	398
19	20	21	37	0.7	46	92	50	16	0.04	0.05	0.3	Tr	399
6	291	513	570	10.8	1,562	1,733	0	0	0.86	1.03	7.4	1	400
1	32	57	63	1.2	173	192	0	0	0.09	0.11	0.8	Tr	401

[35] Excepting angelfood cake, cakes were made from mixes containing vegetable shortening and frostings were made with margarine.

(Tr indicates nutrient present in trace amount.)

Item No.	Foods, approximate measures, units, and weight (weight of edible portion only)		Grams	Water	Food energy	Pro- tein	Fat	Fatty acids		
								Satu- rated	Mono- unsatu- rated	Poly- unsatu- rated
	Grain Products—Con.		Grams	Per- cent	Cal- ories	Grams	Grams	Grams	Grams	Grams
	Cakes prepared from cake mixes with enriched flour:[35] Yellow with chocolate frosting:									
402	Whole, 2-layer cake, 8- or 9-in diam.	1 cake	1,108	26	3,735	45	125	47.8	48.8	21.8
403	Piece, 1/16 of cake	1 piece	69	26	235	3	8	3.0	3.0	1.4
	Cakes prepared from home recipes using enriched flour: Carrot, with cream cheese frosting:[36]									
404	Whole cake, 10-in diam. tube cake	1 cake	1,536	23	6,175	63	328	66.0	135.2	107.5
405	Piece, 1/16 of cake	1 piece	96	23	385	4	21	4.1	8.4	6.7
	Fruitcake, dark:[36]									
406	Whole cake, 7-1/2-in diam., 2-1/4-in high tube cake	1 cake	1,361	18	5,185	74	228	47.6	113.0	51.7
407	Piece, 1/32 of cake, 2/3-in arc	1 piece	43	18	165	2	7	1.5	3.6	1.6
	Plain sheet cake:[37] Without frosting:									
408	Whole cake, 9-in square	1 cake	777	25	2,830	35	108	29.5	45.1	25.6
409	Piece, 1/9 of cake	1 piece	86	25	315	4	12	3.3	5.0	2.8
	With uncooked white frosting:									
410	Whole cake, 9-in square	1 cake	1,096	21	4,020	37	129	41.6	50.4	26.3
411	Piece, 1/9 of cake	1 piece	121	21	445	4	14	4.6	5.6	2.9
	Pound:[38]									
412	Loaf, 8-1/2 by 3-1/2 by 3-1/4 in	1 loaf	514	22	2,025	33	94	21.1	40.9	26.7
413	Slice, 1/17 of loaf	1 slice	30	22	120	2	5	1.2	2.4	1.6
	Cakes, commercial, made with en- riched flour: Pound:									
414	Loaf, 8-1/2 by 3-1/2 by 3 in	1 loaf	500	24	1,935	26	94	52.0	30.0	4.0
415	Slice, 1/17 of loaf	1 slice	29	24	110	2	5	3.0	1.7	0.2
	Snack cakes:									
416	Devil's food with creme filling (2 small cakes per pkg)	1 small cake	28	20	105	1	4	1.7	1.5	0.6
417	Sponge with creme filling (2 small cakes per pkg)	1 small cake	42	19	155	1	5	2.3	2.1	0.5
	White with white frosting:									
418	Whole, 2-layer cake, 8- or 9-in diam.	1 cake	1,140	24	4,170	43	148	33.1	61.6	42.2
419	Piece, 1/16 of cake	1 piece	71	24	260	3	9	2.1	3.8	2.6
	Yellow with chocolate frosting:									
420	Whole, 2-layer cake, 8- or 9-in diam.	1 cake	1,108	23	3,895	40	175	92.0	58.7	10.0
421	Piece, 1/16 of cake	1 piece	69	23	245	2	11	5.7	3.7	0.6
	Cheesecake:									
422	Whole cake, 9-in diam.	1 cake	1,110	46	3,350	60	213	119.9	65.5	14.4
423	Piece, 1/12 of cake	1 piece	92	46	280	5	18	9.9	5.4	1.2
	Cookies made with enriched flour: Brownies with nuts:									
424	Commercial, with frosting, 1-1/2 by 1-3/4 by 7/8 in	1 brownie	25	13	100	1	4	1.6	2.0	0.6
425	From home recipe, 1-3/4 by 1-3/4 by 7/8 in[36]	1 brownie	20	10	95	1	6	1.4	2.8	1.2
	Chocolate chip:									
426	Commercial, 2-1/4-in diam., 3/8 in thick	4 cookies	42	4	180	2	9	2.9	3.1	2.6

[35] Excepting angelfood cake, cakes were made from mixes containing vegetable shortening and frostings were made with margarine.
[36] Made with vegetable oil.

| | | | | | | | Nutrients in Indicated Quantity | | | | | | |

Cho-les-terol	Carbo-hydrate	Calcium	Phos-phorus	Iron	Potas-sium	Sodium	Vitamin A value		Thiamin	Ribo-flavin	Niacin	Ascorbic acid	Item No.
							(IU)	(RE)					
Milli-grams	Grams	Milli-grams	Milli-grams	Milli-grams	Milli-grams	Milli-grams	Inter-national units	Retinol equiva-lents	Milli-grams	Milli-grams	Milli-grams	Milli-grams	
576	638	1,008	2,017	15.5	1,208	2,515	1,550	465	1.22	1.66	11.1	1	402
36	40	63	126	1.0	75	157	100	29	0.08	0.10	0.7	Tr	403
1183	775	707	998	21.0	1,720	4,470	2,240	246	1.83	1.97	14.7	23	404
74	48	44	62	1.3	108	279	140	15	0.11	0.12	0.9	1	405
640	783	1,293	1,592	37.6	6,138	2,123	1,720	422	2.41	2.55	17.0	504	406
20	25	41	50	1.2	194	67	50	13	0.08	0.08	0.5	16	407
552	434	497	793	11.7	614	2,331	1,320	373	1.24	1.40	10.1	2	408
61	48	55	88	1.3	68	258	150	41	0.14	0.15	1.1	Tr	409
636	694	548	822	11.0	669	2,488	2,190	647	1.21	1.42	9.9	2	410
70	77	61	91	1.2	74	275	240	71	0.13	0.16	1.1	Tr	411
555	265	339	473	9.3	483	1,645	3,470	1,033	0.93	1.08	7.8	1	412
32	15	20	28	0.5	28	96	200	60	0.05	0.06	0.5	Tr	413
1100	257	146	517	8.0	443	1,857	2,820	715	0.96	1.12	8.1	0	414
64	15	8	30	0.5	26	108	160	41	0.06	0.06	0.5	0	415
15	17	21	26	1.0	34	105	20	4	0.06	0.09	0.7	0	416
7	27	14	44	0.6	37	155	30	9	0.07	0.06	0.6	0	417
46	670	536	1,585	15.5	832	2,827	640	194	3.19	2.05	27.6	0	418
3	42	33	99	1.0	52	176	40	12	0.20	0.13	1.7	0	419
609	620	366	1,884	19.9	1,972	3,080	1,850	488	0.78	2.22	10.0	0	420
38	39	23	117	1.2	123	192	120	30	0.05	0.14	0.6	0	421
2053	317	622	977	5.3	1,088	2,464	2,820	833	0.33	1.44	5.1	56	422
170	26	52	81	0.4	90	204	230	69	0.03	0.12	0.4	5	423
14	16	13	26	0.6	50	59	70	18	0.08	0.07	0.3	Tr	424
18	11	9	26	0.4	35	51	20	6	0.05	0.05	0.3	Tr	425
5	28	13	41	0.8	68	140	50	15	0.10	0.23	1.0	Tr	426

[37]Cake made with vegetable shortening; frosting with margarine.
[38]Made with margarine.

(Tr indicates nutrient present in trace amount.)

Item No.	Foods, approximate measures, units, and weight (weight of edible portion only)		Water	Food energy	Pro-tein	Fat	Fatty acids		
							Satu-rated	Mono-unsatu-rated	Poly-unsatu-rated
		Grams	Per-cent	Cal-ories	Grams	Grams	Grams	Grams	Grams
	Grain Products—Con.								
	Cookies made with enriched flour:								
	Chocolate chip:								
427	From home recipe, 2-1/3-in diam.[25]	4 cookies	40	3	185	2	11	3.9	4.3	2.0
428	From refrigerated dough, 2-1/4-in diam., 3/8 in thick	4 cookies	48	5	225	2	11	4.0	4.4	2.0
429	Fig bars, square, 1-5/8 by 1-5/8 by 3/8 in or rectangular, 1-1/2 by 1-3/4 by 1/2 in	4 cookies	56	12	210	2	4	1.0	1.5	1.0
430	Oatmeal with raisins, 2-5/8-in diam., 1/4 in thick	4 cookies	52	4	245	3	10	2.5	4.5	2.8
431	Peanut butter cookie, from home recipe, 2-5/8-in diam.[25]	4 cookies	48	3	245	4	14	4.0	5.8	2.8
432	Sandwich type (chocolate or vanilla), 1-3/4-in diam., 3/8 in thick	4 cookies	40	2	195	2	8	2.0	3.6	2.2
	Shortbread:								
433	Commercial	4 small cookies	32	6	155	2	8	2.9	3.0	1.1
434	From home recipe[38]	2 large cookies	28	3	145	2	8	1.3	2.7	3.4
435	Sugar cookie, from refrigerated dough, 2-1/2-in diam., 1/4 in thick	4 cookies	48	4	235	2	12	2.3	5.0	3.6
436	Vanilla wafers, 1-3/4-in diam., 1/4 in thick	10 cookies	40	4	185	2	7	1.8	3.0	1.8
437	Corn chips	1-oz package	28	1	155	2	9	1.4	2.4	3.7
	Cornmeal:								
438	Whole-ground, unbolted, dry form	1 cup	122	12	435	11	5	0.5	1.1	2.5
439	Bolted (nearly whole-grain), dry form	1 cup	122	12	440	11	4	0.5	0.9	2.2
	Degermed, enriched:								
440	Dry form	1 cup	138	12	500	11	2	0.2	0.4	0.9
441	Cooked	1 cup	240	88	120	3	Tr	Tr	0.1	0.2
	Crackers:[39]								
	Cheese:								
442	Plain, 1 in square	10 crackers	10	4	50	1	3	0.9	1.2	0.3
443	Sandwich type (peanut butter)	1 sandwich	8	3	40	1	2	0.4	0.8	0.3
444	Graham, plain, 2-1/2 in square	2 crackers	14	5	60	1	1	0.4	0.6	0.4
445	Melba toast, plain	1 piece	5	4	20	1	Tr	0.1	0.1	0.1
446	Rye wafers, whole-grain, 1-7/8 by 3-1/2 in	2 wafers	14	5	55	1	1	0.3	0.4	0.3
447	Saltines[40]	4 crackers	12	4	50	1	1	0.5	0.4	0.2
448	Snack-type, standard	1 round cracker	3	3	15	Tr	1	0.2	0.4	0.1
449	Wheat, thin	4 crackers	8	3	35	1	1	0.5	0.5	0.4
450	Whole-wheat wafers	2 crackers	8	4	35	1	2	0.5	0.6	0.4
451	Croissants, made with enriched flour, 4-1/2 by 4 by 1-3/4 in	1 croissant	57	22	235	5	12	3.5	6.7	1.4
	Danish pastry, made with enriched flour:								
	Plain without fruit or nuts:								
452	Packaged ring, 12 oz	1 ring	340	27	1,305	21	71	21.8	28.6	15.6
453	Round piece, about 4-1/4-in diam., 1 in high	1 pastry	57	27	220	4	12	3.6	4.8	2.6
454	Ounce	1 oz	28	27	110	2	6	1.8	2.4	1.3
455	Fruit, round piece	1 pastry	65	30	235	4	13	3.9	5.2	2.9
	Doughnuts, made with enriched flour:								
456	Cake type, plain, 3-1/4-in diam., 1 in high	1 doughnut	50	21	210	3	12	2.8	5.0	3.0
457	Yeast-leavened, glazed, 3-3/4-in diam., 1-1/4 in high	1 doughnut	60	27	235	4	13	5.2	5.5	0.9
458	English muffins, plain, enriched	1 muffin	57	42	140	5	1	0.3	0.2	0.3
459	Toasted	1 muffin	50	29	140	5	1	0.3	0.2	0.3

[25]Made with vegetable shortening.
[38]Made with margarine.

	Nutrients in Indicated Quantity												
Cho-les-terol	Carbo-hydrate	Calcium	Phos-phorus	Iron	Potas-sium	Sodium	Vitamin A value (IU)	Vitamin A value (RE)	Thiamin	Ribo-flavin	Niacin	Ascorbic acid	Item No.
Milli-grams	Grams	Milli-grams	Milli-grams	Milli-grams	Milli-grams	Milli-grams	Inter-national units	Retinol equiva-lents	Milli-grams	Milli-grams	Milli-grams	Milli-grams	
18	26	13	34	1.0	82	82	20	5	0.06	0.06	0.6	0	427
22	32	13	34	1.0	62	173	30	8	0.06	0.10	0.9	0	428
27	42	40	34	1.4	162	180	60	6	0.08	0.07	0.7	Tr	429
2	36	18	58	1.1	90	148	40	12	0.09	0.08	1.0	0	430
22	28	21	60	1.1	110	142	20	5	0.07	0.07	1.9	0	431
0	29	12	40	1.4	66	189	0	0	0.09	0.07	0.8	0	432
27	20	13	39	0.8	38	123	30	8	0.10	0.09	0.9	0	433
0	17	6	31	0.6	18	125	300	89	0.08	0.06	0.7	Tr	434
29	31	50	91	0.9	33	261	40	11	0.09	0.06	1.1	0	435
25	29	16	36	0.8	50	150	50	14	0.07	0.10	1.0	0	436
0	16	35	52	0.5	52	233	110	11	0.04	0.05	0.4	1	437
0	90	24	312	2.2	346	1	620	62	0.46	0.13	2.4	0	438
0	91	21	272	2.2	303	1	590	59	0.37	0.10	2.3	0	439
0	108	8	137	5.9	166	1	610	61	0.61	0.36	4.8	0	440
0	26	2	34	1.4	38	0	140	14	0.14	0.10	1.2	0	441
6	6	11	17	0.3	17	112	20	5	0.05	0.04	0.4	0	442
1	5	7	25	0.3	17	90	Tr	Tr	0.04	0.03	0.6	0	443
0	11	6	20	0.4	36	86	0	0	0.02	0.03	0.6	0	444
0	4	6	10	0.1	11	44	0	0	0.01	0.01	0.1	0	445
0	10	7	44	0.5	65	115	0	0	0.06	0.03	0.5	0	446
4	9	3	12	0.5	17	165	0	0	0.06	0.05	0.6	0	447
0	2	3	6	0.1	4	30	Tr	Tr	0.01	0.01	0.1	0	448
0	5	3	15	0.3	17	69	Tr	Tr	0.04	0.03	0.4	0	449
0	5	3	22	0.2	31	59	0	0	0.02	0.03	0.4	0	450
13	27	20	64	2.1	68	452	50	13	0.17	0.13	1.3	0	451
292	152	360	347	6.5	316	1,302	360	99	0.95	1.02	8.5	Tr	452
49	26	60	58	1.1	53	218	60	17	0.16	0.17	1.4	Tr	453
24	13	30	29	0.5	26	109	30	8	0.08	0.09	0.7	Tr	454
56	28	17	80	1.3	57	233	40	11	0.16	0.14	1.4	Tr	455
20	24	22	111	1.0	58	192	20	5	0.12	0.12	1.1	Tr	456
21	26	17	55	1.4	64	222	Tr	Tr	0.28	0.12	1.8	0	457
0	27	96	67	1.7	331	378	0	0	0.26	0.19	2.2	0	458
0	27	96	67	1.7	331	378	0	0	0.23	0.19	2.2	0	459

[39]Crackers made with enriched flour except for rye wafers and whole-wheat wafers.
[40]Made with lard.

(Tr indicates nutrient present in trace amount.)

Item No.	Foods, approximate measures, units, and weight (weight of edible portion only)		Water	Food energy	Pro-tein	Fat	Fatty acids		
							Satu-rated	Mono-unsatu-rated	Poly-unsatu-rated
		Grams	Per-cent	Cal-ories	Grams	Grams	Grams	Grams	Grams
	Grain Products—Con.								
460	French toast, from home recipe--- 1 slice---------	65	53	155	6	7	1.6	2.0	1.6
	Macaroni, enriched, cooked (cut lengths, elbows, shells):								
461	Firm stage (hot)-------------- 1 cup-----------	130	64	190	7	1	0.1	0.1	0.3
	Tender stage:								
462	Cold------------------------ 1 cup----------	105	72	115	4	Tr	0.1	0.1	0.2
463	Hot------------------------- 1 cup----------	140	72	155	5	1	0.1	0.1	0.2
	Muffins made with enriched flour, 2-1/2-in diam., 1-1/2 in high:								
	From home recipe:								
464	Blueberry[25]------------------ 1 muffin--------	45	37	135	3	5	1.5	2.1	1.2
465	Bran[36] --------------------- 1 muffin--------	45	35	125	3	6	1.4	1.6	2.3
466	Corn (enriched, degermed cornmeal and flour)[25] ------ 1 muffin--------	45	33	145	3	5	1.5	2.2	1.4
	From commercial mix (egg and water added):								
467	Blueberry-------------------- 1 muffin--------	45	33	140	3	5	1.4	2.0	1.2
468	Bran------------------------ 1 muffin--------	45	28	140	3	4	1.3	1.6	1.0
469	Corn------------------------ 1 muffin--------	45	30	145	3	6	1.7	2.3	1.4
470	Noodles (egg noodles), enriched, cooked---------------------- 1 cup-----------	160	70	200	7	2	0.5	0.6	0.6
471	Noodles, chow mein, canned------- 1 cup-----------	45	11	220	6	11	2.1	7.3	0.4
	Pancakes, 4-in diam.:								
472	Buckwheat, from mix (with buck-wheat and enriched flours), egg and milk added---------- 1 pancake-------	27	58	55	2	2	0.9	0.9	0.5
	Plain:								
473	From home recipe using enriched flour------------- 1 pancake-------	27	50	60	2	2	0.5	0.8	0.5
474	From mix (with enriched flour), egg, milk, and oil added--------------------- 1 pancake-------	27	54	60	2	2	0.5	0.9	0.5
	Piecrust, made with enriched flour and vegetable shorten-ing, baked:								
475	From home recipe, 9-in diam.--- 1 pie shell-----	180	15	900	11	60	14.8	25.9	15.7
476	From mix, 9-in diam.----------- Piecrust for 2-crust pie-----	320	19	1,485	20	93	22.7	41.0	25.0
	Pies, piecrust made with enriched flour, vegetable shortening, 9-in diam.:								
	Apple:								
477	Whole----------------------- 1 pie----------	945	48	2,420	21	105	27.4	44.4	26.5
478	Piece, 1/6 of pie----------- 1 piece--------	158	48	405	3	18	4.6	7.4	4.4
	Blueberry:								
479	Whole----------------------- 1 pie----------	945	51	2,285	23	102	25.5	44.4	27.4
480	Piece, 1/6 of pie----------- 1 piece--------	158	51	380	4	17	4.3	7.4	4.6
	Cherry:								
481	Whole----------------------- 1 pie----------	945	47	2,465	25	107	28.4	46.3	27.4
482	Piece, 1/6 of pie----------- 1 piece--------	158	47	410	4	18	4.7	7.7	4.6
	Creme:								
483	Whole----------------------- 1 pie----------	910	43	2,710	20	139	90.1	23.7	6.4
484	Piece, 1/6 of pie----------- 1 piece--------	152	43	455	3	23	15.0	4.0	1.1
	Custard:								
485	Whole----------------------- 1 pie----------	910	58	1,985	56	101	33.7	40.0	19.1
486	Piece, 1/6 of pie----------- 1 piece--------	152	58	330	9	17	5.6	6.7	3.2
	Lemon meringue:								
487	Whole----------------------- 1 pie----------	840	47	2,140	31	86	26.0	34.4	17.6
488	Piece, 1/6 of pie----------- 1 piece--------	140	47	355	5	14	4.3	5.7	2.9
	Peach:								
489	Whole----------------------- 1 pie----------	945	48	2,410	24	101	24.6	43.5	26.5
490	Piece, 1/6 of pie----------- 1 piece--------	158	48	405	4	17	4.1	7.3	4.4

[25] Made with vegetable shortening.

							Nutrients in Indicated Quantity						

Nutrients in Indicated Quantity

Cholesterol	Carbohydrate	Calcium	Phosphorus	Iron	Potassium	Sodium	Vitamin A value		Thiamin	Riboflavin	Niacin	Ascorbic acid	Item No.
							(IU)	(RE)					
Milligrams	Grams	Milligrams	Milligrams	Milligrams	Milligrams	Milligrams	International units	Retinol equivalents	Milligrams	Milligrams	Milligrams	Milligrams	
112	17	72	85	1.3	86	257	110	32	0.12	0.16	1.0	Tr	460
0	39	14	85	2.1	103	1	0	0	0.23	0.13	1.8	0	461
0	24	8	53	1.3	64	1	0	0	0.15	0.08	1.2	0	462
0	32	11	70	1.7	85	1	0	0	0.20	0.11	1.5	0	463
19	20	54	46	0.9	47	198	40	9	0.10	0.11	0.9	1	464
24	19	60	125	1.4	99	189	230	30	0.11	0.13	1.3	3	465
23	21	66	59	0.9	57	169	80	15	0.11	0.11	0.9	Tr	466
45	22	15	90	0.9	54	225	50	11	0.10	0.17	1.1	Tr	467
28	24	27	182	1.7	50	385	100	14	0.08	0.12	1.9	0	468
42	22	30	128	1.3	31	291	90	16	0.09	0.09	0.8	Tr	469
50	37	16	94	2.6	70	3	110	34	0.22	0.13	1.9	0	470
5	26	14	41	0.4	33	450	0	0	0.05	0.03	0.6	0	471
20	6	59	91	0.4	66	125	60	17	0.04	0.05	0.2	Tr	472
16	9	27	38	0.5	33	115	30	10	0.06	0.07	0.5	Tr	473
16	8	36	71	0.7	43	160	30	7	0.09	0.12	0.8	Tr	474
0	79	25	90	4.5	90	1,100	0	0	0.54	0.40	5.0	0	475
0	141	131	272	9.3	179	2,602	0	0	1.06	0.80	9.9	0	476
0	360	76	208	9.5	756	2,844	280	28	1.04	0.76	9.5	9	477
0	60	13	35	1.6	126	476	50	5	0.17	0.13	1.6	2	478
0	330	104	217	12.3	945	2,533	850	85	1.04	0.85	10.4	38	479
0	55	17	36	2.1	158	423	140	14	0.17	0.14	1.7	6	480
0	363	132	236	9.5	992	2,873	4,160	416	1.13	0.85	9.5	0	481
0	61	22	40	1.6	166	480	700	70	0.19	0.14	1.6	0	482
46	351	273	919	6.8	796	2,207	1,250	391	0.36	0.89	6.4	0	483
8	59	46	154	1.1	133	369	210	65	0.06	0.15	1.1	0	484
1010	213	874	1,028	9.1	1,247	2,612	2,090	573	0.82	1.91	5.5	0	485
169	36	146	172	1.5	208	436	350	96	0.14	0.32	0.9	0	486
857	317	118	412	8.4	420	2,369	1,430	395	0.59	0.84	5.0	25	487
143	53	20	69	1.4	70	395	240	66	0.10	0.14	0.8	4	488
0	361	95	274	11.3	1,408	2,533	6,900	690	1.04	0.95	14.2	28	489
0	60	16	46	1.9	235	423	1,150	115	0.17	0.16	2.4	5	490

[36] Made with vegetable oil.

(Tr indicates nutrient present in trace amount.)

Item No.	Foods, approximate measures, units, and weight (weight of edible portion only)		Water	Food energy	Protein	Fat	Fatty acids Saturated	Mono-unsaturated	Poly-unsaturated
		Grams	Per-cent	Cal-ories	Grams	Grams	Grams	Grams	Grams
	Grain Products—Con.								
	Pies, piecrust made with enriched flour, vegetable shortening, 9-inch diam.:								
	Pecan:								
491	Whole----------------------- 1 pie----------	825	20	3,450	42	189	28.1	101.5	47.0
492	Piece, 1/6 of pie------------ 1 piece---------	138	20	575	7	32	4.7	17.0	7.9
	Pumpkin:								
493	Whole---------------------- 1 pie----------	910	59	1,920	36	102	38.2	40.0	18.2
494	Piece, 1/6 of pie------------ 1 piece---------	152	59	320	6	17	6.4	6.7	3.0
	Pies, fried:								
495	Apple------------------------ 1 pie----------	85	43	255	2	14	5.8	6.6	0.6
496	Cherry----------------------- 1 pie----------	85	42	250	2	14	5.8	6.7	0.6
	Popcorn, popped:								
497	Air-popped, unsalted---------- 1 cup----------	8	4	30	1	Tr	Tr	0.1	0.2
498	Popped in vegetable oil, salted 1 cup----------	11	3	55	1	3	0.5	1.4	1.2
499	Sugar syrup coated------------ 1 cup----------	35	4	135	2	1	0.1	0.3	0.6
	Pretzels, made with enriched flour:								
500	Stick, 2-1/4 in long---------- 10 pretzels-----	3	3	10	Tr	Tr	Tr	Tr	Tr
501	Twisted, dutch, 2-3/4 by 2-5/8 in------------------------- 1 pretzel-------	16	3	65	2	1	0.1	0.2	0.2
502	Twisted, thin, 3-1/4 by 2-1/4 by 1/4 in-------------------- 10 pretzels-----	60	3	240	6	2	0.4	0.8	0.6
	Rice:								
503	Brown, cooked, served hot------ 1 cup----------	195	70	230	5	1	0.3	0.3	0.4
	White, enriched:								
	Commercial varieties, all types:								
504	Raw-------------------------- 1 cup----------	185	12	670	12	1	0.2	0.2	0.3
505	Cooked, served hot--------- 1 cup----------	205	73	225	4	Tr	0.1	0.1	0.1
506	Instant, ready-to-serve, hot 1 cup----------	165	73	180	4	0	0.1	0.1	0.1
	Parboiled:								
507	Raw-------------------------- 1 cup----------	185	10	685	14	1	0.1	0.1	0.2
508	Cooked, served hot--------- 1 cup----------	175	73	185	4	Tr	Tr	Tr	0.1
	Rolls, enriched:								
	Commercial:								
509	Dinner, 2-1/2-in diam., 2 in high--------------------- 1 roll----------	28	32	85	2	2	0.5	0.8	0.6
510	Frankfurter and hamburger (8 per 11-1/2-oz pkg.)-------- 1 roll----------	40	34	115	3	2	0.5	0.8	0.6
511	Hard, 3-3/4-in diam., 2 in high--------------------- 1 roll----------	50	25	155	5	2	0.4	0.5	0.6
512	Hoagie or submarine, 11-1/2 by 3 by 2-1/2 in----------- 1 roll----------	135	31	400	11	8	1.8	3.0	2.2
	From home recipe:								
513	Dinner, 2-1/2-in diam., 2 in high--------------------- 1 roll----------	35	26	120	3	3	0.8	1.2	0.9
	Spaghetti, enriched, cooked:								
514	Firm stage, "al dente," served hot------------------------- 1 cup----------	130	64	190	7	1	0.1	0.1	0.3
515	Tender stage, served hot------- 1 cup----------	140	73	155	5	1	0.1	0.1	0.2
516	Toaster pastries----------------- 1 pastry--------	54	13	210	2	6	1.7	3.6	0.4
517	Tortillas, corn------------------ 1 tortilla------	30	45	65	2	1	0.1	0.3	0.6
	Waffles, made with enriched flour, 7-in diam.:								
518	From home recipe--------------- 1 waffle--------	75	37	245	7	13	4.0	4.9	2.6
519	From mix, egg and milk added--- 1 waffle--------	75	42	205	7	8	2.7	2.9	1.5
	Wheat flours:								
	All-purpose or family flour, enriched:								
520	Sifted, spooned-------------- 1 cup----------	115	12	420	12	1	0.2	0.1	0.5
521	Unsifted, spooned------------ 1 cup----------	125	12	455	13	1	0.2	0.1	0.5
522	Cake or pastry flour, enriched, sifted, spooned------------ 1 cup----------	96	12	350	7	1	0.1	0.1	0.3
523	Self-rising, enriched, unsifted, spooned----------- 1 cup----------	125	12	440	12	1	0.2	0.1	0.5
524	Whole-wheat, from hard wheats, stirred---------------------- 1 cup----------	120	12	400	16	2	0.3	0.3	1.1

Nutrients in Indicated Quantity

Cho-les-terol	Carbo-hydrate	Calcium	Phos-phorus	Iron	Potas-sium	Sodium	Vitamin A value		Thiamin	Ribo-flavin	Niacin	Ascorbic acid	Item No.
							(IU)	(RE)					
Milli-grams	Grams	Milli-grams	Milli-grams	Milli-grams	Milli-grams	Milli-grams	Inter-national units	Retinol equiva-lents	Milli-grams	Milli-grams	Milli-grams	Milli-grams	
569	423	388	850	27.2	1,015	1,823	1,320	322	1.82	0.99	6.6	0	491
95	71	65	142	4.6	170	305	220	54	0.30	0.17	1.1	0	492
655	223	464	628	8.2	1,456	1,947	22,480	2,493	0.82	1.27	7.3	0	493
109	37	78	105	1.4	243	325	3,750	416	0.14	0.21	1.2	0	494
14	31	12	34	0.9	42	326	30	3	0.09	0.06	1.0	1	495
13	32	11	41	0.7	61	371	190	19	0.06	0.06	0.6	1	496
0	6	1	22	0.2	20	Tr	10	1	0.03	0.01	0.2	0	497
0	6	3	31	0.3	19	86	20	2	0.01	0.02	0.1	0	498
0	30	2	47	0.5	90	Tr	30	3	0.13	0.02	0.4	0	499
0	2	1	3	0.1	3	48	0	0	0.01	0.01	0.1	0	500
0	13	4	15	0.3	16	258	0	0	0.05	0.04	0.7	0	501
0	48	16	55	1.2	61	966	0	0	0.19	0.15	2.6	0	502
0	50	23	142	1.0	137	0	0	0	0.18	0.04	2.7	0	503
0	149	44	174	5.4	170	9	0	0	0.81	0.06	6.5	0	504
0	50	21	57	1.8	57	0	0	0	0.23	0.02	2.1	0	505
0	40	5	31	1.3	0	0	0	0	0.21	0.02	1.7	0	506
0	150	111	370	5.4	278	17	0	0	0.81	0.07	6.5	0	507
0	41	33	100	1.4	75	0	0	0	0.19	0.02	2.1	0	508
Tr	14	33	44	0.8	36	155	Tr	Tr	0.14	0.09	1.1	Tr	509
Tr	20	54	44	1.2	56	241	Tr	Tr	0.20	0.13	1.6	Tr	510
Tr	30	24	46	1.4	49	313	0	0	0.20	0.12	1.7	0	511
Tr	72	100	115	3.8	128	683	0	0	0.54	0.33	4.5	0	512
12	20	16	36	1.1	41	98	30	8	0.12	0.12	1.2	0	513
0	39	14	85	2.0	103	1	0	0	0.23	0.13	1.8	0	514
0	32	11	70	1.7	85	1	0	0	0.20	0.11	1.5	0	515
0	38	104	104	2.2	91	248	520	52	0.17	0.18	2.3	4	516
0	13	42	55	0.6	43	1	80	8	0.05	0.03	0.4	0	517
102	26	154	135	1.5	129	445	140	39	0.18	0.24	1.5	Tr	518
59	27	179	257	1.2	146	515	170	49	0.14	0.23	0.9	Tr	519
0	88	18	100	5.1	109	2	0	0	0.73	0.46	6.1	0	520
0	95	20	109	5.5	119	3	0	0	0.80	0.50	6.6	0	521
0	76	16	70	4.2	91	2	0	0	0.58	0.38	5.1	0	522
0	93	331	583	5.5	113	1,349	0	0	0.80	0.50	6.6	0	523
0	85	49	446	5.2	444	4	0	0	0.66	0.14	5.2	0	524

(Tr indicates nutrient present in trace amount.)

Item No.	Foods, approximate measures, units, and weight (weight of edible portion only)		Grams	Water Per-cent	Food energy Cal-ories	Pro-tein Grams	Fat Grams	Fatty acids Satu-rated Grams	Mono-unsatu-rated Grams	Poly-unsatu-rated Grams
	Legumes, Nuts, and Seeds									
	Almonds, shelled:									
525	Slivered, packed	1 cup	135	4	795	27	70	6.7	45.8	14.8
526	Whole	1 oz	28	4	165	6	15	1.4	9.6	3.1
	Beans, dry:									
	Cooked, drained:									
527	Black	1 cup	171	66	225	15	1	0.1	0.1	0.5
528	Great Northern	1 cup	180	69	210	14	1	0.1	0.1	0.6
529	Lima	1 cup	190	64	260	16	1	0.2	0.1	0.5
530	Pea (navy)	1 cup	190	69	225	15	1	0.1	0.1	0.7
531	Pinto	1 cup	180	65	265	15	1	0.1	0.1	0.5
	Canned, solids and liquid:									
	White with:									
532	Frankfurters (sliced)	1 cup	255	71	365	19	18	7.4	8.8	0.7
533	Pork and tomato sauce	1 cup	255	71	310	16	7	2.4	2.7	0.7
534	Pork and sweet sauce	1 cup	255	66	385	16	12	4.3	4.9	1.2
535	Red kidney	1 cup	255	76	230	15	1	0.1	0.1	0.6
536	Black-eyed peas, dry, cooked (with residual cooking liquid)	1 cup	250	80	190	13	1	0.2	Tr	0.3
537	Brazil nuts, shelled	1 oz	28	3	185	4	19	4.6	6.5	6.8
538	Carob flour	1 cup	140	3	255	6	Tr	Tr	0.1	0.1
	Cashew nuts, salted:									
539	Dry roasted	1 cup	137	2	785	21	63	12.5	37.4	10.7
540		1 oz	28	2	165	4	13	2.6	7.7	2.2
541	Roasted in oil	1 cup	130	4	750	21	63	12.4	36.9	10.6
542		1 oz	28	4	165	5	14	2.7	8.1	2.3
543	Chestnuts, European (Italian), roasted, shelled	1 cup	143	40	350	5	3	0.6	1.1	1.2
544	Chickpeas, cooked, drained	1 cup	163	60	270	15	4	0.4	0.9	1.9
	Coconut:									
	Raw:									
545	Piece, about 2 by 2 by 1/2 in	1 piece	45	47	160	1	15	13.4	0.6	0.2
546	Shredded or grated	1 cup	80	47	285	3	27	23.8	1.1	0.3
547	Dried, sweetened, shredded	1 cup	93	13	470	3	33	29.3	1.4	0.4
548	Filberts (hazelnuts), chopped	1 cup	115	5	725	15	72	5.3	56.5	6.9
549		1 oz	28	5	180	4	18	1.3	13.9	1.7
550	Lentils, dry, cooked	1 cup	200	72	215	16	1	0.1	0.2	0.5
551	Macadamia nuts, roasted in oil, salted	1 cup	134	2	960	10	103	15.4	80.9	1.8
552		1 oz	28	2	205	2	22	3.2	17.1	0.4
	Mixed nuts, with peanuts, salted:									
553	Dry roasted	1 oz	28	2	170	5	15	2.0	8.9	3.1
554	Roasted in oil	1 oz	28	2	175	5	16	2.5	9.0	3.8
555	Peanuts, roasted in oil, salted	1 cup	145	2	840	39	71	9.9	35.5	22.6
556		1 oz	28	2	165	8	14	1.9	6.9	4.4
557	Peanut butter	1 tbsp	16	1	95	5	8	1.4	4.0	2.5
558	Peas, split, dry, cooked	1 cup	200	70	230	16	1	0.1	0.1	0.3
559	Pecans, halves	1 cup	108	5	720	8	73	5.9	45.5	18.1
560		1 oz	28	5	190	2	19	1.5	12.0	4.7
561	Pine nuts (pinyons), shelled	1 oz	28	6	160	3	17	2.7	6.5	7.3
562	Pistachio nuts, dried, shelled	1 oz	28	4	165	6	14	1.7	9.3	2.1
563	Pumpkin and squash kernels, dry, hulled	1 oz	28	7	155	7	13	2.5	4.0	5.9
564	Refried beans, canned	1 cup	290	72	295	18	3	0.4	0.6	1.4
565	Sesame seeds, dry, hulled	1 tbsp	8	5	45	2	4	0.6	1.7	1.9
566	Soybeans, dry, cooked, drained	1 cup	180	71	235	20	10	1.3	1.9	5.3
	Soy products:									
567	Miso	1 cup	276	53	470	29	13	1.8	2.6	7.3
568	Tofu, piece 2-1/2 by 2-3/4 by 1 in	1 piece	120	85	85	9	5	0.7	1.0	2.9
569	Sunflower seeds, dry, hulled	1 oz	28	5	160	6	14	1.5	2.7	9.3
570	Tahini	1 tbsp	15	3	90	3	8	1.1	3.0	3.5

[41] Cashews without salt contain 21 mg sodium per cup or 4 mg per oz.
[42] Cashews without salt contain 22 mg sodium per cup or 5 mg per oz.
[43] Macadamia nuts without salt contain 9 mg sodium per cup or 2 mg per oz.

Nutrients in Indicated Quantity

Cholesterol	Carbohydrate	Calcium	Phosphorus	Iron	Potassium	Sodium	Vitamin A value (IU)	Vitamin A value (RE)	Thiamin	Riboflavin	Niacin	Ascorbic acid	Item No.
Milligrams	Grams	Milligrams	Milligrams	Milligrams	Milligrams	Milligrams	International units	Retinol equivalents	Milligrams	Milligrams	Milligrams	Milligrams	
0	28	359	702	4.9	988	15	0	0	0.28	1.05	4.5	1	525
0	6	75	147	1.0	208	3	0	0	0.06	0.22	1.0	Tr	526
0	41	47	239	2.9	608	1	Tr	Tr	0.43	0.05	0.9	0	527
0	38	90	266	4.9	749	13	0	0	0.25	0.13	1.3	0	528
0	49	55	293	5.9	1,163	4	0	0	0.25	0.11	1.3	0	529
0	40	95	281	5.1	790	13	0	0	0.27	0.13	1.3	0	530
0	49	86	296	5.4	882	3	Tr	Tr	0.33	0.16	0.7	0	531
30	32	94	303	4.8	668	1,374	330	33	0.18	0.15	3.3	Tr	532
10	48	138	235	4.6	536	1,181	330	33	0.20	0.08	1.5	5	533
10	54	161	291	5.9	536	969	330	33	0.15	0.10	1.3	5	534
0	42	74	278	4.6	673	968	10	1	0.13	0.10	1.5	0	535
0	35	43	238	3.3	573	20	30	3	0.40	0.10	1.0	0	536
0	4	50	170	1.0	170	1	Tr	Tr	0.28	0.03	0.5	Tr	537
0	126	390	102	5.7	1,275	24	Tr	Tr	0.07	0.07	2.2	Tr	538
0	45	62	671	8.2	774	[41]877	0	0	0.27	0.27	1.9	0	539
0	9	13	139	1.7	160	[41]181	0	0	0.06	0.06	0.4	0	540
0	37	53	554	5.3	689	[42]814	0	0	0.55	0.23	2.3	0	541
0	8	12	121	1.2	150	[42]177	0	0	0.12	0.05	0.5	0	542
0	76	41	153	1.3	847	3	30	3	0.35	0.25	1.9	37	543
0	45	80	273	4.9	475	11	Tr	Tr	0.18	0.09	0.9	0	544
0	7	6	51	1.1	160	9	0	0	0.03	0.01	0.2	1	545
0	12	11	90	1.9	285	16	0	0	0.05	0.02	0.4	3	546
0	44	14	99	1.8	313	244	0	0	0.03	0.02	0.4	1	547
0	18	216	359	3.8	512	3	80	8	0.58	0.13	1.3	1	548
0	4	53	88	0.9	126	1	20	2	0.14	0.03	0.3	Tr	549
0	38	50	238	4.2	498	26	40	4	0.14	0.12	1.2	0	550
0	17	60	268	2.4	441	[43]348	10	1	0.29	0.15	2.7	0	551
0	4	13	57	0.5	93	[43]74	Tr	Tr	0.06	0.03	0.6	0	552
0	7	20	123	1.0	169	[44]190	Tr	Tr	0.06	0.06	1.3	0	553
0	6	31	131	0.9	165	[44]185	10	1	0.14	0.06	1.4	Tr	554
0	27	125	734	2.8	1,019	[45]626	0	0	0.42	0.15	21.5	0	555
0	5	24	143	0.5	199	[45]122	0	0	0.08	0.03	4.2	0	556
0	3	5	60	0.3	110	75	0	0	0.02	0.02	2.2	0	557
0	42	22	178	3.4	592	26	80	8	0.30	0.18	1.8	0	558
0	20	39	314	2.3	423	1	140	14	0.92	0.14	1.0	2	559
0	5	10	83	0.6	111	Tr	40	4	0.24	0.04	0.3	1	560
0	5	2	10	0.9	178	20	10	1	0.35	0.06	1.2	1	561
0	7	38	143	1.9	310	2	70	7	0.23	0.05	0.3	Tr	562
0	5	12	333	4.2	229	5	110	11	0.06	0.09	0.5	Tr	563
0	51	141	245	5.1	1,141	1,228	0	0	0.14	0.16	1.4	17	564
0	1	11	62	0.6	33	3	10	1	0.06	0.01	0.4	0	565
0	19	131	322	4.9	972	4	50	5	0.38	0.16	1.1	0	566
0	65	188	853	4.7	922	8,142	110	11	0.17	0.28	0.8	0	567
0	3	108	151	2.3	50	8	0	0	0.07	0.04	0.1	0	568
0	5	33	200	1.9	195	1	10	1	0.65	0.07	1.3	Tr	569
0	3	21	119	0.7	69	5	10	1	0.24	0.02	0.8	1	570

[44]Mixed nuts without salt contain 3 mg sodium per oz.
[45]Peanuts without salt contain 22 mg sodium per cup or 4 mg per oz.

(Tr indicates nutrient present in trace amount.)

Item No.	Foods, approximate measures, units, and weight (weight of edible portion only)			Water	Food energy	Pro-tein	Fat	Fatty acids		
								Satu-rated	Mono-unsatu-rated	Poly-unsatu-rated
			Grams	Per-cent	Cal-ories	Grams	Grams	Grams	Grams	Grams
	Legumes, Nuts, and Seeds—Con.									
	Walnuts:									
571	Black, chopped-----------------	1 cup----------	125	4	760	30	71	4.5	15.9	46.9
572		1 oz------------	28	4	170	7	16	1.0	3.6	10.6
573	English or Persian, pieces or									
	chips---------------------	1 cup----------	120	4	770	17	74	6.7	17.0	47.0
574		1 oz------------	28	4	180	4	18	1.6	4.0	11.1
	Meat and Meat Products									
	Beef, cooked:[46]									
	Cuts braised, simmered, or pot roasted:									
	Relatively fat such as chuck blade:									
575	Lean and fat, piece, 2-1/2 by 2-1/2 by 3/4 in-------	3 oz------------	85	43	325	22	26	10.8	11.7	0.9
576	Lean only from item 575----	2.2 oz----------	62	53	170	19	9	3.9	4.2	0.3
	Relatively lean, such as bottom round:									
577	Lean and fat, piece, 4-1/8 by 2-1/4 by 1/2 in-------	3 oz------------	85	54	220	25	13	4.8	5.7	0.5
578	Lean only from item 577----	2.8 oz----------	78	57	175	25	8	2.7	3.4	0.3
	Ground beef, broiled, patty, 3 by 5/8 in:									
579	Lean------------------------	3 oz------------	85	56	230	21	16	6.2	6.9	0.6
580	Regular---------------------	3 oz------------	85	54	245	20	18	6.9	7.7	0.7
581	Heart, lean, braised-------	3 oz------------	85	65	150	24	5	1.2	0.8	1.6
582	Liver, fried, slice, 6-1/2 by 2-3/8 by 3/8 in[47]-----------	3 oz------------	85	56	185	23	7	2.5	3.6	1.3
	Roast, oven cooked, no liquid added:									
	Relatively fat, such as rib:									
583	Lean and fat, 2 pieces, 4-1/8 by 2-1/4 by 1/4 in	3 oz------------	85	46	315	19	26	10.8	11.4	0.9
584	Lean only from item 583----	2.2 oz----------	61	57	150	17	9	3.6	3.7	0.3
	Relatively lean, such as eye of round:									
585	Lean and fat, 2 pieces, 2-1/2 by 2-1/2 by 3/8 in	3 oz------------	85	57	205	23	12	4.9	5.4	0.5
586	Lean only from item 585----	2.6 oz----------	75	63	135	22	5	1.9	2.1	0.2
	Steak:									
	Sirloin, broiled:									
587	Lean and fat, piece, 2-1/2 by 2-1/2 by 3/4 in-------	3 oz------------	85	53	240	23	15	6.4	6.9	0.6
588	Lean only from item 587----	2.5 oz----------	72	59	150	22	6	2.6	2.8	0.3
589	Beef, canned, corned------------	3 oz------------	85	59	185	22	10	4.2	4.9	0.4
590	Beef, dried, chipped------------	2.5 oz----------	72	48	145	24	4	1.8	2.0	0.2
	Lamb, cooked:									
	Chops, (3 per lb with bone):									
	Arm, braised:									
591	Lean and fat---------------	2.2 oz----------	63	44	220	20	15	6.9	6.0	0.9
592	Lean only from item 591----	1.7 oz----------	48	49	135	17	7	2.9	2.6	0.4
	Loin, broiled:									
593	Lean and fat---------------	2.8 oz----------	80	54	235	22	16	7.3	6.4	1.0
594	Lean only from item 593----	2.3 oz----------	64	61	140	19	6	2.6	2.4	0.4
	Leg, roasted:									
595	Lean and fat, 2 pieces, 4-1/8 by 2-1/4 by 1/4 in---------	3 oz------------	85	59	205	22	13	5.6	4.9	0.8
596	Lean only from item 595------	2.6 oz----------	73	64	140	20	6	2.4	2.2	0.4
	Rib, roasted:									
597	Lean and fat, 3 pieces, 2-1/2 by 2-1/2 by 1/4 in---------	3 oz------------	85	47	315	18	26	12.1	10.6	1.5
598	Lean only from item 597------	2 oz------------	57	60	130	15	7	3.2	3.0	0.5

[46] Outer layer of fat was removed to within approximately 1/2 inch of the lean. Deposits of fat within the cut were not removed.
[47] Fried in vegetable shortening.

							Vitamin A value						
Cho-les-terol	Carbo-hydrate	Calcium	Phos-phorus	Iron	Potas-sium	Sodium	(IU)	(RE)	Thiamin	Ribo-flavin	Niacin	Ascorbic acid	Item No.
Milli-grams	Grams	Milli-grams	Milli-grams	Milli-grams	Milli-grams	Milli-grams	Inter-national units	Retinol equiva-lents	Milli-grams	Milli-grams	Milli-grams	Milli-grams	
0	15	73	580	3.8	655	1	370	37	0.27	0.14	0.9	Tr	571
0	3	16	132	0.9	149	Tr	80	8	0.06	0.03	0.2	Tr	572
0	22	113	380	2.9	602	12	150	15	0.46	0.18	1.3	4	573
0	5	27	90	0.7	142	3	40	4	0.11	0.04	0.3	1	574
87	0	11	163	2.5	163	53	Tr	Tr	0.06	0.19	2.0	0	575
66	0	8	146	2.3	163	44	Tr	Tr	0.05	0.17	1.7	0	576
81	0	5	217	2.8	248	43	Tr	Tr	0.06	0.21	3.3	0	577
75	0	4	212	2.7	240	40	Tr	Tr	0.06	0.20	3.0	0	578
74	0	9	134	1.8	256	65	Tr	Tr	0.04	0.18	4.4	0	579
76	0	9	144	2.1	248	70	Tr	Tr	0.03	0.16	4.9	0	580
164	0	5	213	6.4	198	54	Tr	Tr	0.12	1.31	3.4	5	581
410	7	9	392	5.3	309	90	[48]30,690	[48]9,120	0.18	3.52	12.3	23	582
72	0	8	145	2.0	246	54	Tr	Tr	0.06	0.16	3.1	0	583
49	0	5	127	1.7	218	45	Tr	Tr	0.05	0.13	2.7	0	584
62	0	5	177	1.6	308	50	Tr	Tr	0.07	0.14	3.0	0	585
52	0	3	170	1.5	297	46	Tr	Tr	0.07	0.13	2.8	0	586
77	0	9	186	2.6	306	53	Tr	Tr	0.10	0.23	3.3	0	587
64	0	8	176	2.4	290	48	Tr	Tr	0.09	0.22	3.1	0	588
80	0	17	90	3.7	51	802	Tr	Tr	0.02	0.20	2.9	0	589
46	0	14	287	2.3	142	3,053	Tr	Tr	0.05	0.23	2.7	0	590
77	0	16	132	1.5	195	46	Tr	Tr	0.04	0.16	4.4	0	591
59	0	12	111	1.3	162	36	Tr	Tr	0.03	0.13	3.0	0	592
78	0	16	162	1.4	272	62	Tr	Tr	0.09	0.21	5.5	0	593
60	0	12	145	1.3	241	54	Tr	Tr	0.08	0.18	4.4	0	594
78	0	8	162	1.7	273	57	Tr	Tr	0.09	0.24	5.5	0	595
65	0	6	150	1.5	247	50	Tr	Tr	0.08	0.20	4.6	0	596
77	0	19	139	1.4	224	60	Tr	Tr	0.08	0.18	5.5	0	597
50	0	12	111	1.0	179	46	Tr	Tr	0.05	0.13	3.5	0	598

[48] Value varies widely.

(Tr indicates nutrient present in trace amount.)

Item No.	Foods, approximate measures, units, and weight (weight of edible portion only)		Water	Food energy	Pro-tein	Fat	Fatty acids		
							Satu-rated	Mono-unsatu-rated	Poly-unsatu-rated
		Grams	Per-cent	Cal-ories	Grams	Grams	Grams	Grams	Grams
	Meat and Meat Products—Con.								
	Pork, cured, cooked:								
	Bacon:								
599	Regular---------------------- 3 medium slices	19	13	110	6	9	3.3	4.5	1.1
600	Canadian-style--------------- 2 slices--------	46	62	85	11	4	1.3	1.9	0.4
	Ham, light cure, roasted:								
601	Lean and fat, 2 pieces, 4-1/8 by 2-1/4 by 1/4 in-------- 3 oz------------	85	58	205	18	14	5.1	6.7	1.5
602	Lean only from item 601------ 2.4 oz----------	68	66	105	17	4	1.3	1.7	0.4
603	Ham, canned, roasted, 2 pieces, 4-1/8 by 2-1/4 by 1/4 in----- 3 oz------------	85	67	140	18	7	2.4	3.5	0.8
	Luncheon meat:								
604	Canned, spiced or unspiced, slice, 3 by 2 by 1/2 in---- 2 slices--------	42	52	140	5	13	4.5	6.0	1.5
605	Chopped ham (8 slices per 6 oz pkg)-------------------- 2 slices--------	42	64	95	7	7	2.4	3.4	0.9
	Cooked ham (8 slices per 8-oz pkg):								
606	Regular--------------- 2 slices--------	57	65	105	10	6	1.9	2.8	0.7
607	Extra lean------------- 2 slices--------	57	71	75	11	3	0.9	1.3	0.3
	Pork, fresh, cooked:								
	Chop, loin (cut 3 per lb with bone):								
	Broiled:								
608	Lean and fat--------------- 3.1 oz----------	87	50	275	24	19	7.0	8.8	2.2
609	Lean only from item 608---- 2.5 oz----------	72	57	165	23	8	2.6	3.4	0.9
	Pan fried:								
610	Lean and fat--------------- 3.1 oz----------	89	45	335	21	27	9.8	12.5	3.1
611	Lean only from item 610---- 2.4 oz----------	67	54	180	19	11	3.7	4.8	1.3
	Ham (leg), roasted:								
612	Lean and fat, piece, 2-1/2 by 2-1/2 by 3/4 in----------- 3 oz------------	85	53	250	21	18	6.4	8.1	2.0
613	Lean only from item 612------ 2.5 oz----------	72	60	160	20	8	2.7	3.6	1.0
	Rib, roasted:								
614	Lean and fat, piece, 2-1/2 by 3/4 in---------------------- 3 oz------------	85	51	270	21	20	7.2	9.2	2.3
615	Lean only from item 614------ 2.5 oz----------	71	57	175	20	10	3.4	4.4	1.2
	Shoulder cut, braised:								
616	Lean and fat, 3 pieces, 2-1/2 by 2-1/2 by 1/4 in--------- 3 oz------------	85	47	295	23	22	7.9	10.0	2.4
617	Lean only from item 616------ 2.4 oz----------	67	54	165	22	8	2.8	3.7	1.0
	Sausages (See also Luncheon meats, items 604-607):								
618	Bologna, slice (8 per 8-oz pkg) 2 slices--------	57	54	180	7	16	6.1	7.6	1.4
619	Braunschweiger, slice (6 per 6-oz pkg)-------------------- 2 slices--------	57	48	205	8	18	6.2	8.5	2.1
620	Brown and serve (10-11 per 8-oz pkg), browned-------- 1 link----------	13	45	50	2	5	1.7	2.2	0.5
621	Frankfurter (10 per 1-lb pkg), cooked (reheated)------------ 1 frankfurter---	45	54	145	5	13	4.8	6.2	1.2
622	Pork link (16 per 1-lb pkg), cooked[50]--------------------- 1 link----------	13	45	50	3	4	1.4	1.8	0.5
	Salami:								
623	Cooked type, slice (8 per 8-oz pkg)------------------ 2 slices--------	57	60	145	8	11	4.6	5.2	1.2
624	Dry type, slice (12 per 4-oz pkg)---------------------- 2 slices--------	20	35	85	5	7	2.4	3.4	0.6
625	Sandwich spread (pork, beef)--- 1 tbsp----------	15	60	35	1	3	0.9	1.1	0.4
626	Vienna sausage (7 per 4-oz can) 1 sausage-------	16	60	45	2	4	1.5	2.0	0.3
	Veal, medium fat, cooked, bone removed:								
627	Cutlet, 4-1/8 by 2-1/4 by 1/2 in, braised or broiled----- 3 oz----------	85	60	185	23	9	4.1	4.1	0.6
628	Rib, 2 pieces, 4-1/8 by 2-1/4 by 1/4 in, roasted----------- 3 oz----------	85	55	230	23	14	6.0	6.0	1.0

[49]Contains added sodium ascorbate. If sodium ascorbate is not added, ascorbic acid content is negligible.

	Nutrients in Indicated Quantity												
Cho-les-terol	Carbo-hydrate	Calcium	Phos-phorus	Iron	Potas-sium	Sodium	Vitamin A value		Thiamin	Ribo-flavin	Niacin	Ascorbic acid	Item No.
							(IU)	(RE)					
Milli-grams	Grams	Milli-grams	Milli-grams	Milli-grams	Milli-grams	Milli-grams	Inter-national units	Retinol equiva-lents	Milli-grams	Milli-grams	Milli-grams	Milli-grams	
16	Tr	2	64	0.3	92	303	0	0	0.13	0.05	1.4	6	599
27	1	5	136	0.4	179	711	0	0	0.38	0.09	3.2	10	600
53	0	6	182	0.7	243	1,009	0	0	0.51	0.19	3.8	0	601
37	0	5	154	0.6	215	902	0	0	0.46	0.17	3.4	0	602
35	Tr	6	188	0.9	298	908	0	0	0.82	0.21	4.3	[49]19	603
26	1	3	34	0.3	90	541	0	0	0.15	0.08	1.3	Tr	604
21	0	3	65	0.3	134	576	0	0	0.27	0.09	1.6	[49]8	605
32	2	4	141	0.6	189	751	0	0	0.49	0.14	3.0	[49]16	606
27	1	4	124	0.4	200	815	0	0	0.53	0.13	2.8	[49]15	607
84	0	3	184	0.7	312	61	10	3	0.87	0.24	4.3	Tr	608
71	0	4	176	0.7	302	56	10	1	0.83	0.22	4.0	Tr	609
92	0	4	190	0.7	323	64	10	3	0.91	0.24	4.6	Tr	610
72	0	3	178	0.7	305	57	10	1	0.84	0.22	4.0	Tr	611
79	0	5	210	0.9	280	50	10	2	0.54	0.27	3.9	Tr	612
68	0	5	202	0.8	269	46	10	1	0.50	0.25	3.6	Tr	613
69	0	9	190	0.8	313	37	10	3	0.50	0.24	4.2	Tr	614
56	0	8	182	0.7	300	33	10	2	0.45	0.22	3.8	Tr	615
93	0	6	162	1.4	286	75	10	3	0.46	0.26	4.4	Tr	616
76	0	5	151	1.3	271	68	10	1	0.40	0.24	4.0	Tr	617
31	2	7	52	0.9	103	581	0	0	0.10	0.08	1.5	[49]12	618
89	2	5	96	5.3	113	652	8,010	2,405	0.14	0.87	4.8	[49]6	619
9	Tr	1	14	0.1	25	105	0	0	0.05	0.02	0.4	0	620
23	1	5	39	0.5	75	504	0	0	0.09	0.05	1.2	[49]12	621
11	Tr	4	24	0.2	47	168	0	0	0.10	0.03	0.6	Tr	622
37	1	7	66	1.5	113	607	0	0	0.14	0.21	2.0	[49]7	623
16	1	2	28	0.3	76	372	0	0	0.12	0.06	1.0	[49]5	624
6	2	2	9	0.1	17	152	10	1	0.03	0.02	0.3	0	625
8	Tr	2	8	0.1	16	152	0	0	0.01	0.02	0.3	0	626
109	0	9	196	0.8	258	56	Tr	Tr	0.06	0.21	4.6	0	627
109	0	10	211	0.7	259	57	Tr	Tr	0.11	0.26	6.6	0	628

[50] One patty (8 per pound) of bulk sausage is equivalent to 2 links.

(Tr indicates nutrient present in trace amount.)

Item No.	Foods, approximate measures, units, and weight (weight of edible portion only)		Water	Food energy	Pro-tein	Fat	Fatty acids		
							Satu-rated	Mono-unsatu-rated	Poly-unsatu-rated
	Mixed Dishes and Fast Foods	Grams	Per-cent	Cal-ories	Grams	Grams	Grams	Grams	Grams
	Mixed dishes:								
629	Beef and vegetable stew, from home recipe----------------- 1 cup-----------	245	82	220	16	11	4.4	4.5	0.5
630	Beef potpie, from home recipe, baked, piece, 1/3 of 9-in diam. pie[51] ----------------- 1 piece---------	210	55	515	21	30	7.9	12.9	7.4
631	Chicken a la king, cooked, from home recipe------------- 1 cup-----------	245	68	470	27	34	12.9	13.4	6.2
632	Chicken and noodles, cooked, from home recipe------------- 1 cup-----------	240	71	365	22	18	5.1	7.1	3.9
	Chicken chow mein:								
633	Canned-------------------- 1 cup-----------	250	89	95	7	Tr	0.1	0.1	0.8
634	From home recipe------------- 1 cup-----------	250	78	255	31	10	4.1	4.9	3.5
635	Chicken potpie, from home recipe, baked, piece, 1/3 of 9-in diam. pie[51] ------------- 1 piece---------	232	57	545	23	31	10.3	15.5	6.6
636	Chili con carne with beans, canned--------------------- 1 cup-----------	255	72	340	19	16	5.8	7.2	1.0
637	Chop suey with beef and pork, from home recipe------------- 1 cup-----------	250	75	300	26	17	4.3	7.4	4.2
	Macaroni (enriched) and cheese:								
638	Canned[52] --------------------- 1 cup-----------	240	80	230	9	10	4.7	2.9	1.3
639	From home recipe[38] ----------- 1 cup-----------	200	58	430	17	22	9.8	7.4	3.6
640	Quiche Lorraine, 1/8 of 8-in diam. quiche[51] --------------- 1 slice---------	176	47	600	13	48	23.2	17.8	4.1
	Spaghetti (enriched) in tomato sauce with cheese:								
641	Canned--------------------- 1 cup-----------	250	80	190	6	2	0.4	0.4	0.5
642	From home recipe------------- 1 cup-----------	250	77	260	9	9	3.0	3.6	1.2
	Spaghetti (enriched) with meat-balls and tomato sauce:								
643	Canned--------------------- 1 cup-----------	250	78	260	12	10	2.4	3.9	3.1
644	From home recipe------------- 1 cup-----------	248	70	330	19	12	3.9	4.4	2.2
	Fast food entrees:								
	Cheeseburger:								
645	Regular--------------------- 1 sandwich------	112	46	300	15	15	7.3	5.6	1.0
646	4 oz patty------------------- 1 sandwich------	194	46	525	30	31	15.1	12.2	1.4
	Chicken, fried. See Poultry and Poultry Products (items 656-659).								
647	Enchilada--------------------- 1 enchilada-----	230	72	235	20	16	7.7	6.7	0.6
648	English muffin, egg, cheese, and bacon-------------------- 1 sandwich------	138	49	360	18	18	8.0	8.0	0.7
	Fish sandwich:								
649	Regular, with cheese-------- 1 sandwich------	140	43	420	16	23	6.3	6.9	7.7
650	Large, without cheese------- 1 sandwich------	170	48	470	18	27	6.3	8.7	9.5
	Hamburger:								
651	Regular--------------------- 1 sandwich------	98	46	245	12	11	4.4	5.3	0.5
652	4 oz patty------------------- 1 sandwich------	174	50	445	25	21	7.1	11.7	0.6
653	Pizza, cheese, 1/8 of 15-in diam. pizza[51] ---------------- 1 slice---------	120	46	290	15	9	4.1	2.6	1.3
654	Roast beef sandwich------------ 1 sandwich------	150	52	345	22	13	3.5	6.9	1.8
655	Taco------------------------- 1 taco----------	81	55	195	9	11	4.1	5.5	0.8

[38] Made with margarine.
[51] Crust made with vegetable shortening and enriched flour.

							Vitamin A value						
Cho-les-terol	Carbo-hydrate	Calcium	Phos-phorus	Iron	Potas-sium	Sodium	(IU)	(RE)	Thiamin	Ribo-flavin	Niacin	Ascorbic acid	Item No.
Milli-grams	Grams	Milli-grams	Milli-grams	Milli-grams	Milli-grams	Milli-grams	Inter-national units	Retinol equiva-lents	Milli-grams	Milli-grams	Milli-grams	Milli-grams	
71	15	29	184	2.9	613	292	5,690	568	0.15	0.17	4.7	17	629
42	39	29	149	3.8	334	596	4,220	517	0.29	0.29	4.8	6	630
221	12	127	358	2.5	404	760	1,130	272	0.10	0.42	5.4	12	631
103	26	26	247	2.2	149	600	430	130	0.05	0.17	4.3	Tr	632
8	18	45	85	1.3	418	725	150	28	0.05	0.10	1.0	13	633
75	10	58	293	2.5	473	718	280	50	0.08	0.23	4.3	10	634
56	42	70	232	3.0	343	594	7,220	735	0.32	0.32	4.9	5	635
28	31	82	321	4.3	594	1,354	150	15	0.08	0.18	3.3	8	636
68	13	60	248	4.8	425	1,053	600	60	0.28	0.38	5.0	33	637
24	26	199	182	1.0	139	730	260	72	0.12	0.24	1.0	Tr	638
44	40	362	322	1.8	240	1,086	860	232	0.20	0.40	1.8	1	639
285	29	211	276	1.0	283	653	1,640	454	0.11	0.32	Tr	Tr	640
3	39	40	88	2.8	303	955	930	120	0.35	0.28	4.5	10	641
8	37	80	135	2.3	408	955	1,080	140	0.25	0.18	2.3	13	642
23	29	53	113	3.3	245	1,220	1,000	100	0.15	0.18	2.3	5	643
89	39	124	236	3.7	665	1,009	1,590	159	0.25	0.30	4.0	22	644
44	28	135	174	2.3	219	672	340	65	0.26	0.24	3.7	1	645
104	40	236	320	4.5	407	1,224	670	128	0.33	0.48	7.4	3	646
19	24	322	662	11.0	2,180	4,451	2,720	352	0.18	0.26	Tr	Tr	647
213	31	197	290	3.1	201	832	650	160	0.46	0.50	3.7	1	648
56	39	132	223	1.8	274	667	160	25	0.32	0.26	3.3	2	649
91	41	61	246	2.2	375	621	110	15	0.35	0.23	3.5	1	650
32	28	56	107	2.2	202	463	80	14	0.23	0.24	3.8	1	651
71	38	75	225	4.8	404	763	160	28	0.38	0.38	7.8	1	652
56	39	220	216	1.6	230	699	750	106	0.34	0.29	4.2	2	653
55	34	60	222	4.0	338	757	240	32	0.40	0.33	6.0	2	654
21	15	109	134	1.2	263	456	420	57	0.09	0.07	1.4	1	655

[52] Made with corn oil.

(Tr indicates nutrient present in trace amount.)

Item No.	Foods, approximate measures, units, and weight (weight of edible portion only)		Water	Food energy	Pro-tein	Fat	Fatty acids		
							Satu-rated	Mono-unsatu-rated	Poly-unsatu-rated
		Grams	Per-cent	Cal-ories	Grams	Grams	Grams	Grams	Grams
Poultry and Poultry Products									
	Chicken:								
	Fried, flesh, with skin:[53]								
	Batter dipped:								
656	Breast, 1/2 breast (5.6 oz with bones)-------------- 4.9 oz----------	140	52	365	35	18	4.9	7.6	4.3
657	Drumstick (3.4 oz with bones)------------------- 2.5 oz----------	72	53	195	16	11	3.0	4.6	2.7
	Flour coated:								
658	Breast, 1/2 breast (4.2 oz with bones)-------------- 3.5 oz----------	98	57	220	31	9	2.4	3.4	1.9
659	Drumstick (2.6 oz with bones)------------------- 1.7 oz----------	49	57	120	13	7	1.8	2.7	1.6
	Roasted, flesh only:								
660	Breast, 1/2 breast (4.2 oz with bones and skin)------- 3.0 oz----------	86	65	140	27	3	0.9	1.1	0.7
661	Drumstick, (2.9 oz with bones and skin)------------------ 1.6 oz----------	44	67	75	12	2	0.7	0.8	0.6
662	Stewed, flesh only, light and dark meat, chopped or diced-- 1 cup-----------	140	67	250	38	9	2.6	3.3	2.2
663	Chicken liver, cooked------------ 1 liver---------	20	68	30	5	1	0.4	0.3	0.2
664	Duck, roasted, flesh only-------- 1/2 duck--------	221	64	445	52	25	9.2	8.2	3.2
	Turkey, roasted, flesh only:								
665	Dark meat, piece, 2-1/2 by 1-5/8 by 1/4 in-------------- 4 pieces--------	85	63	160	24	6	2.1	1.4	1.8
666	Light meat, piece, 4 by 2 by 1/4 in---------------------- 2 pieces--------	85	66	135	25	3	0.9	0.5	0.7
	Light and dark meat:								
667	Chopped or diced------------- 1 cup-----------	140	65	240	41	7	2.3	1.4	2.0
668	Pieces (1 slice white meat, 4 by 2 by 1/4 in and 2 slices dark meat, 2-1/2 by 1-5/8 by 1/4 in)-------- 3 pieces--------	85	65	145	25	4	1.4	0.9	1.2
	Poultry food products:								
	Chicken:								
669	Canned, boneless------------- 5 oz-----------	142	69	235	31	11	3.1	4.5	2.5
670	Frankfurter (10 per 1-lb pkg) 1 frankfurter---	45	58	115	6	9	2.5	3.8	1.8
671	Roll, light (6 slices per 6 oz pkg)-------------------- 2 slices--------	57	69	90	11	4	1.1	1.7	0.9
	Turkey:								
672	Gravy and turkey, frozen----- 5-oz package----	142	85	95	8	4	1.2	1.4	0.7
673	Ham, cured turkey thigh meat (8 slices per 8-oz pkg)---- 2 slices--------	57	71	75	11	3	1.0	0.7	0.9
674	Loaf, breast meat (8 slices per 6-oz pkg)-------------- 2 slices--------	42	72	45	10	1	0.2	0.2	0.1
675	Patties, breaded, battered, fried (2.25 oz)------------ 1 patty---------	64	50	180	9	12	3.0	4.8	3.0
676	Roast, boneless, frozen, sea-soned, light and dark meat, cooked------------------------ 3 oz------------	85	68	130	18	5	1.6	1.0	1.4
Soups, Sauces, and Gravies									
	Soups:								
	Canned, condensed:								
	Prepared with equal volume of milk:								
677	Clam chowder, New England-- 1 cup-----------	248	85	165	9	7	3.0	2.3	1.1
678	Cream of chicken----------- 1 cup-----------	248	85	190	7	11	4.6	4.5	1.6
679	Cream of mushroom---------- 1 cup-----------	248	85	205	6	14	5.1	3.0	4.6
680	Tomato-------------------- 1 cup-----------	248	85	160	6	6	2.9	1.6	1.1

[53] Fried in vegetable shortening.

Nutrients in Indicated Quantity

Cho-les-terol	Carbo-hydrate	Calcium	Phos-phorus	Iron	Potas-sium	Sodium	Vitamin A value		Thiamin	Ribo-flavin	Niacin	Ascorbic acid	Item No.
							(IU)	(RE)					
Milli-grams	Grams	Milli-grams	Milli-grams	Milli-grams	Milli-grams	Milli-grams	Inter-national units	Retinol equiva-lents	Milli-grams	Milli-grams	Milli-grams	Milli-grams	
119	13	28	259	1.8	281	385	90	28	0.16	0.20	14.7	0	656
62	6	12	106	1.0	134	194	60	19	0.08	0.15	3.7	0	657
87	2	16	228	1.2	254	74	50	15	0.08	0.13	13.5	0	658
44	1	6	86	0.7	112	44	40	12	0.04	0.11	3.0	0	659
73	0	13	196	0.9	220	64	20	5	0.06	0.10	11.8	0	660
41	0	5	81	0.6	108	42	30	8	0.03	0.10	2.7	0	661
116	0	20	210	1.6	252	98	70	21	0.07	0.23	8.6	0	662
126	Tr	3	62	1.7	28	10	3,270	983	0.03	0.35	0.9	3	663
197	0	27	449	6.0	557	144	170	51	0.57	1.04	11.3	0	664
72	0	27	173	2.0	246	67	0	0	0.05	0.21	3.1	0	665
59	0	16	186	1.1	259	54	0	0	0.05	0.11	5.8	0	666
106	0	35	298	2.5	417	98	0	0	0.09	0.25	7.6	0	667
65	0	21	181	1.5	253	60	0	0	0.05	0.15	4.6	0	668
88	0	20	158	2.2	196	714	170	48	0.02	0.18	9.0	3	669
45	3	43	48	0.9	38	616	60	17	0.03	0.05	1.4	0	670
28	1	24	89	0.6	129	331	50	14	0.04	0.07	3.0	0	671
26	7	20	115	1.3	87	787	60	18	0.03	0.18	2.6	0	672
32	Tr	6	108	1.6	184	565	0	0	0.03	0.14	2.0	0	673
17	0	3	97	0.2	118	608	0	0	0.02	0.05	3.5	[54]0	674
40	10	9	173	1.4	176	512	20	7	0.06	0.12	1.5	0	675
45	3	4	207	1.4	253	578	0	0	0.04	0.14	5.3	0	676
22	17	186	156	1.5	300	992	160	40	0.07	0.24	1.0	3	677
27	15	181	151	0.7	273	1,047	710	94	0.07	0.26	0.9	1	678
20	15	179	156	0.6	270	1,076	150	37	0.08	0.28	0.9	2	679
17	22	159	149	1.8	449	932	850	109	0.13	0.25	1.5	68	680

[54] If sodium ascorbate is added, product contains 11 mg ascorbic acid.

(Tr indicates nutrient present in trace amount.)

Item No.	Foods, approximate measures, units, and weight (weight of edible portion only)		Water	Food energy	Pro-tein	Fat	Satu-rated	Mono-unsatu-rated	Poly-unsatu-rated
		Grams	Per-cent	Cal-ories	Grams	Grams	Grams	Grams	Grams
	Soups, Sauces, and Gravies—Con.								
	Soups:									
	Canned, condensed:									
	Prepared with equal volume of water:									
681	Bean with bacon-----------	1 cup----------	253	84	170	8	6	1.5	2.2	1.8
682	Beef broth, bouillon, consomme----------------	1 cup----------	240	98	15	3	1	0.3	0.2	Tr
683	Beef noodle---------------	1 cup----------	244	92	85	5	3	1.1	1.2	0.5
684	Chicken noodle------------	1 cup----------	241	92	75	4	2	0.7	1.1	0.6
685	Chicken rice--------------	1 cup----------	241	94	60	4	2	0.5	0.9	0.4
686	Clam chowder, Manhattan----	1 cup----------	244	90	80	4	2	0.4	0.4	1.3
687	Cream of chicken----------	1 cup----------	244	91	115	3	7	2.1	3.3	1.5
688	Cream of mushroom---------	1 cup----------	244	90	130	2	9	2.4	1.7	4.2
689	Minestrone----------------	1 cup----------	241	91	80	4	3	0.6	0.7	1.1
690	Pea, green----------------	1 cup----------	250	83	165	9	3	1.4	1.0	0.4
691	Tomato-------------------	1 cup----------	244	90	85	2	2	0.4	0.4	1.0
692	Vegetable beef------------	1 cup----------	244	92	80	6	2	0.9	0.8	0.1
693	Vegetarian----------------	1 cup----------	241	92	70	2	2	0.3	0.8	0.7
	Dehydrated:									
	Unprepared:									
694	Bouillon-----------------	1 pkt----------	6	3	15	1	1	0.3	0.2	Tr
695	Onion--------------------	1 pkt----------	7	4	20	1	Tr	0.1	0.2	Tr
	Prepared with water:									
696	Chicken noodle------------	1 pkt (6-fl-oz)	188	94	40	2	1	0.2	0.4	0.3
697	Onion--------------------	1 pkt (6-fl-oz)	184	96	20	1	Tr	0.1	0.2	0.1
698	Tomato vegetable----------	1 pkt (6-fl-oz)	189	94	40	1	1	0.3	0.2	0.1
	Sauces:									
	From dry mix:									
699	Cheese, prepared with milk---	1 cup----------	279	77	305	16	17	9.3	5.3	1.6
700	Hollandaise, prepared with water----------------	1 cup----------	259	84	240	5	20	11.6	5.9	0.9
701	White sauce, prepared with milk---------------------	1 cup----------	264	81	240	10	13	6.4	4.7	1.7
	From home recipe:									
702	White sauce, medium[55] --------	1 cup----------	250	73	395	10	30	9.1	11.9	7.2
	Ready to serve:									
703	Barbecue-----------------	1 tbsp---------	16	81	10	Tr	Tr	Tr	0.1	0.1
704	Soy----------------------	1 tbsp---------	18	68	10	2	0	0.0	0.0	0.0
	Gravies:									
	Canned:									
705	Beef---------------------	1 cup----------	233	87	125	9	5	2.7	2.3	0.2
706	Chicken------------------	1 cup----------	238	85	190	5	14	3.4	6.1	3.6
707	Mushroom-----------------	1 cup----------	238	89	120	3	6	1.0	2.8	2.4
	From dry mix:									
708	Brown--------------------	1 cup----------	261	91	80	3	2	0.9	0.8	0.1
709	Chicken------------------	1 cup----------	260	91	85	3	2	0.5	0.9	0.4
	Sugars and Sweets									
	Candy:									
710	Caramels, plain or chocolate---	1 oz-----------	28	8	115	1	3	2.2	0.3	0.1
	Chocolate:									
711	Milk, plain---------------	1 oz-----------	28	1	145	2	9	5.4	3.0	0.3
712	Milk, with almonds--------	1 oz-----------	28	2	150	3	10	4.8	4.1	0.7
713	Milk, with peanuts--------	1 oz-----------	28	1	155	4	11	4.2	3.5	1.5
714	Milk, with rice cereal-------	1 oz-----------	28	2	140	2	7	4.4	2.5	0.2
715	Semisweet, small pieces (60 per oz)---------------------	1 cup or 6 oz---	170	1	860	7	61	36.2	19.9	1.9
716	Sweet (dark)--------------	1 oz-----------	28	1	150	1	10	5.9	3.3	0.3
717	Fondant, uncoated (mints, candy corn, other)-----------	1 oz-----------	28	3	105	Tr	0	0.0	0.0	0.0
718	Fudge, chocolate, plain--------	1 oz-----------	28	8	115	1	3	2.1	1.0	0.1
719	Gum drops-----------------	1 oz-----------	28	12	100	Tr	Tr	Tr	Tr	0.1

[55] Made with enriched flour, margarine, and whole milk.

| | | | | | | | Nutrients in Indicated Quantity | | | | | | | |

Cho-les-terol	Carbo-hydrate	Calcium	Phos-phorus	Iron	Potas-sium	Sodium	Vitamin A value		Thiamin	Ribo-flavin	Niacin	Ascorbic acid	Item No
							(IU)	(RE)					
Milli-grams	Grams	Milli-grams	Milli-grams	Milli-grams	Milli-grams	Milli-grams	Inter-national units	Retinol equiva-lents	Milli-grams	Milli-grams	Milli-grams	Milli-grams	
3	23	81	132	2.0	402	951	890	89	0.09	0.03	0.6	2	681
Tr	Tr	14	31	0.4	130	782	0	0	Tr	0.05	1.9	0	682
5	9	15	46	1.1	100	952	630	63	0.07	0.06	1.1	Tr	683
7	9	17	36	0.8	55	1,106	710	71	0.05	0.06	1.4	Tr	684
7	7	17	22	0.7	101	815	660	66	0.02	0.02	1.1	Tr	685
2	12	34	59	1.9	261	1,808	920	92	0.06	0.05	1.3	3	686
10	9	34	37	0.6	88	986	560	56	0.03	0.06	0.8	Tr	687
2	9	46	49	0.5	100	1,032	0	0	0.05	0.09	0.7	1	688
2	11	34	55	0.9	313	911	2,340	234	0.05	0.04	0.9	1	689
0	27	28	125	2.0	190	988	200	20	0.11	0.07	1.2	2	690
0	17	12	34	1.8	264	871	690	69	0.09	0.05	1.4	66	691
5	10	17	41	1.1	173	956	1,890	189	0.04	0.05	1.0	2	692
0	12	22	34	1.1	210	822	3,010	301	0.05	0.05	0.9	1	693
1	1	4	19	0.1	27	1,019	Tr	Tr	Tr	0.01	0.3	0	694
Tr	4	10	23	0.1	47	627	Tr	Tr	0.02	0.04	0.4	Tr	695
2	6	24	24	0.4	23	957	50	5	0.05	0.04	0.7	Tr	696
0	4	9	22	0.1	48	635	Tr	Tr	0.02	0.04	0.4	Tr	697
0	8	6	23	0.5	78	856	140	14	0.04	0.03	0.6	5	698
53	23	569	438	0.3	552	1,565	390	117	0.15	0.56	0.3	2	699
52	14	124	127	0.9	124	1,564	730	220	0.05	0.18	0.1	Tr	700
34	21	425	256	0.3	444	797	310	92	0.08	0.45	0.5	3	701
32	24	292	238	0.9	381	888	1,190	340	0.15	0.43	0.8	2	702
0	2	3	3	0.1	28	130	140	14	Tr	Tr	0.1	1	703
0	2	3	38	0.5	64	1,029	0	0	0.01	0.02	0.6	0	704
7	11	14	70	1.6	189	117	0	0	0.07	0.08	1.5	0	705
5	13	48	69	1.1	259	1,373	880	264	0.04	0.10	1.1	0	706
0	13	17	36	1.6	252	1,357	0	0	0.08	0.15	1.6	0	707
2	14	66	47	0.2	61	1,147	0	0	0.04	0.09	0.9	0	708
3	14	39	47	0.3	62	1,134	0	0	0.05	0.15	0.8	3	709
1	22	42	35	0.4	54	64	Tr	Tr	0.01	0.05	0.1	Tr	710
6	16	50	61	0.4	96	23	30	10	0.02	0.10	0.1	Tr	711
5	15	65	77	0.5	125	23	30	8	0.02	0.12	0.2	Tr	712
5	13	49	83	0.4	138	19	30	8	0.07	0.07	1.4	Tr	713
6	18	48	57	0.2	100	46	30	8	0.01	0.08	0.1	Tr	714
0	97	51	178	5.8	593	24	30	3	0.10	0.14	0.9	Tr	715
0	16	7	41	0.6	86	5	10	1	0.01	0.04	0.1	Tr	716
0	27	2	Tr	0.1	1	57	0	0	Tr	Tr	Tr	0	717
1	21	22	24	0.3	42	54	Tr	Tr	0.01	0.03	0.1	Tr	718
0	25	2	Tr	0.1	1	10	0	0	0.00	Tr	Tr	0	719

(Tr indicates nutrient present in trace amount.)

Item No.	Foods, approximate measures, units, and weight (weight of edible portion only)			Water	Food energy	Pro- tein	Fat	Fatty acids		
								Satu- rated	Mono- unsatu- rated	Poly- unsatu- rated
			Grams	Per- cent	Cal- ories	Grams	Grams	Grams	Grams	Grams
	Sugars and Sweets—Con.									
	Candy:									
720	Hard------------------------	1 oz------------	28	1	110	0	0	0.0	0.0	0.0
721	Jelly beans--------------------	1 oz------------	28	6	105	Tr	Tr	Tr	Tr	0.1
722	Marshmallows------------------	1 oz------------	28	17	90	1	0	0.0	0.0	0.0
723	Custard, baked------------------	1 cup-----------	265	77	305	14	15	6.8	5.4	0.7
724	Gelatin dessert prepared with gelatin dessert powder and water------------------------	1/2 cup---------	120	84	70	2	0	0.0	0.0	0.0
725	Honey, strained or extracted-----	1 cup-----------	339	17	1,030	1	0	0.0	0.0	0.0
726		1 tbsp----------	21	17	65	Tr	0	0.0	0.0	0.0
727	Jams and preserves--------------	1 tbsp----------	20	29	55	Tr	Tr	0.0	Tr	Tr
728		1 packet--------	14	29	40	Tr	Tr	0.0	Tr	Tr
729	Jellies------------------------	1 tbsp----------	18	28	50	Tr	Tr	Tr	Tr	Tr
730		1 packet--------	14	28	40	Tr	Tr	Tr	Tr	Tr
731	Popsicle, 3-fl-oz size-----------	1 popsicle------	95	80	70	0	0	0.0	0.0	0.0
	Puddings:									
	Canned:									
732	Chocolate--------------------	5-oz can--------	142	68	205	3	11	9.5	0.5	0.1
733	Tapioca----------------------	5-oz can--------	142	74	160	3	5	4.8	Tr	Tr
734	Vanilla----------------------	5-oz can--------	142	69	220	2	10	9.5	0.2	0.1
	Dry mix, prepared with whole milk:									
	Chocolate:									
735	Instant--------------------	1/2 cup---------	130	71	155	4	4	2.3	1.1	0.2
736	Regular (cooked)-----------	1/2 cup---------	130	73	150	4	4	2.4	1.1	0.1
737	Rice-------------------------	1/2 cup---------	132	73	155	4	4	2.3	1.1	0.1
738	Tapioca----------------------	1/2 cup---------	130	75	145	4	4	2.3	1.1	0.1
	Vanilla:									
739	Instant--------------------	1/2 cup---------	130	73	150	4	4	2.2	1.1	0.2
740	Regular (cooked)-----------	1/2 cup---------	130	74	145	4	4	2.3	1.0	0.1
	Sugars:									
741	Brown, pressed down------------	1 cup-----------	220	2	820	0	0	0.0	0.0	0.0
	White:									
742	Granulated-------------------	1 cup-----------	200	1	770	0	0	0.0	0.0	0.0
743		1 tbsp----------	12	1	45	0	0	0.0	0.0	0.0
744		1 packet--------	6	1	25	0	0	0.0	0.0	0.0
745	Powdered, sifted, spooned into cup------------------	1 cup-----------	100	1	385	0	0	0.0	0.0	0.0
	Syrups:									
	Chocolate-flavored syrup or topping:									
746	Thin type--------------------	2 tbsp----------	38	37	85	1	Tr	0.2	0.1	0.1
747	Fudge type-------------------	2 tbsp----------	38	25	125	2	5	3.1	1.7	0.2
748	Molasses, cane, blackstrap-----	2 tbsp----------	40	24	85	0	0	0.0	0.0	0.0
749	Table syrup (corn and maple)---	2 tbsp----------	42	25	122	0	0	0.0	0.0	0.0
	Vegetables and Vegetable Products									
750	Alfalfa seeds, sprouted, raw-----	1 cup-----------	33	91	10	1	Tr	Tr	Tr	0.1
751	Artichokes, globe or French, cooked, drained----------------	1 artichoke-----	120	87	55	3	Tr	Tr	Tr	0.1
	Asparagus, green:									
	Cooked, drained:									
	From raw:									
752	Cuts and tips-------------	1 cup-----------	180	92	45	5	1	0.1	Tr	0.2
753	Spears, 1/2-in diam. at base-------------------	4 spears--------	60	92	15	2	Tr	Tr	Tr	0.1
	From frozen:									
754	Cuts and tips-------------	1 cup-----------	180	91	50	5	1	0.2	Tr	0.3
755	Spears, 1/2-in diam. at base--------------------	4 spears--------	60	91	15	2	Tr	0.1	Tr	0.1
756	Canned, spears, 1/2-in diam. at base--------------------	4 spears--------	80	95	10	1	Tr	Tr	Tr	0.1
757	Bamboo shoots, canned, drained---	1 cup-----------	131	94	25	2	1	0.1	Tr	0.2

[56] For regular pack; special dietary pack contains 3 mg sodium.

Nutrients in Indicated Quantity

Cholesterol	Carbohydrate	Calcium	Phosphorus	Iron	Potassium	Sodium	Vitamin A value (IU)	(RE)	Thiamin	Riboflavin	Niacin	Ascorbic acid	Item No.
Milligrams	Grams	Milligrams	Milligrams	Milligrams	Milligrams	Milligrams	International units	Retinol equivalents	Milligrams	Milligrams	Milligrams	Milligrams	
0	28	Tr	2	0.1	1	7	0	0	0.10	0.00	0.0	0	720
0	26	1	1	0.3	11	7	0	0	0.00	Tr	Tr	0	721
0	23	1	2	0.5	2	25	0	0	0.00	Tr	Tr	0	722
278	29	297	310	1.1	387	209	530	146	0.11	0.50	0.3	1	723
0	17	2	23	Tr	Tr	55	0	0	0.00	0.00	0.0	0	724
0	279	17	20	1.7	173	17	0	0	0.02	0.14	1.0	3	725
0	17	1	1	0.1	11	1	0	0	Tr	0.01	0.1	Tr	726
0	14	4	2	0.2	18	2	Tr	Tr	Tr	0.01	Tr	Tr	727
0	10	3	1	0.1	12	2	Tr	Tr	Tr	Tr	Tr	Tr	728
0	13	2	Tr	0.1	16	5	Tr	Tr	Tr	0.01	Tr	1	729
0	10	1	Tr	Tr	13	4	Tr	Tr	Tr	Tr	Tr	1	730
0	18	0	0	Tr	4	11	0	0	0.00	0.00	0.0	0	731
1	30	74	117	1.2	254	285	100	31	0.04	0.17	0.6	Tr	732
Tr	28	119	113	0.3	212	252	Tr	Tr	0.03	0.14	0.4	Tr	733
1	33	79	94	0.2	155	305	Tr	Tr	0.03	0.12	0.6	Tr	734
14	27	130	329	0.3	176	440	130	33	0.04	0.18	0.1	1	735
15	25	146	120	0.2	190	167	140	34	0.05	0.20	0.1	1	736
15	27	133	110	0.5	165	140	140	33	0.10	0.18	0.6	1	737
15	25	131	103	0.1	167	152	140	34	0.04	0.18	0.1	1	738
15	27	129	273	0.1	164	375	140	33	0.04	0.17	0.1	1	739
15	25	132	102	0.1	166	178	140	34	0.04	0.18	0.1	1	740
0	212	187	56	4.8	757	97	0	0	0.02	0.07	0.2	0	741
0	199	3	Tr	0.1	7	5	0	0	0.00	0.00	0.0	0	742
0	12	Tr	Tr	Tr	Tr	Tr	0	0	0.00	0.00	0.0	0	743
0	6	Tr	Tr	Tr	Tr	Tr	0	0	0.00	0.00	0.0	0	744
0	100	1	Tr	Tr	4	2	0	0	0.00	0.00	0.0	0	745
0	22	6	49	0.8	85	36	Tr	Tr	Tr	0.02	0.1	0	746
0	21	38	60	0.5	82	42	40	13	0.02	0.08	0.1	0	747
0	22	274	34	10.1	1,171	38	0	0	0.04	0.08	0.8	0	748
0	32	1	4	Tr	7	19	0	0	0.00	0.00	0.0	0	749
0	1	11	23	0.3	26	2	50	5	0.03	0.04	0.2	3	750
0	12	47	72	1.6	316	79	170	17	0.07	0.06	0.7	9	751
0	8	43	110	1.2	558	7	1,490	149	0.18	0.22	1.9	49	752
0	3	14	37	0.4	186	2	500	50	0.06	0.07	0.6	16	753
0	9	41	99	1.2	392	7	1,470	147	0.12	0.19	1.9	44	754
0	3	14	33	0.4	131	2	490	49	0.04	0.06	0.6	15	755
0	2	11	30	0.5	122	[56]278	380	38	0.04	0.07	0.7	13	756
0	4	10	33	0.4	105	9	10	1	0.03	0.03	0.2	1	757

(Tr indicates nutrient present in trace amount.)

Item No.	Foods, approximate measures, units, and weight (weight of edible portion only)			Water	Food energy	Pro-tein	Fat	Fatty acids		
								Satu-rated	Mono-unsatu-rated	Poly-unsatu-rated
	Vegetables and Vegetable Products—Con.		Grams	Per-cent	Cal-ories	Grams	Grams	Grams	Grams	Grams
	Beans:									
	Lima, immature seeds, frozen, cooked, drained:									
758	Thick-seeded types (Ford-hooks)------------------	1 cup-----------	170	74	170	10	1	0.1	Tr	0.3
759	Thin-seeded types (baby limas)-------------------	1 cup-----------	180	72	190	12	1	0.1	Tr	0.3
	Snap:									
	Cooked, drained:									
760	From raw (cut and French style)------------------	1 cup-----------	125	89	45	2	Tr	0.1	Tr	0.2
761	From frozen (cut)----------	1 cup-----------	135	92	35	2	Tr	Tr	Tr	0.1
762	Canned, drained solids (cut)	1 cup-----------	135	93	25	2	Tr	Tr	Tr	0.1
	Beans, mature. See Beans, dry (items 527-535) and Black-eyed peas, dry (item 536).									
	Bean sprouts (mung):									
763	Raw-----------------------	1 cup-----------	104	90	30	3	Tr	Tr	Tr	0.1
764	Cooked, drained------------	1 cup-----------	124	93	25	3	Tr	Tr	Tr	Tr
	Beets:									
	Cooked, drained:									
765	Diced or sliced------------	1 cup-----------	170	91	55	2	Tr	Tr	Tr	Tr
766	Whole beets, 2-in diam.------	2 beets---------	100	91	30	1	Tr	Tr	Tr	Tr
767	Canned, drained solids, diced or sliced------------------	1 cup-----------	170	91	55	2	Tr	Tr	Tr	0.1
768	Beet greens, leaves and stems, cooked, drained-------------	1 cup-----------	144	89	40	4	Tr	Tr	0.1	0.1
	Black-eyed peas, immature seeds, cooked and drained:									
769	From raw-----------------	1 cup-----------	165	72	180	13	1	0.3	0.1	0.6
770	From frozen--------------	1 cup-----------	170	66	225	14	1	0.3	0.1	0.5
	Broccoli:									
771	Raw-----------------------	1 spear---------	151	91	40	4	1	0.1	Tr	0.3
	Cooked, drained:									
	From raw:									
772	Spear, medium--------------	1 spear---------	180	90	50	5	1	0.1	Tr	0.2
773	Spears, cut into 1/2-in pieces-------------------	1 cup-----------	155	90	45	5	Tr	0.1	Tr	0.2
	From frozen:									
774	Piece, 4-1/2 to 5 in long--	1 piece---------	30	91	10	1	Tr	Tr	Tr	Tr
775	Chopped-------------------	1 cup-----------	185	91	50	6	Tr	Tr	Tr	0.1
	Brussels sprouts, cooked, drained:									
776	From raw, 7-8 sprouts, 1-1/4 to 1-1/2-in diam.-----------	1 cup-----------	155	87	60	4	1	0.2	0.1	0.4
777	From frozen--------------	1 cup-----------	155	87	65	6	1	0.1	Tr	0.3
	Cabbage, common varieties:									
778	Raw, coarsely shredded or sliced--------------------	1 cup-----------	70	93	15	1	Tr	Tr	Tr	0.1
779	Cooked, drained------------	1 cup-----------	150	94	30	1	Tr	Tr	Tr	0.2
	Cabbage, Chinese:									
780	Pak-choi, cooked, drained------	1 cup-----------	170	96	20	3	Tr	Tr	Tr	0.1
781	Pe-tsai, raw, 1-in pieces------	1 cup-----------	76	94	10	1	Tr	Tr	Tr	0.1
782	Cabbage, red, raw, coarsely shredded or sliced------------	1 cup-----------	70	92	20	1	Tr	Tr	Tr	0.1
783	Cabbage, savoy, raw, coarsely shredded or sliced------------	1 cup-----------	70	91	20	1	Tr	Tr	Tr	Tr

[57] For green varieties; yellow varieties contain 101 IU or 10 RE.
[58] For green varieties; yellow varieties contain 151 IU or 15 RE.
[59] For regular pack; special dietary pack contains 3 mg sodium.

Nutrients in Indicated Quantity

Cho-les-terol	Carbo-hydrate	Calcium	Phos-phorus	Iron	Potas-sium	Sodium	Vitamin A value		Thiamin	Ribo-flavin	Niacin	Ascorbic acid	Item No.
							(IU)	(RE)					
Milli-grams	Grams	Milli-grams	Milli-grams	Milli-grams	Milli-grams	Milli-grams	Inter-national units	Retinol equiva-lents	Milli-grams	Milli-grams	Milli-grams	Milli-grams	
0	32	37	107	2.3	694	90	320	32	0.13	0.10	1.8	22	758
0	35	50	202	3.5	740	52	300	30	0.13	0.10	1.4	10	759
0	10	58	49	1.6	374	4	[57]830	[57]83	0.09	0.12	0.8	12	760
0	8	61	32	1.1	151	18	[58]710	[58]71	0.06	0.10	0.6	11	761
0	6	35	26	1.2	147	[59]339	[60]470	[60]47	0.02	0.08	0.3	6	762
0	6	14	56	0.9	155	6	20	2	0.09	0.13	0.8	14	763
0	5	15	35	0.8	125	12	20	2	0.06	0.13	1.0	14	764
0	11	19	53	1.1	530	83	20	2	0.05	0.02	0.5	9	765
0	7	11	31	0.6	312	49	10	1	0.03	0.01	0.3	6	766
0	12	26	29	3.1	252	[61]466	20	2	0.02	0.07	0.3	7	767
0	8	164	59	2.7	1,309	347	7,340	734	0.17	0.42	0.7	36	768
0	30	46	196	2.4	693	7	1,050	105	0.11	0.18	1.8	3	769
0	40	39	207	3.6	638	9	130	13	0.44	0.11	1.2	4	770
0	8	72	100	1.3	491	41	2,330	233	0.10	0.18	1.0	141	771
0	10	205	86	2.1	293	20	2,540	254	0.15	0.37	1.4	113	772
0	9	177	74	1.8	253	17	2,180	218	0.13	0.32	1.2	97	773
0	2	15	17	0.2	54	7	570	57	0.02	0.02	0.1	12	774
0	10	94	102	1.1	333	44	3,500	350	0.10	0.15	0.8	74	775
0	13	56	87	1.9	491	33	1,110	111	0.17	0.12	0.9	96	776
0	13	37	84	1.1	504	36	910	91	0.16	0.18	0.8	71	777
0	4	33	16	0.4	172	13	90	9	0.04	0.02	0.2	33	778
0	7	50	38	0.6	308	29	130	13	0.09	0.08	0.3	36	779
0	3	158	49	1.8	631	58	4,370	437	0.05	0.11	0.7	44	780
0	2	59	22	0.2	181	7	910	91	0.03	0.04	0.3	21	781
0	4	36	29	0.3	144	8	30	3	0.04	0.02	0.2	40	782
0	4	25	29	0.3	161	20	700	70	0.05	0.02	0.2	22	783

[60] For green varieties; yellow varieties contain 142 IU or 14 RE.
[61] For regular pack; special dietary pack contains 78 mg sodium.

(Tr indicates nutrient present in trace amount.)

Item No.	Foods, approximate measures, units, and weight (weight of edible portion only)			Water	Food energy	Pro-tein	Fat	Fatty acids		
								Satu-rated	Mono-unsatu-rated	Poly-unsatu-rated
			Grams	Per-cent	Cal-ories	Grams	Grams	Grams	Grams	Grams
	Vegetables and Vegetable Products—Con.									
	Carrots:									
	Raw, without crowns and tips, scraped:									
784	Whole, 7-1/2 by 1-1/8 in, or strips, 2-1/2 to 3 in long	1 carrot or 18 strips--------	72	88	30	1	Tr	Tr	Tr	0.1
785	Grated-----------------------	1 cup-----------	110	88	45	1	Tr	Tr	Tr	0.1
	Cooked, sliced, drained:									
786	From raw---------------------	1 cup-----------	156	87	70	2	Tr	0.1	Tr	0.1
787	From frozen------------------	1 cup-----------	146	90	55	2	Tr	Tr	Tr	0.1
788	Canned, sliced, drained solids	1 cup-----------	146	93	35	1	Tr	0.1	Tr	0.1
	Cauliflower:									
789	Raw, (flowerets)--------------	1 cup-----------	100	92	25	2	Tr	Tr	Tr	0.1
	Cooked, drained:									
790	From raw (flowerets)---------	1 cup-----------	125	93	30	2	Tr	Tr	Tr	0.1
791	From frozen (flowerets)------	1 cup-----------	180	94	35	3	Tr	0.1	Tr	0.2
	Celery, pascal type, raw:									
792	Stalk, large outer, 8 by 1-1/2 in (at root end)-------------	1 stalk---------	40	95	5	Tr	Tr	Tr	Tr	Tr
793	Pieces, diced-----------------	1 cup-----------	120	95	20	1	Tr	Tr	Tr	0.1
	Collards, cooked, drained:									
794	From raw (leaves without stems)	1 cup-----------	190	96	25	2	Tr	0.1	Tr	0.2
795	From frozen (chopped)----------	1 cup-----------	170	88	60	5	1	0.1	0.1	0.4
	Corn, sweet:									
	Cooked, drained:									
796	From raw, ear 5 by 1-3/4 in--	1 ear-----------	77	70	85	3	1	0.2	0.3	0.5
	From frozen:									
797	Ear, trimmed to about 3-1/2 in long-----------------	1 ear-----------	63	73	60	2	Tr	0.1	0.1	0.2
798	Kernels---------------------	1 cup-----------	165	76	135	5	Tr	Tr	Tr	0.1
	Canned:									
799	Cream style------------------	1 cup-----------	256	79	185	4	1	0.2	0.3	0.5
800	Whole kernel, vacuum pack----	1 cup-----------	210	77	165	5	1	0.2	0.3	0.5
	Cowpeas. See Black-eyed peas, immature (items 769,770), mature (item 536).									
801	Cucumber, with peel, slices, 1/8 in thick (large, 2-1/8-in diam.; small, 1-3/4-in diam.)--	6 large or 8 small slices	28	96	5	Tr	Tr	Tr	Tr	Tr
802	Dandelion greens, cooked, drained	1 cup-----------	105	90	35	2	1	0.1	Tr	0.3
803	Eggplant, cooked, steamed--------	1 cup-----------	96	92	25	1	Tr	Tr	Tr	0.1
804	Endive, curly (including esca-role), raw, small pieces-------	1 cup-----------	50	94	10	1	Tr	Tr	Tr	Tr
805	Jerusalem-artichoke, raw, sliced	1 cup-----------	150	78	115	3	Tr	0.0	Tr	Tr
	Kale, cooked, drained:									
806	From raw, chopped-------------	1 cup-----------	130	91	40	2	1	0.1	Tr	0.3
807	From frozen, chopped----------	1 cup-----------	130	91	40	4	1	0.1	Tr	0.3
808	Kohlrabi, thickened bulb-like stems, cooked, drained, diced--	1 cup-----------	165	90	50	3	Tr	Tr	Tr	0.1
	Lettuce, raw:									
	Butterhead, as Boston types:									
809	Head, 5-in diam--------------	1 head----------	163	96	20	2	Tr	Tr	Tr	0.2
810	Leaves-----------------------	1 outer or 2 inner leaves--	15	96	Tr	Tr	Tr	Tr	Tr	Tr
	Crisphead, as iceberg:									
811	Head, 6-in diam--------------	1 head----------	539	96	70	5	1	0.1	Tr	0.5
812	Wedge, 1/4 of head-----------	1 wedge---------	135	96	20	1	Tr	Tr	Tr	0.1
813	Pieces, chopped or shredded--	1 cup-----------	55	96	5	1	Tr	Tr	Tr	0.1
814	Looseleaf (bunching varieties including romaine or cos), chopped or shredded pieces---	1 cup-----------	56	94	10	1	Tr	Tr	Tr	0.1

[62]For regular pack; special dietary pack contains 61 mg sodium.
[63]For yellow varieties; white varieties contain only a trace of vitamin A.

							Vitamin A value						
Cho-les-terol	Carbo-hydrate	Calcium	Phos-phorus	Iron	Potas-sium	Sodium	(IU)	(RE)	Thiamin	Ribo-flavin	Niacin	Ascorbic acid	Item No.
Milli-grams	Grams	Milli-grams	Milli-grams	Milli-grams	Milli-grams	Milli-grams	Inter-national units	Retinol equiva-lents	Milli-grams	Milli-grams	Milli-grams	Milli-grams	
0	7	19	32	0.4	233	25	20,250	2,025	0.07	0.04	0.7	7	784
0	11	30	48	0.6	355	39	30,940	3,094	0.11	0.06	1.0	10	785
0	16	48	47	1.0	354	103	38,300	3,830	0.05	0.09	0.8	4	786
0	12	41	38	0.7	231	86	25,850	2,585	0.04	0.05	0.6	4	787
0	8	37	35	0.9	261	[62]352	20,110	2,011	0.03	0.04	0.8	4	788
0	5	29	46	0.6	355	15	20	2	0.08	0.06	0.6	72	789
0	6	34	44	0.5	404	8	20	2	0.08	0.07	0.7	69	790
0	7	31	43	0.7	250	32	40	4	0.07	0.10	0.6	56	791
0	1	14	10	0.2	114	35	50	5	0.01	0.01	0.1	3	792
0	4	43	31	0.6	341	106	150	15	0.04	0.04	0.4	8	793
0	5	148	19	0.8	177	36	4,220	422	0.03	0.08	0.4	19	794
0	12	357	46	1.9	427	85	10,170	1,017	0.08	0.20	1.1	45	795
0	19	2	79	0.5	192	13	[63]170	[63]17	0.17	0.06	1.2	5	796
0	14	2	47	0.4	158	3	[63]130	[63]13	0.11	0.04	1.0	3	797
0	34	3	78	0.5	229	8	[63]410	[63]41	0.11	0.12	2.1	4	798
0	46	8	131	1.0	343	[64]730	[63]250	[63]25	0.06	0.14	2.5	12	799
0	41	11	134	0.9	391	[65]671	[63]510	[63]51	0.09	0.15	2.5	17	800
0	1	4	5	0.1	42	1	10	1	0.01	0.01	0.1	1	801
0	7	147	44	1.9	244	46	12,290	1,229	0.14	0.18	0.5	19	802
0	6	6	21	0.3	238	3	60	6	0.07	0.02	0.6	1	803
0	2	26	14	0.4	157	11	1,030	103	0.04	0.04	0.2	3	804
0	26	21	117	5.1	644	6	30	3	0.30	0.09	2.0	6	805
0	7	94	36	1.2	296	30	9,620	962	0.07	0.09	0.7	53	806
0	7	179	36	1.2	417	20	8,260	826	0.06	0.15	0.9	33	807
0	11	41	74	0.7	561	35	60	6	0.07	0.03	0.6	89	808
0	4	52	38	0.5	419	8	1,580	158	0.10	0.10	0.5	13	809
0	Tr	5	3	Tr	39	1	150	15	0.01	0.01	Tr	1	810
0	11	102	108	2.7	852	49	1,780	178	0.25	0.16	1.0	21	811
0	3	26	27	0.7	213	12	450	45	0.06	0.04	0.3	5	812
0	1	10	11	0.3	87	5	180	18	0.03	0.02	0.1	2	813
0	2	38	14	0.8	148	5	1,060	106	0.03	0.04	0.2	10	814

[64] For regular pack; special dietary pack contains 8 mg sodium.
[65] For regular pack; special dietary pack contains 6 mg sodium.

(Tr indicates nutrient present in trace amount.)

Item No.	Foods, approximate measures, units, and weight (weight of edible portion only)		Water	Food energy	Pro-tein	Fat	Fatty acids		
							Satu-rated	Mono-unsatu-rated	Poly-unsatu-rated
		Grams	Per-cent	Cal-ories	Grams	Grams	Grams	Grams	Grams

Vegetables and Vegetable Products—Con.

	Mushrooms:								
815	Raw, sliced or chopped--------	1 cup-----------	70	92	20	1	Tr	Tr	Tr	0.1
816	Cooked, drained----------------	1 cup-----------	156	91	40	3	1	0.1	Tr	0.3
817	Canned, drained solids---------	1 cup-----------	156	91	35	3	Tr	0.1	Tr	0.2
818	Mustard greens, without stems and midribs, cooked, drained-------	1 cup-----------	140	94	20	3	Tr	Tr	0.2	0.1
819	Okra pods, 3 by 5/8 in, cooked---	8 pods----------	85	90	25	2	Tr	Tr	Tr	Tr
	Onions:								
	Raw:								
820	Chopped----------------------	1 cup-----------	160	91	55	2	Tr	0.1	0.1	0.2
821	Sliced-----------------------	1 cup-----------	115	91	40	1	Tr	0.1	Tr	0.1
822	Cooked (whole or sliced), drained----------------------	1 cup-----------	210	92	60	2	Tr	0.1	Tr	0.1
823	Onions, spring, raw, bulb (3/8-in diam.) and white portion of top	6 onions--------	30	92	10	1	Tr	Tr	Tr	Tr
824	Onion rings, breaded, par-fried, frozen, prepared--------------	2 rings---------	20	29	80	1	5	1.7	2.2	1.0
	Parsley:								
825	Raw--------------------------	10 sprigs-------	10	88	5	Tr	Tr	Tr	Tr	Tr
826	Freeze-dried------------------	1 tbsp----------	0.4	2	Tr	Tr	Tr	Tr	Tr	Tr
827	Parsnips, cooked (diced or 2 in lengths), drained--------------	1 cup-----------	156	78	125	2	Tr	0.1	0.2	0.1
828	Peas, edible pod, cooked, drained	1 cup-----------	160	89	65	5	Tr	0.1	Tr	0.2
	Peas, green:								
829	Canned, drained solids---------	1 cup-----------	170	82	115	8	1	0.1	0.1	0.3
830	Frozen, cooked, drained--------	1 cup-----------	160	80	125	8	Tr	0.1	Tr	0.2
	Peppers:								
831	Hot chili, raw----------------	1 pepper--------	45	88	20	1	Tr	Tr	Tr	Tr
	Sweet (about 5 per lb, whole), stem and seeds removed:								
832	Raw--------------------------	1 pepper--------	74	93	20	1	Tr	Tr	Tr	0.2
833	Cooked, drained--------------	1 pepper--------	73	95	15	Tr	Tr	Tr	Tr	0.1
	Potatoes, cooked:								
	Baked (about 2 per lb, raw):								
834	With skin--------------------	1 potato--------	202	71	220	5	Tr	0.1	Tr	0.1
835	Flesh only-------------------	1 potato--------	156	75	145	3	Tr	Tr	Tr	0.1
	Boiled (about 3 per lb, raw):								
836	Peeled after boiling---------	1 potato--------	136	77	120	3	Tr	Tr	Tr	0.1
837	Peeled before boiling--------	1 potato--------	135	77	115	2	Tr	Tr	Tr	0.1
	French fried, strip, 2 to 3-1/2 in long, frozen:								
838	Oven heated------------------	10 strips-------	50	53	110	2	4	2.1	1.8	0.3
839	Fried in vegetable oil-------	10 strips-------	50	38	160	2	8	2.5	1.6	3.8
	Potato products, prepared:								
	Au gratin:								
840	From dry mix-----------------	1 cup-----------	245	79	230	6	10	6.3	2.9	0.3
841	From home recipe-------------	1 cup-----------	245	74	325	12	19	11.6	5.3	0.7
842	Hashed brown, from frozen------	1 cup-----------	156	56	340	5	18	7.0	8.0	2.1
	Mashed:								
	From home recipe:								
843	Milk added---------------	1 cup-----------	210	78	160	4	1	0.7	0.3	0.1
844	Milk and margarine added---	1 cup-----------	210	76	225	4	9	2.2	3.7	2.5
845	From dehydrated flakes (without milk), water, milk, butter, and salt added---------------------	1 cup-----------	210	76	235	4	12	7.2	3.3	0.5
846	Potato salad, made with mayonnaise--------------------	1 cup-----------	250	76	360	7	21	3.6	6.2	9.3
	Scalloped:								
847	From dry mix-----------------	1 cup-----------	245	79	230	5	11	6.5	3.0	0.5
848	From home recipe-------------	1 cup-----------	245	81	210	7	9	5.5	2.5	0.4

[66] For regular pack; special dietary pack contains 3 mg sodium.
[67] For red peppers; green peppers contain 350 IU or 35 RE.
[68] For green peppers; red peppers contain 4,220 IU or 422 RE.

Nutrients in Indicated Quantity

Cho-les-terol	Carbo-hydrate	Calcium	Phos-phorus	Iron	Potas-sium	Sodium	Vitamin A value		Thiamin	Ribo-flavin	Niacin	Ascorbic acid	Item No.
							(IU)	(RE)					
Milli-grams	Grams	Milli-grams	Milli-grams	Milli-grams	Milli-grams	Milli-grams	Inter-national units	Retinol equiva-lents	Milli-grams	Milli-grams	Milli-grams	Milli-grams	
0	3	4	73	0.9	259	3	0	0	0.07	0.31	2.9	2	815
0	8	9	136	2.7	555	3	0	0	0.11	0.47	7.0	6	816
0	8	17	103	1.2	201	663	0	0	0.13	0.03	2.5	0	817
0	3	104	57	1.0	283	22	4,240	424	0.06	0.09	0.6	35	818
0	6	54	48	0.4	274	4	490	49	0.11	0.05	0.7	14	819
0	12	40	46	0.6	248	3	0	0	0.10	0.02	0.2	13	820
0	8	29	33	0.4	178	2	0	0	0.07	0.01	0.1	10	821
0	13	57	48	0.4	319	17	0	0	0.09	0.02	0.2	12	822
0	2	18	10	0.6	77	1	1,500	150	0.02	0.04	0.1	14	823
0	8	6	16	0.3	26	75	50	5	0.06	0.03	0.7	Tr	824
0	1	13	4	0.6	54	4	520	52	0.01	0.01	0.1	9	825
0	Tr	1	2	0.2	25	2	250	25	Tr	0.01	Tr	1	826
0	30	58	108	0.9	573	16	0	0	0.13	0.08	1.1	20	827
0	11	67	88	3.2	384	6	210	21	0.20	0.12	0.9	77	828
0	21	34	114	1.6	294	[66]372	1,310	131	0.21	0.13	1.2	16	829
0	23	38	144	2.5	269	139	1,070	107	0.45	0.16	2.4	16	830
0	4	8	21	0.5	153	3	[67]4,840	[67]484	0.04	0.04	0.4	109	831
0	4	4	16	0.9	144	2	[68]390	[68]39	0.06	0.04	0.4	[69]95	832
0	3	3	11	0.6	94	1	[70]280	[70]28	0.04	0.03	0.3	[71]81	833
0	51	20	115	2.7	844	16	0	0	0.22	0.07	3.3	26	834
0	34	8	78	0.5	610	8	0	0	0.16	0.03	2.2	20	835
0	27	7	60	0.4	515	5	0	0	0.14	0.03	2.0	18	836
0	27	11	54	0.4	443	7	0	0	0.13	0.03	1.8	10	837
0	17	5	43	0.7	229	16	0	0	0.06	0.02	1.2	5	838
0	20	10	47	0.4	366	108	0	0	0.09	0.01	1.6	5	839
12	31	203	233	0.8	537	1,076	520	76	0.05	0.20	2.3	8	840
56	28	292	277	1.6	970	1,061	650	93	0.16	0.28	2.4	24	841
0	44	23	112	2.4	680	53	0	0	0.17	0.03	3.8	10	842
4	37	55	101	0.6	628	636	40	12	0.18	0.08	2.3	14	843
4	35	55	97	0.5	607	620	360	42	0.18	0.08	2.3	13	844
29	32	103	118	0.5	489	697	380	44	0.23	0.11	1.4	20	845
170	28	48	130	1.6	635	1,323	520	83	0.19	0.15	2.2	25	846
27	31	88	137	0.9	497	835	360	51	0.05	0.14	2.5	8	847
29	26	140	154	1.4	926	821	330	47	0.17	0.23	2.6	26	848

[69]For green peppers; red peppers contain 141 mg ascorbic acid.
[70]For green peppers; red peppers contain 2,740 IU or 274 RE.
[71]For green peppers; red peppers contain 121 mg ascorbic acid.

(Tr indicates nutrient present in trace amount.)

Item No.	Foods, approximate measures, units, and weight (weight of edible portion only)		Grams	Water Per-cent	Food energy Cal-ories	Pro-tein Grams	Fat Grams	Fatty acids		
								Satu-rated Grams	Mono-unsatu-rated Grams	Poly-unsatu-rated Grams
	Vegetables and Vegetable Products—Con.									
849	Potato chips-------------------	10 chips--------	20	3	105	1	7	1.8	1.2	3.6
	Pumpkin:									
850	Cooked from raw, mashed--------	1 cup-----------	245	94	50	2	Tr	0.1	Tr	Tr
851	Canned-------------------------	1 cup-----------	245	90	85	3	1	0.4	0.1	Tr
852	Radishes, raw, stem ends, rootlets cut off--------------	4 radishes------	18	95	5	Tr	Tr	Tr	Tr	Tr
853	Sauerkraut, canned, solids and liquid-------------------------	1 cup-----------	236	93	45	2	Tr	0.1	Tr	0.1
	Seaweed:									
854	Kelp, raw----------------------	1 oz------------	28	82	10	Tr	Tr	0.1	Tr	Tr
855	Spirulina, dried---------------	1 oz------------	28	5	80	16	2	0.8	0.2	0.6
	Southern peas. See Black-eyed peas, immature (items 769,770), mature (item 536).									
	Spinach:									
856	Raw, chopped-------------------	1 cup-----------	55	92	10	2	Tr	Tr	Tr	0.1
	Cooked, drained:									
857	From raw----------------------	1 cup-----------	180	91	40	5	Tr	0.1	Tr	0.2
858	From frozen (leaf)------------	1 cup-----------	190	90	55	6	Tr	0.1	Tr	0.2
859	Canned, drained solids--------	1 cup-----------	214	92	50	6	1	0.2	Tr	0.4
860	Spinach souffle----------------	1 cup-----------	136	74	220	11	18	7.1	6.8	3.1
	Squash, cooked:									
861	Summer (all varieties), sliced, drained---------------------	1 cup-----------	180	94	35	2	1	0.1	Tr	0.2
862	Winter (all varieties), baked, cubes-----------------------	1 cup-----------	205	89	80	2	1	0.3	0.1	0.5
	Sunchoke. See Jerusalem-arti-choke (item 805).									
	Sweetpotatoes:									
	Cooked (raw, 5 by 2 in; about 2-1/2 per lb):									
863	Baked in skin, peeled--------	1 potato--------	114	73	115	2	Tr	Tr	Tr	0.1
864	Boiled, without skin---------	1 potato--------	151	73	160	2	Tr	0.1	Tr	0.2
865	Candied, 2-1/2 by 2-in piece---	1 piece---------	105	67	145	1	3	1.4	0.7	0.2
	Canned:									
866	Solid pack (mashed)----------	1 cup-----------	255	74	260	5	1	0.1	Tr	0.2
867	Vacuum pack, piece 2-3/4 by 1 in----------------------	1 piece---------	40	76	35	1	Tr	Tr	Tr	Tr
	Tomatoes:									
868	Raw, 2-3/5-in diam. (3 per 12 oz pkg.)--------------------	1 tomato--------	123	94	25	1	Tr	Tr	Tr	0.1
869	Canned, solids and liquid------	1 cup-----------	240	94	50	2	1	0.1	0.1	0.2
870	Tomato juice, canned-----------	1 cup-----------	244	94	40	2	Tr	Tr	Tr	0.1
	Tomato products, canned:									
871	Paste--------------------------	1 cup-----------	262	74	220	10	2	0.3	0.4	0.9
872	Puree--------------------------	1 cup-----------	250	87	105	4	Tr	Tr	Tr	0.1
873	Sauce--------------------------	1 cup-----------	245	89	75	3	Tr	0.1	0.1	0.2
874	Turnips, cooked, diced---------	1 cup-----------	156	94	30	1	Tr	Tr	Tr	0.1
	Turnip greens, cooked, drained:									
875	From raw (leaves and stems)----	1 cup-----------	144	93	30	2	Tr	0.1	Tr	0.1
876	From frozen (chopped)----------	1 cup-----------	164	90	50	5	1	0.2	Tr	0.3
877	Vegetable juice cocktail, canned	1 cup-----------	242	94	45	2	Tr	Tr	Tr	0.1
	Vegetables, mixed:									
878	Canned, drained solids---------	1 cup-----------	163	87	75	4	Tr	0.1	Tr	0.2
879	Frozen, cooked, drained--------	1 cup-----------	182	83	105	5	Tr	0.1	Tr	0.1
880	Waterchestnuts, canned---------	1 cup-----------	140	86	70	1	Tr	Tr	Tr	Tr

[1] Value not determined.
[72] With added salt; if none is added, sodium content is 58 mg.
[73] For regular pack; special dietary pack contains 31 mg sodium.
[74] With added salt; if none is added, sodium content is 24 mg.

							Vitamin A value						
Cho-les-terol	Carbo-hydrate	Calcium	Phos-phorus	Iron	Potas-sium	Sodium	(IU)	(RE)	Thiamin	Ribo-flavin	Niacin	Ascorbic acid	Item No.
Milli-grams	Grams	Milli-grams	Milli-grams	Milli-grams	Milli-grams	Milli-grams	Inter-national units	Retinol equiva-lents	Milli-grams	Milli-grams	Milli-grams	Milli-grams	
0	10	5	31	0.2	260	94	0	0	0.03	Tr	0.8	8	849
0	12	37	74	1.4	564	2	2,650	265	0.08	0.19	1.0	12	850
0	20	64	86	3.4	505	12	54,040	5,404	0.06	0.13	0.9	10	851
0	1	4	3	0.1	42	4	Tr	Tr	Tr	0.01	0.1	4	852
0	10	71	47	3.5	401	1,560	40	4	0.05	0.05	0.3	35	853
0	3	48	12	0.8	25	66	30	3	0.01	0.04	0.1	(1)	854
0	7	34	33	8.1	386	297	160	16	0.67	1.04	3.6	3	855
0	2	54	27	1.5	307	43	3,690	369	0.04	0.10	0.4	15	856
0	7	245	101	6.4	839	126	14,740	1,474	0.17	0.42	0.9	18	857
0	10	277	91	2.9	566	[72]163	14,790	1,479	0.11	0.32	0.8	23	858
0	7	272	94	4.9	740	[72]683	18,780	1,878	0.03	0.30	0.8	31	859
184	3	230	231	1.3	201	763	3,460	675	0.09	0.30	0.5	3	860
0	8	49	70	0.6	346	2	520	52	0.08	0.07	0.9	10	861
0	18	29	41	0.7	896	2	7,290	729	0.17	0.05	1.4	20	862
0	28	32	63	0.5	397	11	24,880	2,488	0.08	0.14	0.7	28	863
0	37	32	41	0.8	278	20	25,750	2,575	0.08	0.21	1.0	26	864
8	29	27	27	1.2	198	74	4,400	440	0.02	0.04	0.4	7	865
0	59	77	133	3.4	536	191	38,570	3,857	0.07	0.23	2.4	13	866
0	8	9	20	0.4	125	21	3,190	319	0.01	0.02	0.3	11	867
0	5	9	28	0.6	255	10	1,390	139	0.07	0.06	0.7	22	868
0	10	62	46	1.5	530	[73]391	1,450	145	0.11	0.07	1.8	36	869
0	10	22	46	1.4	537	[74]881	1,360	136	0.11	0.08	1.6	45	870
0	49	92	207	7.8	2,442	[75]170	6,470	647	0.41	0.50	8.4	111	871
0	25	38	100	2.3	1,050	[76]50	3,400	340	0.18	0.14	4.3	88	872
0	18	34	78	1.9	909	[77]1,482	2,400	240	0.16	0.14	2.8	32	873
0	8	34	30	0.3	211	78	0	0	0.04	0.04	0.5	18	874
0	6	197	42	1.2	292	42	7,920	792	0.06	0.10	0.6	39	875
0	8	249	56	3.2	367	25	13,080	1,308	0.09	0.12	0.8	36	876
0	11	27	41	1.0	467	883	2,830	283	0.10	0.07	1.8	67	877
0	15	44	68	1.7	474	243	18,990	1,899	0.08	0.08	0.9	8	878
0	24	46	93	1.5	308	64	7,780	778	0.13	0.22	1.5	6	879
0	17	6	27	1.2	165	11	10	1	0.02	0.03	0.5	2	880

[75] With no added salt; if salt is added, sodium content is 2,070 mg.
[76] With no added salt; if salt is added, sodium content is 998 mg.
[77] With salt added.

(Tr indicates nutrient present in trace amount.)

Item No.	Foods, approximate measures, units, and weight (weight of edible portion only)		Grams	Water Per-cent	Food energy Cal-ories	Pro-tein Grams	Fat Grams	Fatty acids		
								Satu-rated Grams	Mono-unsatu-rated Grams	Poly-unsatu-rated Grams
	Miscellaneous Items									
	Baking powders for home use:									
	Sodium aluminum sulfate:									
881	With monocalcium phosphate monohydrate	1 tsp	3	2	5	Tr	0	0.0	0.0	0.0
882	With monocalcium phosphate monohydrate, calcium sulfate	1 tsp	2.9	1	5	Tr	0	0.0	0.0	0.0
883	Straight phosphate	1 tsp	3.8	2	5	Tr	0	0.0	0.0	0.0
884	Low sodium	1 tsp	4.3	1	5	Tr	0	0.0	0.0	0.0
885	Catsup	1 cup	273	69	290	5	1	0.2	0.2	0.4
886		1 tbsp	15	69	15	Tr	Tr	Tr	Tr	Tr
887	Celery seed	1 tsp	2	6	10	Tr	1	Tr	0.3	0.1
888	Chili powder	1 tsp	2.6	8	10	Tr	Tr	0.1	0.1	0.2
	Chocolate:									
889	Bitter or baking	1 oz	28	2	145	3	15	9.0	4.9	0.5
	Semisweet, see Candy, (item 715).									
890	Cinnamon	1 tsp	2.3	10	5	Tr	Tr	Tr	Tr	Tr
891	Curry powder	1 tsp	2	10	5	Tr	Tr	(1)	(1)	(1)
892	Garlic powder	1 tsp	2.8	6	10	Tr	Tr	Tr	Tr	Tr
893	Gelatin, dry	1 envelope	7	13	25	6	Tr	Tr	Tr	Tr
894	Mustard, prepared, yellow	1 tsp or individual packet	5	80	5	Tr	Tr	Tr	0.2	Tr
	Olives, canned:									
895	Green	4 medium or 3 extra large	13	78	15	Tr	2	0.2	1.2	0.1
896	Ripe, Mission, pitted	3 small or 2 large	9	73	15	Tr	2	0.3	1.3	0.2
897	Onion powder	1 tsp	2.1	5	5	Tr	Tr	Tr	Tr	Tr
898	Oregano	1 tsp	1.5	7	5	Tr	Tr	Tr	Tr	0.1
899	Paprika	1 tsp	2.1	10	5	Tr	Tr	Tr	Tr	0.2
900	Pepper, black	1 tsp	2.1	11	5	Tr	Tr	Tr	Tr	Tr
	Pickles, cucumber:									
901	Dill, medium, whole, 3-3/4 in long, 1-1/4-in diam.	1 pickle	65	93	5	Tr	Tr	Tr	Tr	0.1
902	Fresh-pack, slices 1-1/2-in diam., 1/4 in thick	2 slices	15	79	10	Tr	Tr	Tr	Tr	Tr
903	Sweet, gherkin, small, whole, about 2-1/2 in long, 3/4-in diam.	1 pickle	15	61	20	Tr	Tr	Tr	Tr	Tr
	Popcorn. See Grain Products, (items 497-499).									
904	Relish, finely chopped, sweet	1 tbsp	15	63	20	Tr	Tr	Tr	Tr	Tr
905	Salt	1 tsp	5.5	0	0	0	0	0.0	0.0	0.0
906	Vinegar, cider	1 tbsp	15	94	Tr	Tr	0	0.0	0.0	0.0
	Yeast:									
907	Baker's, dry, active	1 pkg	7	5	20	3	Tr	Tr	0.1	Tr
908	Brewer's, dry	1 tbsp	8	5	25	3	Tr	Tr	Tr	0.0

[1] Value not determined.

							Vitamin A value						
Cho-les-terol	Carbo-hydrate	Calcium	Phos-phorus	Iron	Potas-sium	Sodium	(IU)	(RE)	Thiamin	Ribo-flavin	Niacin	Ascorbic acid	Item No.
Milli-grams	Grams	Milli-grams	Milli-grams	Milli-grams	Milli-grams	Milli-grams	Inter-national units	Retinol equiva-lents	Milli-grams	Milli-grams	Milli-grams	Milli-grams	
0	1	58	87	0.0	5	329	0	0	0.00	0.00	0.0	0	881
0	1	183	45	0.0	4	290	0	0	0.00	0.00	0.0	0	882
0	1	239	359	0.0	6	312	0	0	0.00	0.00	0.0	0	883
0	1	207	314	0.0	891	Tr	0	0	0.00	0.00	0.0	0	884
0	69	60	137	2.2	991	2,845	3,820	382	0.25	0.19	4.4	41	885
0	4	3	8	0.1	54	156	210	21	0.01	0.01	0.2	2	886
0	1	35	11	0.9	28	3	Tr	Tr	0.01	0.01	0.1	Tr	887
0	1	7	8	0.4	50	26	910	91	0.01	0.02	0.2	2	888
0	8	22	109	1.9	235	1	10	1	0.01	0.07	0.4	0	889
0	2	28	1	0.9	12	1	10	1	Tr	Tr	Tr	1	890
0	1	10	7	0.6	31	1	20	2	0.01	0.01	0.1	Tr	891
0	2	2	12	0.1	31	1	0	0	0.01	Tr	Tr	Tr	892
0	0	1	0	0.0	2	6	0	0	0.00	0.00	0.0	0	893
0	Tr	4	4	0.1	7	63	0	0	Tr	0.01	Tr	Tr	894
0	Tr	8	2	0.2	7	312	40	4	Tr	Tr	Tr	0	895
0	Tr	10	2	0.2	2	68	10	1	Tr	Tr	Tr	0	896
0	2	8	7	0.1	20	1	Tr	Tr	0.01	Tr	Tr	Tr	897
0	1	24	3	0.7	25	Tr	100	10	0.01	Tr	0.1	1	898
0	1	4	7	0.5	49	1	1,270	127	0.01	0.04	0.3	1	899
0	1	9	4	0.6	26	1	Tr	Tr	Tr	0.01	Tr	0	900
0	1	17	14	0.7	130	928	70	7	Tr	0.01	Tr	4	901
0	3	5	4	0.3	30	101	20	2	Tr	Tr	Tr	1	902
0	5	2	2	0.2	30	107	10	1	Tr	Tr	Tr	1	903
0	5	3	2	0.1	30	107	20	2	Tr	Tr	0.0	1	904
0	0	14	3	Tr	Tr	2,132	0	0	0.00	0.00	0.0	0	905
0	1	1	1	0.1	15	Tr	0	0	0.00	0.00	0.0	0	906
0	3	3	90	1.1	140	4	Tr	Tr	0.16	0.38	2.6	Tr	907
0	3	[78]17	140	1.4	152	10	Tr	Tr	1.25	0.34	3.0	Tr	908

[78]Value may vary from 6 to 60 mg.

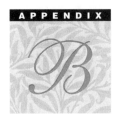

Recommended Dietary Allowances

Food and Nutrition Board, Natural Academy of Sciences—National Research Council
Recommended Dietary Allowances,[a] Revised 1989

Designed for the maintenance of good nutrition of practically all healthy people in the United States.

Category	Age (years) or Condition	Weight[b] (kg)	Weight[b] (lb)	Height[b] (cm)	Height[b] (in)	Protein (g)	Fat-Soluble Vitamins Vitamin A (μg RE)[c]	Vitamin D (μg)[d]	Vitamin E (mg α-TE)[e]	Vitamin K (μg)
Infants	0.0-0.5	6	13	60	24	13	375	7.5	3	5
	0.5-1.0	9	20	71	28	14	375	10	4	10
Children	1-3	13	29	90	35	16	400	10	6	15
	4-6	20	44	112	44	24	500	10	7	20
	7-10	28	62	132	52	28	700	10	7	30
Males	11-14	45	99	157	62	45	1,000	10	10	45
	15-18	66	145	176	69	59	1,000	10	10	65
	19-24	72	160	177	70	58	1,000	10	10	70
	25-50	79	174	176	70	63	1,000	5	10	80
	51+	77	170	173	68	63	1,000	5	10	80
Females	11-14	46	101	157	62	46	800	10	8	45
	15-18	55	120	163	64	44	800	10	8	55
	19-24	58	128	164	65	46	800	10	8	60
	25-50	63	138	163	64	50	800	5	8	65
	51 +	65	143	160	63	50	800	5	8	65
Pregnant						60	800	10	10	65
Lactating	1st 6 months					65	1,300	10	12	65
	2nd 6 months					62	1,200	10	11	65

[a]The allowances, expressed as average daily intakes over time, are intended to provide for individual variations among most normal persons as they live in the United States under usual environmental stresses. Diets should be based on a variety of common foods in order to provide other nutrients for which human requirements have been less well defined. See text for detailed discussion of allowances and of nutrients not tabulated.

[b]Weights and heights of Reference Adults are actual medians for the U.S population of the designated age, as reported by NHANES II. The median weights and heights of those under 19 years of age were taken from Hamill et al. (1979). The use of these figures does not imply that the height-to-weight ratios are ideal.

Water-Soluble Vitamins							Minerals						
Vitamin C (mg)	Thiamin (mg)	Riboflavin (mg)	Niacin (mg NE)[f]	Vitamin B6 (mg)	Folate (µg)	Vitamin B$_{12}$ (µg)	Calcium (mg)	Phosphorus (mg)	Magnesium (mg)	Iron (mg)	Zinc (mg)	Iodine (µg)	Selenium (µg)
30	0.3	0.4	5	0.3	25	0.3	400	300	40	6	5	40	10
40	0.7	0.8	9	1.0	50	0.7	800	800	80	10	10	70	20
45	0.9	1.1	12	1.1	75	1.0	800	800	120	10	10	90	20
45	1.0	1.2	13	1.4	100	1.4	800	800	170	10	10	120	30
50	1.3	1.5	17	1.7	150	2.0	1,200	1,200	270	12	15	150	40
60	1.5	1.8	20	2.0	200	2.0	1,200	1,200	400	12	15	150	50
60	1.5	1.7	19	2.0	200	2.0	1,200	1,200	350	10	15	150	70
60	1.5	1.7	19	2.0	200	2.0	800	800	350	10	15	150	70
60	1.2	1.4	15	2.0	200	2.0	800	800	350	10	15	150	70
50	1.1	1.3	15	1.4	150	2.0	1,200	1,200	280	15	12	150	45
60	1.1	1.3	15	1.5	180	2.0	1,200	1,200	300	15	12	150	50
60	1.1	1.3	15	1.6	180	2.0	1,200	1,200	280	15	12	150	55
60	1.1	1.3	15	1.6	180	2.0	800	800	280	15	12	150	55
60	1.0	1.2	13	1.6	180	2.0	800	800	280	10	12	150	55
70	1.5	1.6	17	2.2	400	2.2	1,200	1,200	320	30	15	175	65
95	1.6	1.8	20	2.1	280	2.6	1,200	1,200	355	15	19	200	75
90	1.6	1.7	20	2.1	260	2.6	1,200	1,200	340	15	16	200	75

[c] Retinol equivalent. 1 retinol equivalent = 1 µg retinol or 6 µg ß = carotene.
[d] As cholecalciferol. 10 µg cholecalciferol = 400 IU of vitamin D.
[e] a-Tocopherol equivalents. 1 mg d-α tocopherol = 1 α-TE.
[f] 1 NE (niacin equivalent) is equal to 1 mg of niacin or 60 mg of dietary tryptophan.

Source: Recommended Dietary Allowances. ©1989 by the National Academy of Sciences, National Academy Press, Washington, DC.

Median heights and weights and recommended energy intake.

Category	Age (years) or Condition	Weight (kg)	Weight (lb)	Height (cm)	Height (in)	REE[a] (kcal/day)	Multiples of REE	Average Energy Allowance (kcal)[b] Per kg	Average Energy Allowance (kcal)[b] Per day[c]
Infants	0.0–0.5	6	13	60	24	320		108	650
	0.5–1.0	9	20	71	28	500		98	850
Children	1–3	13	29	90	35	740		102	1,300
	4–6	20	44	442	44	950		90	1,800
	7–10	28	62	132	52	1,430		70	2,000
Males	11–14	45	99	157	62	1,440	1.70	55	2,500
	15–18	66	145	176	69	1,760	1.67	45	3,000
	19–24	72	160	177	70	1,780	1.67	40	2,900
	25–50	79	174	176	70	1,800	1.60	37	2,900
	51+	77	170	173	68	1,530	1.50	30	2,300
Females	11–14	46	101	157	62	1,340	1.67	47	2,200
	15–18	55	120	163	64	1,370	1.60	40	2,200
	19–24	58	128	164	65	1,350	1.60	38	2,200
	25–50	63	138	163	64	1,380	1.55	36	2,200
	51+	65	143	160	63	1,280	1.50	30	1,900
Pregnant	1st trimester								+0
	2nd trimester								+300
	3rd trimester								+300
Lactating	1st 6 months								+500
	2nd 6 months								+500

[a]Calculations based on FAO equations then rounded.
[b]In the range of light to moderate activity, the coefficient of vavariation is ±20%.
[c]Figure is rounded.

Source: Recommended Dietary Allowances. ©1989 by the National Academy of Sciences, National Academy Press, Washington, DC.

Estimated safe and adequate daily dietary intakes of selected vitamins and minerals.[a]

Category	Age (years)	Vitamins	
		Biotin (µg)	Pantothenic Acid (mg)
Infants	0–0.5	10	2
	0.5–1	15	3
Children and adolescents	1–3	20	3
	4–6	25	3–4
	7–10	30	4–5
	11 +	30–100	4–7
Adults	30–100	4–7	

Category	Age (years)	Trace Elements[b]				
		Copper (mg)	Manganese (mg)	Fluoride (mg)	Chromium (µg)	Molybdenum (µg)
Infants	0–0.5	0.4–0.6	0.3–0.6	0.1–0.5	10–10	15–30
	0.5–1	0.6–0.7	0.6–1.0	0.2–1.0	20–60	20–10
Children and adolescents	1–3	0.7–1.0	1.0–1.5	0.5–1.5	20–80	25–30
	4–6	1.0–1.5	1.5–2.0	1.0–2.5	30–120	30–75
	7–10	1.0–2.0	2.0–3.0	1.5–2.5	50–200	50–150
	11 +	1.5–2.5	2.0–5.0	1.5–2.5	50–200	75–250
Adults		1.5–3.0	2.0–5.0	1.5–4.0	50–200	75–250

[a]Because there is less information on which to base allowances, these figures are not given in the main table of RDA and are provided here in the form of ranges of recommended intakes.
[b]Since thetoxic levels for many trace elements may be only several times usual intakes, the upper levels for the trace elelents given in this table should not be habitually exceeded.
given in this table should not be habitually exceeded
Source: Recommended Dietary Allowances. ©1989 by the National Academy of Sciences, National Academy Press, Washington, DC.

Estimated sodium, chloride, and potassium minimum requirements of healthy persons.[a]

Age	Weight (kg)[a]	Sodium (mg)[a]1[b]	Chloride (mg)[a]1[b]	Potassium (mg)[c]
Months				
0–5	4.5	120	180	500
6–11	8.9	200	300	700
Years				
1	11.0	225	350	1,000
2–5	16.0	300	500	1,400
6–9	25.0	400	600	1,600
10–18	50.0	500	750	2,000
>18d	70.0	500	750	2,000

[a] No allowance has been included for large, prolonged losses from the skin through sweat.
[b] There is no evidence that higher intakes confer any health benefit.
[c] Desirable intakes of potassium may considerably exceed these values (~3,500 mg for adults).
[d] No allowance included for growth.
Source: Recommended Dietary Allowances. ©1989 by the National Academy of Sciences, National Academy Press, Washington, DC.

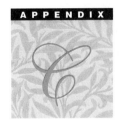

APPENDIX

Fiber Content of Food

Abbreviations

c	— cup
ckd	— cooked
cnd	— canned
dk	— dark
GF	— General Foods
GM	— grams
G.M.	— General Mills
K	— Kellogg
lrg	— large
lt	—light
med	— medium
nd	— not determined
oz	— ounce
P	— Post
Q	— Quaker
SF	— soluble fiber
sml	— small
SVG	— serving
Tbsp	— tablespoon
TF	— total fiber
tr	— trace (<0.01)
tsp	— teaspoon
unckd	— uncooked
unswt	— unsweetened
w	— with

*Source: Anderson, James W., M.D. *Plant Fiber in Foods* (2nd ed.). HCF Nutrition Research Foundation, Inc., P.O. Box 22129, Lexington, KY 40522. 1990. Phone (1-800-727-4423). Reprinted with the permission of Dr. James W. Anderson.

Item	*Serving Size*	*GM/Svg*	*TF/Svg*
Cereals			
All Bran, K.	⅓ c	28	8.6
All Bran with Extra Fiber, K.	½ c	28	13.8
Benefit, G.M.	¾ c	28	5.0
Cheerios, G.M.	1¼ c	28	2.5
Common Sense, K.	⅔ c	28	2.7
Cornflakes, K.	1 c	28	0.5
Cream of Wheat, regular, unckd	2½ Tbsp	28	1.1
Crispy Oats, Kolln	½ c	28	2.4
Fiber One, G.M.	½ c	28	11.9
40% Bran Flakes	⅔ c	28	4.3
Fruit and Fitness, Health Valley	⅓ c	19	2.9
Grapenuts, P.	¼ c	28	2.8
Grits, corn, quick, unckd	3 Tbsp	28	0.6
Heartwise, K.	1 c	28	5.7
Just Right with Fiber Nuggets, K.	⅔ c	28	1.1
Nutri-Grain Wheat, K.	⅔ c	28	2.7
Oat bran, ckd, Q.	¾ c	224	4.0
Oatbran, unckd. Q.	⅓ c	28	4.0
Oat Bran Cereal, (cold) Q.	¾ c	28	2.9
Oat Bran Crunch, Kolln	½ c	28	4.6
Oat Bran Flakes, Health Valley	½ c	28	2.1
Oat Bran Hot Cereal, Apples & Cinnamon, unckd, HealthValley	¼ c	28	2.5
Oat Bran O's, HealthValley	¾ c	28	1.6
Oat Flakes, P.	⅔ c	28	2.1
Oatbran and Oatgerm	⅓ c	28	3.8
Oatmeal, unckd, Q.	⅓ c	28	2.7
Product 19, K.	1 c	28	1.2
Puffed Rice	1 c	14	0.2
Puffed Wheat	1 c	14	1.0
Quaker Oat Squares	½ c	28	2.2
Raisin Bran	¾ c	39	5.3
Real Oat Bran Cereal, Almond Crunch, Health Valley	¼ c	28	2.0
Rice Krispies, K.	1 c	28	0.3
Shredded Wheat	⅔ c	28	3.5
Shredded Wheat & Bran, N.	⅔ c	28	2.5
Special K, K.	1 c	28	0.9
Total, Whole Wheat, G.M.	1 c	28	2.6
Wheat Flakes	¾ c	22	2.3
Wheaties, G.M.	⅔ c	28	2.3

Item	Serving Size	GM/Svg	TF/Svg
Grains			
Arrowroot	2 Tbsp	16	tr
Barley, pearl, unckd	2 Tbsp	25	3.0
Corn bran, unckd	⅓ c	25	20.4
Corn bran, unckd			
JR Short Milling Co.	⅓ c	25	18.4
Cornmeal	2 ½ Tbsp	20	0.4
Cornmeal, blue,			
Arrowhead Mills	3 ½ Tbsp	28	2.2
Flour, buck wheat	2 ½ Tbsp	20	0.5
corn	2 ½ Tbsp	19	tr
oat	2 ½ Tbsp	19	1.8
rye	2 ½ Tbsp	20	2.6
white	2 ½ Tbsp	18	0.6
Flour, whole wheat	2 ½ Tbsp	19	2.1
Grits, corn, quick, unckd	3 Tbsp	28	0.6
Macaroni, white, ckd	½ c	70	0.7
white, unckd	¼ c	21	0.6
whole wheat, ckd	½ c	70	2.1
whole wheat, unckd	¼ c	26	2.3
Millet, unckd	1 ½ Tbsp	18	0.4
Noodles, egg, ckd	½ c	80	1.4
egg, unckd	½ c	28	1.1
spinach, ckd	½ c	80	1.1
Oatmeal, unckd	⅓ c	28	2.7
Popcorn, popped	3 c	18	2.0
Rice, brown, long grain, unckd	⅙ c	28	nd
white, ckd	⅓ c	68	0.5
white, unckd	⅙ c	31	0.4
wild, ckd	⅓ c	55	0.4
Semolina, unckd	2 Tbsp	20	0.5
Spaghetti, white, ckd	½ c	70	0.9
Spaghetti, white, unckd	¼ c	21	0.7
whole wheat, ckd	½ c	70	2.7
whole wheat, unckd	¼ c	21	2.0
Tapioca, unckd	2 Tbsp	19	0.1
Wheat bran	½ c	30	12.3
Wheat germ	3 Tbsp	22	3.9

Item	Serving Size	GM/Svg	TF/Svg
Breads & Crackers			
Bagel, plain	½	28	0.7
Bagel, plain, microwaved	½	28	0.7
Biscuit, baked	1	28	0.5
Bread, bran	1 slice	28	1.5
cellulose	2 slices	46	4.6
cornbread	1-2" cube	56	1.4
cracked wheat	1 slice	28	1.9
French	1 slice	28	0.9
mixed grain	1 slice	28	1.9
mixed grain "lite"	2 slices	46	6.3
oatmeal	½ slice	30	1.2
Bread, pita, white	½ pocket	19	0.5
pumpernickel	1 slice	32	2.7
raisin	1 slice	28	1.2
rye	1 slice	28	1.8
rye (German)	1 slice	28	2.3
sourdough	1 slice	28	0.8
wheat "lite"	2 slices	46	5.6
white	1 slice	28	0.6
white "lite"	2 slices	46	5.9
whole-wheat	1 slice	28	1.5
Bread sticks	2	19	0.6
Bun, hamburger	½	25	0.7
Crackers, matzo	1	30	1.0
round, butter-type	6	21	0.4
saltine	6	17	0.5
saltine, wheat	5	14	0.5
snack, whole-wheat	4	18	2.0
wheat	5	14	0.6
English muffin	½	28	0.8
Melba toast, wheat	5 slices	20	1.8
Melba toast, white	5 slices	20	1.2
Pretzels, hard	¾ oz	21	0.8
Roll, brown and serve	1 roll	28	0.8
Roll, French	1 roll	28	0.9
Taco shell	2	22	1.4
Tortilla, corn	1	30	1.4
Tortilla, flour	1	30	0.7
Waffle, toasted	1	36	0.7

Item	Serving Size	GM/Svg	TF/Svg
Fruits & Juices			
Apple, Golden Delicious,	1 sml	128	2.3
fresh, flesh only	1 sml	128	2.3
Golden Delicious, fresh w skin	1 sml	138	2.8
Granny Smith, fresh, flesh only	1 sml	128	2.3
Granny Smith, fresh w skin	1 sml	138	2.8
red, fresh, flesh only	1 sml	128	2.4
red, fresh w skin	1 sml	138	2.8
Applesauce, cnd, unswt	½ c	122	2.0
Apricots, cnd, drained	4 halves	84	1.2
dried	7 halves	25	2.0
fresh w skin	4	141	3.5
Avocado, fresh, flesh only	⅛	25	1.2
Banana, fresh	½ sml	57	1.1
Blackberries, fresh	¾ c	108	3.7
Blueberries, fresh	¾ c	109	1.4
Cherries, black, fresh	12 lrg	84	1.3
Cherries, red, cnd	½ c	122	1.8
Cranberries, fresh	½ c	48	1.6
Currants, black, fresh	1 c	112	4.4
dried	2 Tbsp	18	0.4
red, fresh	1 c	112	4.1
Dates, dried	2 ½ med	21	0.9
Figs, dried	1 ½	28	2.3
Figs, fresh	2	100	3.0
Fruit cocktail, cnd	1/2 c	123	2.0
Gooseberries, fresh w skin	3/4 c	113	2.9
Grapefruit, cnd	½ c	122	1.3
Florida, yellow, fresh	½ med	118	1.4
fresh	½ med	120	1.6
Grapes, red, fresh w skin	15 sml	60	0.4
Grapes, white, fresh w skin	15 sml	75	0.6
Guava, fresh	1 ⅓	120	6.2
Kiwi fruit, fresh, flesh only	1 lrg	91	1.7
Lemon juice, fresh squeezed	2 Tbsp	30	tr
Loganberries, cnd	¾ c	110	3.5
Lychees, cnd	10	96	1.1
Mango, fresh, flesh only	½ sml	104	2.9
Melon, cantaloupe	1 c cubed	160	1.1
honeydew	1 c cubed	170	0.9
watermelon	1 ¼ c cubed	200	0.6

Item	Serving Size	GM/Svg	TF/Svg
Nectarine, fresh w skin	1	136	1.8
Orange, CA navel, fresh, flesh only	1 sml	140	2.0
Orange, fresh, flesh only	1 sml	131	2.9
Orange, mandarin, cnd	¾ c	186	0.7
Orange juice, in carton, unswt	½ c	125	0.1
Passion fruit, fresh, flesh & juice	3	54	0.4
Peaches, cnd, unswt	½ c	122	2.0
dried	⅙ c	19	1.5
fresh w skin	1 med or ¾ c	128	2.0
Pear, cnd	½ c	122	3.7
Comice, fresh, flesh only	½ lrg or 1 sml	83	1.4
Comice, fresh w skin	½ lrg or 1 sml	83	1.9
fresh w skin	½ lrg or 1 sml	83	2.9
Pineapple, cnd	⅓ c	82	1.4
Pineapple, fresh	¾ c	116	1.4
Plum, Greengages, fresh w skin	2 med	132	3.2
purple, cnd	½ c	125	2.8
red, fresh	2 med	132	2.4
Sicoval, fresh	2 med	132	2.4
Plum, Victoria, fresh	2 med	132	2.6
Pomegranate, fresh, flesh, seeds & juice	½	77	2.8
Prunes, dried	3 med	25	1.7
Prunes, stewed, unswt, drained	¼ c	53	1.6
Raisins, dried	2 Tbsp	18	0.4
Raspberries, cnd	½ c	128	3.8
Raspberries, fresh	1 c	123	3.3
Rhubarb, fresh	2 c	244	4.1
Strawberries, cnd	½ c	127	1.8
Strawberries, fresh	1¼ c	186	2.8
V-8 Juice	½ c	121	0.7

Item	Serving Size	GM/Svg	TF/Svg
Vegetables			
Asparagus, ckd	½ c	90	1.8
Asparagus, cnd	½ c	121	2.9
Bean sprouts, fresh	1 c	104	1.6
Beets, cnd	½ c	85	2.2
Beets, flesh only, ckd	½ c	68	1.8
Broccoli, ckd	½ c	78	2.4
Broccoli spears, frozen	½ c	78	2.2
Brussels sprouts, ckd	½ c	78	3.8
fresh	1 c	88	5.0
frozen	½ c	78	3.5
Cabbage, fresh	1 c	70	1.5
red, ckd	½ c	75	2.6
red, fresh	1 c	70	2.7
winter, savoy, ckd	½ c	73	2.4
winter, savoy, fresh	1 c	70	2.7
Carrots, cnd	½ c	73	1.5
fresh	1-7½" long	72	2.3
sliced, ckd	½ c	78	2.0
Cauliflower, ckd	½ c	62	1.0
fresh	1 c	100	1.8
frozen	½ c	66	1.7
Celeriac, fresh	½ c	78	3.1
Celery, fresh	1 c chopped	120	1.7
Chicory, fresh	½ c chopped	90	1.2
Corn, whole kernel, cnd	½ c	82	1.6
Corn on the cob, sweet, ckd	1–6" long	82	2.4
Cress, fresh	1 ½ c	75	0.9
Cucumber, fresh	1 c	104	0.5
Eggplant, fresh	1 c	82	1.8
Eggplant, fresh, microwaved	½ c	48	0.9
Endive, fresh	1 c	50	1.1
Fennel, fresh	1 tsp	2	0.1
Creen beans, cnd	½ c	68	2.0
French style, ckd	½ c	86	2.8
frozen, microwaved	½ c	68	1.6
runners, ckd	½ c	62	1.6
Kale, chopped, frozen	½ c	65	2.5
Leeks, sliced, ckd	½ c	52	1.3
Lettuce, butterhead	1 c	30	0.4
Lettuce, iceberg	1 c	56	0.5
Mushrooms, fresh	1 c pieces	70	0.8
Okra, fresh, trimmed pods	1 c slices	100	7.3
Okra, frozen, ckd	½ c	92	4.1
Olives, cnd	10 sml	33	1.0

Item	Serving Size	GM/Svg	TF/Svg
Onion, ckd	½ c chopped	105	2.0
Onion, fresh	½ c chopped	80	1.7
Parsley, fresh	1 tsp	4	0.2
Parsnip, ckd	½ c	78	3.3
Peas, green, cnd	½ c	85	3.2
green, fresh, ckd	½ c	80	2.4
green, frozen, ckd	½ c	80	4.3
Pepper, green, fresh	1 c chopped	100	1.7
Plantain, flesh only, ckd	½ c	77	1.0
Potato, sweet, cnd	⅓ c	67	0.8
sweet, flesh only, ckd	⅓ c	109	2.7
white, fresh w skin	½ c	75	1.5
Pumpkin, fresh, ckd	1 c	107	1.2
Radish, fresh	1 c slices	116	1.3
Snow peas, fresh, microwaved	½ c	80	1.4
Spinach, ckd	½ c	90	1.6
Spinach, frozen	½ c	78	1.7
Squash, yellow, crookneck, frozen	½ c	65	0.7
Tomato, cnd	½ c	120	1.3
fresh	1 med	123	1.0
sauce	⅓ c	82	1.1
Turnip, ckd	½ c	78	4.8
Watercress, fresh	1 c	34	0.6
Yam, flesh only, ckd	⅓ c	45	0.5
Yam, flesh only, fresh	⅓ c	50	0.7
Zucchini, fresh	1 c	130	1.6
Zucchini, sliced, ckd	½ c	90	1.2
Legumes			
Black beans, ckd	½ c	86	6.1
Black-eyed peas, cnd	½ c	120	4.7
Broad beans, no pods, ckd	½ c	85	5.1
Butter beans, dried, ckd	½ c	94	6.9
Butter beans, dried, unckd	⅙ c	30	5.1
Chick peas, dried, ckd	½ c	82	4.3
Chick peas, dried, unckd	⅙ c	33	3.9
Cranberry beans, dried, ckd	½ c	88	5.4
Garbanzo beans, cnd	⅓ c	80	2.8
Kidney beans, dk red, dried, ckd	½ c	88	6.9
dk red, dried, unckd	⅙ c	30	5.5
lt red, cnd	½ c	128	7.9

Item	Serving Size	GM/Svg	TF/Svg
Lentils, dried, ckd	½ c	99	5.2
dried, unckd	⅙ c	32	3.7
red, dried, ckd	½ c	99	2.3
red, dried, unckd	⅙ c	32	1.8
Lima beans, cnd	½ c	120	4.3
Mung beans, dried, ckd	½ c	101	3.3
Mungbeans, dried, unckd	⅙ c	35	3.9
Navy beans, dried, ckd	½ c	91	6.5
Pinto beans, cnd	½ c	120	6.1
dried, ckd	½ c	85	5.9
dried, unckd	⅙ c	32	6.2
Pork & beans w sauce, cnd	½ c	128	5.4
Soybeans, dried, unckd	⅙ c	31	5.4
Split peas, dried, ckd	½ c	98	3.1
Split peas, dried, unckd	⅙ c	33	2.4
White beans, Great Northern, cnd	½ c	131	7.2
Great Northern, dried, ckd	½ c	90	5.0
Great Northern, dried, unckd	⅙ c	34	6.0
Nuts & Seeds			
Almonds	6 whole	7	0.6
Brazilnuts	1 Tbsp	9	0.5
Chestnuts, microwaved	2 Tbsp	18	0.9
Coconut, dried	1½ Tbsp	9	1.5
Coconut, fresh	2 Tbsp	13	1.1
Hazelnuts (filberts)	1 Tbsp	7	0.5
Peanut butter, smooth	1 Tbsp	16	1.0
Peanuts, fresh	10 lrg	8	0.6
Peanuts, roasted	10 lrg	8	0.6
Sesame seeds	1 Tbsp	9	0.8
Sunflower seeds	1 Tbsp	9	0.5
Walnuts	2 whole	8	0.3
Miscellaneous foods			
Angel food cake	¹⁄₁₂ cake	60	0.5
Blueberry muffln, store-bought	½	20	0.3
Bran muffin, store-bought	½	20	0.7
Gingersnaps	3	21	0.3
Craham crackers	3–2 ½" squares	11	0.3
Oat Bran Animal Cookies, Health Valley	9	28	2.1
Oat Bran Fancy Fruit Muffin, Health Valley	½	28	1.7

Item	Serving Size	GM/Svg	TF/Svg
Oat Bran Fruit Jumbo Cookies, Health Valley	1	16	1.2
Oat Bran Fruit and Nut Cookies, HealthValley	2	28	1.7
Oat Bran Graham Crackers, Health Valley	3–2½" squares	16	1.3
Oat Bran Jumbo Fruit Bar, HealthValley	½	21	1.1
Oat bran muffin, store-bought	½	31	0.5
Oat bran raisin muffin, Dr. Anderson's recipe	½	33	1.6
Tomato ketchup	1 Tbsp	15	0.1
Vanilla wafers	6	24	0.4
Concentrated fibers			
Citrucel	1 Tbsp	6	2.0
Citrus pectin	1 Tbsp	10	5.5
Corn bran, unckd	⅓ c	25	20.4
Corn bran, unckd JR Short Milling Co.	⅓ c	25	18.4
Effer-syllium	1 tsp	7	2.5
Fibrim, Protein Technologies International, Inc.	1 tsp	4	2.9
Flax fiber (Nutri-Flax), Omega Nutrition	2 Tbsp	17	5.7
Konsyl	1 packet	6	4.6
Metamucil	1 tsp	7	2.7
Metamucil, sugar-free	1 tsp	4	3.0
Oat bran, unckd, Q.	⅓ c	28	4.0
Oat fiber (Advanced Tan #770), Williamson	1⅛ Tbsp	3	2.9
Oat fiber (Advanced White #780), Williamson	1⅛ Tbsp	3	2.9
Oat gum	3⅓ Tbsp	10	5.0
Per Diem	1 tsp	6	4.3
Rice bran	⅛ c	10	2.1
Wheat bran	½ c	30	12.3

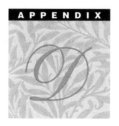

APPENDIX

Exchange Lists for Meal Planning

The exchange lists are the basis of a meal planning system designed by a committee of the American Diabetes Association and The American Diabetic Association. While designed primarily for people with diabetes and others who must follow special diets, the exchange lists are based on principles of good nutrition that apply to everyone.

STARCH LIST

Cereals, grains, pasta, breads, crackers, snacks, starchy vegetables, and cooked dried beans, peas, and lentils are starches. In general, one starch is:

- ½ cup of cereal, grain, pasta, or starchy vegetable
- 1 ounce of a bread product, such as 1 slice of bread
- ¾ to 1 ounce of most snack foods (Some snack foods may also have added fat.)

Nutrition Tips
1. Most starch choices are good sources of B vitamins.
2. Foods made from whole grains are good sources of fiber.
3. Dried beans and peas are a good source of protein and fiber.

Selection Tips
1. Choose starches made with little fat as often as you can.
2. Starchy vegetables prepared with fat count as one starch and one fat.
3. Bagels or muffins can be 2, 3, or 4 ounces in size, and can therefore, count as 2, 3, or 4 starch choices. Check the size you eat.
4. Dried beans, peas, and lentils are also found on the Meat and Meat Substitutes list.
5. Regular potato chips and tortilla chips are found on the Other Carbohydrates list.
6. Most of the serving sizes are measured after cooking.
7. Always check Nutrition Facts on the food label.

One starch exchange equals
15 grams carbohydrate,
3 grams protein,
0–1 grams fat, and
80 calories.

Bread

Bagel	½ (1 oz)
Bread, reduced-calorie	2 slices (1½ oz)
Bread, white, whole-wheat, pumpernickel, rye	1 slice (1 oz)
Bread sticks, crisp, 4 in. long x ½ in.	2 (⅔ oz)
English muffin	1/2
Hot dog or hamburger bun	½ (1 oz)
Pita, 6 in. across	½
Roll, plain, small	1 (1 oz)
Raisin bread, unfrosted	1 slice (1 oz)
Tortilla, corn, 6 in. across	1
Tortilla, flour, 7–8 in. across	1
Waffle, 4½ in. square, reduced-fat	1

Cereals and Grains

Bran cereals	½ cup
Bulgur	½ cup
Cereals	½ cup
Cereals, unsweetened, ready-to-eat	¾ cup
Cornmeal (dry)	3 Tbsp
Couscous	⅓ cup
Flour (dry)	3 Tbsp
Granola, low-fat	¼ cup
Grape-Nuts	¼ cup
Grits	½ cup
Kasha	½ cup
Millet	¼ cup
Muesli	¼ cup
Oats	½ cup
Pasta	½ cup
Puffed cereal	1½ cups
Rice milk	½ cup
Rice, white or brown	⅓ cup
Shredded Wheat	½ cup
Sugar-frosted cereal	½ cup
Wheat germ	3 Tbsp

One starch exchange equals
15 grams carbohydrate,
3 grams protein,
0–1 grams fat, and
80 calories.

Starchy Vegetables

Baked beans	⅓ cup
Corn	½ cup
Corn on cob, medium..	1 (5 oz)
Mixed vegetables with corn, peas, or pasta	1 cup
Peas, green	½ cup
Plantain...	½ cup
Potato, baked or boiled	1 small (3 oz)
Potato, mashed	½ cup
Squash, winter (acorn, butternut)	1 cup
Yam, sweet potato, plain	½ cup

Crackers and Snacks

Animal crackers...	8
Graham crackers, 2 ½ in. square	3
Matzoh	¾ oz
Melba toast..	4 slices
Oyster crackers	24
Popcorn (popped, no fat added or low-fat microwave)	3 cups
Pretzels	¾ oz
Rice cakes, 4 in. across...	2
Saltine-type crackers	6
Snack chips, fat-free (tortilla, potato)	15-20 (¾ oz)
Whole-wheat crackers, no fat added	2-5 (¾ oz)

Dried Beans, Peas, and Lentils
(Count as 1 starch exchange, plus 1 very lean meat exchange.)

Beans and peas (garbanzo, pinto, kidney, white, split, black-eyed)	½ cup
Lima beans..	⅔ cup
Lentils...	½ cup
Miso*	3 Tbsp

* = 400 mg or more of sodium per serving.

One starch exchange equals
15 grams carbohydrate,
3 grams protein,
0–1 grams fat, and
80 calories.

Starchy Foods Prepared with Fat
(Count as 1 starch exchange, plus 1 fat exchange.)

Biscuit, 2 ½ in. across	1
Chow mein noodles	½ cup
Corn bread, 2 in. cube	1 (2 oz)
Crackers, round butter type	6
Croutons	1 cup
French-fried potatoes	16-25 (3 oz)
Granola	¼ cup
Muffin, small	1 (1½ oz)
Pancake, 4 in. across	2
Popcorn, microwave	3 cups
Sandwich crackers, cheese or peanut butter filling	3
Stuffing, bread (prepared)	⅓ cup
Taco shell, 6 in. across	2
Waffle, 4 ½ in. square	1
Whole-wheat crackers, fat added	4–6 (1 oz)

Some food you buy uncooked will weigh less after you cook it. Starches often swell in cooking, so a small amount of uncooked starch will become a much larger amount of cooked food. The following table shows some of the changes.

Food (Starch Group):	*Uncooked*	*Cooked*
Oatmeal	3 Tbsp	½ cup
Cream of Wheat	2 Tbsp	½ cup
Grits	3 Tbsp	½ cup
Rice	2 Tbsp	⅓ cup
Spaghetti	¼ cup	½ cup
Noodles	⅓ cup	½ cup
Macaroni	¼ cup	½ cup
Dried beans	¼ cup	½ cup
Dried peas	¼ cup	½ cup
Lentils	3 Tbsp	½ cup

Common Measurements

3 tsp = 1 Tbsp	4 ounces = ½ cup
4 Tbsp = ¼ cup	8 ounces = 1 cup
5⅓ Tbsp = ⅓ cup	1 cup = ½ pint

FRUIT LIST

Fresh, frozen, canned, and dried fruits and fruit juices are on this list. In general, one fruit exchange is:

- 1 small to medium fresh fruit,
- ½ cup of canned or fresh fruit or fruit juice,
- ¼ cup of dried fruit.

Nutrition Tips

1. Fresh, frozen, and dried fruits have about 2 grams of fiber per choice. Fruit juices contain very little fiber.
2. Citrus fruits, berries, and melons are good sources of vitamin C.

Selection Tips

1. Count ½ cup cranberries or rhubarb sweetened with sugar substitutes as free foods.
2. Read the Nutrition Facts on the food label. If one serving has more than 15 grams of carbohydrate, you will need to adjust the size of the serving you eat or drink.
3. Portion sizes for canned fruits are for the fruit and a small amount of juice.
4. Whole fruit is more filling than fruit juice and may be a better choice.
5. Food labels for fruits may contain the words "no sugar added" or "unsweetened." This means that no sucrose (table sugar) has been added.
6. Generally, fruit canned in extra light syrup has the same amount of carbohydrate per serving as the "no sugar added" or the juice pack. All canned fruits on the fruit list are based on one of these three types of pack.

One fruit exchange equals
15 grams carbohydrate and
60 calories.
The weight includes skin, core, seeds, and rind.

Fruit

Apple, unpeeled, small	1 (4 oz)
Applesauce, unsweetened	½ cup
Apples, dried	4 rings
Apricots, fresh	4 whole (5 ½ oz)
Apricots, dried	8 halves
Apricots, canned	½ cup
Banana, small	1 (4 oz)
Blackberries	¾ cup
Blueberries	¾ cup
Cantaloupe, small	⅓ melon (11 oz) or 1 cup cubes
Cherries, sweet, fresh	12 (3 oz)
Cherries, sweet, canned	½ cup
Dates	3
Figs, fresh	1 ½ large or 2 medium (3 ½ oz)
Figs, dried	1 ½
Fruit cocktail	½ cup
Grapefruit, large	½ (11 oz)
Grapefruit sections, canned	¾ cup
Grapes, small	17 (3 oz)
Honeydew melon	1 slice (10 oz) or 1 cup cubes
Kiwi	1 (3 ½ oz)
Mandarin oranges, canned	¾ cup
Mango, small	½ fruit (5 ½ oz) or ½ cup
Nectarine, small	1 (5 oz)
Orange, small	1 (6 ½ oz)
Papaya	½ fruit (8 oz) or 1 cup cubes
Peach, medium, fresh	1 (6 oz)
Peaches, canned	½ cup
Pear, large, fresh	½ (4 oz)
Pears, canned	½ cup
Pineapple, fresh	¾ cup
Pineapple, canned	½ cup
Plums, small	2 (5 oz)
Plums, canned	½ cup
Prunes, dried	3
Raisins	2 Tbsp
Raspberries	1 cup
Strawberries	1 ¼ cup whole berries
Tangerines, small	2 (8 oz)
Watermelon	1 slice (13 ½ oz) or 1 ¼ cup cubes

Fruit Juice

Apple juice/cider	½ cup	Grape juice	⅓ cup
Cranberry juice cocktail	⅓ cup	Grapefruit juice	½ cup
Cranberry juice cocktail, reduced-calorie	1 cup	Orange juice	½ cup
		Pineapple juice	½ cup
Fruit juice blends, 100% juice	⅓ cup	Prune juice	⅓ cup

MILK LIST

Different types of milk and milk products are on this list. Cheeses are on the Meat list and cream and other dairy fats are on the Fat list. Based on the amount of fat they contain, milks are divided into skim/very low-fat milk, low-fat milk, and whole milk. One choice of these includes:

	Carbohydrate (grams)	Protein (grams)	Fat (grams)	Calories
Skim/very low-fat	12	8	0–3	90
Low-fat	12	8	5	120
Whole	12	8	8	150

Nutrition Tips
1. Milk and yogurt are good sources of calcium and protein. Check the food label.
2. The higher the fat content of milk and yogurt, the greater the amount of saturated fat and cholesterol. Choose lower-fat varieties .
3. For those who are lactose intolerant, look for lactose-reduced or lactose-free varieties of milk.

Selection Tips
1. One cup equals 8 fluid ounces or ½ pint.
2. Look for chocolate milk, frozen yogurt, and ice cream on the Other Carbohydrates list.
3. Nondairy creamers are on the Free Foods list.
4. Look for rice milk on the Starch list.
5. Look for soy milk on the Medium-fat Meat list.

One milk exchange equals
12 grams carbohydrate and
8 grams protein.

Skim and Very Low-fat Milk

(0–3 grams fat per serving)

Skim milk ....1 cup

½ % milk ....1 cup

1% milk ....1 cup

Nonfat or low-fat buttermilk ....1 cup

Evaporated skim milk ....½ cup

Nonfat dry milk ....⅓ cup dry

Plain nonfat yogurt ....¾ cup

Nonfat or low-fat fruit-flavored yogurt sweetened
   with aspartame or with a nonnutritive sweetener ....1 cup

Low-fat

(5 grams fat per serving)

2% milk ....1 cup

Plain low-fat yogurt ....¾ cup

Sweet acidophilus milk ....1 cup

Whole Milk

(8 grams fat per serving)

Whole milk..1 cup

Evaporated whole milk ....½ cup

Goat's milk ....1 cup

Kefir ....1 cup

OTHER CARBOHYDRATES LIST

You can substitute food choices from this list for a starch, fruit, or milk choice on your meal plan. Some choices will also count as one or more fat choices.

Nutrition Tips

1. These foods can be substituted in your meal plan, even though they contain added sugars or fat. However, they do not contain as many important vitamins and minerals as the choices on the Starch, Fruit, or Milk list.
2. When planning to include these foods in your meal, be sure to include foods from all the lists to eat a balanced meal.

Selection Tips

1. Because many of these foods are concentrated sources of carbohydrates and fat, the portion sizes are often very small.
2. Always check Nutrition Facts on the food label. It will be your most accurate source of information.
3. Many fat-free or reduced-fat products made with fat replacers contain carbohydrate. When eaten in large amounts, they may need to be counted. Talk with your dietitian to determine how to count these in your meal plan.
4. Look for fat-free salad dressings in smaller amounts on the Free Foods list.

One exchange equals
15 grams carbohydrate, or 1 starch, or 1 fruit, or 1 milk.

Food	Serving Size	Exchanges Per Serving
Angel food cake, unfrosted	½₂ cake	2 carbohydrates
Brownie, small, unfrosted	2 in. square	1 carbohydrate, 1 fat
Cake, unfrosted	2 in. square	1 carbohydrate, 1 fat
Cake, frosted	2 in. square	2 carbohydrates, 1 fat
Cookie, fat-free	2 small	1 carbohydrate
Cookie or sandwich cookie with creme filling	2 small	1 carbohydrate, 1 fat
Cupcake, frosted	1 small	2 carbohydrates, 1 fat
Cranberry sauce, jellied	¼ cup	2 carbohydrates
Doughnut, plain cake	1 medium (1½ oz)	1 ½ carbohydrates, 2 fats
Doughnut, glazed	3 ¾ in. across (2 oz)	2 carbohydrates, 2 fats
Fruit juice bars, frozen, 100% juice	1 bar (3 oz)	1 carbohydrate
Fruit snacks, chewy (pureed fruit concentrate)	1 roll (¾ oz)	1 carbohydrate
Fruit spreads, 100% fruit	1 Tbsp	1 carbohydrate
Gelatin, regular	½ cup	1 carbohydrate
Gingersnaps	3	1 carbohydrate

One exchange equals
15 grams carbohydrate, or 1 starch, or 1 fruit, or 1 milk.

Food	*Serving Size*	*Exchanges Per Serving*
Granola bar	1 bar	1 carbohydrate, 1 fat
Granola bar, fat-free	1 bar	2 carbohydrates
Hummus	⅓ cup	1 carbohydrate, 1 fat
Ice cream	½ cup	1 carbohydrate, 2 fats
Ice cream, light	½ cup	1 carbohydrate, 1 fat
Ice cream, fat-free, no sugar added	½ cup	1 carbohydrate
Jam or jelly, regular	1 Tbsp	1 carbohydrate
Milk, chocolate, whole	1 cup	2 carbohydrates, 1 fat
Pie, fruit, 2 crusts	⅙ pie	3 carbohydrate, 2 fats
Pie, pumpkin or custard	⅛ pie	1 carbohydrate, 2 fats
Potato chips	12-18 (1 oz)	1 carbohydrate, 2 fats
Pudding, regular (made with low-fat milk)	½ cup	2 carbohydrates
Pudding, sugar-free (made with low-fat milk)	½ cup	1 carbohydrate
Salad dressing, fat-free*	¼ cup	1 carbohydrate
Sherbet, sorbet	½ cup	2 carbohydrates
Spaghetti or pasta sauce, canned*	½ cup	1 carbohydrate, 1 fat
Sweet roll or Danish	1 (2 ½ oz)	2 ½ carbohydrates, 2 fats
Syrup, light	2 Tbsp	1 carbohydrate
Syrup, regular	1 Tbsp	1 carbohydrate
Syrup, regular	¼ cup	4 carbohydrates
Tortilla chips	6–12(1 oz)	1 carbohydrate, 2 fats
Yogurt, frozen, low-fat, fat-free	⅓ cup	1 carbohydrate, 0–1 fat
Yogurt, frozen, fat-free, no sugar added	½ cup	1 carbohydrate
Yogurt, low-fat with fruit	1 cup	3 carbohydrates, 0–1 fat
Vanilla wafers	5	1 carbohydrate, 1 fat

* = 400 mg or more of sodium per serving.

VEGETABLE LIST

Vegetables that contain small amounts of carbohydrates and calories are on this list. Vegetables contain important nutrients. Try to eat at least 2 or 3 vegetable choices each day. In general, one vegetable exchange is:

- ½ cup of cooked vegetables or vegetable juice,
- 1 cup of raw vegetables.

If you eat 1 to 2 vegetable choices at a meal or snack, you do not have to count the calories or carbohydrates because they contain small amounts of these nutrients.

Nutrition Tips

1. Fresh and frozen vegetables have less added salt than canned vegetables. Drain and rinse canned vegetables if you want to remove some salt.
2. Choose more dark green and dark yellow vegetables, such as spinach, broccoli, romaine, carrots, chilies, and peppers.
3. Broccoli, brussels sprouts, cauliflower, greens, peppers, spinach, and tomatoes are good sources of vitamin C.
4. Vegetables contain 1 to 4 grams of fiber per serving.

Selection Tips

1. A 1-cup portion of broccoli is a portion about the size of a light bulb.
2. Tomato sauce is different from spaghetti sauce, which is on the Other Carbohydrates list.
3. Canned vegetables and juices are available without added salt.
4. If you eat more than 4 cups of raw vegetables or 2 cups of cooked vegetables at one meal, count them as 1 carbohydrate choice.
5. Starchy vegetables such as corn, peas, winter squash, and potatoes that contain larger amounts of calories and carbohydrates are on the Starch list.

One vegetable exchange equals
5 grams carbohydrate,
2 grams protein,
0 grams fat, and
25 calories.

Artichoke

Artichoke hearts

Asparagus

Beans (green, wax, Italian)

Bean sprouts

Beets

Broccoli

Brussels sprouts

Cabbage

Carrots

Cauliflower

Celery

Cucumber

Eggplant

Green onions or scallions

Greens (collard, kale, mustard, turnip)

Kohlrabi

Leeks

Mixed vegetables
  (without corn, peas, or pasta)

Mushrooms

Okra

Onions

Pea pods

Peppers (all varieties)

Radishes

Salad greens (endive, escarole, lettuce,
  romaine, spinach)

Sauerkraut*

Spinach

Summer squash

Tomato

Tomatoes, canned

Tomato sauce*

Tomato/vegetable juice*

Turnips

Water chestnuts

Watercress

Zucchini

* = 400 mg or more sodium per exchange.

MEAT AND MEAT SUBSTITUTES LIST

Meat and meat substitutes that contain both protein and fat are on this list. In general, one meat exchange is:

- 1 oz meat, fish, poultry, or cheese,
- ½ cup dried beans.

Based on the amount of fat they contain, meats are divided into very lean, lean, medium-fat, and high-fat lists. This is done so you can see which ones contain the least amount of fat. One ounce (one exchange) of each of these includes:

	Carbohydrate (grams)	Protein (grams)	Fat (grams)	Calories
Very lean	0	7	0–1	35
Lean	0	7	3	55
Medium-fat	0	7	5	75
High-fat	0	7	8	100

1. Choose very lean and lean meat choices whenever possible. Items from the high-fat group are high in saturated fat, cholesterol, and calories and can raise blood cholesterol levels.
2. Meats do not have any fiber.
3. Dried beans, peas, and lentils are good sources of fiber.
4. Some processed meats, seafood, and soy products may contain carbohydrates when consumed in large amounts. Check the Nutrition Facts on the label to see if the amount is close to 15 grams. If so, count it as a carbohydrate choice as well as a meat choice.

Selection Tips

1. Weigh meat after cooking and removing bones and fat. Four ounces of raw meat is equal to 3 ounces of cooked meat. Some examples of meat portions are:

   - 1 ounce cheese = 1 meat choice and is about the size of a 1-inch cube
   - 2 ounces meat = 2 meat choices, such as
       1 small chicken leg or thigh
       ½ cup cottage cheese or tuna
   - 3 ounces meat = 3 meat choices and is about the size of a deck of cards, such as
       1 medium pork chop
       1 small hamburger
       ½ of a whole chicken breast
       1 unbreaded fish fillet

2. Limit your choices from the high-fat group to three times per week or less.
3. Most grocery stores stock Select and Choice grades of meat. Select grades of meat are the leanest meats. Choice grades contain a moderate amount of fat, and Prime cuts of meat have the highest amount of fat. Restaurants usually serve Prime cuts of meat.
5. "Hamburger" may contain added seasoning and fat, but ground beef does not.
6. Read labels to find products that are low in fat and cholesterol (5 grams or less of fat per serving).
7. Dried beans, peas, and lentils are also found on the Starch list.
8. Peanut butter, in smaller amounts, is also found on the Fats list.
9. Bacon, in smaller amounts, is also found on the Fats list.

Meal Planning Tips

1. Bake, roast, broil, grill, poach, steam, or boil these foods rather than frying.
2. Place meat on a rack so the fat will drain off during cooking.
3. Use a nonstick spray and a nonstick pan to brown or fry foods.
4. Trim off visible fat before or after cooking.
5. If you add flour, bread crumbs, coating mixes, fat, or marinades when cooking, ask your dietitian how to count it in your meal plan.

Very Lean Meat and Substitutes List
One exchange equals 0 grams carbohydrate,
7 grams protein, 0–1 grams fat, and 35 calories.

One very lean meat exchange is equal to any one of the following items.

Poultry: Chicken or turkey (white meat, no skin),
Cornish hen (no skin) ....1 oz

Fish: Fresh or frozen cod, flounder, haddock,
halibut, trout; tuna fresh or canned in water ....1 oz

Shellfish: Clams, crab, lobster, scallops, shrimp,
imitation shellfish ....1 oz

Game: Duck or pheasant (no skin), venison,
buffalo, ostrich ....1 oz

Cheese with 1 gram or less fat per ounce:
Nonfat or low-fat cottage cheese ....¼ cup
Fat-free cheese..1 oz

Other: Processed sandwich meats with 1 gram or less fat per ounce,
such as deli thin, shaved meats, chipped beef*, turkey ham.....................1 oz
Egg whites...2
Egg substitutes, plain ....¼ cup
Hot dogs with 1 gram or less fat per ounce* ....1 oz
Kidney (high in cholesterol) ....1 oz
Sausage with 1 gram or less fat per ounce ....1 oz

Count as one very lean meat and one starch exchange.

Dried beans, peas, lentils (cooked) ....½ cup

* = 400 mg or more sodium per exchange.

Lean Meat and Substitutes List
One exchange equals 0 grams carbohydrate,
7 grams protein, 3 grams fat, and 55 calories.

One lean meat exchange is equal to any one of the following items.

Beef: USDA Select or Choice grades of lean beef trimmed of fat,
such as round, sirloin, and flank steak; tenderloin; roast
(rib, chuck, rump); steak (T-bone, porterhouse, cubed),
ground round ....1 oz

Pork: Lean pork, such as fresh ham; canned, cured, or boiled ham;
Canadian bacon*; tenderloin, center loin chop ....1 oz

Lamb: Roast, chop, leg ....1 oz

Veal: Lean chop, roast ....1 oz

Poultry: Chicken, turkey (dark meat, no skin),
chicken white meat (with skin), domestic duck or goose
(well-drained of fat, no skin) ....1 oz

Fish:
Herring (uncreamed or smoked) ....1 oz
Oysters...6 medium
Salmon (fresh or canned), catfish...1 oz
Sardines (canned) ....2 medium
Tuna (canned in oil, drained) ....1 oz

Game: Goose (no skin), rabbit..1 oz

Cheese:
4.5%-fat cottage cheese...¼ cup
Grated Parmesan ....2 Tbsp
Cheeses with 3 grams or less fat per ounce ....1 oz

Other:
Hot dogs with 3 grams or less fat per ounce* ....1½ oz
Processed sandwich meat with 3 grams or less
fat per ounce, such as turkey pastrami or kielbasa...................1 oz
Liver, heart (high in cholesterol) ....1 oz

* = 400 mg or more sodium per exchange.

Medium-Fat Meat and Substitutes List
One exchange equals 0 grams carbohydrate,
7 grams protein, 5 grams fat, and 75 calories.

One medium-fat meat exchange is equal to any one of the following items.

Beef: Most beef products fall into this category (ground beef, meatloaf, corned beef, short ribs, Prime grades of meat trimmed of fat, such as prime rib) ....1 oz

Pork: Top loin, chop, Boston butt, cutlet ....1 oz

Lamb: Rib roast, ground...1 oz

Veal: Cutlet (ground or cubed, unbreaded)...1 oz

Poultry: Chicken dark meat (with skin), ground turkey or ground chicken, fried chicken (with skin) ....1 oz

Fish: Any fried fish product ....1 oz

Cheese: With 5 grams or less fat per ounce
Feta ....1 oz
Mozzarella...1 oz
Ricotta ....¼ cup (2 oz)

Other:
Egg (high in cholesterol, limit to 3 per week) 1
Sausage with 5 grams or less fat per ounce ....1 oz
Soy milk...1 cup
Tempeh ....¼ cup
Tofu ....4 oz or ½ cup

High-Fat Meat and Substitutes List
One exchange equals 0 grams carbohydrate,
7 grams protein, 8 grams fat, and 100 calories.

Remember these items are high in saturated fat, cholesterol, and calories and may raise blood cholesterol levels if eaten on a regular basis. One high-fat meat exchange is equal to any one of the following items.

Pork: Spareribs, ground pork, pork sausage ....1 oz

Cheese: All regular cheeses, such as American*, Cheddar,
   Monterey Jack, Swiss ....1 oz

Other: Processed sandwich meats with 8 grams or less fat
   per ounce, such as bologna, pimiento loaf, salami. ....1 oz
   Sausage, such as bratwurst, Italian,
   knockwurst, Polish, smoked ....1 oz
   Hot dog (turkey or chicken)* 1 (10/lb)
   Bacon...3 slices (20 slices/lb)

Count as one high-fat meat plus one fat exchange.

Hot dog (beef, pork, or combination* 1 (10/lb)
Peanut butter (contains unsaturated fat) ....2 Tbsp

* = 400 mg or more sodium per exchange.

FAT LIST

Fats are divided into three groups, based on the main type of fat they contain: monounsaturated, polyunsaturated, and saturated. Small amounts of monounsaturated and polyunsaturated fats in the foods we eat are linked with good health benefits. Saturated fats are linked with heart disease and cancer. In general, one fat exchange is:

- 1 teaspoon of regular margarine or vegetable oil,
- 1 tablespoon of regular salad dressings.

Nutrition Tips

1. All fats are high in calories. Limit serving sizes for good nutrition and health.
2. Nuts and seeds contain small amounts of fiber, protein, and magnesium.
3. If blood pressure is a concern, choose fats in the unsalted form to help lower sodium intake, such as unsalted peanuts.

Selection Tips

1. Check the Nutrition Facts on food labels for serving sizes. One fat exchange is based on a serving size containing 5 grams of fat.
2. When selecting regular margarine, choose those with liquid vegetable oil as the first ingredient. Soft margarines are not as saturated as stick margarines. Soft margarines are more healthful choices. Avoid those listing hydrogenated or partially hydrogenated fat as the first ingredient.
3. When selecting low-fat margarines, look for liquid vegetable oil as the second ingredient. Water is usually the first ingredient.
4. When used in smaller amounts, bacon and peanut butter are counted as fat choices. When used in larger amounts, they are counted as high-fat meat choices.
5. Fat-free salad dressings are on the Other Carbohydrates list and the Free Foods list.
6 See the Free Foods list for nondairy coffee creamers, whipped topping, and fat-free products, such as margarines, salad dressings, mayonnaise, sour cream, cream cheese, and nonstick cooking spray.

Monounsaturated Fats List
One fat exchange equals 5 grams fat and 45 calories.

Avocado, medium ....⅛ (1 oz)
Oil (canola, olive, peanut) ....1 tsp
Olives: ripe (black) ....8 large
   green, stuffed* ....10 large
Nuts
   almonds, cashews ....6 nuts
   mixed (50% peanuts)..6 nuts
   peanuts ....10 nuts
   pecans..4 halves
Peanut butter, smooth or crunchy ....2 tsp
Sesame seeds ....1 Tbsp
Tahini paste ....2 tsp

Polyunsaturated Fats List
One fat exchange equals 5 grams fat and 45 calories.

Margarine: stick, tub, or squeeze ....1 tsp
   lower-fat (30% to 50% vegetable oil) ....1 Tbsp
Mayonnaise: regular ....1 tsp
   reduced-fat ....1 Tbsp
Nuts, walnuts, English ....4 halves
Oil (corn, safflower, soybean) ....1 tsp
Salad dressing: regular* ....1 Tbsp
   reduced-fat ....2 Tbsp
Miracle Whip Salad Dressing® regular...2 tsp
   reduced-fat ....1 Tbsp
Seeds: pumpkin, sunflower ....1 Tbsp

* = 400 mg or more sodium per exchange.

Saturated Fats List**
One fat exchange equals 5 grams fat and 45 calories.

Bacon, cooked...1 slice (20 slices/lb)
Bacon, grease..1 tsp
Butter: stick ....1 tsp
   whipped ....2 tsp
   reduced-fat ....1 Tbsp
Chitterlings, boiled..2 Tbsp (½ oz)
Coconut, sweetened, shredded..2 Tbsp
Cream, half and half ....2 Tbsp
Cream cheese: regular ....1 Tbsp (½ oz)
   reduced-fat ....2 Tbsp (1 oz)
Fatback or salt pork, see below†
Shortening or lard ....1 tsp
Sour cream: regular...2 Tbsp
   reduced-fat ....3 Tbsp

†Use a piece 1 in. x 1 in. x 1/4 in. if you plan to eat the fatback cooked with vegetables. Use a piece 2 in. x 1 in. x 1/2 in. when eating only the vegetables with the fatback removed.
**Saturated fats can raise blood cholesterol levels.

FREE FOODS LIST

A *free food* is any food or drink that contains less than 20 calories or less than 5 grams of carbohydrate per serving. Foods with a serving size listed should be limited to three servings per day. Be sure to spread them out throughout the day. If you eat all three servings at one time, it could affect your blood glucose level. Foods listed without a serving size can be eaten as often as you like.

Fat-free or Reduced-fat Foods

Cream cheese, fat-free ....1 Tbsp
Creamers, nondairy, liquid ....1 Tbsp
Creamers, nondairy, powdered ....2 tsp
Mayonnaise, fat-free...1 Tbsp
Mayonnaise, reduced-fat...1 tsp
Margarine, fat-free..4 Tbsp
Margarine, reduced-fat ....1 tsp
Miracle Whip®, nonfat...1 Tbsp
Miracle Whip®, reduced-fat ....1 tsp
Nonstick cooking spray
Salad dressing, fat-free ....1 Tbsp
Salad dressing, fat-free, Italian ....2 Tbsp
Salsa ....¼ cup
Sour cream, fat-free, reduced-fat ....1 Tbsp
Whipped topping, regular or light..2 Tbsp

Sugar-free or Low-sugar Foods

Candy, hard, sugar-free ....1 candy
Gelatin dessert, sugar-free
Gelatin, unflavored
Gum, sugar-free
Jam or jelly, low-sugar or light ....2 tsp
Sugar substitutes†
Syrup, sugar-free ....2 Tbsp

†Sugar substitutes, alternatives, or replacements that are approved by the Food and Drug Administration (FDA) are safe to use. Common brand names include:

Equal® (aspartame)
Sprinkle Sweet® (saccharin)
Sweet One® (acesulfame K)
Sweet-10® (saccharin)
Sugar Twin® (saccharin)
Sweet 'n Low®(saccharin)

Drinks

Bouillon, broth, consommé*
Bouillon or broth, low-sodium
Carbonated or mineral water
Cocoa powder, unsweetened..1 Tbsp
Coffee
Club soda
Diet soft drinks, sugar-free
Drink mixes, sugar-free
Tea
Tonic water, sugar-free

Condiments

Catsup...1 Tbsp
Horseradish
Lemon Juice
Lime juice
Mustard
Pickles, dill* ....1 ½ large
Soy sauce, regular or light*
Taco sauce ....1 Tbsp
Vinegar

Seasonings

Be careful with seasonings that contain sodium or are salts, such as garlic or celery salt, and lemon pepper.

Flavoring extracts
Garlic
Herbs, fresh or dried
Pimiento
Spices
Tabasco* or hot pepper sauce
Wine, used in cooking
Worcestershire sauce

* = 400 mg or more of sodium per choice.

COMBINATION FOODS LIST

Many of the foods we eat are mixed together in various combinations. These combination foods do not fit into any one exchange list. Often it is hard to tell what is in a
casserole dish or prepared food item. This is a list of exchanges for some typical combination foods. This list will help you fit these foods into your meal plan. Ask your
dietitian for information about any other combination foods you would like to eat.

Food	Serving Size	Exchanges per Serving
Entrees		
Tuna noodle casserole, lasagna, spaghetti with meatballs, chili with beans, macaroni and cheese*	1 cup (8 oz)	2 carbohydrates, 2 medium-fat meats
Chow mein (without noodles or rice)	2 cups (16 oz)	1 carbohydrate, 2 lean meats
Pizza, cheese, thin crust*	¼ of 10 in (5 oz)	2 carbohydrates, 2 medium-fat meats, 1 fat
Pizza, meat topping, thin crust*	¼ of 10 in (5 oz)	2 carbohydrates, 2 medium-fat meats, 2 fats
Pot pie*	1 (7 oz)	2 carbohydrates, 1 medium-fat meat, 4 fats
Frozen entrees		
Salisbury steak with gravy, mashed potato*	1 (11 oz)	2 carbohydrates, 3 medium-fat meats, 3–4 fats
Turkey with gravy, mashed potato, dressing*	1 (11 oz)	2 carbohydrates, 2 medium-fat meats, 2 fats
Entree with less than 300 calories*	1 (8 oz)	2 carbohydrates, 3 lean meats
Soups		
Bean*	1 cup	1 carbohydrate, 1 very lean meat
Cream (made with water)*	1 cup (8 oz)	1 carbohydrate, 1 fat
Split pea (made with water)*	½ cup (4 oz)	1 carbohydrate
Tomato (made with water)*	1 cup (8 oz)	1 carbohydrate
Vegetable beef, chicken noodle, or other broth-type*	1 cup (8 oz)	1 carbohydrate

* = 400 mg or more sodium per exchange.

FAST FOODS**

Food	Serving Size	Exchanges per Serving
Burritos with beef*	2	4 carbohydrates, 2 medium-fat meats, 2 fats
Chicken nuggets*	6	1 carbohydrate, 2 medium-fat meats, 1 fat
Chicken breast and wing, breaded and fried*	1 each	1 carbohydrate, 4 medium-fat meats, 2 fats
Fish sandwich/tartar sauce*	1	3 carbohydrates, 1 medium-fat meat, 3 fats
French fries, thin	20–25	2 carbohydrates, 2 fats
Hamburger, regular	1	2 carbohydrates, 2 medium-fat meats
Hamburger, large*	1	2 carbohydrates, 3 medium-fat meats, 1 fat
Hot dog with bun*	1	1 carbohydrate, 1 high-fat meat, 1 fat
Individual pan pizza*	1	5 carbohydrates, 3 medium-fat meats, 3 fats
Soft-serve cone	1 medium	2 carbohydrates, 1 fat
Submarine sandwich*	1 sub (6 in.)	3 carbohydrates, 1 vegetable, 2 medium-fat meats, 1 fat
Taco, hard shell*	1 (6 oz)	2 carbohydrates, 2 medium-fat meats, 2 fats
Taco, soft shell*	1 (3 oz)	1 carbohydrate, 1 medium-fat meat, 1 fat

* = 400 mg or more of sodium per serving.
**Ask at your fast-food restaurant for nutrition information about your favorite fast foods.

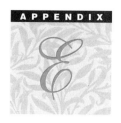

Resources for Developing Healthy Menu Items

RESOURCES FOR DEVELOPING A NUTRITION PROGRAM

1. American Culinary Federation, P.O. Box 3466, St. Augustine, Florida, 904-824-4468. The ACF, which certifies chefs, requires a nutrition course for certification or recertification. Some local chapters offer the nutrition course, often through a community college, or it is available as a self-study course through the ACF.

2. American Dietetic Association, 430 North Michigan Avenue, Chicago, Illinois, 312-280-5000. The ADA maintains a directory of consulting nutritionists who can help develop and implement a nutrition program.

3. American Heart Association, National Center, 7320 Greenville Avenue, Dallas, Texas, 214-748-7212. The local chapter of the AHA can give you much help in some or all phases of developing and marketing a nutrition program. They are an excellent resource for recipes and will work with you to develop a "Dine to Your Heart's Content" program that meets AHA nutritional goals as well as your marketing needs.

4. Culinary Institute of America, Hyde Park, New York, 914-452-9600. The CIA offers a nutrition class that covers the basics of light cooking.

5. Johnson and Wales College, Department of Continuing Education, 8 Abbott Park Place, Providence, Rhode Island, 401-456-1120. Johnson and Wales offers a nutrition course that can be taken during the week or on weekends.

6. Check with local colleges and cooking schools to see if they offer any classes in nutritious cooking.

7. Two publications on public relations:

Media Resource Guide
Foundation for American
  Communications
3800 Barham Blvd, Suite 409
Los Angeles, CA 90068

The New, Revised Restaurateur's Easy
  Guide to Do-It-Yourself Public Relations
Traina-Bessell Communications
676 W. Dana Street
Mountain View, CA 94041

FOR RECIPES

Nutritious Recipes

American Heart Association
  7320 Greenville Avenue
  Dallas, TX 75231
  214-750-5362
  Creative Cuisine Recipes

American Spice Trade Association
  Box 1267
  Englewood Cliffs, NJ 07632
  201-568-2163
  Information and recipes using spices

Beef Industry Council
  A Division of the National Live Stock
    and Meat Board
  444 North Michigan Avenue
  Chicago, IL 60611
  312-467-5520
  The Lighter Side of Beef recipes,
    recipes for barbecuing beef

General Foods
  250 North Street
  White Plains, NY 10625
  914-335-3381
  Recipes using sugar-free Jell-O and
    puddings

Idaho Potato Commission
  P.O. Box 1068
  Boise, ID 83701
  208-334-2350
  Spa Series calorie-controlled quantity
    recipes

Nabisco Brands
  Foodservice Division
  Marketing Department
  100 DeForest Avenue
  East Hanover, NJ 07936
  Recipes using Egg Beater,
    Cholesterol-free 99% Real Egg
    Product

National Fisheries Institute, Inc.
  2000 M Street, N.W., Suite 580
  Washillgton, DC 20036
  202-296-3428
  Recipes using nutritious fish

National Turkey Federation
  11319 Sunset Hills Road
  Reston, VA 22090
  703-135-7206
  Recipe cards using turkey

Product Marketing Association
  700 Barksdale Plaza
  Newark, DE 19711
  302-738-7100
  Food For You Series includes
    nutritious recipes

For Drink and Food Ideas

California Strawberry Advisory Board
   P.O. Box 269
   Watsonville, CA 95077
   408-724-1301

Canada Dry Corp.
   2600 Century Highway
   Atlanta, GA 30345
   404-982-8871

Del Monte Corp. (Hawaiian Punch)
   P.O. Box 3575
   San Francisco, CA 94119-3575
   415-442-4906

Foods and Wine from France
   24 East 21st Street
   New York, NY 10010

E & J Gallo Winery
   600 Yosemite Blvd.
   Modesto, CA 95354
   209-579-4059

Miller Brewing Co.
   3939 W. Highland Blvd.
   Milwaukee, WI 53201
   414-931-2785

Moore's Food Products (appetizers)
   1221 Broadway
   Oakland, CA 94612
   800-556-1234

National Cherry Foundation
   190 Queen Anne N.
   Seattle, WA 98109
   206-285-7082

North American Blueberry Council
   P.O. Box 166
   Marmora, NJ 08223
   609-399-1559

Ocean Spray Cranberry
   Water St.
   Plymouth, MA 02360
   617-747-1000

Joseph E. Seagram & Sons
   375 Park Avenue
   New York, NY 10152-0192
   212-572-7137

Welchs Grape Juice
   100 Main St.
   Concord, MA 01742
   617-371-1000

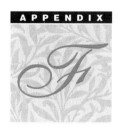

Metric Conversion of Recipes

Metric Equivalents

Capacity or Volume	*Weight*
1000 milliliters (ml) = 1 liter (1)	1000 grams (g) = 1 kilogram (kg)

Conversion Table: English to Metric

Capacity		*Weight*	
English	*Metric*	*English*	*Metric*
1 quart	= 946 milliliters	2.2 pounds	= 1 kilogram
34 fluid ounces	= 1 liter	1 pound	= 454 grams
1 cup	= 240 milliliters	1/2 pound	= 226 grams
1/2 cup	= 120 milliliters	1/4 pound	= 113 grams
1/4 cup	= 60 milliliters	1 ounce	= 28 grams
1 fluid ounce	= 30 milliliters		
3 tablespoons	= 45 milliliters		
2 tablespoons	= 30 milliliters		
1 tablespoon	= 15 milliliters		
2 teaspoons	= 10 milliliters		
1 teaspoon	= 5 milliliters		
1/2 teaspoon	= 2 ½ milliliters		

Conversion Table: Metric to English

Capacity		*Weight*	
Metric	*English*	*Metric*	*English*
4 liters	= 1.06 gallons	1 kilogram	= 2.2 pounds
1 liter	= 1.06 quarts	500 grams	= 1.1 pounds
500 milliliters	= 1.06 pints	250 grams	= 8.8 ounces
240 milliliters	= 1 cup	100 grams	= 3.5 ounces
15 milliliters	= 1 tablespoon	30 grams	= 1.1 ounces
5 milliliters	= 1 teaspoon	28 grams	= 1 ounce

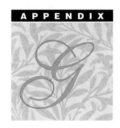

APPENDIX

Nutrient Analysis Programs

CBORD DIET ANALYZER SYSTEM
CBORD Group, Inc.
61 Brown Road
Ithaca, NY 14850

TELEPHONE: (607) 257-2410
TYPE OF PROGRAM: Nutrient Analysis
COST: $995
HARDWARE: IBM Compatible
VERSION: 3.0.3
TARGET AUDIENCE: Dietitians
PROGRAM INFORMATION CURRENT AS OF: 8/4/94
DESCRIPTION: Part of CBORD's Menu Management Family of Systems, this program is a tool for nutrition counseling, recipe and menu analysis. Database can include up to 2400 food items, and analyzes up to 32 nutritive components. Includes on-line help, nutrition guidelines, diaries, recalls, histograms, and graphs.

COMPREHENSIVE NUTRITION CONSULTANT
Carolina Nutritionworks, Inc.
5248 Inverness Drive
Durham, NC 27712

TELEPHONE: (919) 383-2570
TYPE OF PROGRAM: Nutrient Analysis
COST: $79.95
HARDWARE: IBM Compatible
VERSION: 1.1
TARGET AUDIENCE Dietitians
PROGRAM INFORMATION CURRENT AS OF: 8/4/94
DESCRIPTION: Calculates energy requirements, analyzes diet histories and recipes for 20 nutritive components. Database includes 2800 foods and can be expanded. Prints up to one month's individualized menus.

COMPUTRITION: NUTRITIONAL SOFTWARE LIBRARY (NSL) III
Computrition, Inc.
9121 Oakdale Avenue
Suite 201
Chatsworth, CA 91311

TELEPHONE: (818) 701-5544
             (800) 222-4488
TYPE OF PPOGRAM: Nutrient Analysis, Menu Planning
COST: $295 to $695 (for modules 1 to 3)
HARDWARE: IBM Compatible
TARGET AUDIENCE: Health Professionals
PROGRAM INFORMATION CURRENT AS OF: 9/12/94
DESCRIPTION: Analyzes intakes and recipes, creates menus based on preferences, and includes weight control plans. Available on Government Services Administration (GSA) list. Program with larger 17,000 food database also available for both single and multi users. Price ranges from $3,500 to $6,500 plus annual fee.

DIET BALANCER, THE
Nutridata Software Corporation
P.O. Box 769
Wappinger Falls, NY 12590

TELEPHONE: (800) 922-2988
TYPE OF PPOGRAM: Nutrient Analysis, Menu Planning
COST: $59.95 for IBM version; $69.95 for MacIntosh version
HARDWARE: IBM; MacIntosh
VERSION: 3.0
TARGET AUDIENCE: Health Professionals, Dietitians
PROGRAM INFORMATION CURRENT AS OF: 8/8/94
DESCRIPTION: Analyzes diets for 26 nutritive components in over 1700 foods. Foods can be added. Highlights excess fat, sodium, and cholesterol. Includes exercise plan. Supplemental disk containing meal plans for modified diets, including low fat, diabetic, and calorie is available.

DIET EASY
First Databank Division
The Hearst Corporation
1111 Bayhill Drive
San Bruno, CA 94066

TELEPHONE: (415) 266-8016
             (800) 289-1701
TYPE OF PROGRAM: Nutrient Analysis
COST: $49 for 2,025 foods; $249 for 5,000 foods; $349 for 8,500
HARDWARE: IBM compatible, requires graphics driver for Food Guide Pyramid and

pie chart graphics. Requires 640K RAM (550K available); 3 MB hard drive space (6 MB for installation only), and a parallel printer.
VERSION: 1.0
TARGET AUDIENCE: Consumers, Health Professionals, Dietitans
PROGRAM INFORMATION CURRENT AS OF: 1/3/95
DESCRIPTION: 2,025; 5,000; or 8,500 foods. Ready-to-Cook (RTC) foods included with 5,000 and 8,500 food versions. Foods can be added. 30 nutritive components, including alcohol. Analyzes diets, foods, and recipes. Creates Food Guide Pyramid graphic, circular graphs (pie charts), recipe cards, and bar graphs. Calculates exchanges, energy expenditure, and food costs. Includes exercise/activity component, weight control component, and text editor. Sorts foods by nutrient. Compares intake to RDA, USRDA, and RNI (Canada).

DIETARY ANALYSIS PROGRAM
USDA/Human Nutrition Information Service
5285 Port Royal Road
Springfield, VA 22161

TELEPHONE: (703) 487-4650
TYPE OF PROGRAM: Nutrient Analysis
COST: $60
HARDWARE: IBM Compatible
VERSION: 1.41
TARGET AUDIENCE: Consumers
PROGRAM INFORMATION CURRENT AS OF: 8/8/94
DESCRIPTION: Analyzes diets of up to 3 days for 27 nutritive components and 850 foods. Available from National Technical Information Service. Use accession #PB90-501826 (low density) for 5¼"; 360K disks; PB90-504101 (high density) for 5¼", 1.2 MB disks; PB90-504085 (low density) for 3½", 720K disks; and PB90-504093 (high density) for 3½", 1.44 MB disks. Also, available at no charge for the Nurtient Data Bank Bulletin Board. Access with a modem and communications software at (301) 436-5078. Time to download is 20 minutes.

DINE FOR WINDOWS
DINE Systems, Inc.
586 N. French Road
Amherst, NY 14228

TELEPHONE: (716) 688-2400
TYPE OF PROGRAM: Nutrient Analysis
COST: $295 for DINE FOR WINDOWS version 3.4; call for other prices
HARDWARE: IBM Compatible, Apple IIc, IIc+, IIgs, lie. Requires mouse.
VERSION: IBM: 3.4; Apple: 1.0
TARGET AUDIENCE: Health Professionals, Dietitians
PROGRAM INFORMATION CURRENT AS OF: 8/8/94
DESCRIPTION: Analyzes diets and recipes for 26 nutritive components from over

5600 foods and gives "DINE score" for intake. Includes 194 item database, food and nutrient search function, choice of standards (U.S., Canadian, National Cholesterol Education Program, pregnant or lactating). Includes Nutrition Guide Book and Activity and Food Record Book.

DINE HEALTHY
DINE Systems, Inc.
586 N. French Road
Amherst, NY 14228

TELEPHONE: (716) 688-2400
TYPE OF PROGRAM: Nutrient Analysis, Menu Planning
COST: $99
HARDWARE: IBM Compatible with at least a 496DX-33 with Windows 3.1 or later; or Macintosh with System 6.0.4 or later. Both versions require 2MB RAM and 7MB hard drive space.
VERSION: 1.0.6 for Macintosh; 1.2.1 for IBM
TARGET AUDIENCE: Consumers, Some Health Professionals
PROGRAM INFORMATION CURRENT AS OF: 11/1/94
DESCRIPTION: Program focus: low-fat eating. 7,000 foods. Foods can be added in either standard or food label format. 26 nutritive components, including animal protein, plant protein, aspartame, caffeine, water, and alcohol, with no missing values. Analyzes foods, diets, recipes, and menus. Creates bar charts. Calculates DINE Score. Includes exercise activity component. Weight control component, diet record form, and sample 7-day menu plans at three calorie levels. Sorts foods by nutritive components. Compares foods in food label format.

FOOD PROCESSOR—BASIC VERSION
ESHA Research
P.O. Box 13028
Salem, OR 97309

TELEPHONE: (503) 585-6242
         (800) 659-ESHA
TYPE OF PROGRAM: Nutrient Analysis
COST: $295
HARDWARE: Macintosh; IBM Compatible
VERSION: 2.1 (version 6.0 now available)
TARGET AUDIENCE: Dieticians, Health Professionals
PROGRAM INFORMATION CURRENT AS OF: 11/17/94
DESCRIPTION: Analyzes daily intakes, recipes, and menus. 37 nutritive components in over 2500 foods. (Basic version 6.0) 54 nutritive components in over 5800 foods. Nutrient excesses or deficiencies are shown in numeric/graphic form. Compares analysis to U.S. or Canadian dietary guidelines. Foods can be added and additional databases containing a total of over 11,000 foods are available. IBM version includes 300 exercises that can be used for the personal profile. Free demonstration disk is available from producer.

FOOD PROCESSOR—PLUS
ESHA Research
P.O. Box 13028
Salem, OR 97309

TELEPHONE: (503) 585-6242
            (800) 659-ESHA
TYPE OF PROGRAM: Nutrient Analysis
COST: $495
HARDWARE: IBM Compatible
VERSION: 6.0
TARGET AUDIENCE: Dietitians, Health Professionals
PROGRAM INFORMATION CURRENT AS OF: 11/17/94
DESCRIPTION: Analyzes diets, recipes, and menus. 114 nutritive components

MACDIET
Drexel University/Nutrition Program
32nd & Chestnut Sts.
Philadelphia, PA 19104

TELEPHONE: (215) 895-2418
TYPE OF PROGRAM: Nutrient Analysis
COST: $99 for MacDiet; $129 for MacDiet Academic
HARDWARE: MacIntosh
TARGET AUDIENCE: Dietitians, Health Professionals
PROGRAM INFORMATION CURRENT AS OF: 8/3/94
DESCRIPTION: Program focus: analyzes foods and diets for 24 nutritive components in 5200 foods. Foods can be added. Intake is compared to recommended servings of food groups in the Food Guide Pyramid. Program includes on-screen documentation in Hypercard.

NUTRIENT ANALYSIS SYSTEM 2
DDA Software
P.O. Box 477
Long Valley, NJ 07853

TELEPHONE: (908) 876-5580
TYPE OF PROGRAM: Nutrient Analysis
COST: $289.95
HARDWARE: IBM Compatible or MacIntosh
VERSION: 5.0 for IBM; 4.0 for MacIntosh
TARGET AUDIENCE: Nutritionists, Registered Dieticians, Educators, Health Professionals, Food Service Operations.
PROGRAM INFORMATION CURRENT AS OF: 3/22/95
DESCRIPTION: 2700 foods. Foods and nutrients can be added. 24 nutritive components. Analyzes diets, meals, menus, and recipes. Calculates calorie expenditure.

Compares intake to five dietary standards. Creates spreadsheets, tabular graphs, client printouts, and bar graphs. Version 5.0 has pull down menus, creates nutrient labels, gives food units by weight or serving size, and features entry of food costs while selecting foods for analysis.

NUTRIFIT

Colorado State University Cooperative Extension
Department of Food Science and Human Nutrition
200 Gifford Building
Fort Collins, CO 80523

TELEPHONE: (303) 491-7334
TYPE OF PROGRAM: Nutrient Analysis
COST: $95 (Discount to Cooperative Extension staff)
HARDWARE: IBM Compatible, 640K RAM, Hard Disk, Printer required.
VERSION: 2.0
TARGET AUDIENCE: Nutritionists, Educators, Researchers, Physicians, and Organizations with Cycle Menus.
PROGRAM INFORMATION CURRENT AS OF: 3/22/96
DESCRIPTION: 3000 foods. 26 nutritive components. Analyzes diets, cycle menus, and recipes. Prints nutrient density table, total nutrient content for ingredients or food items, nutrient and caloric distribution profile, comparison with recommended ranges, and foods to choose more or less often to improve diet quality.

NUTRITION PRO!

ESHA Research
P.O. Box 13028
Salem, OR 97309

TELEPHONE: (503) 585-6242
　　　　　　(800) 659-ESHA
TYPE OF PROGRAM: Nutrient Analysis, Nutrition Education
COST: $79 for full version; $29 for student version
HARDWARE: IBM compatible
VERSION: 1.1
TARGET AUDIENCE: Consumers, Students
PROGRAM INFORMATION CURRENT AS OF: 1/4/95
DESCRIPTION: Consumer version of The Food Processor. 2000 foods. Foods can be added in the full version only. Includes fast foods, convenience foods, and vegetarian foods. 18 nutritive components. Analyzes diets, menus, and recipes. Averages one week's intake. Can search for foods high or low in a nutrient. Calculates exchanges. Creates reports and graphs. Includes exercise/activity plan and weight control plan. Student version has fewer food selections and exercises/activities and does not include the food exchanges or nutrient search.

NUTRITIONIST IV - DIET ANALYSIS
First Databank Division
The Hearst Corporation
1111 Bayhill Drive
San Bruno, CA 94066

Telephone: (415) 266-8016
         (800) 289-1701
Type of Program: Nutrient Analysis
Cost: $495
Hardware: IBM Compatible. DOS version: 640 KB RAM, 6 MB hard disk space; DOS 3.3 or later, HP or compatible laser printer. Windows version: 386 processor or greater, 10 MB hard disk space, 4 MB RAM; DOS 5.0 or later, Windows 3.1, a mouse.
Version: DOS 3.5; Windows 3.5
Target Audience: Health Professionals
Program Information Current as of: 3/22/95
Description: 12,000 foods (foods can be added). 76 nutritive componets (including amino acids, omega-3 fatty acids). Analyzes foods, diets, recipes, food frequencies. Calculates exchanges, ideal body weight, calories expended from activities. Creates pie charts, spreadsheets, bar graphs, cycle menus, shopping lists, Food Guide Pyramid graphic. Includes exercise/activity component, weight control component, text editor. Interfaces with mouse systems and optical scanners.

SANTE CD-ROM
Hopkins Technology
421 Hazel Lane
Hopkins, MN 55343-7117

Telephone: (612) 931-9376
Type of Program: Nutrient Analysis
Cost: $59.95
Hardware: IBM compatible; requires CD-ROM drive
Version: 3.0
Target Audience: Consumers
Program Information Current as of: 7/11/94
Description: 18,000 foods and foods can be added. 30 nutritive components. Analyzes foods, diets, menus, and recipes. Creates menu plans, shopping lists, and pie charts. Calculates food costs, recipe size adjustments, ratios, and calorie expenditure. Includes recipe files, exercise/activity and weight control components, food buying and storage tips, and nutrition and health guidelines.

Glossary

ABSORPTION The passage of digested nutrients through the walls of the intestines into the intestinal cells. Nutrients are then transported through the body via the blood or lymph systems. A few nutrients are absorbed elsewhere in the gastrointestinal tract, such as the stomach.

ACID-BASE BALANCE The process by which the body buffers the acids and bases normally produced in the body so the blood is neither too acidic nor basic.

ACIDOSIS A dangerous condition in which the blood is too acidic.

ADEQUATE DIET A diet that provides enough of the essential nutrients and calories.

ALKALOSIS A dangerous condition in which the blood is too basic.

AMINO ACIDS The building blocks of protein. There are 20 different amino acids, each consisting of a backbone to which a side chain is attached.

AMINO ACID POOL The overall amount of amino acids distributed in the blood, organs, and body cells. Amino acids from foods, as well as amino acids from body proteins that have been dismantled, stock these pools.

AMNIOTIC SAC The protective bag, or sac, that cushions and protects the fetus during pregnancy.

ANABOLISM The metabolic process by which body tissues and substances are built. Metabolism has two functions: building up (anabolism) and breaking down (catabolism).

ANGINA Symptoms of pressing, intense pain in the heart area because the heart muscle gets insufficient blood. Sometimes stress or exertion can cause angina.

ANOREXIA Lack of appetite.

ANOREXIA NERVOSA An eating disorder most prevalent in adolescent females who starve themselves.

ANTIBODIES Proteins in the blood that bind with foreign bodies or invaders.

ANTIGENS Foreign invaders in the body.

ANTIOXIDENT A compound that combines with oxygen to prevent oxygen from oxidizing, or destroying, important substances. Antioxidants prevent the oxidation of unsaturated fatty acids in the cell membrane, DNA (the genetic code), and other cell parts that substances called free radicals try to destroy.

ANUS The opening of the digestive tract through which feces travels out of the body.

ARTERIAL BLOOD PRESSURE The pressure of blood within arteries as it is pumped through the body by the heart.

ATHEROSCLEROSIS The most common form of artery disease, characterized by plaque buildup along artery walls.

BABY BOTTLE TOOTH DECAY Serious tooth decay in babies caused by letting a baby go to bed with a bottle of juice, formula, cow's milk, or breast milk.

BALANCED DIET A diet that does not overemphasize certain foods at the expense of other foods. For example, if you drink a lot of soft drinks, you may not be drinking much milk, a rich source of the mineral calcium.

BALSAMIC VINEGAR A dark brown vinegar with a rich sweet-sour flavor, made from the juice of a very sweet white grape and aged for at least ten years.

BASAL METABOLIC NEEDS The energy needs of your body when at rest and awake.

BASAL METABOLISM The minimum energy needed by the body for vital functions when at rest and awake.

BASIC FOUR FOOD GROUPS An outmoded food-group system based on four groups of foods.

BETA-CAROTENE A precursor of vitamin A that functions as an antioxidant in the body. Beta-carotene is the most abundant carotenoid.

BILE A yellow-green liver secretion that is stored in the gallbladder and released when fat enters the small intestine because it emulsifies fats.

BILE ACIDS A component of bile that aids in the digestion and absorption of fats in the duodenum of the small intestine.

BINGE EATING DISORDER An eating disorder characterized by episodes of uncontrolled eating or binging.

BIOTECHNOLOGY The use of genetic engineering to create an abundant supply of better tasting and more nutritious foods.

BLOOD CHOLESTEROL Cholesterol circulating in the bloodstream. The blood carries it for use by all parts of the body. A high level of blood cholesterol leads to atherosclerosis and an increased risk of heart disease.

BODY MASS INDEX (BMI) A method used to estimate ideal body weight, calculated as follows:

$$\text{BMI} = \frac{body\ weight\ (in\ kilograms)}{\text{height (in meters)}^2}$$

BOLUS A ball of chewed food that travels from the mouth through the esophagus to the stomach.

BOTTLED WATER Water that is bottled and sold.

BRANDY A distilled spirit made from wine or other fermented fruit juice.

BRIOCHE A French bread made with eggs.

BULIMIA NERVOSA An eating disorder characterized by a destructive pattern of excessive overeating followed by vomiting or other "purging" behaviors to control weight.

CAFE LATTE Espresso coffee with 75 percent steamed milk.

CALORIE A measure of the energy in food, specifically the energy-yielding nutrients. The correct name for calorie is kilocalorie.

CANCER A group of diseases characterized by unrestrained cell division and growth that can disrupt the normal functioning of an organ and also spread beyond the tissue in which it started.

CARBOHYDRATE OR GLYCOGEN LOADING A regimen involving both decreased exercise and increased consumption of carbohydrates before an event to increase the amount of glycogen stores.

CARBOHYDRATES A nutrient group containing carbon, hydrogen, and oxygen that includes sugars, starch, and fibers.

CARCINOGENS Substances that initiate cancer.

CARDIAC SPHINCTER A muscle that relaxes and contracts to move food from the esophagus into the stomach.

CARDIOVASCULAR DISEASE (CVD) A general term for diseases of the heart and blood vessels.

CAROTENOIDS A class of pigments that contribute red, orange, or yellow color to fruits and vegetables. Beta-carotene is the most abundant.

CATABOLISM The metabolic processes by which large, complex molecules are converted to a smaller set of simpler ones.

CEREBRAL HEMORRHAGE A stroke due to a ruptured brain artery.

CHLOROPHYLL A pigment in plants that convert energy from sunlight into energy stored in carbohydrate.

CHOLESTEROL The most abundant sterol (a category of lipids). Cholesterol is a soft, waxy substance present only in foods of animal origin. The body makes enough cholesterol to meet its needs. Cholesterol has a number of important functions in the body and is present in all body parts.

CHUTNEY A condiment of Indian origin made from fruits, vegetables, and herbs.

CHYLOMICRON The lipoprotein responsible for carrying mostly triglycerides, and some cholesterol, from the intestines through the lymph system to the bloodstream.

CHYME A liquid mixture in the stomach that contains partially digested food and stomach secretions.

CIDER VINEGAR A vinegar made from apples.

CIRRHOSIS The final stage of liver disease, seen mostly in alcoholics.

CLUB SODA Filtered, carbonated tap water to which mineral salts are added to give it a unique taste.

COLLAGEN The most abundant protein in the human body. Collagen is a fibrous protein that is a component of skin, bone, teeth, ligaments, tendons, and other connective structures.

COLON The large intestine.

COLOSTRUM A yellowish fluid that is the first secretion to come from the breast a day or so after delivery of a baby. It is rich in proteins, antibodies, and other factors that protect against infectious disease.

COMPLEMENTARY PROTEINS The ability of two protein foods to make up for the lack of certain amino acids in each other.

COMPLETE PROTEINS Food proteins that provide all of the essential amino acids in the proportions needed.

COMPLEX CARBOHYDRATES Long chains of many sugars that include starches and fibers.

CORONARY HEART DISEASE (CHD) Damage to or malfunction of the heart caused by narrowing or blockage of the coronary arteries.

COULIS A sauce consisting primarily of a thick puree, usually of vegetables, but also of fruit. Flavorings such as fresh herbs, and a liquid, such as broth, give it taste and body.

CROISSANTS French breads containing much fat.

CRUCIFEROUS VEGETABLES Members of the cabbage family that contain phytochemicals that might help prevent cancer.

DAILY VALUE A food-label guide to the total daily nutrient amount needed based on a 2000-calorie diet.

DEALCOHOLIZED WINE Wine that contains up to 0.5 percent alcohol.

DENATURATION Alteration of a proteins's three-dimensional form that renders it useless; can be caused by high temperatures, ultraviolet radiation, acids, and bases, agitation or whipping, and high salt concentration.

DENTAL CARIES Tooth decay. To prevent dental caries, you should brush your teeth often, floss your teeth once a day, and try to limit sweets to mealtime.

DEOXYRIBONUCLEIC ACID (DNA) The protein carrier of the genetic code in the cells.

DESIGNER FOODS Foods that are supplemented with ingredients thought to help prevent disease or improve health.

DIABETES MELLITUS A disorder of carbohydrate metabolism characterized by high blood sugar levels and inadequate or nonfunctioning insulin.

DIASTOLIC PRESSURE The pressure in the arteries when the heart is resting between beats—the bottom number in blood pressure.

DIETARY GUIDELINES FOR AMERICANS A periodically revised government booklet that gives dietary advice for Americans.

DIETARY RECOMMENDATIONS Guidelines that discuss specific foods and food groups to eat for optimal health.

DIGESTION The breakdown of food into its components in the mouth, stomach, and small intestine with the help of digestive enzymes. Complex proteins are digested, or broken, down into their amino acid building blocks; complicated sugars are reduced to simple sugars such as glucose; and fat molecules are broken down into fatty acids and glycerol.

DISACCHARIDES Double sugars such as sucrose (table sugar) and lactose (milk sugar).

DIURETICS A category of drugs frequently used to treat hypertension. Diuretics stimulate urination and some may deplete potassium.

DIVERTICULOSIS A disease of the large intestine in which the intestinal walls become weakened, bulge out into pockets, and at times become inflamed.

DOCOSAHEXAENOIC ACID (DHA) An omega-3 fatty acid found in seafood that may reduce the risk of heart disease.

DRAMSHOP ACTS State acts that define liability for liquor sales to customers who injure or kill third parties.

DUODENUM The first segment of the small intestine, about one foot long.

EDEMA Swelling due to an abnormal accumulation of fluid in the intercellular spaces.

EICOSAPENTAENOIC ACID (EPA) An omega-3 fatty acid found in seafood that may reduce the risk of heart disease.

ELECTROLYTES Chemical elements or compounds that ionize in solution and can carry an electric current. The most common electrolytes in the blood are sodium, potassium, and chloride.

EMBRYO The name of the fertilized egg from conception to the eighth week. After the eighth week, it is called a fetus.

EMPYY CALORIES Foods that provide few nutrients for the number of calories they contain.

ENERGY-YIELDING NUTRIENTS Nutrients that can be burned as fuel to provide energy for the body, including carbohydrates, fats, and protein.

ENRICHED FOODS Refined foods, such as white bread, to which nutrients have been added to make up for some of the nutrients lost in processing.

ENZYMES Catalysts in the body.

EPIGLOTTIS The flap that covers the larynx and the opening to the trachea so that food does not enter during swallowing.

ESSENTIAL OR INDISPENSABLE AMINO ACIDS Amino acids that either cannot be made in the body or cannot be made in the quantities needed by the body. These amino acids must therefore be obtained in foods for the body to function properly.

ESSENTIAL FATTY ACIDS Fatty acids that the body cannot produce, making them necessary in the diet: linoleic acid and linolenic acid.

ESSENTIAL HYPERTENSION High blood pressure.

ESOPHAGUS The approximately ten-inch muscular tube that is the part of the gastrointestinal tract that connects the pharynx to the stomach. At the bottom of it is the lower esohageal sphincter.

ESTIMATED MINIMUM REQUIREMENTS National Academy of Sciences' Food and Nutrition Board nutrient requirements for sodium, chloride, and potassium. They are based on what is needed for growth and for replacement of normal daily losses.

ESTIMATED SAFE AND ADEQUATE DAILY DIETARY INTAKE National Academy of Sciences' Food and Nutrition Board nutrient intake recommendations in cases where there is not enough scientific evidence to develop an RDA.

EXCHANGE LISTS FOR MEAL PLANNING A menu-planning guide that groups foods by their calorie, carbohydrate, fat, and protein content. Each listed food has approximately the same amount of calories, carbohydrates, fat, and protein as another listed food, so that any food can be exchanged for any other food on the same list. The Exchange Lists for Meal Planning, developed by the American Diabetes and American Dietetic Association, are used primarily by diabetics, who need to regulate what and how much they eat.

FASTING HYPOGLYCEMIA A type of hypoglycemia in which symptoms occur after not eating for eight or more hours, so it usually occurs during the night or before breakfast.

FAT A nutrient that provides 9 calories a gram. The total fat in food is the sum of the saturated, monounsaturated, and polyunsaturated fats present in food.

FAT-OFF LADLE A ladle that skims fat off the surface of a soup, for instance.

FAT-SEPARATOR PITCHER A pitcher that allows you to pour out the fat from the bottom of the pitcher, where it settles.

FAT-SOLUBLE VITAMINS A group of vitamins that include vitamins A, D, E, and K. They generally occur in foods containing fats and are stored in the body either in the liver or in adipose (fatty) tissue until they are needed.

FAT SUBSTITUTES Ingredients that mimic the functions of fat in foods, and either contain fewer calories than fat or no calories.

FATTY ACIDS Acids found in fats; three fatty acids are present in each triglyceride; may be saturated or unsaturated.

FATTY LIVER The first stage of liver deterioration seen in heavy drinkers.

FETAL ALCOHOL SYNDROME (FAS) A set of symptoms occuring in new-born babies due to alcohol use of the mother during pregnancy. FAS children may show signs of mental retardation, growth retardation, brain damage, and facial deformities.

FETUS The infant in the mother's uterus from 8 weeks after conception until birth.

FIBER Material from plant cells that resists digestion by our digestive enzymes.

FIRST TRIMESTER The first 13 weeks of pregnancy.

FLAVORED OILS Oils that are infused or flavored with ingredients such as fresh herbs, ground spices, and fresh roots.

FLAVORED VINEGARS Vinegars that are infused or flavored with ingredients such as chili peppers, roasted garlic, or any herbs, vegetables, and fruits.

FLAVORINGS Substances that add a new flavor to a dish or modify the original flavor.

FLUOROSIS A condition in which the teeth become mottled and discolored due to high fluoride ingestion.

FOOD ALLERGENS Those parts of food causing allergic reactions.

FOOD ALLERGY An abnormal response of the immune system to an otherwise harmless food.

FOOD GUIDE PYRAMID The most recent food guidance system developed by the U.S. Department of Agriculture.

FOOD INTOLERANCE Symptoms of gas, bloating, constipation, dizziness, or difficulty sleeping after eating certain foods.

FOOD JAG A habit of young children in which they have favorite foods they want to eat frequently.

FOOD PRODUCTS Food that contain parts of whole foods and often have ingredients such as sugars, sugar or fat substitutes, and nutrients added to them.

FREE RADICALS An unstable compound that reacts quickly with other molecules in the body.

FRESH FOODS Raw foods that have not been frozen, processed (such as canned or frozen), or heated, or contain any preservatives.

FROMAGE BLANC A fat-free cheese that can be substituted for ricotta or cottage cheese.

FRUCTOSE A monosaccharide found in fruits and honey. Fructose is the sweetest natural sugar.

FRUIT SMOOTHIES Frozen blends of fruit, milk, and/or fresh or frozen yogurt.

FUSION COOKING The blending of ingredients, flavors, and techniques from various cuisines.

GAG REFLEX A normal reflex stimulated by touching the back of the throat. The gag reflex pulls the tongue back and contracts the throat muscles. If something gets stuck in the back of the throat, the gag reflex often results in vomiting of the food so that the food does not obstruct the windpipe.

GASTROINTESTINAL TRACT A hollow tube running down the middle of the body in which digestion of food and absorption of nutrients takes place. At the top of the tube is the mouth, which connects in turn to the pharynx, esophagus, stomach, small intestine, large intestine, rectum, and anus, where solid wastes leave the body.

GALACTOSE A monosaccharide found linked to glucose to form lactose, or milk sugar.

GELATINIZATION A process in which starches, when heated in liquid, absorb some of the water and swell in size.

GENETIC ENGINEERING A process that allows plant breeders to modify the genetic makeup of a plant species precisely and predictably, creating improved varieties faster and easier than can be done using more traditional plant-breeding techniques.

GLUCOSE The most significant monosaccharide. Glucose is the human body's primary source of energy. Also called dextrose.

GLYCEROL A derivative of carbohydrate that is part of triglycerides.

GLYCOGEN The storage form of glucose in the body.

GRAM A unit of weight. There are 28 grams in 1 ounce.

GROWTH SPURTS Periods of rapid growth.

HEALTHY PEOPLE 2000 A 1990 report from the U.S. Department of Health and Human Services, Public Health Services, designed to improve health-promotion and disease-prevention efforts. Objectives listed in this report aim for specific, measurable changes in what Americans eat, as well as increased accessibility to healthier foods and healthy choices in areas other than nutrition.

HEARTBURN A painful burning sensation in the esophagus caused by acidic stomach contents flowing back into the lower esophagus.

HEIGHT/WEIGHT TABLES Tables that show an appropriate weight for a given height.

HEME IRON The predominant form of iron in animal foods, heme iron is absorbed and used twice as readily as iron in plant foods, called nonheme iron. Animal foods also contain some nonheme iron.

HEMOGLOBIN A conjugated protein in red blood cells made up of two parts: heme and globin. Heme is an iron-containing red pigment that carries oxygen. Globin is the protein part. Hemoglobin enables red blood cells to carry oxygen.

HEMORRHOIDS Enlarged veins in the lower rectum.

HERBS Leaves of certain plants grown in temperate climates.

HIGH-DENSITY LIPOPROTEIN (HDL) Lipoproteins that contain a small amount of cholesterol and carry cholesterol away from body cells and tissues to the liver for excretion from the body. A low HDL level increases the risk of heart disease, so the higher the HDL level, the better. HDL is sometimes called "good" cholesterol.

HIGH-FRUCTOSE CORN SYRUP Corn syrup that has been treated with an enzyme that converts part of the glucose it contains to fructose to make it sweeter.

HOMEOSTASIS A constant internal environment in the body.

HORMONE A chemical messenger in the body.

HUMMUS A chickpea-based dip or spread.

HYDROCHLORIC ACID A strong acid made by the stomach that aids in protein digestion, destroys harmful bacteria, and increases the ability of calcium and iron to be absorbed.

HYDROGENATION A process in which liquid vegetable oils are converted into solid fats (such as margarine) by the use of heat, hydrogen, and certain metal catalysts.

HYPERGLYCEMIA High blood sugar levels.

HYPERTENSION High blood pressure.

HYPOGLYCEMIA Low blood sugar levels.

ICE MILK A type of ice cream with less fat.

ILEUM The final segment of the small intestine.

IMMUNE RESPONSE The body's response to a foreign substance, such as a virus, in the body.

INCOMPLETE PROTEINS Food proteins that contain at least one limiting amino acid.

INSULIN A hormone that pushes sugar from the blood into the body's cells, resulting in lower, more normal blood sugar levels.

INTRINSIC FACTOR A protein secreted by stomach cells that is necessary for the absorption of vitamin B_{12}.

IONS Charged atoms that have lost or gained electrons and no longer have the same number of electrons as proteins.

IRON-DEFICIENCY ANEMIA A condition in which the size and number of red blood cells are reduced. This condition may result from inadequate iron intake or from blood loss. Symptoms of iron-deficiency anemia include fatigue, pallor, irritability, and lethargy.

IRON OVERLOAD A common genetic disease in which individuals absorb about twice as much iron from their food and supplements as other people. Also called hemochromatosis.

JEJUNUM The second portion of the small intestine between the duodenum and the ileum. The jejunum is about 8 feet long.

KETONE BODIES A group of organic compounds including acetone, acetoacetic acid, and B-hydroxybutyric acid, that occur as intermediate products of fat metabolism. When fat is burned for energy without any carbohydrate present (as can occur during starvation or a complication of diabetes mellitus), the process is incomplete and ketone bodies are produced. An excessive level of ketone bodies can cause the blood to become too acidic (called ketosis).

KWASHIORKOR A type of protein-energy malnutrition characterized by retarded growth and development, a protruding abdomen due to edema (swelling), peeling skin, a loss of normal hair color, irritability, and sadness. Kwashiorkor is associated with poor protein intake and late weaning.

LACTASE An enzyme needed to split lactose into its components in the intestines.

LACTATION The process of producing and secreting milk in the mammary glands.

LACTO-OVOVEGETARIAN Vegetarians who do not eat meat, poultry, or fish but do consume animal products in the form of eggs (ovo) and milk and milk products.

LACTOSE A disaccharide found in milk and milk products that is made of glucose and galactose.

LACTOSE INTOLERANCE An intolerance to milk and most milk products due to a deficiency of the enzyme lactase. Symptoms often include flatulence and diarrhea.

LACTOVEGETARIANS Vegetarians who do not eat meat, poultry, or fish but do consume animal products in the form of milk and milk products.

LANUGO Downy hair on the skin.

LARGE INTESTINE The part of the gastrointestinal tract between the small intestine and the rectum. The large intestine is about 2½ inches wide and 5 feet long.

LECITHIN A phospholipid and a vital component of cell membranes that acts as an emulsifier (a substitute that keeps fats in solution). Lecithin is not an essential nutrient.

LEGUMES Dried beans, peas, and lentils.

LIGHT BEERS Beers with one-third to one-half less alcohol and calories than regular beers.

LIMITING AMINO ACID An essential amino acid in lowest concentration in a protein.

LINEOLIC ACID An essential fatty acid.

LINOLENIC ACID An essential fatty acid.

LIPID A group of fatty substances, including cholesterol and triglycerides, present in blood and body tissues.

LIPOPROTEIN LIPASE An enzyme that breaks down triglycerides in the blood into fatty acids and glycerol so they can be absorbed into the body's cells.

LIPOPROTEINS Protein-coated packages that carry fat and cholesterol through the bloodstream. They are classified according to their density.

LIQUEURS Brandies or other spirits sweetened and flavored with natural flavors.

LOW BIRTH WEIGHT BABY A newborn who weighs less than 5½ pounds. These babies are at higher risk for disease and experience more difficulties surviving the first year.

LOW-DENSITY LIPOPROTEIN (LDL) Lipoproteins that contain most of the cholesterol in the blood. LDL carries cholesterol to body tissues, including the arteries. For this reason, a high LDL level increases the risk of heart disease.

MAJOR MINERALS. *See* **MINERALS.**

MALTOSE A disaccharide made of two glucose units bonded together.

MANNITOL A sugar alcohol.

MARASMUS A type of protein-energy malnutrition characterized by gross underweight, no fat stores, and wasting away of muscles. Marasmus is usually associated with severe food shortage, prolonged semistarvation, or early weaning.

MARINADES Liquids in which meat, poultry, or fish are soaked to soften them and give them flavor.

MARKETING Ascertaining the needs and wants of the consumer, creating the product-service mix that satisfies these needs and wants, and promoting and selling the product-service mix in order to generate a level of income satisfactory to the management and stockholders of an organization (Reid, 1989).

MARKETING CYCLE A cycle encompassing the following steps.
- Ascertaining the needs and wants of the consumer
- Creating the product-service mix that satisfies these needs and wants
- Promoting and selling the product-service mix in order to generate a level of income satisfactory to the management and stockholders of the organization (Reid, 1989).

MEGADOSE A supplement intake of 10 times the RDA of a vitamin or mineral.

MEGALOBLASTIC ANEMIA A form of anemia caused by a deficiency of vitamin B_{12} and folate and characterized by large, immature red blood cells.

METABOLISM All the chemical processes by which nutrients are used to support life.

MILD FLUOROSIS A condition in which small, white, virtually invisible opaque areas appear on the teeth due to intake of too much fluoride.

MILD OBESITY 20 to 40 percent over desirable weight.

MILK LETDOWN The process by which milk comes out of the mother's breast to feed the baby. Sucking causes the release of a hormone (oxytocin) that allows milk letdown.

MINERALS Naturally occurring, inorganic chemical elements that form a class of nutrients. Some minerals are needed in relatively large amounts in the diet—over 100 milligrams daily. These minerals are called major minerals and include calcium, chloride, magnesium, phosphorus, potassium, sodium, and sulfur. Other minerals, called trace minerals or trace elements, are needed in smaller amounts—less than 100 milligrams daily. The trace minerals include chromium, cobalt, copper, fluoride, iodine, iron, manganese, molybdenum, selenium, and zinc.

MINERAL WATER Water that must come from a protected underground source and contain at least 250 parts per million in total dissolved solids.

MOCKTAILS Drinks made to resemble mixed alcoholic drinks but containing no alcohol.

MODERATE DIET A diet that avoids excessive amounts of calories or any particular food or nutrient.

MODERATE OBESITY 10 to 19 percent over desirable weight.

MONOGLYCERIDES Triglycerides with only one fatty acid.

MONOSACCHARIDES Single sugars such as glucose or fructose. The monosaccharides are the building blocks of other carbohydrates.

MONOUNSATURATED FAT A monounsaturated triglyceride containing at least one monounsaturated fatty acid. Monounsaturated fats are found in greatest amounts in plant foods, including olive and canola oil.

MONOUNSATURATED FATTY ACID A fatty acid that contains only one double bond in the chain (*mono* means one).

MORNING SICKNESS Symptoms, especially nausea and vomiting, that occur in some women during the first half of pregnancy. Morning sickness is really a misnomer, since the symptoms can occur at any time of the day.

MYOCARDIAL ISCHEMIA A temporary injury to heart cells caused by a lack of blood flow and oxygen.

MYOGLOBIN An iron-containing protein found in muscles that stores and carries oxygen.

NEGATIVE NITROGEN BALANCE A condition in which the body excretes more protein than is taken in. Negative nitrogen balance can occur during starvation and certain illnesses.

NEURAL TUBE The embryonic tissue that develops into the brain and spinal cord.

NEURAL TUBE DEFECTS A group of defects of the brain and/or spinal cord that are caused by failure of the neural tube to close during early pregnancy. Such defects include spina bifida and meningocele.

NEUROTRANSMITTERS Chemical messengers released at the end of the nerve cell to stimulate or inhibit a second cell, which may be another nerve cell, a muscle cell, or a gland cell.

NIGHT BLINDNESS A condition caused by insufficient vitamin A in which it takes longer to adjust to dim lights after seeing a bright flash of light (such as oncoming car headlights) at night. This is an early sign of vitamin A deficiency.

NITROGEN BALANCE The amount of nitrogen taken in by mouth compared with the amount excreted in a given period of time.

NONALCOHOLIC BEERS Beers that contain one-half of 1 percent or less of alcohol.

NONHEME IROM A form of iron found in all plant sources of iron and also as part of the iron in animal food sources. Nonheme iron is less readily absorbed than heme iron.

NONNUTRITIVE SWEETENERS Sweeteners such as aspartame that contain either no or very few calories.

NONSTICK PANS Pans that require little or no oil for cooking or baking.

NUTRIENT The nourishing substances in food. They provide energy and promote body growth and maintenance. In addition, nutrients regulate the many body processes, such as heart rate and digestion, and support the bodys' optimum health and growth. The six groups of nutrients are **carbohydrates**, **lipids**, **proteins**, **vitamins**, **minerals**, and **water**.

NUTRIENT CONTENT CLAIMS Claims about the nutrient composition of a food that are written on food labels.

NUTRIENT-DENSE FOODS Foods that contain many nutrients for the calories they provide.

NUTRIENT DENSITY The nutrient content of a food expressed in relation to its calories.

NUTRITION A science that studies nutrients in foods and the body and their action, interaction, and balance in relation to health and disease. Nutrition also examines the processes by which an organism ingests, digests, absorbs, transports, utilizes, and excretes food substances. Nutrition looks at how you select foods and the type of diet you eat.

OBESITY Body weight of 20 percent or more over desirable weight. Obesity is classified into three categories: mild, moderate, and severe.

OLIGOSACCHARIDES A chain of 4 to 10 glucose units.

OILS A form of fat. Oils are usually liquid at room temperature.

ORAL CAVITY The mouth.

ORGANIC FOODS Foods that have been grown without nearly all synthetic insecticides, fungicides, herbicides, and fertilizers.

OSTEOMALACIA A disease of vitamin D deficiency in adults in which the leg and spinal bones soften and may bend. Osteomalacia may be seen in elderly individuals with poor milk intake and little exposure to the sun.

OSTEOPOROSIS The most common bone disease, characterized by loss of bone density and strength. Osteoporosis is associated with debilitating fractures, especially in people 45 and older. It is caused by either a failure of the body to build strong bones during the time bones are being built (up to about age 30 to 35) or to a tremendous loss of bone tissue in midlife.

OVERWEIGHT Body weight between 10 and 19 percent over desirable weight.

OXALIC ACID A substance found in some plant foods, such as spinach, beet greens, Swiss chard, sorrel, and parsley, that prevents calcium absorption. Oxalic acid is also in tea and cocoa.

PALMAR GRASP The ability of a baby from about 6 months of age to grab objects with the palm of the hand.

PEPSIN The principal digestive enzyme of the stomach.

PEPTIDE BONDS The bonds that form between adjoining amino acids.

PERISTALSIS Involuntary muscular contraction that forces food through the entire digestive system.

PERNICIOUS ANEMIA A type of anemia caused by a deficiency of vitamin B_{12} and characterized by macrocytic anemia and deterioration in the functioning of the nervous system that, if untreated, could cause significant and sometimes irreversible damage.

PESCOVEGETARIANS Vegetarians who will eat seafood.

PESTICIDES Chemicals used on crops to protect them from insects, disease, weeds, and fungi.

PHOTOSYNTHESIS A process during which plants convert energy from sunlight into energy stored in carbohydrate.

PHYTOCHEMICALS Minute, cancer-fighting compounds found in plants.

PINCER GRASP The ability of a baby at about 8 months to use the thumb and forefinger together to pick things up.

PLACENTA The organ that develops during the first month of pregnancy that provides for exchange of nutrients and wastes between fetus and mother and secretes the hormones necessary to maintain pregnancy.

PLAQUE (1) Deposits on arterial walls that contains cholesterol, fat, fibrous scar tissue, calcium, and other biological debris. (2) Deposits of bacteria, protein, and polysaccharides found on teeth.

POINT OF UNSATURATION The location of the double bond on unsaturated fatty acids.

POLTPEPTIDES Protein fragments with ten or more amino acids.

POLYSACCHARIDE Another name for complex carbohydrate or long chains of many sugars including starch and fiber.

POLYUNSATURATED FAT A polyunsaturated triglyercide, also called a saturated fat, made of at least one polyunsaturated fatty acid. Polyunsaturated fats are found in greatest amounts in foods from plants, including safflower, sunflower, and corn oil.

POLYUNSATURATED FATTY ACID A fatty acid that contains two or more double bonds in the chain.

POSITIVE NITROGEN BALANCE A condition in which the body excretes less protein than is taken in. Positive nitrogen balance occurs during growth and pregnancy.

POSTPRANDIAL HYPOGLYCEMIA A type of hypoglycemia that occurs generally 2 to 4 hours after meals. This condition has symptoms such as quick heartbeats, shakiness, weakness, anxiety, sweating, and dizziness that mimic anxiety or stress symptoms.

PRECOMPETITION MEAL The meal closest to the time of a competition or athletic event.

PRECURSORS Forms of vitamins that the body changes chemically to active vitamin forms.

PREFORMED VITAMIN A The form of vitamin A called retinol.

PRESS RELEASE A written statement sent out to various news media for publicity purposes. The first paragraph often tells the who, what, when, where, and why of your story.

PRIMARY HYPERTENSION A form of hypertension whose cause is unknown.

PRIMARY STRUCTURE The number and sequence of the amino acids in the protein chain.

PROCESSED FOODS Foods prepared using a certain procedure: cooking (such as frozen pancakes), freezing (frozen dinners), canning (canned vegetables), dehydrating (dried fruits), milling (white flour), culturing with bacteria (yogurt), or adding vitamins and minerals (enriched foods).

PROMOTERS Substances such as fat that advance the development of mutated cells into a tumor.

PROTEINS Major structural parts of animal tissue made up of nitrogen-containing amino acids. Proteins are nutrients that yield 4 calories per gram.

PROTEIN-ENERGY MALNUTRITION A broad spectrum of malnutrition from mild to much more serious cases.

PROVITAMIN A Precursors of vitamin A such as beta carotene.

PUBERTY The time period in which children start to develop secondary sex characteristics and the beginning of the fertile period when gametes (sperm or ovum) are produced.

PUBLICITY Obtaining free space or time in various media to get public notice of a program, book, and so on.

RANCIDITY The deterioration of fat, resulting in undesirable flavors and odors.

REBOUND SCURVY A scurvy-like condition caused by a period of excessive intake of vitamin C supplements followed by a period of normal or low intake of vitamin C.

RECOMMENDED DIETARY ALLOWANCE The levels of intake of essential nutrients that, on the basis of scientific knowledge, are judged by the Food and Nutrition Board to be adequate to meet the known nutrient needs of practically all healthy persons in the United States.

RECTUM The last part of the large intestine in which feces, the waste products of digestion, is stored until elimination.

RELISH A spicy condiment, often made from pickles but also made with other ingredients.

RESETTING THE AMERICAN TABLE: CREATING A NEW ALLIANCE OF TASTE & HEALTH A project sponsored by the American Institute of Wine and Food that works on bridging the gap between taste and nutrition and between culinary professionals and health professionals.

RETINOL One of the active forms of vitamin A. *See also* VITAMIN A.

RETINOL EQUIVALENT The unit of measure for vitamin A activity in both its forms (retinol and beta-carotene). 1 RE = 1ug retinol or 6 ug beta-carotene.

R PROTEIN A compound produced in most body fluids. R protein is particularly important in vitamin B_{12} absorption because it attaches to the vitamin in the stomach and is then released in the small intestine, where it complexes with the intrinsic factor.

RICKETS A childhood disease in which bones do not grow normally, resulting in bowed legs and knock knees. Rickets is generally caused by a vitamin D deficiency.

RISK FACTORS Habits, traits, or conditions of an individual that are associated with an increased chance of developing a disease.

RUBS Dry spices, such as cinnamon, and finely cut herbs such as cilantro, that are put on raw meat to give it flavor. Rubs may be wet or dry.

SALIVA A fluid secreted into the mouth from the salivary glands, that contains important digestive enzymes and lubricates the food so that it may readily pass down the esophagus.

SALSA A sauce made from tomatoes, onions, hot peppers, garlic, and herbs.

SATIETY VALUE The ability of foods to make you feel full.

SATURATED FAT A type of fat containing three saturated fatty acids. Saturated fats are found in greatest amounts in foods from animals, such as fatty cuts of meat, poultry with the skin, whole-milk dairy products, lard, and in some vegetable oils, including coconut, palm kernel, and palm oils. Saturated fat raises blood cholesterol more than any other types of foods.

SATURATED FATTY ACID A type of fatty acid that is filled to capacity with hydrogens.

Scurvy Vitamin C deficiency disease. Scurvy is marked by bleeding gums, weakness, loose teeth, and broken capillaries (small blood vessels) under the skin.

Seasonings Substances used to bring out flavor that is already present in a dish.

Secondary Hypertension Persistently elevated blood pressure caused by a medical problem, such as hormonal abnormality or an inherited narrowing of the aorta (the largest artery leading from the heart).

Secondary Structure The bending and coiling of the protein chain.

Seltzer Filtered, artificially carbonated tap water that generally has no added mineral salts.

Severe Obesity 100 percent or more over desirable weight.

Sherry A fortified wine.

Simple Carbohdyrate Sugars including monosaccharides and disaccharides.

Slurry Flour and water mixed together and then used to thicken.

Small Intestine The digestive tract organ that extends from the stomach to the opening of the large intestine.

Sorbitol A sugar alcohol used in such products as sugarless hard and soft candies, chewing gums, jams and jellies. Excessive amounts of sorbitol can cause diarrhea.

Spices Dried bits of bark, leaves, and berries from tropical plants.

Spina Bifida A birth defect in which parts of the spinal cord are not fused together properly so gaps are present where the spinal cord has little or no protection. Spina bifida is a type of neural tube defect.

Spring water Water collected as it flows naturally to the surface, or when pumped through a hole from the spring source.

Starch A complex carbohydrate made up of a long chain of hundreds to thousands of glucoses linked together; found in grains, legumes, vegetables, and some fruits.

STOMACH A digestive tract organ that prepares food chemically and mechanically so that it can be further digested and absorbed in the small intestine.

STROKE Damage to brain cells resulting from an interruption of blood flow to the brain.

SUCROSE A disaccharide commonly called cane sugar, table sugar, granulated sugar, or simply sugar. Sucrose is made of glucose and fructose.

SUGAR A form of carbohydrate.

SUGAR ALCOHOLS Forms of sugar that contain an alcohol group. They include sorbitol, xylitol, and mannitol.

SYSTOLIC PRESSURE The pressure of blood within arteries when the heart is pumping—the top blood pressure number.

TASTE BUDS Clusters of cells found on the tongue, cheeks, throat, and roof of the mouth. Each taste bud houses 60 to 100 receptor cells. The body regenerates taste buds about every three days. These cells bind food molecules dissolved in saliva and alert the brain to interpret them.

TEAM NUTRITION A project of the U.S. Department of Agriculture to implement the School Meals Initiative for Healthy Children.

TERTIARY STRUCTURE The folding of the protein chain.

THERMIC EFFECT OF FOOD The energy needed to digest and absorb food. The thermic effect of food is the smallest contributor to your energy needs—from 5 to 10 percent. In other words, for every 100 calories consumed, about 5 to 10 calories are used for digestion, absorption, and metabolism of nutrients.

THYROID GLAND A gland found on either side of the trachea that produces and secretes two important hormones that regulate the level of metabolism.

TOFU Soybean curd.

TRACE MINERALS. *See* **MINERALS.**

TRANS FATTY ACIDS Unsaturated fatty acids that lose a natural bend or kink so they become straight (like saturated fatty acids) after being hydrogenated.

TRANSITIONAL MILK The type of breast milk produced from about the third to the tenth day after childbirth, when mature milk appears.

TRIGLYCERIDES The major form of lipid in food and in the body. Triglycerides are made of three fatty acids attached to a glycerol backbone.

TRYPTOPHAN An amino acid that can be converted to make the vitamin niacin.

TYPE I DIABETES MELLITUS A form of diabetes seen mostly in children and adolescents. These patients make no insulin at all and therefore require frequent injections of insulin to maintain a normal level of blood glucose. Also called *insulin-dependent diabetes.*

TYPE II DIABETES MELLITUS A form of diabetes seen most often in older, overweight adults. The diabetic makes insulin but his or her tissues aren't sensitive enough to the hormone and so use it inefficiently. Also called *noninsulin-dependent diabetes.*

UNSATURATED FAT A type of fat that is usually liquid at refrigerator temperature. Monounsaturated fat and polyunsaturated fat are two kinds of unsaturated fat. When used in place of saturated fat, monounsaturated and polyunsaturated fats help lower blood cholesterol levels.

UNSATURATED FATTY ACID A fatty acid ith at least one double bond.

VARIED DIET A diet that includes many different foods.

VEGANS Individuals eating a type of vegetarian diet in which no eggs or dairy products are eaten. The diet relies exclusively on plant foods to meet protein and other nutrient needs. Vegans are a small group, and it is estimated that only 4 percent of vegetarians are vegans. Vegans are also called strict vegetarians.

VERY LOW DENSITY LIPOPROTEIN (VLDL) The liver's version of chylomicrons. Triglycerides, and some cholesterol, are carried through the body by VLDL, which releases triglycerides throughout the body, with the help of lipoprotein lipase. Once the majority of triglycerides are removed, VLDLs are converted in the blood into another type of lipoprotein called low density lipoprotein (LDL).

VITAMINS Noncaloric, organic nutrients found in foods that are essential in small quantities for growth and good health.

WATER BALANCE The process of maintaining the proper amount of water in each of three bodily "compartments": inside the cells, outside the cells, and in the blood vessels.

WATER-INSOLUBLE FIBER A classification of fiber that includes cellulose, lignin, and the remaining hemicelluloses. They generally form the structural parts of plants.

WATER-SOLUBLE FIBER A classification of fiber that includes gums, mucilages, pectin, and some hemicelluloses. They are generally found around and inside plant cells. This type of fiber swells in water.

WATER-SOLUBLE VITAMINS The vitamins that are soluble in water and are not stored appreciably in the body: vitamin C, thiamin, riboflavin, niacin, vitamin B_6, folate, vitamin B_{12}, pantothenic acid, and biotin.

WHITE WHOLE-WHEAT FLOUR A flour made from a variety of wheat with the same nutritional value as regular whole wheat but with a much lighter taste. Milled from hard white winter wheat, it lacks the strong, almost bitter, flavor associated with the types of wheat used for classic whole-wheat flour.

WHOLE FOODS Foods as we get them from nature.

WINE COOLERS Mixes of wine, fruit flavor, and carbonated water or plain water.

WINE SPRITZERS Drinks made with wine and club soda.

WINE VINEGARS Vinegars made from wine, sherry, or champagne.

WOK A round-bottom metal pan that fits over a gas or electric burner.

XEROSIS A condition in which the cornea of the eye becomes dry and cloudy. A lack of vitamin A often causes this condition. Xerosis also refers to dryness of other body parts, such as the skin.

XEROPHTHALMIA Hardening and thickening of the cornea that can lead to blindness. A deficiency of vitamin A usually causes this medical problem.

XYLITOL A sugar alcohol.

ZESTS The grated skins of citrus fruits.

Index